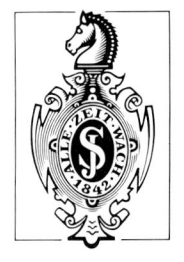

Paul G.J. Maquet

Biomechanics of the Hip

As Applied to Osteoarthritis and
Related Conditions

With a Foreword by William H. Harris

With 651 Figures, Some in Color

Springer-Verlag
Berlin Heidelberg NewYork Tokyo 1985

Docteur Paul G.J. Maquet
25, Thier Bosset, B-4070 Aywaille

ISBN 3-540-13257-0 Springer-Verlag Berlin Heidelberg New York Tokyo
ISBN 0-387-13257-0 Springer-Verlag New York Heidelberg Berlin Tokyo

Library of Congress Cataloging in Publication Data

Maquet, Paul G.J., 1928- Biomechanics of the hip. Bibliography: p. Includes index. 1. Hip joint-Surgery. 2. Osteoarthritis-Surgery. 3. Hip joint. 4. Human mechanics. I. Title. [DNLM: 1. Biomechanics. 2. Hip Joint-physiology. 3. Osteoarthritis-etiology. 4. Osteoarthritis-surgery. WE 860 M297b] RD549.M325 1984 617′.581059 84-14041

This work is subject to copyright. All rights are reserved, whether the whole or part of the material is concerned, specifically those of translation, reprinting, re-use of illustrations, broadcasting, reproduction by photocopying machine or similar means, and storage in data banks. Under §54 of the German Copyright Law where copies are made for other than private use a fee is payable to "Verwertungsgesellschaft Wort", Munich.

© by Springer-Verlag Berlin Heidelberg 1985
Printed in Germany

The use of registered names, trademarks, etc. in this publication does not imply, even in the absence of a specific statement, that such names are exempt from the relevant protective laws and regulations and therefore free for general use.

Product Liability: The publisher can give no guarantee for information about drug dosage and application thereof contained in this book. In every individual case the respective user must check its accuracy by consulting other pharmaceutical literature.

Typesetting, printing, and bookbinding: Universitätsdruckerei H. Stürtz AG, D-Würzburg.
2124/3130-543210

Foreword

Dr. MAQUET, the foremost disciple of Professor PAUWELS' and the orthopaedic heir to the PAUWELS' concepts of osteotomy of the hip for arthritis, has assembled in this one book the strongest and most lucid contemporary statement of the principles and practice of this very important school of hip surgery. Professor PAUWELS' contributions to the understanding of the biomechanics of the hip and to the concepts and execution of osteotomy of the hip for arthritis are outstanding and timeless. With clarity, Dr. MAQUET articulates this position and refines it further in the light of his own investigation.

While other investigators, of course, differ on individual concepts or principles in this book or disagree with specific positions, assumptions, or conclusions, it is clear to all that this book is a benchmark work.

Dr. MAQUET, as Professor PAUWELS always did, illustrates his text lavishly with beautiful examples of individual cases illuminating the principles advanced. But in addition, he has gone further and presents long-term follow-up data, quantifying the results of these surgical precepts as experienced in his own practice.

It is a work that has been long sought and is richly received.

Boston, Massachusetts, 1984   WILLIAM H. HARRIS, M.D.

Preface

Towards the end of his life, Pauwels (1973) summarized his views on the surgical treatment of three different conditions of the hip — pseudarthrosis of the femoral neck, congenital coxa vara and osteoarthritis of the hip — in a superb atlas, magnificently illustrated with long-term follow-up results. He taught me his concepts. He used to check the planning of my hip operations, and he critically evaluated the postoperative X-rays. The results repeatedly confirmed his theories.

Having had the privilege of discussing these theories in many parts of the world, I have frequently been asked the same questions and been confronted with the same objections. The questions have dealt primarily with the technical procedures and postoperative care. The primary objection was that Pauwels never published a statistical analysis of his results.

In the meantime I had devised new instruments and implants which facilitate the Pauwels' operations and enable any orthopaedic surgeon to carry them out with accuracy. I also developed surgical procedures which fulfilled the basic principles by other means. I achieved the same good results which Pauwels obtained from his own operations. On the other hand, I repeatedly observed poor results whenever an operation failed to ensure congruence of the joint surfaces. All these facts seem to indicate that correct application of the principles is essential.

These considerations led me to review my own experience of joint-preserving operations on the osteoarthritic hip. This may seem preposterous in the present era of total replacement. However, in spite of the initial universal enthusiasm for this new method, the potential complications of total arthroplasty of the hip cause many surgeons to reflect before opting finally for this drastic solution. Although I implant a total prosthesis when I find it necessary, I remain convinced that it makes more sense for the patient to heal with living tissues than to be subjected to the definitive ablation of the joint which a total replacement arthroplasty implies. If the result of a joint-preserving operation deteriorates after some years, as does sometimes occur, the hip can still be replaced and the patient has gained some years. The reverse is not true. After a failed total replacement, there are really no possibilities other than another replacement in poorer conditions or a Girdlestone operation.

In the course of my fruitful monthly scientific meetings, kindly organized by Mrs. Pauwels, with my good friends Professor Benno Kummer and Dr. Willy Baumann, they persuaded me to write about my clinical experience along the guide-lines laid down by our famous teacher, Professor Friedrich Pauwels. In this book, pre-operative planning and surgical techniques have been emphasized more than in Pauwels' work and, after reviewing all the patients I could, I have attempted to analyse the results. Therefore, the present book should be regarded as a modest complement to Pauwels' atlas.

Aywaille, Autumn 1984   PAUL G.J. MAQUET

Acknowledgements

I am deeply indebted to the many other individuals who made this monograph possible, and first of all to my wife, Josette, who traced the patients and did all the exacting secretarial work. Mrs. Germaine Pelzer and Mr. François de Lamotte of the Laboratoire de Photoélasticité of the University of Liège carefully analysed photoelastic models which we had designed after a thorough study of the mechanics of the hip. Mr. Vu Anh Tuan, of the Institut de Mathématiques of the University of Liège, solved the difficult problem of analysing in three dimensions the forces exerted on the hip when walking. Drs. Marcel Watillon and Francis Hoet analysed short-term results of the osteotomies after Drs. Hugues Hachez, Franz Langlais, Philippe Roure and Pierre Thomas had computerized my medical records. Last but not least, my friend Mr. Ronald Furlong, FRCS, very competently edited the final version of the text. For his infinite patience and for his innumerable questions I am very grateful.

Contents

Chapter I. Biomechanics of the Hip 1

    I. Previous Works 1
   II. Forces Exerted on a Normal Hip 2
       A. When the Subject Is Standing on Both Legs 2
       B. When the Subject Is Standing on One Leg 2
       C. During the Single-Support Period of Gait 3
          1. Problem 3
             a) Co-ordinates of the Centre of the Femoral Head in the System of Axes Originating in S_5 4
             b) Force $\vec{K}$ 6
             c) Plane of the Forces 6
             d) Force M 8
                α) Direction of $\vec{M}$ Using the First Approach 8
                β) Direction of $\vec{M}$ Using the Second Approach 8
             e) Reaction $\vec{R}$ 11
          2. Discussion 14
          3. Conclusion 15
  III. Mechanical Stressing of the Normal Hip Joint 16
  IV. Mechanical Stressing of the Normal Femoral Neck 16
   V. Cartilage Reaction to the Articular Compressive Stresses . . 22
  VI. Bone Reaction to the Articular Compressive Stresses 22
 VII. Mechanical Significance of the Neck-Shaft Angle 24
       A. Hip Joint 24
       B. Growth Plate 27
       C. Femoral Neck 30
       D. Conclusion 34
VIII. Significance of the Subchondral Sclerosis in the Acetabulum . . 37
       A. Normal Hip Joint 37
       B. Primary Osteoarthritis 37
       C. Osteoarthritis with Subluxation 39
       D. Osteoarthritis with Protrusio Acetabuli 41
       E. Different Types of Osteoarthritis 42
  IX. Conclusion 45

Chapter II. Principles of a Biomechanical Treatment of Osteoarthritis of the Hip. Critical Analysis of Different Surgical Procedures. Instinctive Attempts to Relieve Stress in the Joint 47

    I. Modifying the Biology of the Tissues 47
   II. Reducing Joint Pressure 47

A. McMurray Osteotomy 47
　　　B. Multiple Tenotomy 50
　　　C. Shelf Operation 50
　　　D. Pauwels' Approach to Osteoarthritis of the Hip 50
　　　E. Remarks on Bombelli's Concepts 50

　III. Instinctive Attempts to Reduce the Stress on the Affected Hip 52
　　　A. Limping 52
　　　B. Using a Walking Stick 53

　IV. Conclusion 56

Chapter III. Surgical Treatment of Osteoarthritis of the Hip 57

　　I. X-rays 57
　　　A. Before the Operation 57
　　　　1. Overall Anteroposterior View of the Pelvis 57
　　　　2. Anteroposterior Views of the Affected Hip 57
　　　　3. Lateral View of the Femoral Neck
　　　　　 and Three-quarter View 60
　　　　4. Anteroposterior View of the Lower Limbs 60
　　　B. During the Operation 62
　　　C. After the Operation 62

　　II. Hanging-Hip Procedure 64
　　　A. Rationale 64
　　　B. Experimental Study 64
　　　　1. Material and Method 64
　　　　2. Results 64
　　　　3. Discussion 67
　　　C. Indications 68
　　　D. Operative Procedure 68
　　　E. Postoperative Care 70
　　　F. Postoperative Evolution 70
　　　G. Incorrect Indications 74
　　　H. Conclusion 75

　III. Varus Intertrochanteric Osteotomy (Pauwels I) 76
　　　A. Rationale 76
　　　B. Indications 77
　　　C. Pre-operative X-rays 78
　　　D. Pre-operative Planning 78
　　　E. Instruments 79
　　　F. Operative Procedure (Adults) 84
　　　　1. Position 84
　　　　2. Approach 84
　　　　3. Delineation of the Wedge to Be Resected 85
　　　　4. Resection of the Wedge 85
　　　　5. Derotation 85
　　　　6. Positioning the Compression-hook 86
　　　　7. Suture 88
　　　　8. Using the Resected Wedge 88

	G. Postoperative Care	89
	H. Postoperative Evolution	89
	I. Incorrect Indications	101
	J. Procedure in Children	101
	K. Conclusion	101

IV. Valgus Intertrochanteric Osteotomy and Tenotomy (Pauwels II)   102

    A. Rationale 102
    B. Indications 107
    C. Pre-operative Planning 107
    D. Operative Procedure 111
        1. Standard Procedure 111
            a) Delineating the Wedge to Be Resected 111
            b) Tenotomy of the Abductor Muscles 111
            c) Resection of the Wedge 111
            d) Derotation 111
            e) Fixing the Fragments 112
            f) Suture 114
        2. Valgus Osteotomy Combined with a Shortening of the Leg 115
        3. Correction of a Flexion Contracture 117
        4. Correction of an Adduction Contracture or Deformity . . 117
        5. Too Much Valgum 118
    E. Postoperative Care 118
    F. Postoperative Evolution 121
    G. Reducing the Compressive Stresses in the Joint
       Rather than Restoring Normal Anatomical Shape 129
    H. Conclusion 133

V. Lateral Displacement of the Greater Trochanter 134

    A. Rationale 134
    B. Indications 136
    C. Pre-operative Planning 139
    D. Operative Procedure 140
    E. Postoperative Care 140
    F. Postoperative Evolution 141
    G. Lateral Displacement of the Greater Trochanter Complementing a Varus Intertrochanteric Osteotomy 144
    H. Lateral Displacement of the Greater Trochanter Complementing a Valgus Intertrochanteric Osteotomy 148
    I. Conclusion 149

VI. Shortening of the Opposite Leg 150

    A. Rationale 150
    B. Pre-operative Planning 151
    C. Surgical Procedure 151
    D. Results 155
    E. Conclusion 159

VII. Changing Indication 163
VIII. No Indication for Any of the Operations Previously Described 166
IX. Reoperations 170

    A. After a Hanging-Hip Operation 170
    B. After a Varus Osteotomy 175

C. After a Valgus Osteotomy	182
D. Conclusion	185
X. Age of the Patients and Duration of the Postoperative Results	186
XI. Long-term Results	189
A. Lasting Positive Results	189
B. Secondary Deterioration	191
XII. Osteotomies Distal to the Lesser Trochanter (Lorenz, Schanz, Milch)	201
A. Rationale	201
B. Indications	204
C. Pre-operative Planning	205
D. Operative Procedure	205
E. Postoperative Care	205
F. Postoperative Evolution	208
G. Additional Procedures	209
H. Conclusion	210

Chapter IV. Osteoarthritis with Protrusio acetabuli 213

I. Rationale	213
II. Indications	214
III. Abduction Contracture	218
IV. Conclusion	220

Chapter V. Avascular Necrosis of the Femoral Head 221

I. Legg-Calvé-Perthes' Disease	221
II. Avascular Necrosis of the Femoral Head in Adults	238
A. Rationale	238
B. Hanging-Hip Procedure	240
C. Varus Intertrochanteric Osteotomy	244
D. Lateral Displacement of the Greater Trochanter	244
E. Valgus Intertrochanteric Osteotomy	244
F. Conclusion	252

Chapter VI. Dysplastic Hips 253

I. Introduction	253
II. In Infants	256
A. Innominate Osteotomy	256
B. Lowering the Lateral Aspect of the Acetabulum	258
C. Varus Intertrochanteric Osteotomy	260
D. Combining Different Surgical Procedures	260
E. Spontaneous Recurrence of the Valgus Deformity of the Femoral Neck	269
III. In Children and Adolescents	270
A. Colonna Procedure	270
B. Varus Intertrochanteric Osteotomy	272
C. Varus Intertrochanteric Osteotomy Supplemented by Lateral Displacement of the Greater Trochanter	274

    IV. In Adults 278
        A. Dysplastic Hips with Osteoarthritis 278
        B. Unreduced Congenital High Dislocation 281

    V. Conclusion 282

Chapter VII. Results 283

    I. Hanging-Hip Procedure 283
        A. As Procedure of Choice 283
        B. As Temporary Palliative Measure 285
        C. Complications 286

    II. Varus and Valgus Intertrochanteric Osteotomy 286
        A. Three-Year Follow-up 286
        B. Ten-Year Follow-up 290
            1. Varus Intertrochanteric Osteotomy (Pauwels I) 290
            2. Valgus Intertrochanteric Osteotomy (Pauwels II) 293
            3. Comment 294

    III. Lateral Displacement of the Greater Trochanter 295
        A. Single Procedure 295
        B. As a Complement to an Intertrochanteric Osteotomy . . . 297

    IV. Schanz Osteotomy 297
    V. Conclusion 297

Chapter VIII. General Conclusions 299

Appendix: Fixation of the Fragments After Intertrochanteric Osteotomy   302

References 305

Subject Index 309

XIII

Chapter I. Biomechanics of the Hip

I. Previous Works

In 1935 PAUWELS published an analysis of the forces acting on the hip in a subject standing on both legs, in a subject standing on one leg and in a subject walking. Using the data of BRAUNE and FISCHER (1889, 1895) and FISCHER (1899, 1900, 1901, 1903, 1904), he calculated the successive positions of the centre of gravity S_5 of that part of the body acting on the hip during the single-support period of gait. This includes the head, the trunk, the upper limbs and the swinging leg. For each phase[1] of this single-support period, PAUWELS entered S_5 in the same rectangular network of three-dimensional co-ordinates as that described by BRAUNE and FISCHER in their classic work *Der Gang des Menschen* (1895). From the displacement of S_5 during gait, PAUWELS deduced the velocities and the accelerations of S_5 by means of graphical differentiations. From these accelerations, he calculated the force of inertia exerted by the part of the body acting on the hip. First he determined its vertical component, which he added to the partial body weight. The sum of these forces acts eccentrically on the hip and is counterbalanced by the abductor muscles. The resultant or overall force transmitted across the hip joint reaches a peak of more than four times the body weight at the beginning of the single-support period of gait. Secondly, PAUWELS calculated the horizontal component of the force of inertia. This component also acts eccentrically on the hip, in a horizontal plane. According to PAUWELS, it is counterbalanced by the external rotator muscles of the thigh. The moments of inertia of the body segments supported by the hip were ignored, since they must be small in relation to the calculated forces and in effect they counterbalance each other. This solution of the problem is simple and didactic. However, the transverse component of the resultant force calculated by PAUWELS in the horizontal plane does not correspond to the projection on this plane of the resultant force acting in the coronal plane, as it should. This mismatching results from an oversimplification of the problem. The forces acting on the hip should first be considered in space and only then projected on to the three planes of the system of co-ordinates.

KUMMER (1963, 1968, 1969, 1978, 1979) and his co-workers (AMTMANN 1968; KNIEF 1967; KURRAT 1977; MOLZBERGER 1973; OBERLÄNDER 1973, 1977; TILLMANN 1969) have carried out the most thorough analysis of the hip joint up to the present time. They confirm the guide-lines given by PAUWELS and we shall refer to their results.

Several authors have measured the force exerted by the foot on the ground during gait and from this they have deduced the force transmitted across the hip joint. It is certainly possible to calculate the force acting on the hip using the reaction force of the ground as long as the muscular forces and the accelerations of the moving parts are taken into account.

PAUL (1966), experimenting on 12 living subjects walking on a force plate, calculated that the force transmitted across the hip varies from 2.3 times body weight "for a female walking very slowly with a short stride" to 5.8 times body weight "for a heavy male subject walking very energetically". For his 12 subjects, aged 18–36, the average value of the ratio of the force to body weight was 5.0. This is very similar to PAUWELS' figures. PAUL (1974) also calculated that 7–7.5 times body weight acts on the hip during fast walking and walking up or down stairs.

PAUWELS started his research from the other end, that is to say, the weight and the accelerations of that part of the body supported by the joint. He relied on anatomical works in order to evaluate the position of the muscular forces necessary to ensure equilibrium. Using all these data, he calculated the force transmitted across the hip joint. From a mathematical point of view, both approaches are correct. In the present chapter we shall test PAUWELS' calculations by improving the mathematical solution of the problem.

---
[1] BRAUNE and FISCHER divided the period of walking into 31 phases. Phases 12–23 corresponded to the right single-support period. Pauwels and I have retained the same subdivisions.

II. Forces Exerted on a Normal Hip

A. When the Subject Is Standing on Both Legs

When a subject stands on both legs, the hips support the head, the trunk and the upper limbs (Fig. 1). This represents 62% of the body weight. The centre of gravity of this part of the body lies in or close to the vertical plane through the centres of the femoral heads, above the mid-point of the axis joining these two centres. Theoretically, little or no muscular force is necessary to maintain equilibrium, but it is unstable. If the support is symmetrical, each hip carries 31% of the body weight. This force acts vertically on the joint. In the subject of BRAUNE and FISCHER (weight 58.7 kg) used by PAUWELS, each hip is subjected to a vertical force of 18.41 kg.

B. When the Subject Is Standing on One Leg

When a subject stands on one leg, the loaded hip supports the mass of the head, trunk, upper limbs and the other leg. This mass can be imagined as concentrated at its centre of gravity S_5, and acts on the hip with its weight K (Fig. 2). Weight K represents 81% of the total body weight (47.76 kg in the subject of BRAUNE and FISCHER). The centre of gravity S_6 of the whole body lies on the perpendicular through the supporting foot on the ground. The partial centre of gravity S_5 lies further away from the loaded hip. Weight K acts eccentrically on the hip and tends to tilt the pelvis in adduction on the femur. It is counterbalanced by the abductor muscles acting with the force M. The lever arm of force K is h' and the lever arm of M is h. The moments of the two forces are equal, since there is equilibrium:

$$K h' = M h$$

The hip supports the resultant or vectorial sum R of the two forces K and M.

$$R = \sqrt{K^2 + M^2 + 2 KM \cos(\widehat{KM})}$$

$$\sin(\widehat{KR}) = \frac{M \sin(\widehat{KM})}{R}$$

in which $\widehat{KM}$ is the angle formed by the lines of action of the forces K and M, and $\widehat{KR}$ is the angle formed by the lines of action of the forces K and R. The lever arm of force K is normally about three times as long as that of force M. Therefore, R is a little less than four times the partial body weight or a little more than three times the total body weight.

The line of action of force R passes through the intersection of the lines of action of the forces K and M and through the centre of the femoral head. Since the coefficient of friction of two cartilage layers is extremely low (RADIN et al. 1970), the line of action of R must be normal to the tangent to the articular surfaces at its intersection with the latter. Force R thus acts on the hip obliquely from above downwards and from inside outwards. The inclination of the line of action of force R to the perpendicular is about 16° in a normal hip, according to PAUWELS (1935).

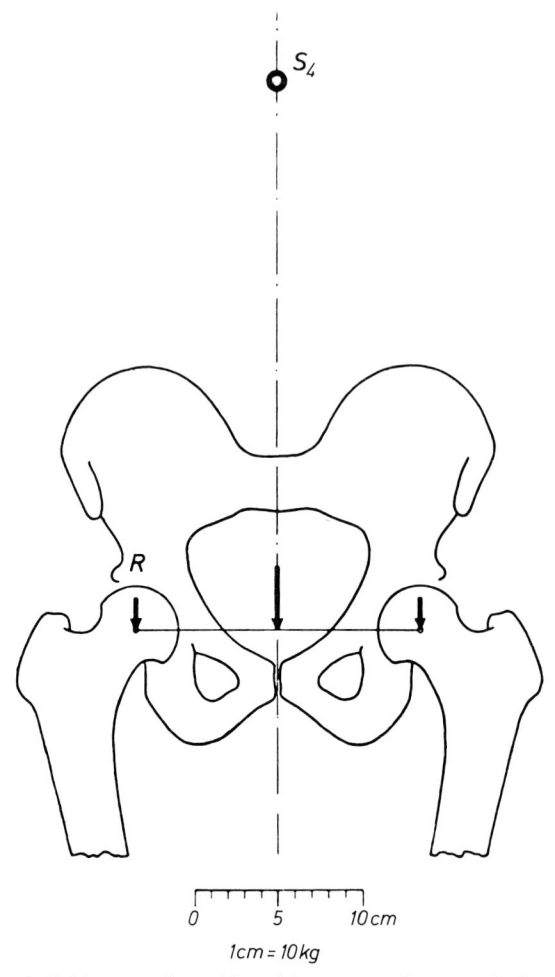

Fig. 1. Subject standing with weight supported symmetrically on both legs. S_4, centre of gravity of the head, trunk and upper limbs; R, force exerted on one hip. (After PAUWELS 1935)

C. During the Single-Support Period of Gait

When a subject is walking, each hip alternately supports the part of the body mass constituted by the head, trunk, upper limbs and swinging leg during the successive single-support periods. We have calculated again the co-ordinates of the centre of gravity S_5 of this part of the body for the successive phases of one single-support period of gait for the subject of BRAUNE and FISCHER, whom PAUWELS uses for his study (Table 1). Some of our results are slightly different from those of PAUWELS. We have then plotted the successive z co-ordinates as the ordinate and the phases and the times as the abscissa. This enabled us to draw the curve of the vertical displacement of S_5 during the single-support period. Graphical differentiation of this curve gave the curve of velocity, and differentiation of the latter led to the curve of acceleration. Displacement, velocity and acceleration of S_5 in the direction of gait and in a horizontal direction normal to that of gait were found in the same way, from the x and y co-ordinates of S_5.

Up to now we have repeated the process used by PAUWELS. Further on, the approach is different.

1. Problem

During the single-support period of gait, the hip is subjected eccentrically to the partial body weight $\vec{P}$ (47.760 kg')[2] acting at the centre of gravity S_5 and to the force of inertia $\vec{D}$ resulting from the

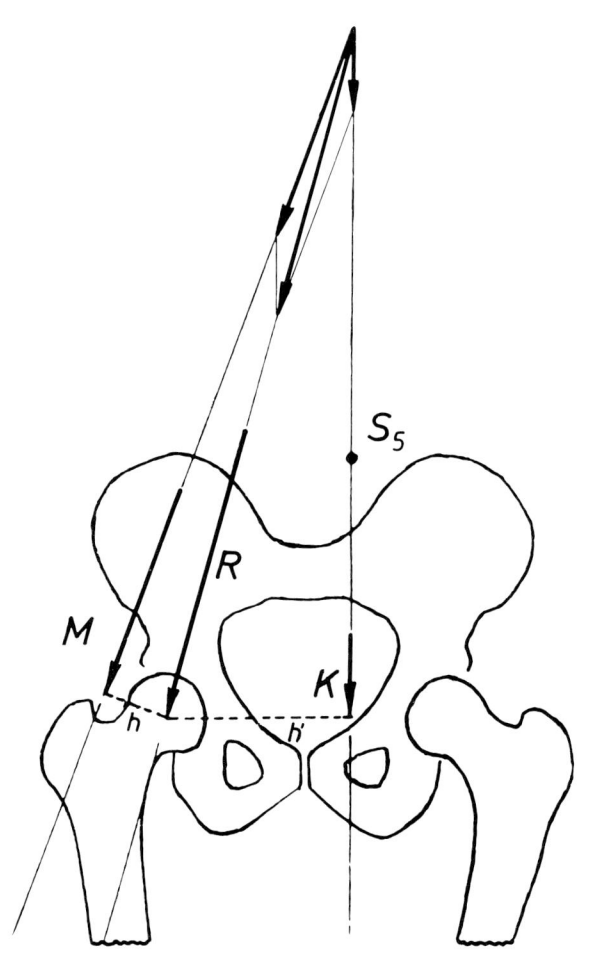

Fig. 2. Forces exerted on the hip when the subject is standing on one leg. S_5, centre of gravity of the mass of the body acting on the hip (head, trunk, upper limbs and opposite leg); K, force exerted by this partial body mass; h', lever arm of force K; M, force exerted by the abductor muscles to counterbalance K; h, lever arm of force M; R, resultant of forces K and M. (After PAUWELS 1976)

[2] kg' = kilogram force

Table 1. Co-ordinates of S_5 and H for the successive phases of the right single-support period of gait (cm)

Phase	X_S	Y_S	Z_S	X_H	Y_H	Z_H	x_H	y_H	z_H
12	102.44	−1.47	98.28	107.73	8.35	82.27	5.29	9.82	16.01
13	109.69	−1.12	98.67	113.92	9.19	82.83	4.23	10.31	15.84
14	116.41	−0.89	99.58	119.90	9.78	83.97	3.49	10.67	15.61
15	123.35	−0.75	101.03	125.38	10.16	85.28	2.03	10.91	15.75
16	129.43	−0.71	102.09	130.40	10.28	85.95	0.97	10.99	16.14
17	136.17	−0.72	102.81	135.39	10.20	86.32	−0.78	10.92	16.49
18	142.34	−0.82	102.76	140.41	10.01	86.16	−1.93	10.83	16.60
19	148.89	−0.88	102.18	145.87	9.92	85.42	−3.02	10.80	16.76
20	155.21	−1.00	101.19	151.32	9.78	84.31	−3.89	10.78	16.88
21	161.45	−1.17	100.09	156.90	9.63	83.30	−4.55	10.80	16.79
22	167.83	−1.50	99.25	162.91	9.25	82.78	−4.92	10.75	16.47
23	174.26	−2.00	98.64	169.40	8.70	82.56	−4.86	10.70	16.08

X_S, co-ordinate x of the partial centre of gravity S_5; Y_S, co-ordinate y of the partial centre of gravity S_5; Z_S, co-ordinate z of the partial centre of gravity S_5; X_H, co-ordinate x of the centre of the hip; Y_H, co-ordinate y of the centre of the hip; Z_H, co-ordinate z of the centre of the hip; x_H, co-ordinate x of the centre of the hip in relation to S_5 considered as the origin of the co-ordinates; y_H, co-ordinate y of the centre of the hip in relation to S_5 considered as the origin of the co-ordinates; z_H, co-ordinate z of the centre of the hip in relation to S_5 considered as the origin of the co-ordinates

accelerations of S_5. Since $\vec{P}$ and $\vec{D}$ are exerted at S_5, they can be combined into one force, called $\vec{K}$ (Fig. 3). Since there is equilibrium, muscular forces (the resultant of which is designated $\vec{M}$) and the reaction $\vec{R}$ of the femoral head must be involved. They counterbalance force $\vec{K}$ (Fig. 4). Consequently, the femoral head is stressed by the reaction to force $\vec{R}$, which acts in the opposite direction. The reaction force is equal to $\vec{R}$. These three forces, $\vec{K}$, $\vec{M}$ and $\vec{R}$, act in one plane and intersect each other at one point.

We wish to calculate $\vec{R}$. To this end, the balance of the forces will be considered in a system of rectangular axes, the origin of which is S_5. We choose:

The axis x, horizontal in the direction of gait
The axis y, horizontal and normal to the direction of gait
The axis z, vertical from above downwards (Fig. 4).

a) Co-ordinates of the Centre of the Femoral Head in the System of Axes Originating in S_5 (Fig. 5)

Knowing the co-ordinates of S_5 (X_S, Y_S, Z_S) (Table 1) and those of H, the centre of the femoral

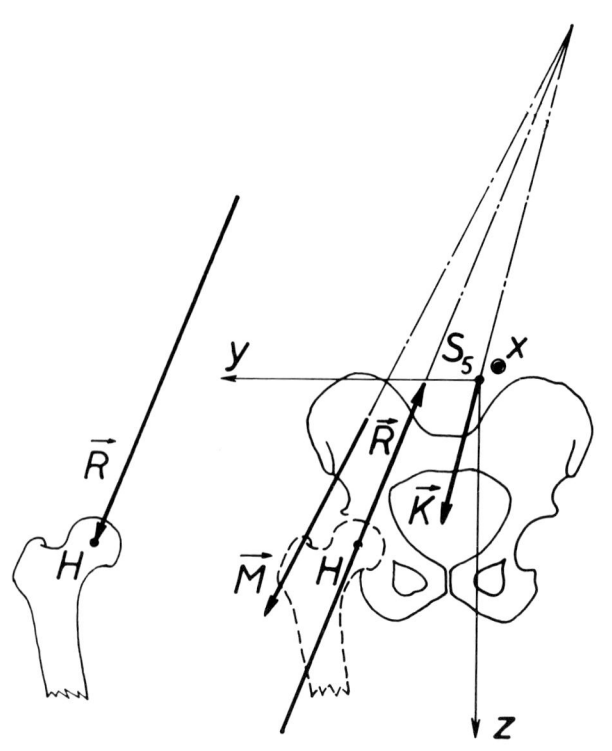

Fig. 4. Forces acting on the hip during the single-support period of gait. *Axis x*, horizontal in the direction of gait; *axis y*, horizontal and normal to the direction of gait; *axis z*, vertical from above downwards; S_5, centre of gravity of the part of the body supported by the loaded hip (the body minus the swinging leg); K, force exerted by this part of the body; M, force exerted by the abductor muscles; R, reaction to the resultant of forces K and M; H, centre of the femoral head

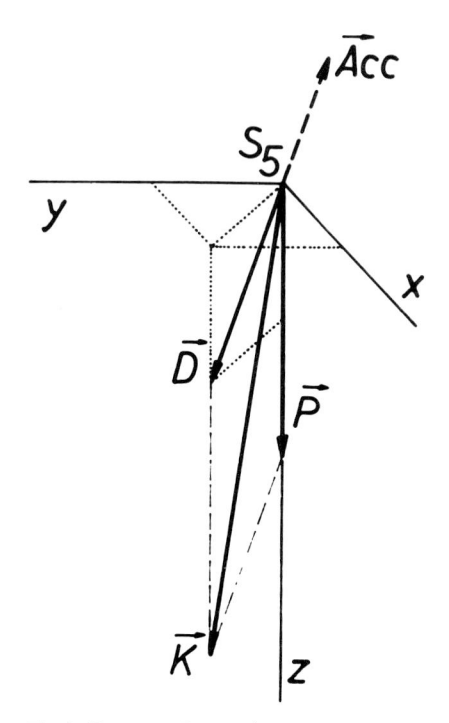

Fig. 3. Forces acting at the centre of gravity, S_5, of the part of the body supported by the loaded hip: P, partial body weight (weight of the body minus that of the swinging leg); D, force of inertia; *Acc*, acceleration of S_5; K, resultant of forces P and D. *Axis x*, horizontal in the direction of gait; *axis y*, horizontal and normal to the direction of gait; *axis z*, vertical from above downwards

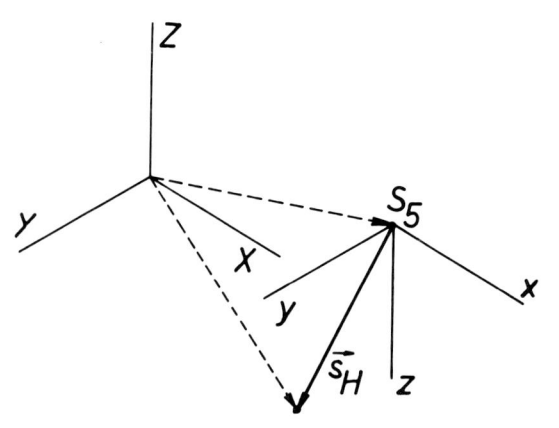

Fig. 5. Entering the point H, centre of the femoral head, into a system of co-ordinates parallel to the initial ones and originating at S_5, the centre of gravity of the part of the body supported by the loaded hip. s_H, distance from S_5 to H. *Axis x*, horizontal in the direction of gait; *axis y*, horizontal and normal to the direction of gait; *axis z*, vertical from above downwards

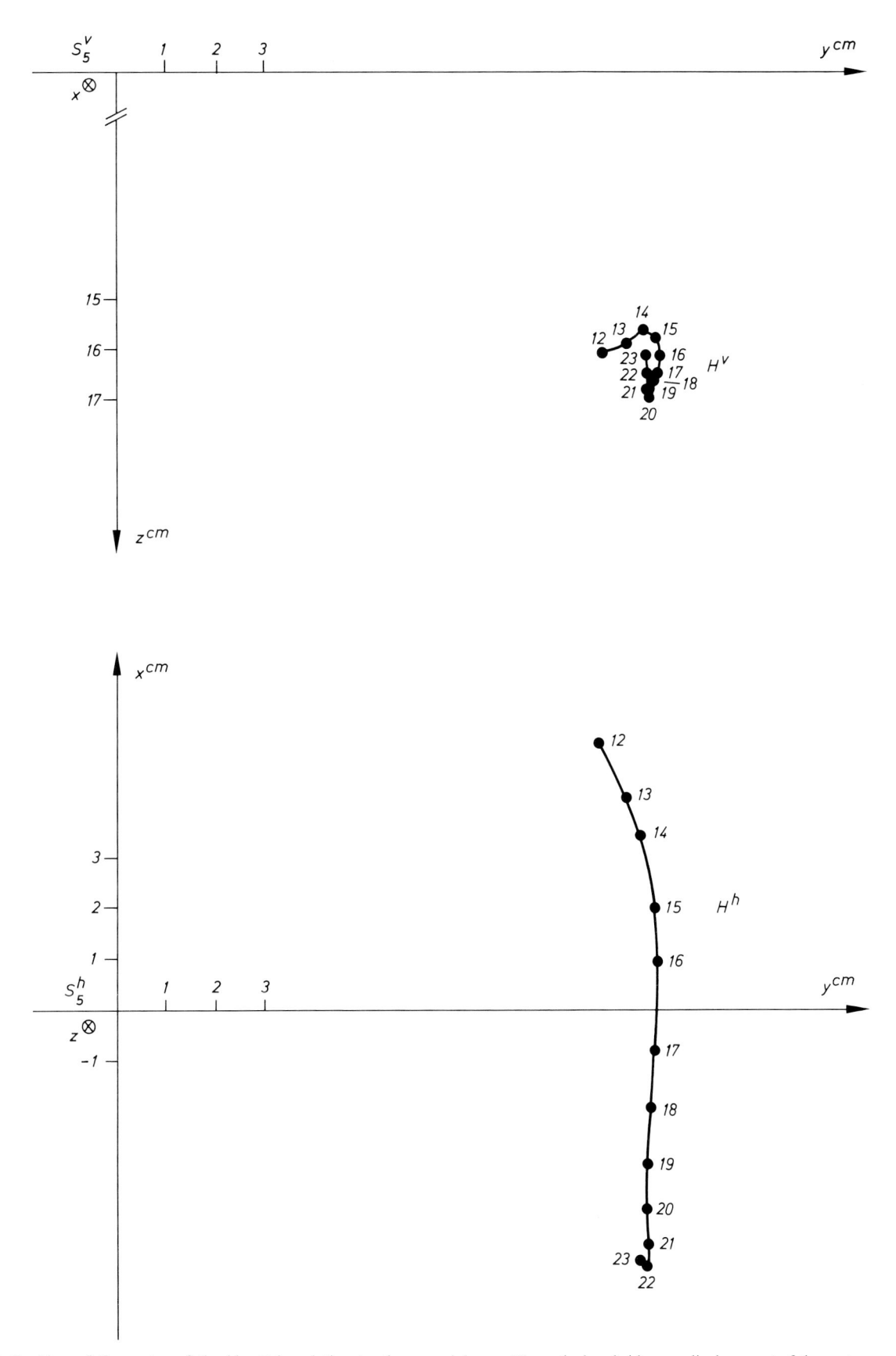

Fig. 6. Position of the centre of the hip H in relation to the partial centre of gravity S_5 in a coronal projection (*above*) and in a horizontal projection (*below*). S_5^v, S_5 moving vertically up and down; H^v, vertical and sideways displacement of the centre of the hip; S_5^h, S_5 moving horizontally forwards and backwards; H^h horizontal displacement of the centre of the hip

head (X_H, Y_H, Z_H) (Table 1), in the initial system of axes (BRAUNE and FISCHER 1895; PAUWELS 1935), we can find the co-ordinates x_H, y_H, z_H in the system of axes parallel to the initial axes but originating in S_5. It must be noticed that the system X, Y, Z is retrograde, whereas x, y, z is direct.

The position of H in relation to the partial centre of gravity S_5 has been entered into the system of co-ordinates x, y, z in a coronal projection z, y and in a horizontal projection x, y (Fig. 6):

$$x_H = X_H - X_S$$
$$y_H = Y_H - Y_S$$
$$z_H = -(Z_H - Z_S)$$

b) *Force $\vec{K}$ (Fig. 7)*

The resultant $\vec{K}$ of forces $\vec{P}$ and $\vec{D}$ can be resolved following the three axes x, y, z originating in S_5. Then:

Along axis x: $K_x = D_x = -m\,\mathrm{Acc}_x$
Along axis y: $K_y = D_y = -m\,\mathrm{Acc}_y$
Along axis z: $K_z = P + D_z = P - m\,\mathrm{Acc}_z$

Acc_x, Acc_y, Acc_z are the components of the acceleration of S_5. Their magnitudes are read on the curves mentioned above (Table 2); m represents the partial mass the centre of gravity of which is at S_5, and is deduced from P:

$$m = \frac{P}{g} = \frac{47.760 \text{ kg}'}{981 \text{ cm/s}^2} = 0.048685 \frac{\text{kg}'/\text{s}^2}{\text{cm}}$$

We can thus calculate the magnitude and the directional cosines of force $\vec{K}$, its projection on the horizontal plane (Oxy), on the coronal plane (Oyz) and on the sagittal plane (Oxz), and the angles formed by these projections and the axes x, y, z (Table 2). In Table 2, $\vec{e}_x$, $\vec{e}_y$, $\vec{e}_z$ represent the unitary vectors. O is the origin of the axes x, y and z and corresponds to S_5.

c) *Plane of the Forces*

The forces $\vec{K}$, $\vec{R}$ and $\vec{M}$ are in equilibrium, in one plane, and intersect each other at one point. The

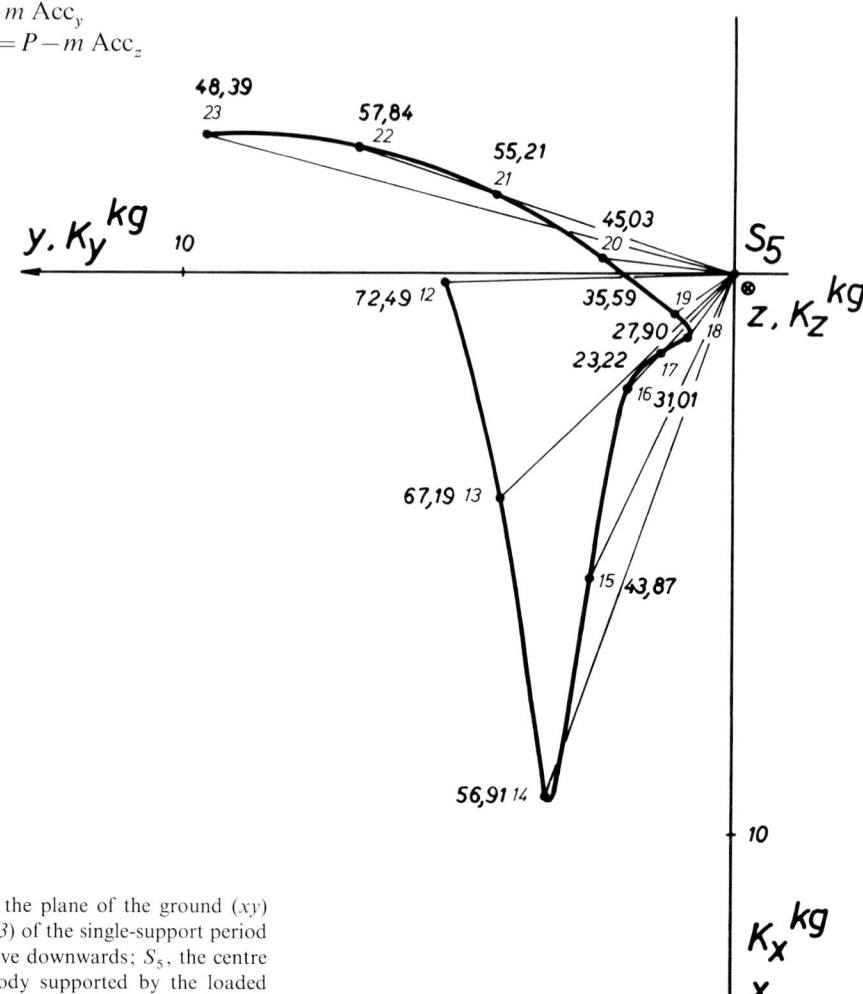

Fig. 7. Projection of force K on the plane of the ground (xy) during the different phases *(12–23)* of the single-support period of gait. Axis z, vertical from above downwards; S_5, the centre of gravity of the part of the body supported by the loaded hip

Table 2. Force exerted by the mass of the body supported by the hip

Phase	Acc_x	Acc_y	Acc_z	D_x kg'	D_y kg'	D_z kg'	Weight+D_z kg'	K kg'	$\cos(\vec{K},\vec{e}_x)$	$\cos(\vec{K},\vec{e}_y)$	$\cos(\vec{K},e_z)$
12	− 3	− 108	− 508	0.146	5.258	24.732	72.492	72.683	0.0020	0.0723	0.9974
13	− 82	− 88	− 399	3.992	4.284	19.425	67.185	67.440	0.5292	0.0635	0.9962
14	− 191	− 71	− 188	9.299	3.457	9.153	56.913	57.771	0.1610	0.0598	0.9851
15	− 112	− 54	+ 80	5.453	2.629	− 3.895	43.865	44.281	0.1231	0.0594	0.9906
16	− 42	− 40	+ 344	2.045	1.947	− 16.748	31.012	31.141	0.0657	0.0625	0.9959
17	− 30	− 28	+ 504	1.461	1.363	− 24.537	23.223	23.308	0.0627	0.0585	0.9953
18	− 24	− 18	+ 408	1.168	0.876	− 19.863	27.896	27.935	0.0418	0.0314	0.9986
19	− 13	− 23	+ 250	0.633	1.120	− 12.171	35.589	35.612	0.0178	0.0314	0.9993
20	+ 6	− 50	+ 56	−0.292	2.434	− 2.726	45.034	45.100	−0.0065	0.0540	0.9985
21	+ 29	− 89	− 153	−1.412	4.333	7.449	55.209	55.397	−0.0255	0.0782	0.9966
22	+ 46	− 140	− 207	−2.239	6.816	10.078	57.838	58.281	−0.0384	0.1169	0.9924
23	+ 50	− 197	− 13	−2.434	9.591	0.633	48.393	49.394	−0.0493	0.1942	0.9797

Phase	K_{xy} kg'	$\vec{e}_y, \vec{K}_{xy}$ +towards e_x	K_{yz} kg'	$\vec{e}_z, \vec{K}_{yz}$ +towards e_y	K_{zx} kg'	$\vec{e}_z, \vec{K}_{zx}$ +towards e_x
12	5.260	1° 35′	72.682	4° 09′	72.492	0° 07′
13	5.856	42° 59′	67.322	3° 39′	67.304	3° 24′
14	9.920	69° 37′	57.018	3° 29′	57.667	9° 17′
15	6.053	64° 16′	43.944	3° 26′	44.203	7° 05′
16	2.824	46° 24′	31.073	3° 36′	31.080	3° 46′
17	1.998	46° 58′	23.263	3° 22′	23.269	3° 36′
18	1.461	53° 08′	27.910	1° 48′	27.921	2° 24′
19	1.286	29° 29′	35.606	1° 48′	35.594	1° 01′
20	2.452	− 6° 51′	45.099	3° 06′	45.035	−0° 22′
21	4.557	−18° 03′	55.379	4° 29′	55.227	−1° 28′
22	7.174	−18° 11′	58.238	6° 43′	57.881	−2° 13′
23	9.895	−14° 14′	49.334	11° 13′	48.454	−2° 53′

plane π of these forces is determined by the line of action of $\vec{K}$ and by the centre of the femoral head H, through which the line of action of $\vec{R}$ must pass. $\vec{K}$ and H are known.

The directional cosines of plane π are:

$$p_x = \frac{q_x}{q}, \; p_y = \frac{q_y}{q} \text{ and } p_z = \frac{q_z}{q}$$

in which

$$q_x = y_H K_z - z_H K_y$$
$$q_y = z_H K_x - x_H K_z$$
$$q_z = x_H K_y - y_H K_x$$
$$q = \sqrt{q_x^2 + q_y^2 + q_z^2}$$

where q is equal to the moment of force $\vec{K}$ in relation to point H (Table 3).

Table 3. Calculation of the directional cosines of plane π and moment of the muscular force M

Phase	q_x (kg' cm)	q_y	q_z	q (kg' cm)	$(\sqrt{p_x^2+p_y^2+p_z^2}=1)$ p_x	p_y	p_z	$M=\frac{q}{4}$ (kg')
12	627.6909	− 381.1436	26.3801	734.8212	0.8542	−0.5187	0.0359	183.705
13	624.8171	− 220.9574	23.0370	663.136	0.9422	−0.3332	−0.0347	165.784
14	553.3021	− 53.4714	−87.1547	562.6707	0.9833	−0.0950	−0.1549	140.668
15	437.1626	− 3.1663	−54.1521	440.5151	0.9124	−0.0072	−0.1229	110.129
16	309.3952	2.9210	−20.5834	310.0929	0.9978	0.0094	−0.0664	77.523
17	231.1138	42.1991	−17.0130	235.5580	0.9812	0.1792	−0.0722	58.888
18	287.5725	73.2357	−14.3450	297.0980	0.9679	0.2465	−0.0483	74.274
19	365.5901	118.0853	−10.2171	384.3236	0.9513	0.3073	−0.0266	96.081
20	444.3712	170.2501	− 6.3206	475.9105	0.9337	0.3577	−0.0133	118.978
21	523.5840	227.4942	− 4.4666	570.7988	0.9171	0.3186	−0.0078	142.700
22	509.4985	247.6774	− 9.4596	566.5883	0.8992	0.4371	−0.0167	141.647
23	363.5824	196.0460	−20.5648	413.5808	0.8791	0.4740	−0.0497	103.395

d) Force $\vec{M}$

Relying on the work of FICK (1860, 1879), PAUWELS found that the resultant $\vec{M}$ of the forces exerted by the abductor muscles, when projected on the coronal plane, forms an angle of 21° with the perpendicular and acts with a lever arm of 4 cm in relation to H, the centre of the femoral head. The first of these data will be used to find the direction of $\vec{M}$ and the second to calculate the magnitude of $\vec{M}$.

Because $\vec{K}$, $\vec{M}$ and $\vec{R}$ are in equilibrium, the moment of $\vec{M}$ in relation to the axis passing through H and normal to the plane π of the forces must be equal and opposite in sign to the moment of $\vec{K}$ in relation to the same axis since $\vec{R}$ passes through H. Since the lever arm of $\vec{M}$ in relation to H is 4 cm, the moment is 4 M kg′cm.

Our assumption is not exactly that of PAUWELS. According to PAUWELS, the lever arm of the coronal projection of vector $\vec{M}$ is equal to 4 cm, whereas for us the lever arm of vector $\vec{M}$ itself is equal to 4 cm. On the other hand, the moment of force $\vec{K}$ is equal to q kg′cm

$$M = \frac{q}{4} \text{ kg}'$$

As far as the direction of $\vec{M}$ is concerned, we can use one of two approaches:

1. Either we can assume that the projection of $\vec{M}$ on the coronal plane O_{yz} forms an angle of 21° with the perpendicular (Fig. 8a)
2. Or we can assume that $\vec{M}$ itself forms an angle of 21° with the perpendicular (Fig. 8b)

α) Direction of $\vec{M}$ Using the First Approach (Fig. 8a). In the system of axes xyz, the force $\vec{M}$ is a vector, and $\vec{m}$ is the vector unit. Since the projection of $\vec{M}$ (and thus also of $\vec{m}$) on the coronal plane Oyz has a given inclination, we deduce that it belongs to the plane normal to plane Oyz the directional cosines of which are 0, cos 21°, $-\sin 21°$. On the other hand, $\vec{m}$ belongs to the plane π, the directional cosines of which are p_x, p_y, p_z. Consequently, the directional cosines of $\vec{M}$ are:

$$m_x = \frac{m'_x}{m'}, \quad m_y = \frac{m'_y}{m'}, \quad m_z = \frac{m'_z}{m'}$$

in which

$$m'_x = -p_y \sin 21° - p_z \cos 21°$$
$$m'_y = p_x \sin 21°$$
$$m'_z = p_x \cos 21° \quad \text{and}$$
$$m' = \sqrt{m'^2_x + m'^2_y + m'^2_z}$$

Knowing the magnitude and directional cosines of $\vec{M}$, we can calculate the components of $\vec{M}$ and its projections on the coronal, sagittal and horizontal planes (Fig. 9 and Table 4).

β) Direction of $\vec{M}$ Using the Second Approach (Fig. 8b). Here the inclination of vector $\vec{M}$ is given. Consequently, $\vec{M}$ belongs to a cone with a vertical axis. The angle of opening of the cone is 42° (21° × 2).

On the other hand, $\vec{M}$ belongs to the plane π, the directional cosines of which are p_x, p_y, p_z. Consequently, the directional cosines of $\vec{M}$ are:

$$m_x = \frac{-1}{1 - p_z^2} (\cos 21° \, p_x p_z + \sqrt{\sin^2 21° - p_z^2} \, p_y)$$

$$m_y = \frac{-1}{1 - p_z^2} (\cos 21° \, p_y p_z - \sqrt{\sin^2 21° - p_z^2} \, p_x)$$

$$m_z = \cos 21°$$

Knowing the magnitude and directional cosines of $\vec{M}$ we can determine the components and pro-

Table 4. Force M, its directional cosines and projections. First approach

Phase	M (kg′)	m_x	m_y	m_z	M_{xy} (kg′)	M_{yz}	M_{zx}
12	183.705	0.1756	0.3528	0.9191	72.396	180.851	171.893
13	165.784	0.1591	0.3538	0.9217	64.312	163.674	165.063
14	140.668	0.1788	0.3520	0.9185	55.612	138.397	131.629
15	110.129	0.1174	0.3559	0.9271	41.272	109.365	102.916
16	77.523	0.0586	0.3578	0.9370	28.107	77.393	72.394
17	58.888	0.0032	0.3584	0.9336	21.106	58.889	64.978
18	74.275	−0.0446	0.3580	0.9326	26.797	74.197	69.348
19	96.081	−0.0893	0.3569	0.9299	35.348	95.700	89.757
20	118.978	−0.1231	0.3556	0.9265	44.772	118.073	111.202
21	142.700	−0.1462	0.3545	0.9235	54.720	141.159	133.424
22	141.647	−0.1550	0.3540	0.9223	54.739	139.934	132.473
23	103.395	−0.1391	0.3549	0.9245	39.413	102.390	96.665

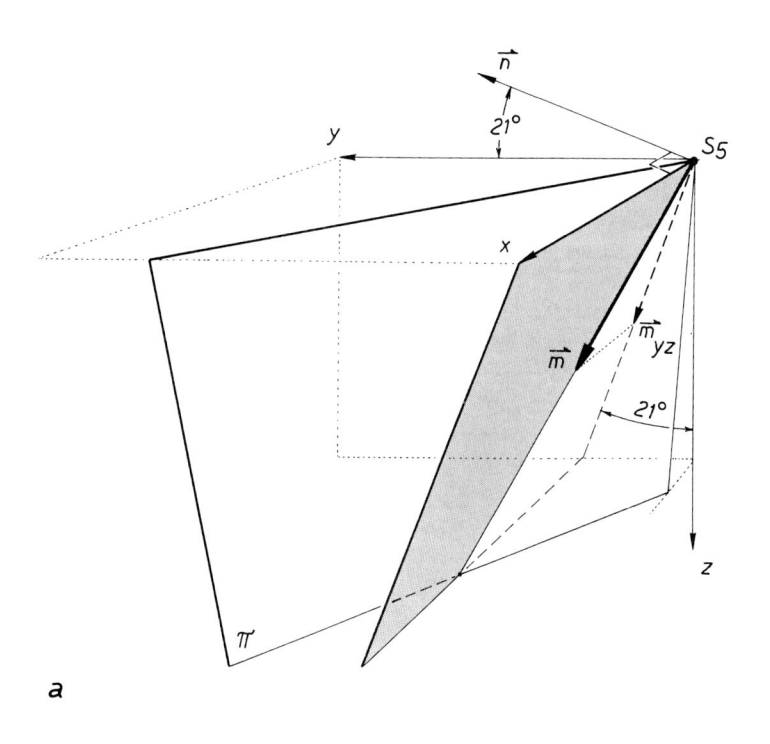

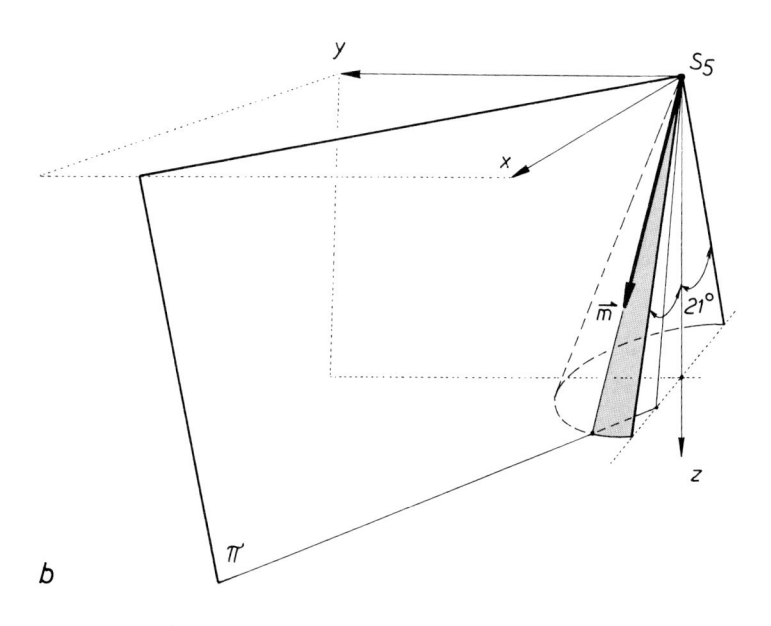

Fig. 8a, b. Direction M of the force M exerted by the abductor muscles. The forces are exerted in plane π. **a** The projection of vector $\vec{M}$ on the coronal plane Oyx forms an angle of 21° with the vertical axis z. The plane determined by M and the axis x intersects plane π. It is *grey* on this side of plane π and *white* beyond. $\vec{n}$ vector normal to the plane normal to plane Oyz. **b** The vector $\vec{M}$ forms an angle of 21° with the vertical axis z. The cone to which $\vec{M}$ belongs intersects plane π. It is *grey* on this side of plane π and *white* beyond. S_5, centre gravity of the part of the body supported by the loaded hip

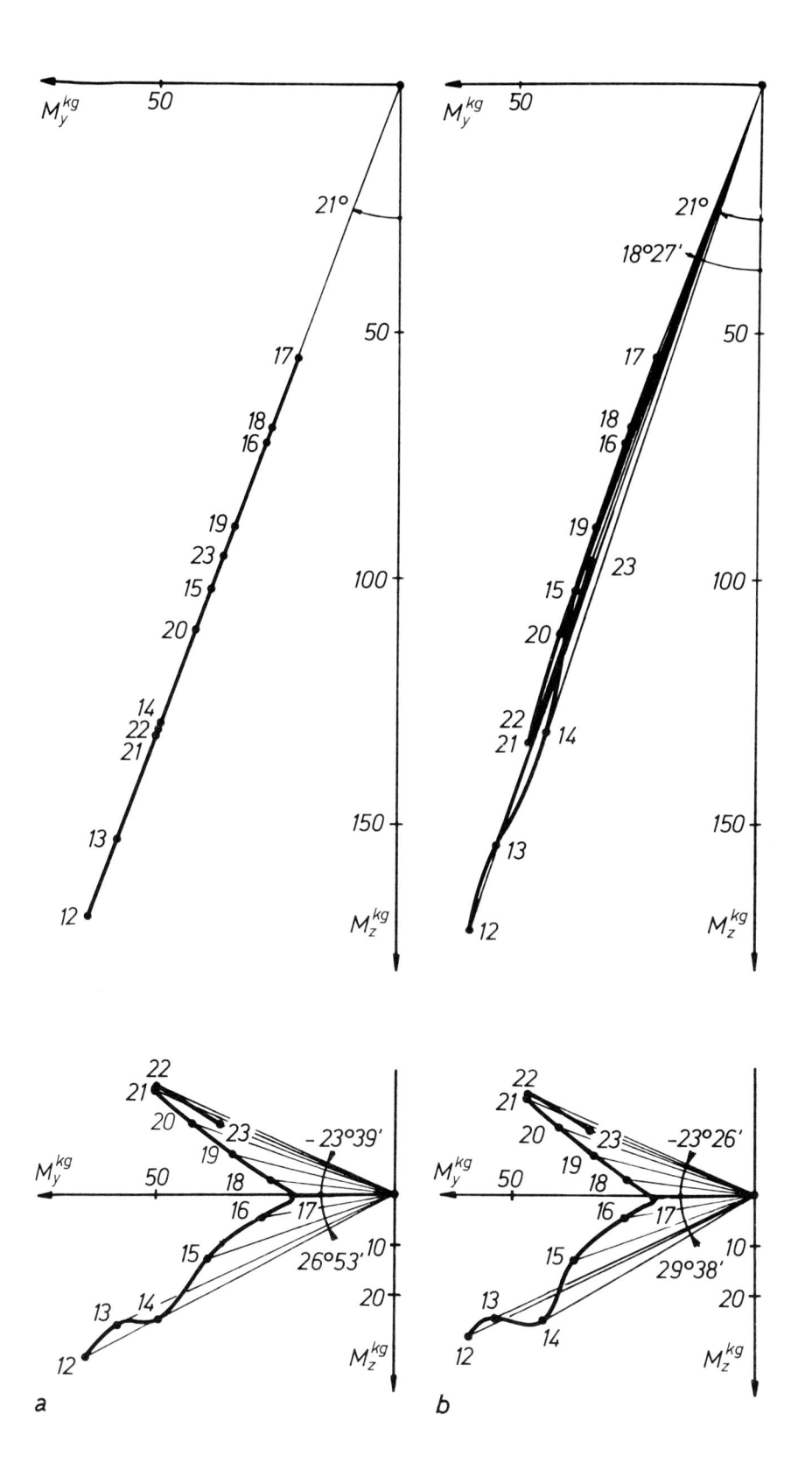

Fig. 9a, b. Projection of force M on the coronal plane (above) and on the horizontal plane (below). **a** for the first hypothesis; **b** for the second hypothesis

jections of $\vec{M}$ on the different planes (Fig. 9 and Table 5).

e) *Reaction $\vec{R}$ (Fig. 10)*

Since there is equilibrium, the geometrical sum of the three vectors $\vec{K}$, $\vec{M}$ and $\vec{R}$ is 0. $\vec{R}$ can thus be calculated:

$$R_x = -K_x - M_x$$
$$R_y = -K_y - M_y$$
$$R_z = -K_z - M_z$$

Knowing the components of $\vec{R}$ we can calculate all the elements of $\vec{R}$: magnitude, directional cosines and projections on the coronal, sagittal and horizontal planes (Table 6).

Table 5. Force M, its directional cosines and projections. Second approach

Phase	M (kg')	m_x	m_y	m_z	M_{xy} (kg')	M_{yz}	M_{zx}
12	183.705	0.1565	0.3224	0.9336	65.834	181.441	173.897
13	165.784	0.1495	0.3257	0.9336	59.411	163.919	156.746
14	140.668	0.1771	0.3115	0.9336	50.408	138.442	133.668
15	110.129	0.1181	0.3384	0.9336	39.467	109.359	103.663
16	77.523	0.0588	0.3535	0.9336	27.783	77.390	72.618
17	58.888	0.0033	0.3584	0.9336	21.104	58.888	54.977
18	74.275	−0.0440	0.3556	0.9336	26.017	74.202	69.418
19	96.081	−0.0863	0.3479	0.9336	34.434	95.723	90.081
20	118.978	−0.1165	0.3389	0.9336	42.636	118.167	111.937
21	142.700	−0.1361	0.3315	0.9336	51.139	171.371	134.631
22	141.647	−0.1425	0.3288	0.9336	50.759	140.101	133.771
23	103.395	−0.1278	0.3348	0.9336	37.053	102.548	97.427

Table 6. Resultant force R, its directional cosines and projections.

Phase	R (kg')	$\cos(\vec{R}, \vec{e}_x)$	$\cos(\vec{R}, e_y)$	$\cos(\vec{R}, e_z)$	R_{xy} (kg')	R_{yz}	R_{zx}
			First approach to M				
12	253.381	−0.1279	−0.2766	−0.9524	77.209	251.300	243.997
13	230.821	−0.1316	−0.2727	−0.9531	69.882	228.815	222.075
14	196.573	−0.1753	−0.2699	−0.9468	63.259	193.531	189.278
15	152.948	−0.1202	−0.2735	−0.9543	45.685	151.839	147.119
16	107.648	−0.0612	−0.2758	−0.9593	30.407	107.446	103.474
17	81.381	−0.0203	−0.2761	−0.9609	22.529	81.364	78.218
18	100.996	0.0212	−0.2720	−0.9621	27.550	100.972	97.189
19	130.099	0.0611	−0.2722	−0.9603	36.292	129.856	125.187
20	162.274	0.0921	−0.2757	−0.9568	47.171	161.584	155.983
21	196.159	0.1136	−0.2800	−0.9533	59.265	194.890	188.314
22	198.379	0.1220	−0.2871	−0.9501	61.885	196.898	190.026
23	152.171	0.1105	−0.3042	−0.9462	49.246	151.239	144.961
			Second approach to M				
12	254.021	−0.1138	−0.2538	−0.9605	70.661	252.372	245.701
13	231.279	−0.1245	−0.2520	−0.9597	64.996	279.480	223.817
14	197.076	−0.1236	−0.2399	−0.9551	58.359	194.083	191.322
15	153.124	−0.1205	−0.2605	−0.9579	43.955	162.007	147.836
16	107.676	−0.0061	−0.2726	−0.9602	30.088	107.473	103.597
17	81.379	−0.0203	−0.2761	−0.9609	22.527	81.362	78.216
18	101.017	0.0208	−0.2782	−0.9626	27.372	100.995	97.260
19	130.188	0.0588	−0.2653	−0.9624	35.380	129.962	125.522
20	162.475	0.0871	−0.2631	−0.9608	45.036	161.857	156.749
21	196.486	0.1061	−0.2628	−0.9590	55.685	195.378	189.579
22	198.702	0.1128	−0.2687	−0.9566	57.907	197.433	191.395
23	152.319	0.1027	−0.2902	−0.9514	46.895	151.514	146.762

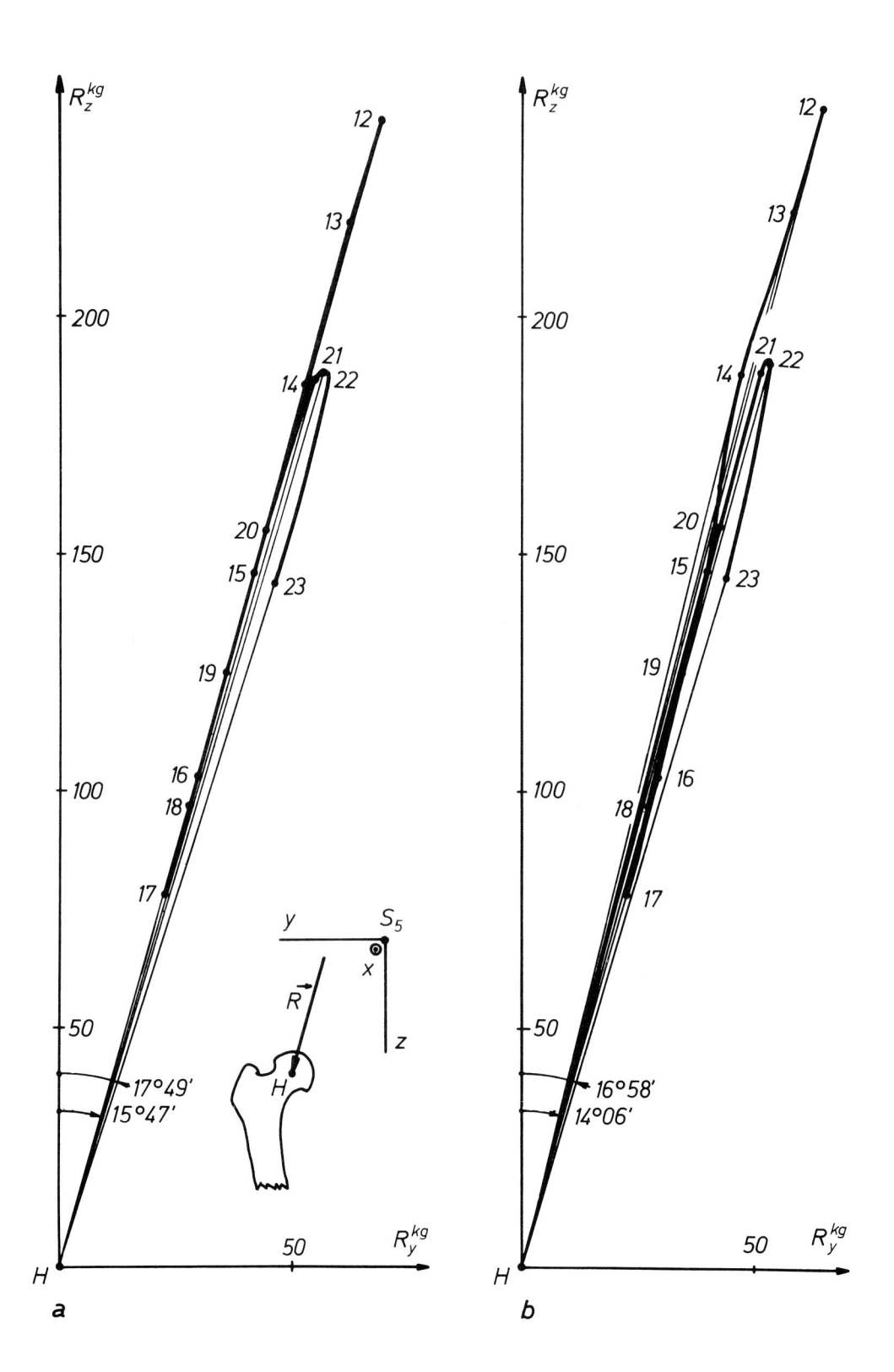

Fig. 10a, b

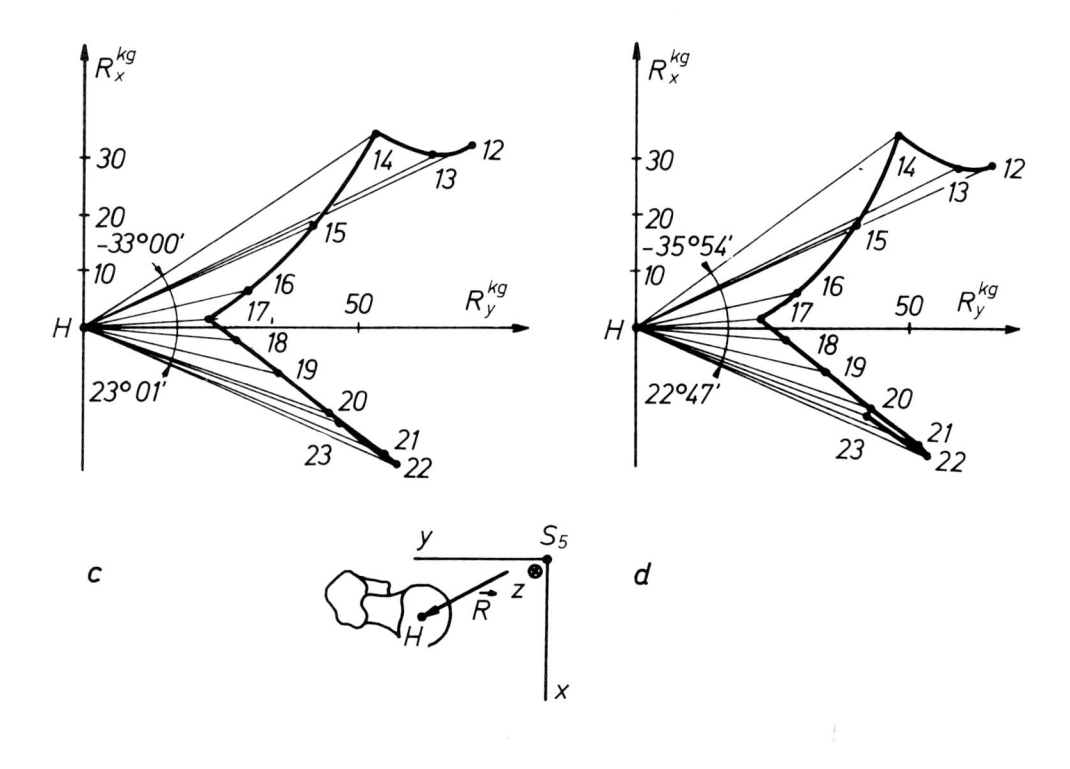

Fig. 10. Projection of the resultant force R on the coronal plane (**a, b**) and on the horizontal plane (**c, d**). **a** and **c** for the first hypothesis; **b** and **d** for the second hypothesis. S_5, centre of gravity of the part of the body acting on the loaded hip; H, centre of the femoral head

2. Discussion

In the coronal projection our curve illustrating the compressive force $\vec{R}$ transmitted from the pelvis to the femur during the single-support period of gait corresponds closely to that of PAUWELS (Fig. 11). However, there exists a significant discrepancy at phases 12 and 13. The inclination of our force $\vec{R}$ to the perpendicular (15°47′ to 17°49′ or 14°06′ to 16°58′, depending on the approach to the problem) is also very close to the 16° assumed by PAUWELS as an average for the phases 12–23.

However, in the horizontal projection our curve attains values nearly twice as great as those found by PAUWELS in this plane (Figs. 12 and 13). It must be noticed that the transverse component (axis y) of the force calculated by PAUWELS in the horizontal plane does not represent the projection on this plane of the force $\vec{R}$ which he finds in the coronal plane, except for phase 23. This is obviously a mistake due to the oversimplification of the solution of the problem which has already been mentioned. On the other hand, the direction of the projection of force $\vec{R}$ in the horizontal plane differs considerably from that given by PAUWELS in this plane. For PAUWELS, the compressive force transmitted from the pelvis to the femur would be directed outwards and always from behind forwards. Its line of action would make with the coronal plane an angle varying from −30°30′ to −2°30′ between phases 12 and 23. For us, the projection of $\vec{R}$ on the horizontal plane runs outwards but at first forwards (phases 12–17) and then backwards (phases 18–23). Its line of action forms with the coronal plane an angle varying from −33° to +23°01′ or from −35°54′ to +22°47′, depending on the solution chosen (Figs. 10 and 13). Since the centre H of the femoral head lies successively in front and then behind the coronal plane through S_5, it seems logical that force $\vec{R}$ should be transmitted from the pelvis to the femur, at first forwards and then backwards.

During all the phases of the single-support period, the resultant force oscillates about a coronal plane in such a way that it never differs much from its projection on this coronal plane. This explains why the anteroposterior view is essential to the study of the mechanical stressing of the hip. The other views are useful but much less important. For the knee the problem is completely different (MAQUET 1976).

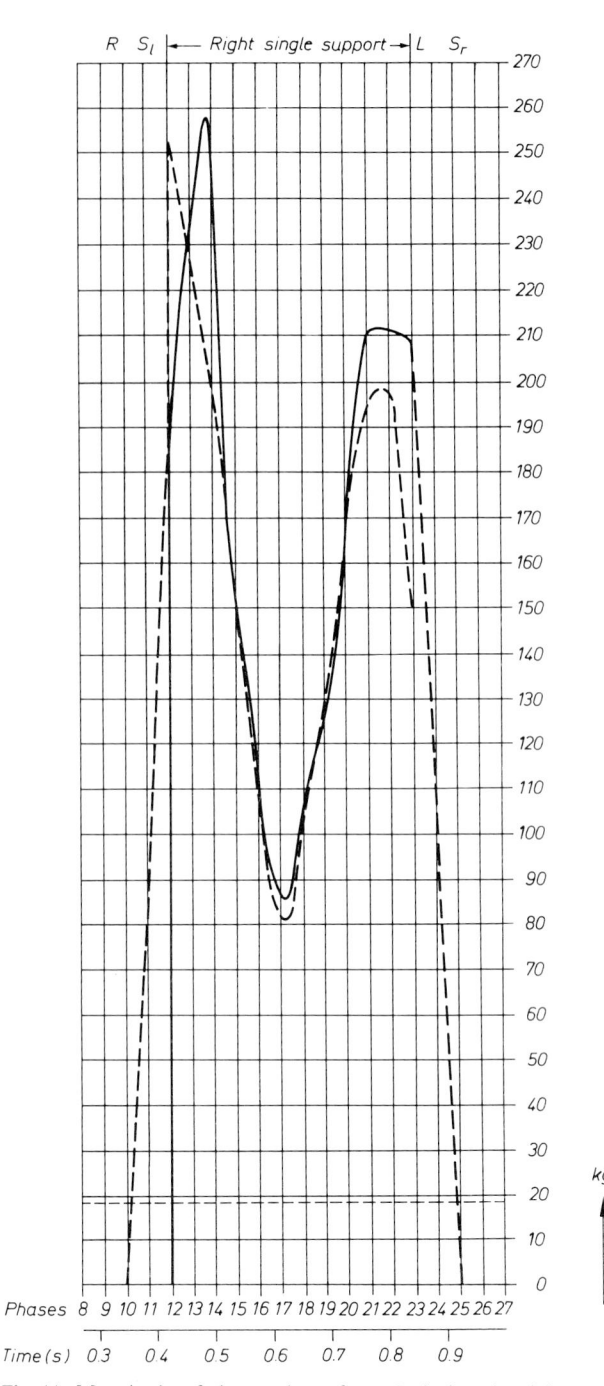

Fig. 11. Magnitude of the resultant force R during the right single-support period of gait in the coronal projection (phases 12–23 of BRAUNE and FISCHER). R, right heel strike; S_l, swinging of the left leg; L, left heel strike; S_r, swinging of the right leg. The *unbroken curve* is that of PAUWELS; the *dotted curve* is the curve for our calculation of muscular force M at 21° to the perpendicular

3. Conclusion

As far as the coronal projection is concerned, our analysis of the force transmitted across the hip joint during the single-support period of gait in the subject of BRAUNE and FISCHER confirms the study on the same subject carried out by PAUWELS using other methods. In the horizontal plane the force exerted on the hip seems to be greater and its direction is different from that described by PAUWELS.

The force exerted on the hip during gait is thus analogous to a continuous hammering, varying between 81 kg and 254 kg for the subject under consideration, whose weight is 58.7 kg. This force oscillates forwards and backwards over the joint, but remains close to the coronal plane. The projection of the resultant force on this coronal plane is very close to the resultant force itself.

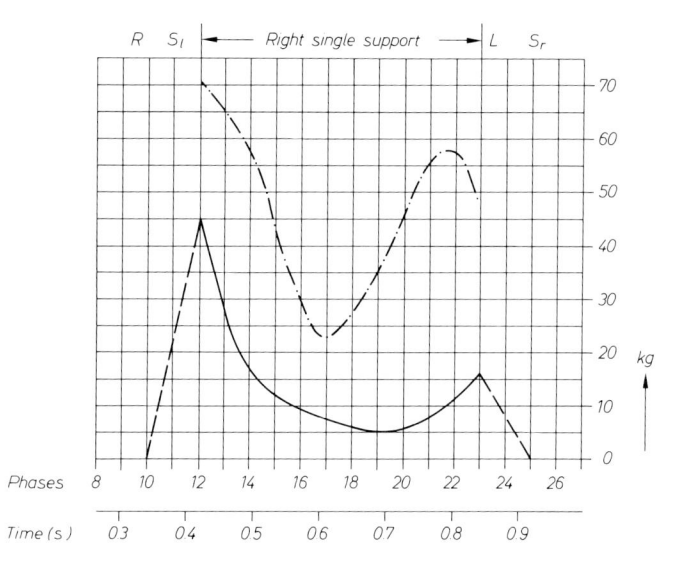

Fig. 12. Projection of the resultant force R on a horizontal plane during the right single-support period of gait. R, right heel strike; S_l, swinging of the left leg; L, left heel strike; S_r, swinging of the right leg. The *continuous curve* is that of PAUWELS. The *broken line* is the curve for our calculation of muscular force M at 21° to the perpendicular

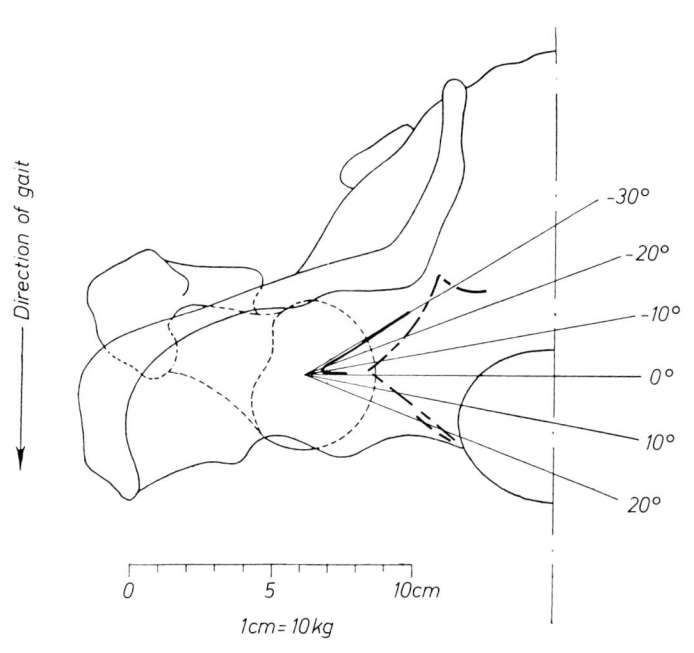

Fig. 13. Direction and magnitude of the horizontal projection of the resultant force R during the right single-support period of gait. The *continuous curve* is that of PAUWELS. The *broken line* is the curve for our calculation of muscular force M at 21° to the perpendicular

III. Mechanical Stressing of the Normal Hip Joint

The resultant force R creates compressive stresses in the joint, the articular pressure. The magnitude and distribution of the articular compressive stresses depend on:

1. The magnitude of R
2. The extent of the weight-bearing surface of the joint
3. The position of R in the weight-bearing area

In a normal individual, R attains more than four times body weight during gait. We shall see, however, that this magnitude can vary depending on the anatomical structure of different individuals. GREENWALD and HAYNES (1972) measured the contact surfaces of the hip joint. In their experiment, the area of full contact, under load, ranged between 22.19 and 33.68 cm^2 (average: 26.77 cm^2).

The weight-bearing area of the contact surfaces was deduced by KUMMER (1968, 1974, 1979) from the shape of the articular components and from the position of the resultant force in the joint. KUMMER calculated the weight-bearing area for different radii of the femoral head (between 15 and 33 mm) for different widths of the facies lunata (10°, 65° and 70°) and for different distances of the resultant force R from the lateral edge of the acetabulum (between 10° and 50°). The wider the facies lunata, the further the resultant force from the edge of the acetabulum and the greater the radius of the femoral head, the larger the weight-bearing surface area. For a femoral head of 25-mm radius, the calculated weight-bearing surface was between 11.4 and 24.5 cm^2. To determine the articular stresses, the resultant force must be divided by the projection of the actual weight-bearing surface on a plane normal to the resultant force. This is reliable as long as the resultant force intersects the centre of the weight-bearing surface area, as seems to be the case in a normal hip.

KUMMER concludes that the maximum compressive stresses in a normal hip attain an order of magnitude of 16–20 kg/cm^2. It is interesting to notice that we arrived at the same order of magnitude for the femorotibial and patellofemoral compressive stresses, although we calculated the latter in a completely different way.

IV. Mechanical Stressing of the Normal Femoral Neck

The resultant force R is exerted on the neck of the femur as well as on the joint, since no muscles are inserted on the neck. The stressing of the bone changes at the next muscular origin, on the greater trochanter. The line of action of R does not coincide with the axis of the femoral neck. They intersect at the centre of the femoral head and then diverge distally (Fig. 14). Force R thus tends to bend the femoral neck. Its line of action soon runs outside the core of the femoral neck, medially. Therefore, R evokes both compressive stresses and tensile stresses in the neck. Since force R acts to compress as well as to bend the femoral neck, however, the compressive stresses are always greater than the tensile stresses. The maximum compressive stresses arise at the medial margin of the neck, the maximum tensile stresses at its lateral margin. They decrease towards the neutral fibre in the centre of the neck. At the neutral fibre there are no compressive or tensile stresses. Since it is exerted obliquely on the femoral neck, the resultant force R also evokes shearing stresses. The magni-

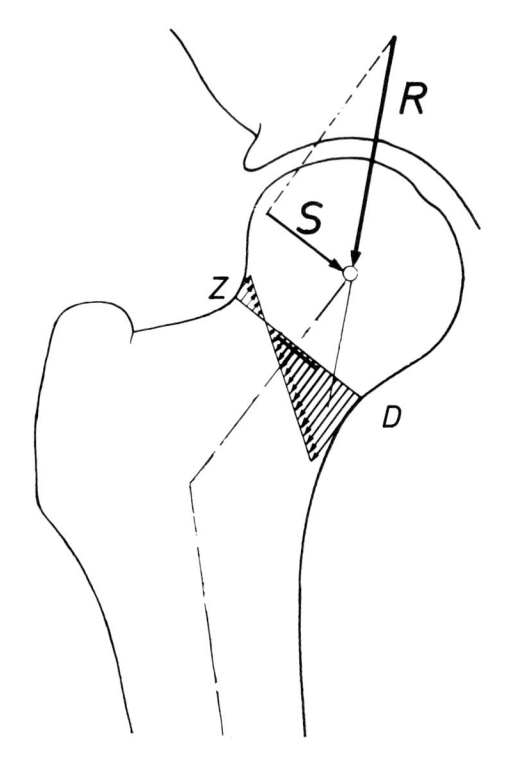

Fig. 14. Stressing of the femoral neck by the resultant force R. D, compression; Z, tension; S, shearing component. The core of the femoral neck is indicated by a heavy line inside the stress diagram

tude of the shearing component S of force R depends on the degree of inclination of the line of action of R to the axis of the femoral neck.

PAUWELS has used photoelastic models in order to demonstrate and analyse the mechanical stressing of the femoral neck. Photoelasticity uses the accidental birefringence which appears in every monorefringent, translucent material when loaded and consequently subjected to internal stresses. Glass has this property to some degree and gelatine more so. Plexiglass, araldite, bakelite, lucite and dekorite are most often used to make the models. When loaded and observed in white polarized light, the model shows continuous black and coloured lines. The black lines are called "isoclinics". From these can be constructed the isostatics, which indicate the flow of forces. The coloured lines, isochromatics, indicate the relative magnitude of the stresses.

The basis of the optical phenomenon has been summarized by KUMMER (1956, 1959), relying on the work of FÖPPL and MÖNCH (1959). Recently, the photoelastic technique has been considerably improved, and it is now possible to solve certain problems by observing a third arrangement, the "pattern of isopachics". Combined isochromatics and isopachics give the absolute magnitude of the stresses in the model. The complete photoelastic effect has been described by PIRARD (1960).

A plane model corresponding to a plane mechanical object can be rigorously analysed by photoelastimetry, which accurately indicates the mechanical state of the object — qualitative as well as quantitative. Projecting from the model to the object is quite legitimate, since the solution assumes isotropic materials. Only the problem of scales (size and force) intervenes, and this can be overcome.

Replacing the body to be analysed by a plane cross section roughly through its diameter gives an accurate solution only for a body with symmetry of rotation, which is not the case in bone. Nevertheless, the pictures have reasonable qualitative value and give a good quantitative approximation.

The experiments in photoelasticity show the direction and the magnitude of the stresses. These can be used in functional anatomy to recognize and study the functional structure and to determine relatively the quantitative distribution of the stresses at several levels of the skeleton.

Since the model is plane and its material homogeneous and isotropic, the experiment will give information about stresses appearing in a cross section of a homogeneous and isotropic body stressed by a force acting in the plane of the cross section.

The only question which can be answered by such an experiment is: Does the direction of the elements of bone (for instance the trabeculae in cancellous bone) correspond to the direction of the trajectories of stresses in a cross section of the model with the same outline as the studied bone?

There exists another possible use of photoelasticity. In some complicated instances it is not possible to analyse with certainty the physiological stress on the studied structure. One must then rely on more or less acceptable hypotheses. If, in such instances, the model shows a trajectorial picture in conditions of loading which agree with the theoretical possibilities, and if the trajectorial picture obtained corresponds to the analysed structure, one can conclude that the studied structure is trajectorial. Most biological structures are complicated and of irregular outline. On the other hand, the trajectorial pattern of the model is far from simple. It is unlikely that a similarity between them is due to chance. The results of the photoelastic study must thus be regarded as an important clue to the solution of the problem.

In the models of PAUWELS the body weight was represented by a weight suspended from the pelvis medially and the abductor muscles were simulated by a cable attached at the greater trochanter and pulling upwards and medially. In fact, some of the abductor muscles are biarticular and do not originate from the greater trochanter. Therefore, we repeated the experiment with photoelastic models in which we simulated two groups of abductor muscles. Plane models of the upper part of the femur were cut and articulated with a model of the pelvis. A layer of rubber was interposed between the femur and the pelvis (Fig. 15). The mass of the body supported by the hip should be represented by a force acting eccentrically on the femoral head, through the pelvis. Actually, we used the reaction P to this force. Reaction P is exerted along the line of action of the force due to the body mass and is equal to this force but is applied at the femur. The abductor muscles, which counterbalance force P, were replaced by two cables. One originated from the pelvis and was attached at the greater trochanter. It was appropriately tightened and corresponded to the monarticular abductor muscles, such as the gluteus medius and minimus. The other ran over the greater trochanter and was tightened by a weight S. It corresponded to the biarticular muscles, such as the tensor fasciae latae and part of the gluteus maximus. The inclination and position of the two cables and the position of the weight S were such

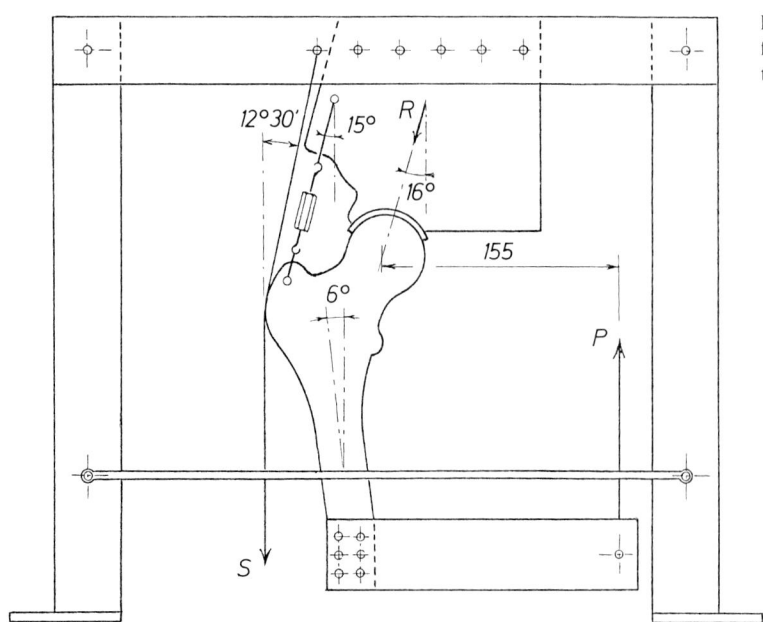

Fig. 15. Loading of the models. *P*, reaction force to the body weight; *R*, compressive articular force; *S*, pull on the lateral cable

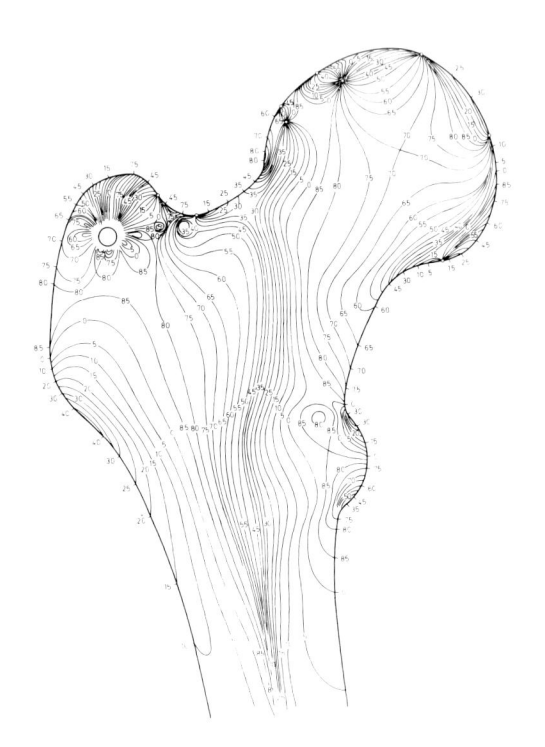

Fig. 16. Pattern of isoclinics

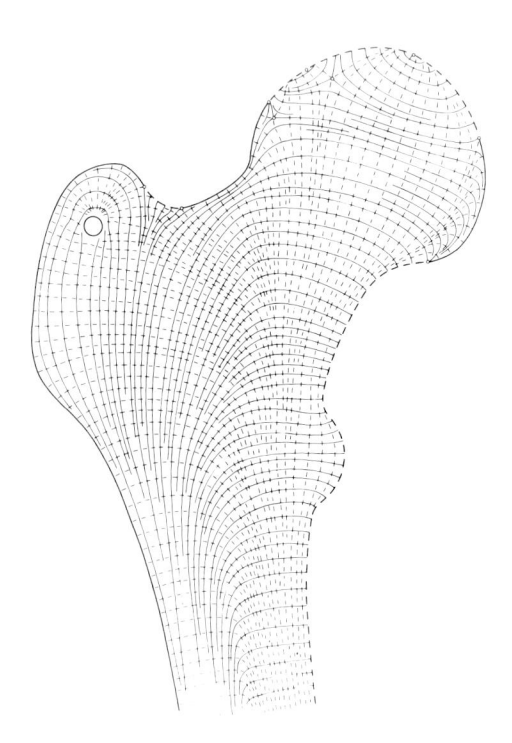

Fig. 17. Pattern of isostatics

that the resultant of the forces exerted by the two cables counterbalanced P exactly and was inclined at 21° to the perpendicular. The resultant R of all the forces exerted on the model formed an angle of 16° with the perpendicular. The neck-shaft angle was 130°. These data correspond to those given by PAUWELS.

Using a plexiglass model we obtained the pattern of isoclinics (Fig. 16) from which the network of isostatics was drawn (Fig. 17). The isostatics illustrate the orientation β of the stresses. β is the angle formed by the direction of the stress and the axis x in a system of rectangular co-ordinates x, y. The pattern of isochromatics appeared in an araldite model (Fig. 18). The isochromatics represent the difference of the principal stresses $(\sigma_1-\sigma_2)$ everywhere in the model. The principal stresses are the maximum (σ_1) and minimum (σ_2) stresses. We used holography to obtain the network of isopachics giving the lines along which the sums of the principal stresses $(\sigma_1+\sigma_2)$ are equal (Fig. 19). Knowing the sum, difference and orientation of the principal stresses, we could calculate the stresses σ_x and σ_y and the shearing stresses τ for any directions (xy) normal to each other.

$$\sigma_x = \sigma_1 \cos^2\beta + \sigma_2 \sin^2\beta$$
$$\sigma_y = \sigma_1 \sin^2\beta + \sigma_2 \cos^2\beta$$
$$\tau = \frac{\sigma_1-\sigma_2}{2} \sin 2\beta$$

The normal stresses and the shearing stresses have been calculated in different cross sections of the femoral neck and head (Fig. 20). These cross sections are normal to the axis of the neck. EF lies at the base of the neck, GH at the narrowest part of the neck, IJ at the border between the neck and the head, and KL coincides with the largest diameter of the head.

The distribution of the normal stresses σ_y over the cross sections is illustrated by Figs. 21–24. The normal stresses are normal to the cross sections. In the diagrams the magnitude of the stresses is indicated by the ordinate and the abscissa corresponds to the cross section. The tensile stresses are positive $(+\sigma_y)$. Their distribution curve lies above the axis of the abscissa. The compressive stresses are negative $(-\sigma_y)$. Their distribution curve lies beneath the axis of the abscissa. The magnitude of the stresses is given in isochromatic fringe orders. Using kg/cm² or any other force/surface unit would be meaningless, since the data thus calculated pertain to the plane model only. They cannot be applied as such to the three-dimensional femoral neck. They must be multiplied by an appropriate factor to give an idea of the actual order of magnitude of the stresses in the upper end of the human femur.

Fig. 18. Pattern of isochromatics

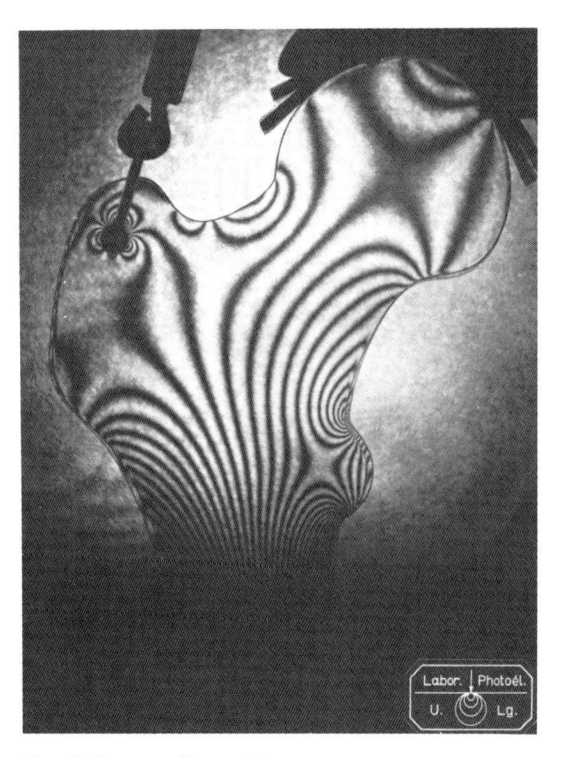

Fig. 19. Pattern of isopachics

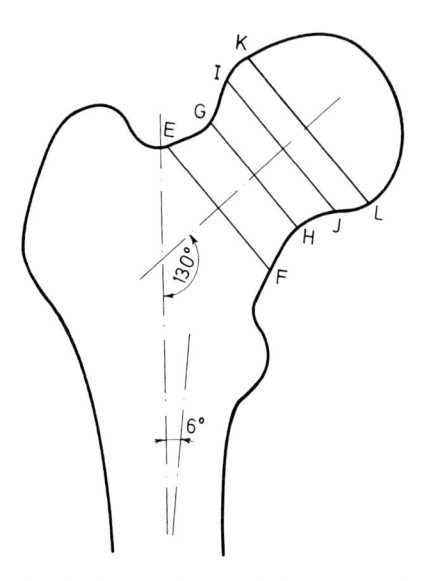

Fig. 20. Cross sections in which the stresses have been calculated

The cross section KL through the femoral head (Fig. 21) is subjected only to compression ($-\sigma_y$). The maximum compressive stress attains the order 3.4 and arises near the centre of the cross section. The compressive stresses decrease towards the two extremities of the cross section. The distribution of the shearing stresses τ is cup-shaped, with a maximum attaining the order 1.25 a little laterally from the centre of the cross section. The distribution curve of the shearing stresses lies above the axis of the abscissa except for its medial extremity.

When the curve lies above the axis of the abscissa the shearing stresses are positive, and the part of the neck proximal to the cross section KL tends to slide downwards over the part of the neck distal to the cross section KL. When the curve lies beneath the axis of the abscissa, the shearing stresses are said to be negative and the proximal part of the neck tends to slide upwards over the distal part.

In the cross section IJ, at the border between the neck and the head (Fig. 22), the maximum tensile stress ($+\sigma_y$) attains the order 0.4 and the maximum compressive stress ($-\sigma_y$) the order 2.2. The neutral fibre lies laterally from the centre of the cross section at a distance equal to 42.2% of the diameter of the cross section. The distribution of the shearing stresses τ is cup-shaped, with a maximum in the centre of the cross section (order 1.6). The curve of the shearing stresses lies above the axis of the abscissa except at the two extremities of the cross section, where it passes beneath the axis. However, this discrepancy is not significant. In general, the shearing stresses are positive, with the proximal part of the head tending to slide downwards over the distal part.

In the cross section GH at the narrowest part of the neck (Fig. 23), the maximum tensile and compressive stresses are greater than in the cross section IJ. They are found at the lateral and at the medial border. The maximum tensile stress ($+\sigma_y$) attains the order 1.25, the maximum compressive stress ($-\sigma_y$) the order 6.5. The neutral fibre lies laterally from the centre of the cross section at a distance equal to 30.8% of the diameter of the cross section. The shearing stresses τ are

Fig. 21. Distribution of the stresses in cross section KL. σ_y, stresses normal to the cross section; τ, shearing stresses

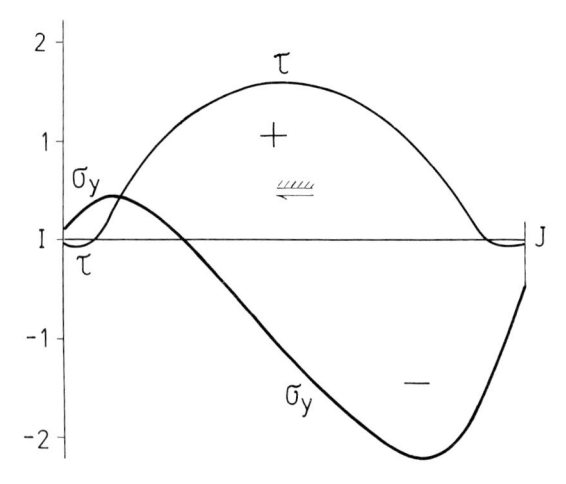

Fig. 22. Distribution of the stresses in cross section IJ. σ_y, stresses normal to the cross section; τ, shearing stresses

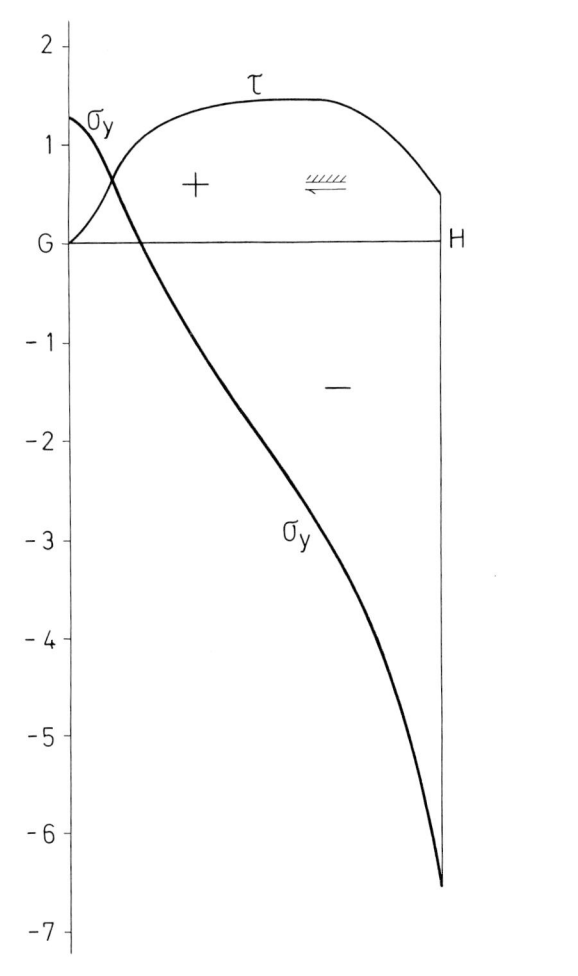

Fig. 23. Distribution of the stresses in cross section GH. σ_y, stresses normal to the cross section; τ, shearing stresses

at their greatest in the centre of the cross section, where they attain the order 1.45. They decrease towards the lateral and the medial borders of the cross section. Their curve lies everywhere above the axis of the abscissa; they are thus positive.

The cross section EF at the base of the femoral neck (Fig. 24) is subjected to tension in its lateral aspect ($+\sigma_y$) and to compression in its medial aspect ($-\sigma_y$). The maximum compressive stress is much greater than the maximum tensile stress. The maximum compressive stress attains almost the order 9 whereas the maximum tensile stress is less than the order 1.5. The neutral fibre lies laterally from the centre of the cross section at a distance equal to 7.9% of the diameter of the cross section. The shearing stresses τ are at their smallest in the lateral third of the cross section. There their curve is partly above and partly beneath the axis of the abscissa.

The distribution of the stresses in the model results from the fact that the load acts obliquely

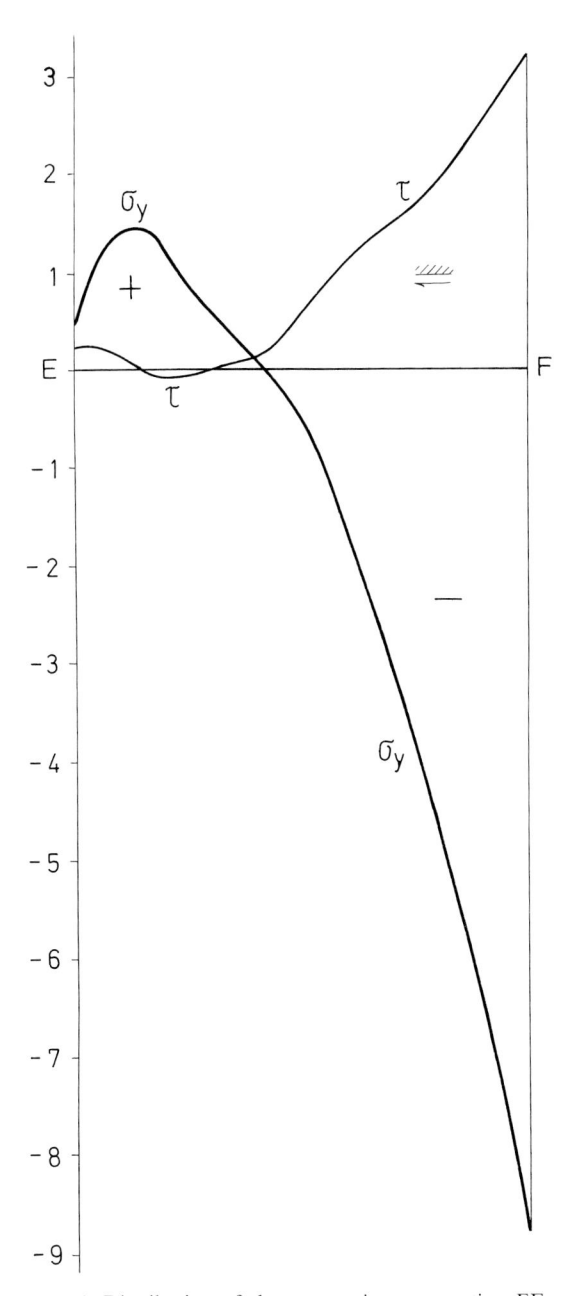

Fig. 24. Distribution of the stresses in cross section EF. σ_y, stresses normal to the cross section; τ, shearing stresses

in relation to the axis of the femoral neck, and from the shape of the model. The femoral neck is thus subjected to bending stress with superimposed compression. The line of action of the load passes further and further away from the axis of the femoral neck from proximally distalwards. Therefore, the maximum stresses increase in the same direction.

Despite the change in the arrangement of the abductor forces in our models, the networks of isostatics and isochromatics which we arrived at were not essentially different from the pictures published by PAUWELS. We can thus confirm the results of his photoelastic experiments.

The structure of the cancellous bone in a normal femoral neck illustrates the distribution and relative magnitude of the principal stresses which have been described (Fig. 25). The X-ray shows a bundle of trabeculae leaving the medial cortex of the metaphysis and fanning upwards into the weight-bearing surface of the femoral head. These trabeculae coincide with the compressive trajectories in the model. Another bundle of trabeculae which runs along the base of the greater trochanter and along the lateral cortex of the neck, intersects the first bundle in the femoral head and fans into the inferior aspect of the head. The trabeculae of this bundle coincide with the tensile trajectories in the models. They are less pronounced than the compressive trabeculae. Both bundles of trabeculae circumscribe a more translucent area, WARD's triangle, in which the stresses are minimal. This architecture of the normal femoral neck conforms with PAUWELS' law (1973b), according to which the quantity of bone depends on the magnitude of the stresses. It is typical of bending stress superimposed on compression.

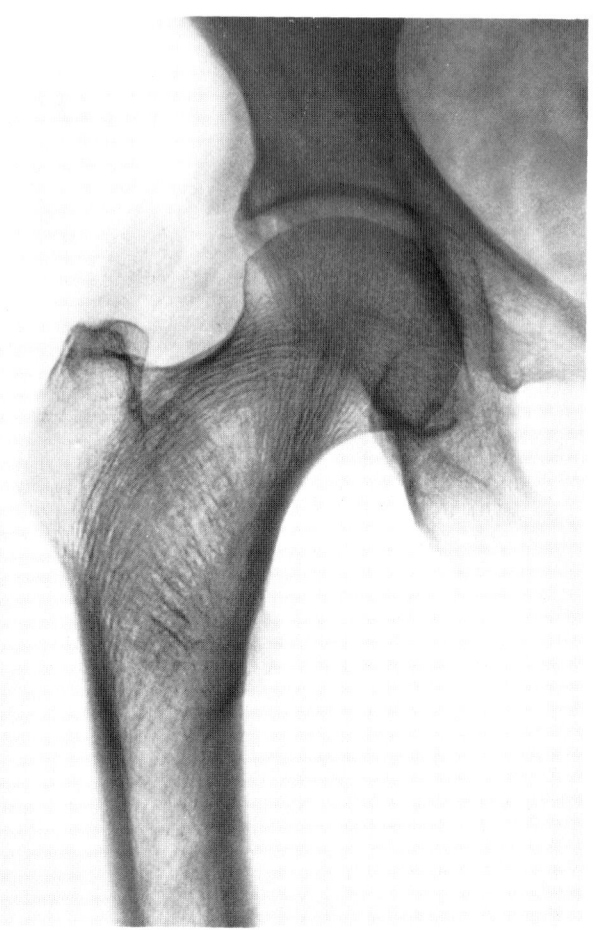

V. Cartilage Reaction to the Articular Compressive Stresses

According to KUMMER (1963, 1978), formation and maintenance of hyaline cartilage in a joint depend on the magnitude of the local compressive stresses. Hyaline cartilage is present where the compressive stresses are between an upper and a lower physiological threshold of magnitude. It disappears where the stresses are below the lower threshold and where they are above the upper threshold. The former condition occurs in the depths of the acetabulum, medial to the facies lunata, and determines the medial border of the facies lunata. This has been beautifully documented by TILLMANN (1978). Exaggerated increase of the compressive stresses destroys cartilage. This occurs in osteoarthritis.

VI. Bone Reaction to the Articular Compressive Stresses

According to PAUWELS (1973), bone is even more sensitive than cartilage to the magnitude of the stresses. Increased stresses stimulate formation of bone and decreased stresses stimulate resorption. The subchondral sclerosis in the roof of the socket clearly demonstrates that the stresses are evenly distributed over the weight-bearing surface of the normal joint (Fig. 25).

This is different from what is calculated in the model of a ball and socket joint. In such a joint, the distribution of the stresses appears cup-shaped if the resultant force intersects the centre of the weight-bearing area. The stresses are maximum along the line of action of the resultant force and decrease towards the periphery of the weight-bearing area (Fig. 26a).

Even distribution of the compressive stresses over the whole weight-bearing area seems to result from the presence of elastic cartilage in the joint. Even distribution of the articular stresses may also result from the fact that the diameter of the femoral head is a little larger than that of the socket.

Fig. 25. A normal hip with the medial bundle of compressive trabeculae and the lateral bundle of tensile trabeculae surrounding Ward's triangle. The subchondral sclerosis in the roof of the socket presents the same width throughout

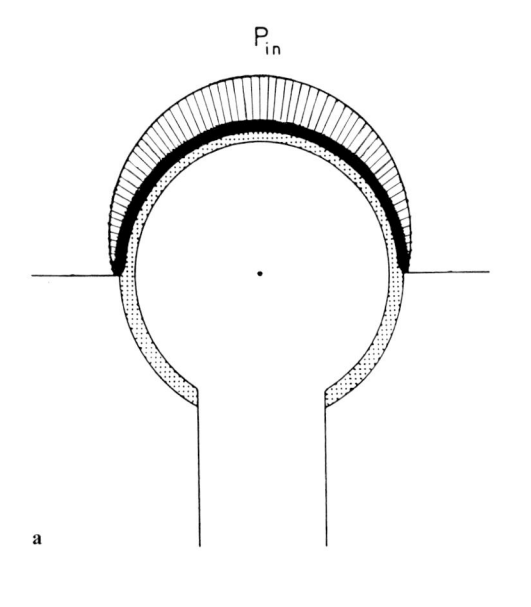

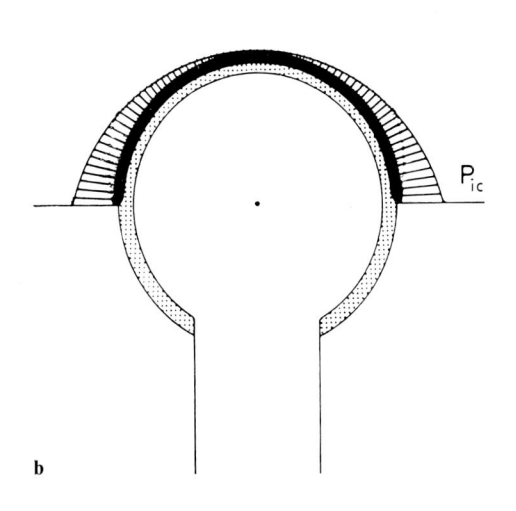

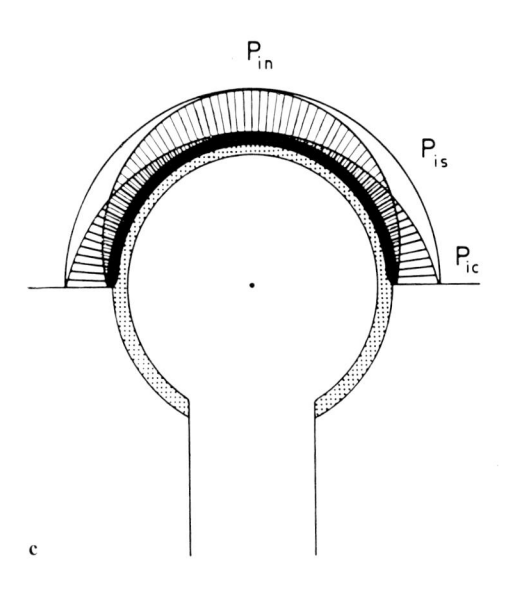

Then, as long as the joint is not loaded or is only slightly loaded, cartilage is compressed at the periphery of the socket where the stresses are increased. The central part of the socket is unloaded (Fig. 26b). When the slightly incongruent joint is loaded, the two previous stress diagrams P_{in} and P_{ic} combine into a resultant stress diagram P_{is}, of even width throughout (Fig. 26c). The observations of GREENWALD and O'CONNOR (1971) confirm this view.

The subchondral sclerosis of even width throughout in the roof of the acetabulum of a normal hip (Fig. 25) demonstrates the even distribution of the compressive stresses in the joint. Therefore, it seems that the line of action of the resultant force should intersect the centre of the subchondral sclerosis. It also passes through the centre of the femoral head. However, the line joining the centre of the subchondral sclerosis in the roof of the acetabulum and the centre of the femoral head appears to be inclined at less than 16° to the vertical in most apparently normal hips. There are two possible explanations of this discrepancy from the results of PAUWELS' fundamental analysis of the forces acting on the hip. One is that the resultant of the forces exerted by the abductor muscles, which was deduced from the work of FICK (1860, 1879), is inclined at less than 21° to the vertical and that the resultant compressive force acting on the hip is in fact closer to the vertical than was calculated by PAUWELS (1935) and more recently by ourselves (MAQUET and VU ANH TUAN 1981). The second is that, as a consequence of the semilunar shape of the facies lunata, the centre of gravity of the actual weight-bearing surface of the joint lies medial to the centre of the radiological picture of the subchondral sclerosis, which corresponds to a projection of only a part of the weight-bearing surface (Fig. 27). This second hypothesis seems more probable. In the diagram, the centre of gravity of the weight-bearing surface of the joint lies at the junction of the medial third and lateral two-thirds of the coronal projection of the proximal width of the weight-bearing surface. The resultant R passing through this point is inclined at 16° to the perpendicular.

Fig. 26. a Stress distribution in a congruent ball and socket joint. The force intersects the centre of the weight-bearing area (diagram P_{in}). **b** Slightly incongruent ball and socket joint. When unloaded, the stresses are at their greatest at the periphery (diagram P_{ic}). **c** Slightly incongruent ball and socket joint. When loaded, the stresses are evenly distributed. Their diagram, P_{is}, is the sum of the two diagrams P_{in} and P_{ic}. (After KUMMER 1978)

VII. Mechanical Significance of the Neck-Shaft Angle

An alteration in the forces acting on the hip will provoke changes in the mechanical stressing of the joint, of the growth plate when present and of the femoral neck. This has been described by PAUWELS (1973). These changes find expression in the X-ray picture.

A. Hip Joint

In a normal hip, the partial mass of the body imagined as concentrated at its centre of gravity S_5 exerts a force K which acts on the hip joint with

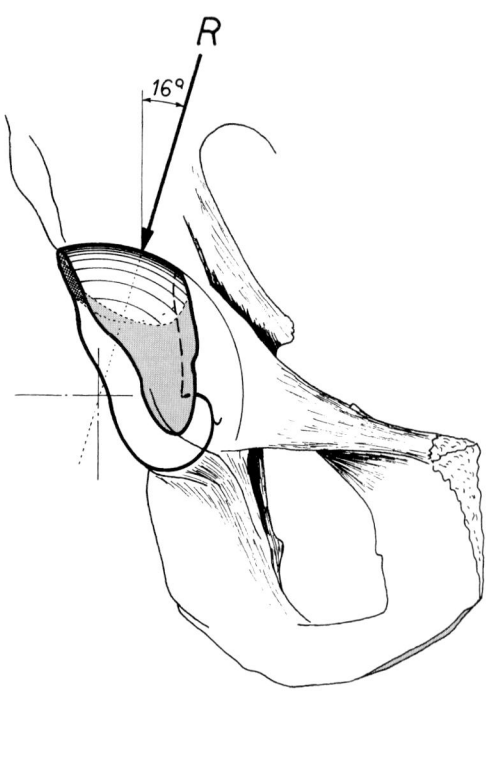

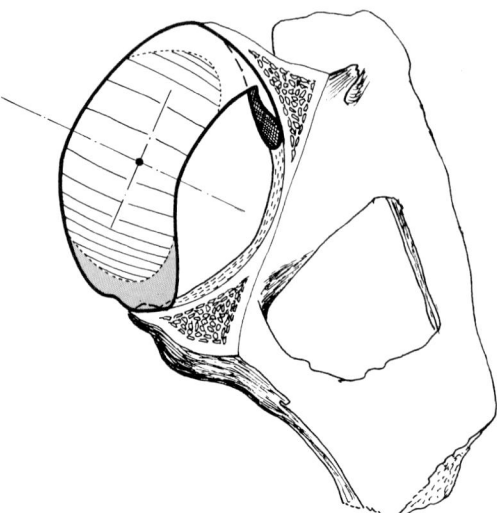

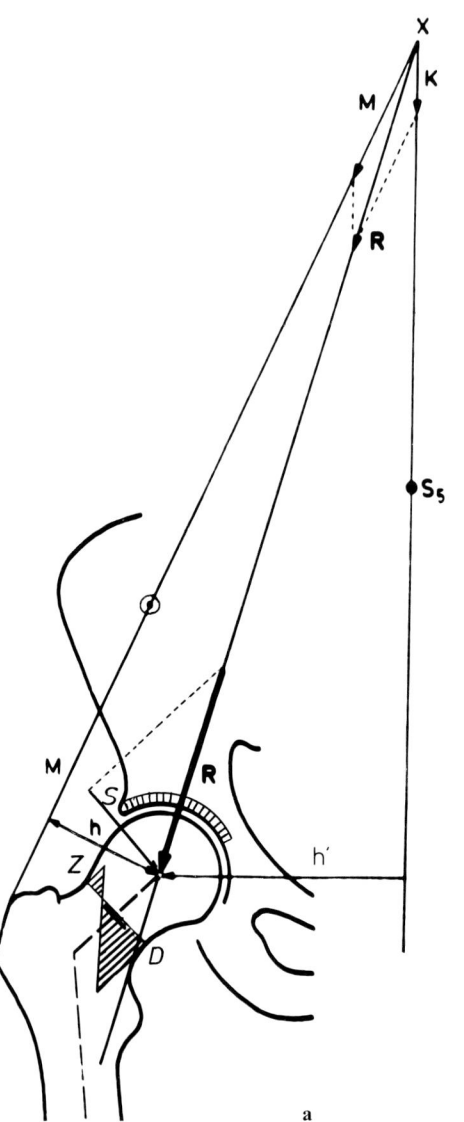

Fig. 27. The line of action of the resultant force R intersects the centre of gravity of the weight-bearing surface of a normal hip. Because of the semilunar shape of the facies lunata this centre of gravity does not lie in the middle of the projection of the facies lunata as seen in the X-ray

a lever arm h' (Fig. 28a). This lever arm originates at the centre of the femoral head. Force K is counterbalanced by force M exerted by the abductor muscles; force M acts with a lever arm h, which is one-third of the length of h'. The resultant R of forces K and M, inclined at 16° to the perpendicular, acts along a line passing through the centre of the femoral head and the intersection X of forces K and M. The resultant R intersects the centre of the weight-bearing area of the joint and creates articular compressive stresses in the joint. According to PAUWELS (1973b), the quantity of bone depends on the magnitude of the stresses. Consequently, the shape of the subchondral sclerosis in the roof of the socket coincides with the outline of the stress diagram. Its width is uniform throughout in a normal hip (Fig. 25). The articular stresses are thus evenly distributed over the weight-bearing surface of the joint.

Let us assume a femoral neck of constant length in a normal hip, in coxa vara and in coxa valga. In coxa vara (Fig. 28b), the greater trochanter lies higher than normal. This lengthens h, the lever arm of the force M exerted by the abductor muscles, and changes the direction of M. Lengthening h enables the abductor muscles to counterbalance K with less force. The change of direction of force M lowers the intersection X of the forces K and M and opens the angle $\widehat{MK}$ formed by the lines of action of forces K and M. Reducing force M and opening the angle $\widehat{MK}$ both decrease the resultant R. Moreover, the line of action of R passing through X and the centre of the femoral head becomes more inclined to the vertical. This displaces

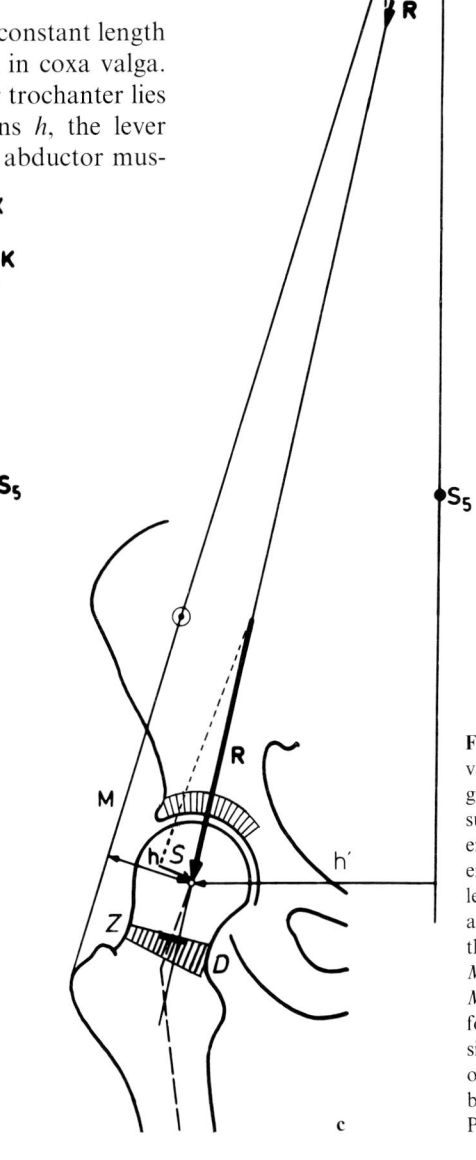

Fig. 28. a Normal hip. **b** Coxa vara. **c** Coxa valga. S_5, centre of gravity of the mass of the body supported by the hip; K, force exerted by this mass; M, force exerted by the abductor muscles; h, lever arm of force M; h', lever arm of force K; X, intersection of the lines of action of forces K and M; R, resultant of forces K and M; S, shearing component of force R; D, compression; Z, tension. The cross section of the core of the femoral neck is represented by a *thick dark line*. (After PAUWELS 1976)

R medially into the acetabulum. As long as the line of action of R continues to pass through the centre of the weight-bearing surface of the joint, the articular compressive stresses remain evenly distributed. They are smaller in coxa vara than in a normal hip because the weight-bearing surface is larger and the compressive force R is less.

In coxa valga (Fig. 28c), the greater trochanter lies lower than normal. This shortens the lever arm h of the force M exerted by the abductor muscles and changes the direction of M. Shortening h compels the abductor muscles to develop more force to counterbalance the force K. The change in direction of the force exerted by the abductor muscles raises the intersection X of the forces K and M, and closes the angle $\widehat{MK}$ formed by the lines of action of the forces K and M. Increasing force M and closing the angle $\widehat{MK}$ both increase the resultant force R, the line of action of which is displaced laterally in the acetabulum. As long as this line of action of R acts at the centre of the weight-bearing surface of the joint, the articular compressive stresses remain evenly distributed. They are greater than in a normal hip because the weight-bearing area of the joint is smaller and the resultant R is greater.

The resultant force R, or rather its counterforce R_1, can be resolved into a longitudinal component L and a transverse component Q (Fig. 29). The longitudinal component L tends to push the femoral head upwards and to provoke subluxation if the socket is shallow. The transverse component Q tends to push the femoral head into the acetabulum. In coxa vara (Fig. 29b), L is smaller and Q is greater than normal. In coxa valga (Fig. 29c), L is greater and Q is smaller than normal.

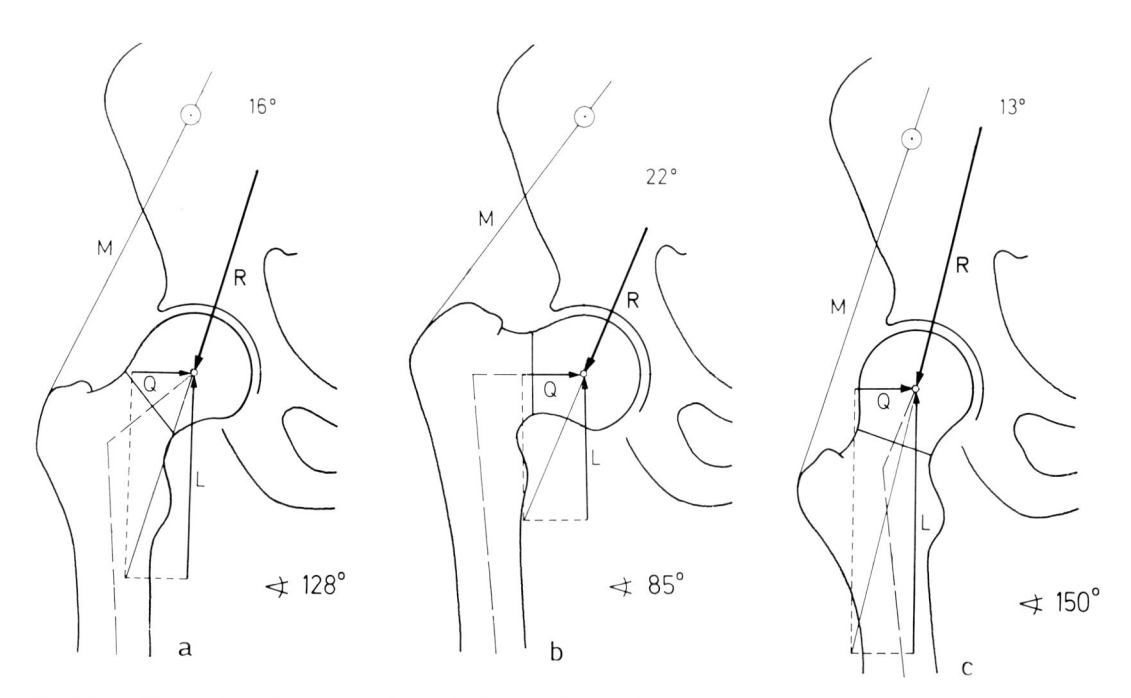

Fig. 29a–c. The resultant force R can be resolved into a longitudinal component L and a transverse component Q. M, force exerted by the abductor muscles. **a** normal hip; **b** coxa vara; **c** coxa valga. (Redrawn after PAUWELS 1976)

B. Growth Plate

Usually, the resultant force R acts normally to the centre of the epiphysial cartilage (Fig. 30a). Being subjected to compressive stresses evenly throughout, this cartilage grows evenly everywhere. When the line of action of the resultant R becomes oblique to the plane of the growth plate, as occurs after a varus intertrochanteric osteotomy or in congenital coxa vara, the medial part of the growth plate is subjected to greater compressive stresses than the lateral part, which may even be subjected to tensile stress (Fig. 30b). As long as the epiphysial cartilage reacts normally, this leads to more active growth in the medial aspect of the plate than in its lateral aspect, until the growth plate is again perpendicular to the line of action of the resultant force R. Then normal growth continues. This has been demonstrated by Pauwels (1958). We have frequently observed this reorientation of the femoral neck due to uneven growth.

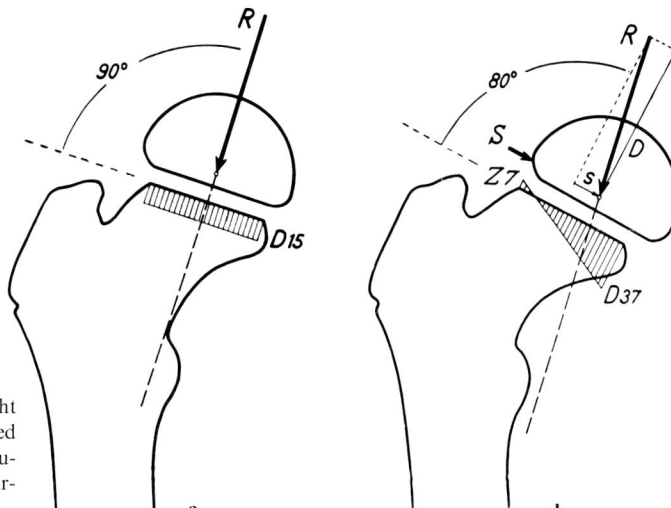

Fig. 30. a The resultant force R normally acts at right angles to the growth plate at its centre. **b** When inclined to the growth plate, force R evokes an uneven distribution of the stresses in the plate. D, compression; S, shearing force; Z, tension. (After Pauwels 1958)

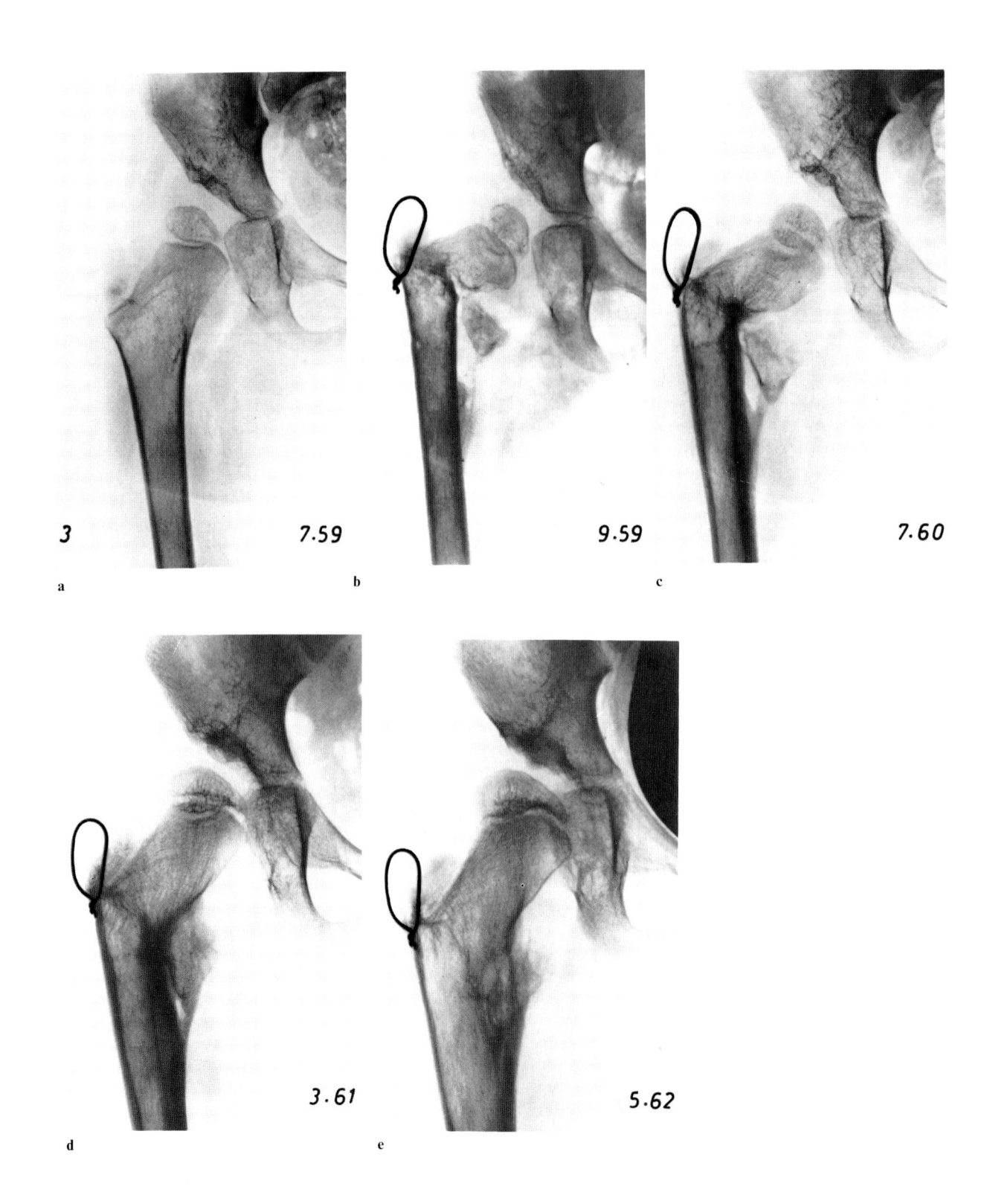

Fig. 31. a Congenitally subluxated hip in a 3-year-old female patient. **b** Varus osteotomy. **c** Twelve months later. **d** Twenty months after the operation. **e** Thirty-four months after the operation. **f** Near the end of growth. **g** New varus osteotomy. **h** Latest follow-up, 13 years after the second varus osteotomy

In a 3-year-old female child who had been born with a subluxation of the hip (Fig. 31a), the growth plate was inclined at 10° to the horizontal plane. She underwent a varus osteotomy, after which the growth plate lay inclined at 54° to the horizontal plane (Fig. 31b). Ten months later the angle formed by the epiphysial cartilage and the horizontal plate was about 36° (Fig. 31c). Eighteen months after the operation, this angle was 18° (Fig. 31d). Thirty-two months after the varus osteotomy the growth plate was nearly horizontal (Fig. 31e). After growth this patient was subjected to a new varus osteotomy (Fig. 31f, g). She was doing very well at the latest follow-up, 13 years after this second osteotomy (Fig. 31h).

If the epiphysial cartilage is unable to react normally, as in congenital coxa vara, the mechanical conditions become worse and worse and the typical picture of the condition develops (PAUWELS 1973a).

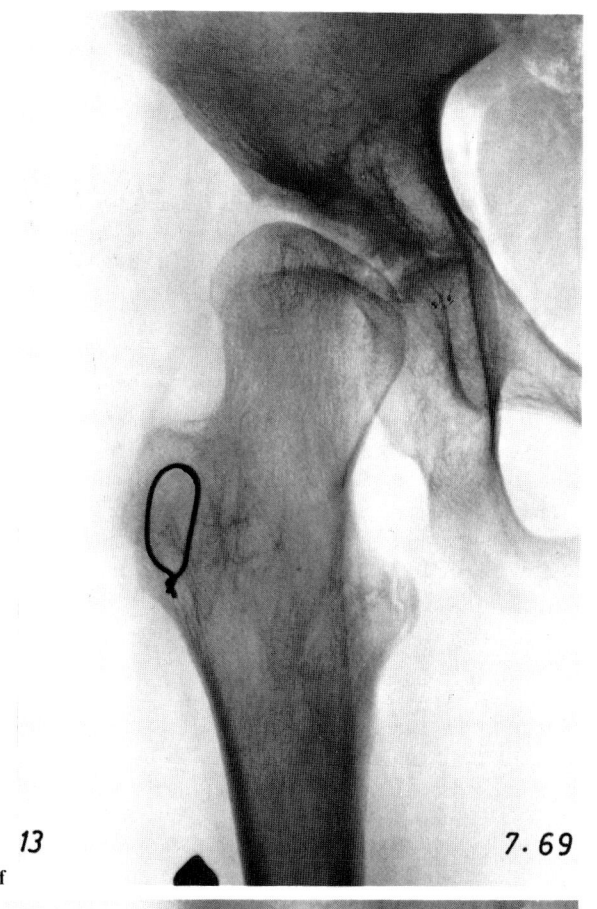

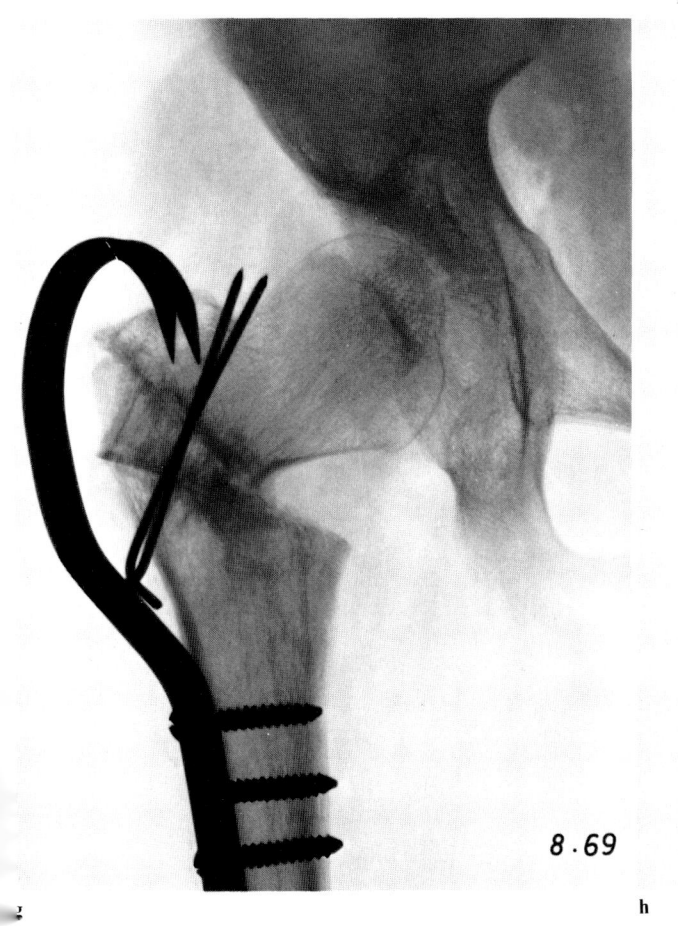

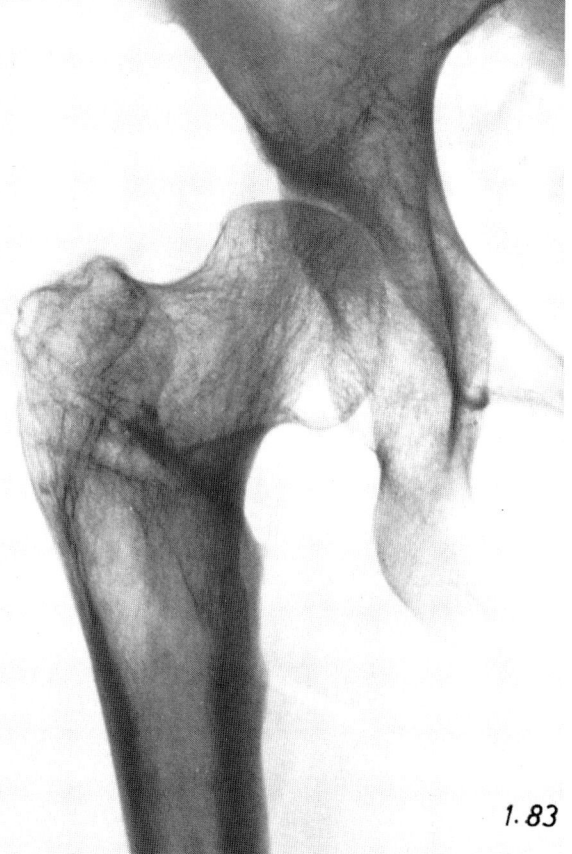

C. Femoral Neck

In a normal hip, the line of action of the resultant force R points away from the axis of the femoral neck from above downwards. The force R thus tends to bend the femoral neck more and more in this direction (Fig. 14). Oblique to the axis of the femoral neck, R evokes shearing stresses in the neck. The more the line of action of R diverges from the axis of the femoral neck, the greater is the shearing component S. S is greater than normal in coxa vara (Fig. 28b) and smaller than normal in coxa valga (Fig. 28c). In coxa valga there is no shearing component if the line of action of force R coincides with the axis of the femoral neck.

When a load acts exactly along the axis of a vertical column of homogeneous material, the load creates compressive stresses of even magnitude throughout the cross section of the column (Fig. 32a). When acting off-centre, the load subjects the column to bending stress. Acting slightly to the right of the axis but still in the core of the column, the load evokes compressive stresses greater in the right aspect of the cross section of the column than in the left (Fig. 32b). The core is the central part of the column delineated by k k in the diagram. If the load acts exactly at the right limit of the core, the maximum compressive stresses arise at the right margin of the column and are twice as great as when the load acts at the centre of the column. They are 0 at the left margin of the column (Fig. 32c). If the load acts outside the core of the column, to the right side, the maximum compressive stresses are higher at the right margin of the column and tensile stresses arise in the left aspect of the column with the maximum at the left margin (Fig. 32d). Further displacement of the load to the right considerably increases the maximum compressive stresses at the right margin and maximum tensile stresses at the left margin of the column (Fig. 32e).

PAUWELS has used photoelastic models to demonstrate the distribution of the stresses in the upper end of the femur. When the model is loaded, with the line of action of force R remaining in the core of the femoral neck, as in coxa valga, only compressive trajectories (isostatics) (Fig. 33a) are observed. They fill in the femoral neck and run nearly parallel to the axis of the neck. The load evokes only compressive stresses everywhere in the femoral neck. The X-ray of coxa valga presents one type of trabeculae corresponding to the compressive isostatics of the model (Fig. 33b).

When the load acts outside the core, as in a normal hip, two types of trajectory (isostatics) appear, compressive medially and tensile laterally (Fig. 34a). Similarly, the X-ray of a normal hip shows two main bundles of cancellous trabeculae, one medial in the compression area and one lateral in the tension area (Fig. 34b). Their directions correspond to the stress trajectories.

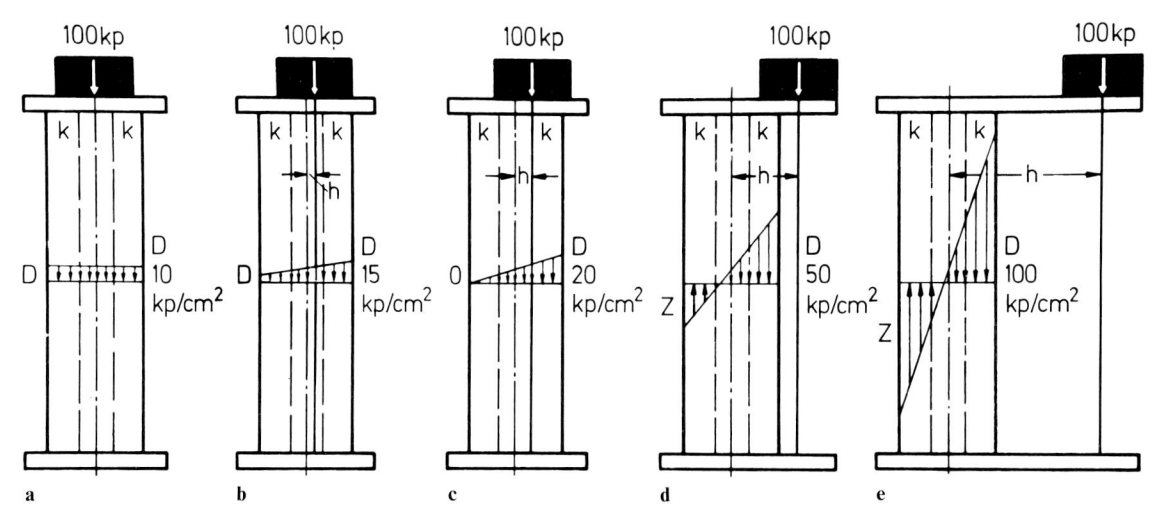

Fig. 32. a Load acting along the axis of the column. **b** Load acting eccentrically but still in the core of the column. **c** Load acting at the limit of the core. **d, e** Load acting outside the core. *KK*, core; *h*, lever arm of the load; *D*, compression; *Z*, tension. (After PAUWELS 1976)

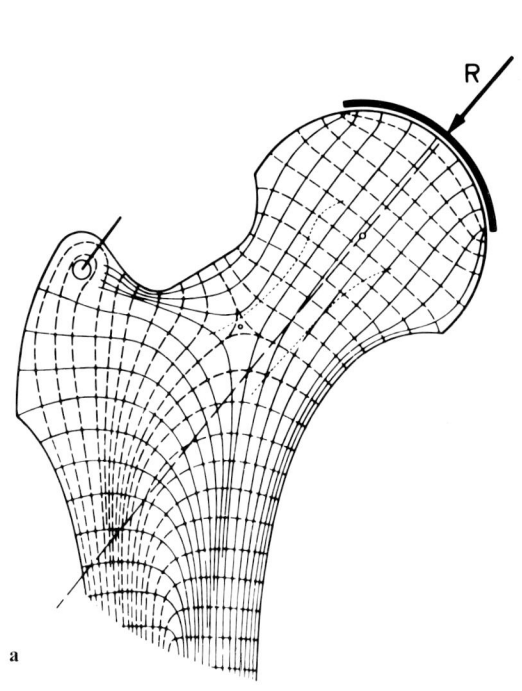

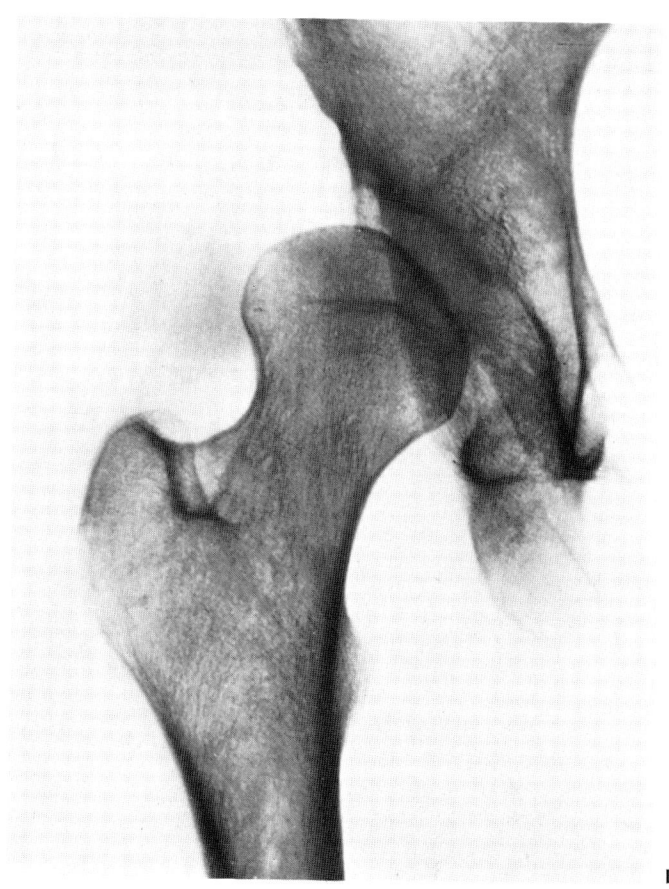

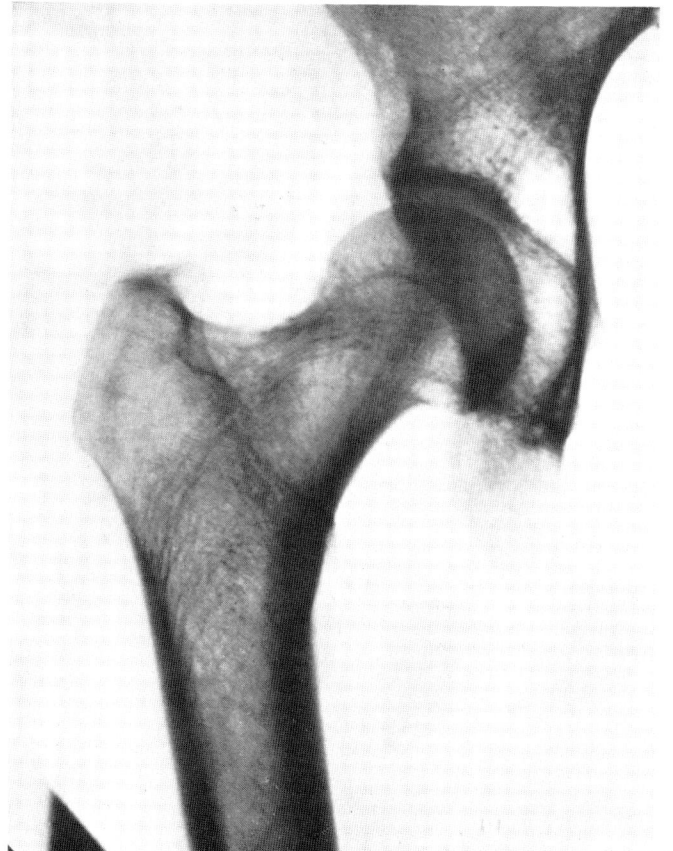

Fig. 33. a Pattern of isostatics in a model stressed as in coxa valga. *R*, resultant force acting on the hip. **b** Coxa valga. (After Pauwels 1976)

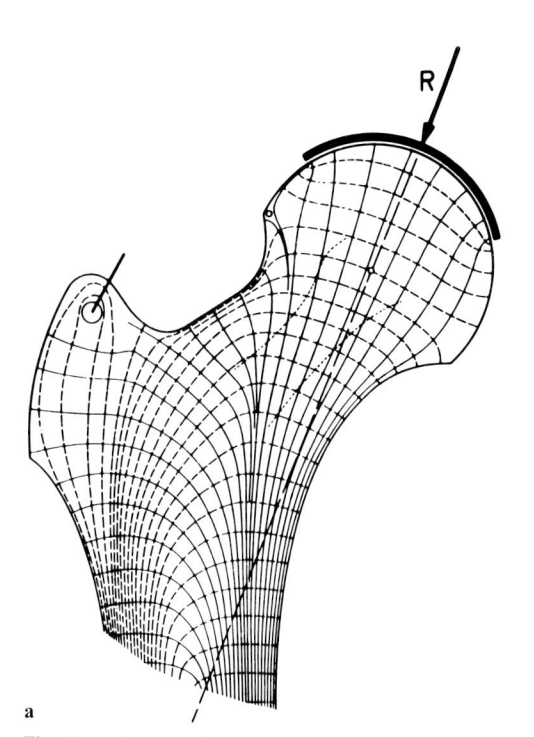

Fig. 34. a Pattern of isostatics in a model stressed as in a normal hip. *R*, resultant force acting on the hip. **b** A normal hip. (After Pauwels 1976)

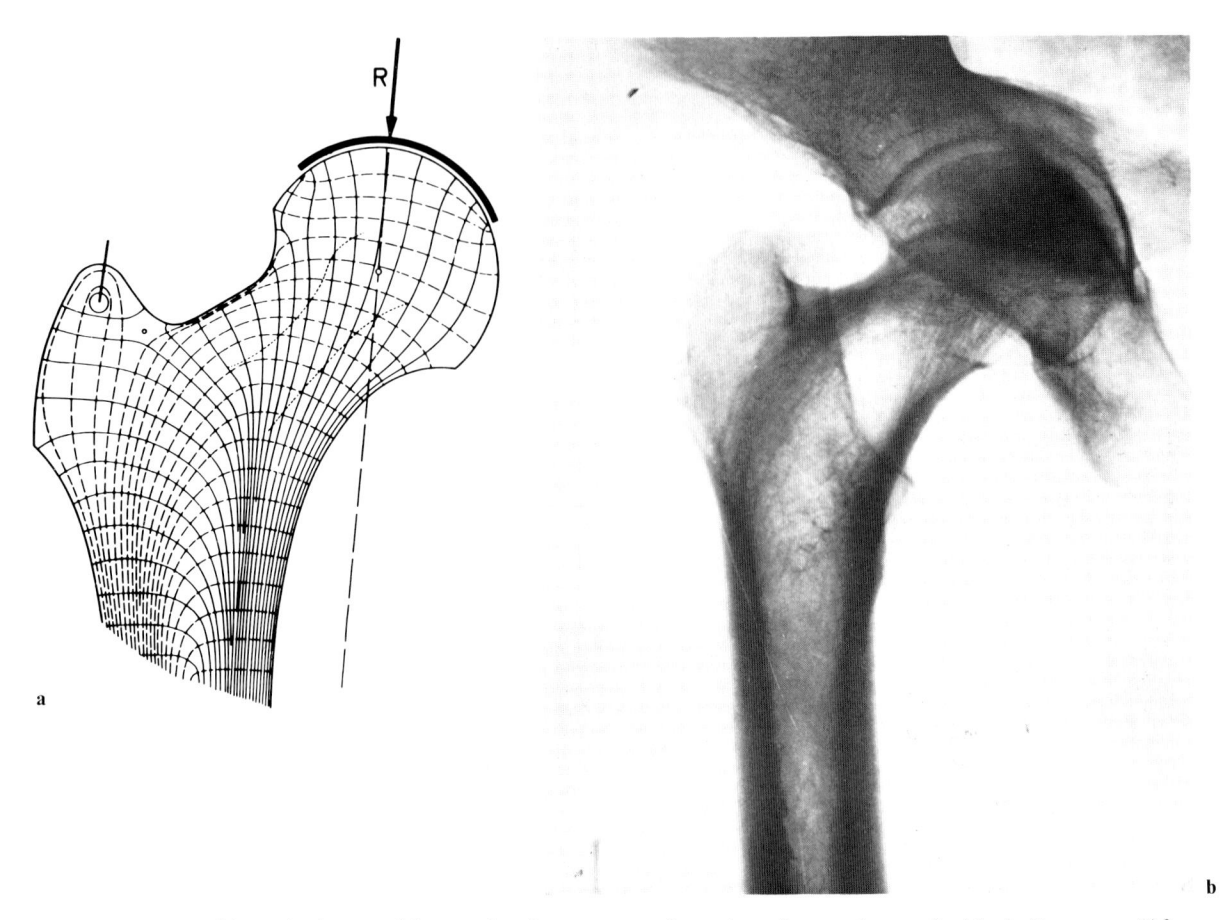

Fig. 35. a Pattern of isostatics in a model stressed as in coxa vara. *R*, resultant force acting on the hip. **b** Coxa vara. (After Pauwels 1976)

When the line of action of the load lies further away from the core of the femoral neck, as in coxa vara, the compressive and tensile trajectories are more arched (Fig. 35a). Other models showing the isochromatics indicate that the compressive and tensile stresses are greater. Similarly, in the X-ray of coxa vara, the compressive and tensile trabeculae appear more pronounced in the femoral neck than in a normal hip. They circumscribe an area which looks empty. This is Ward's triangle, where the stresses are very small (Fig. 35b).

It is interesting to compare the cancellous architecture of coxa valga with that of coxa vara (Figs. 33b and 35b). This architecture gives information on the way the femoral neck is stressed and, by deduction, on the line of action of force *R*. The change in the architecture of the cancellous trabeculae in the neck of femora from a coxa valga type to a coxa vara type and conversely is regularly observed after intertrochanteric osteotomy, especially in children or young adults.

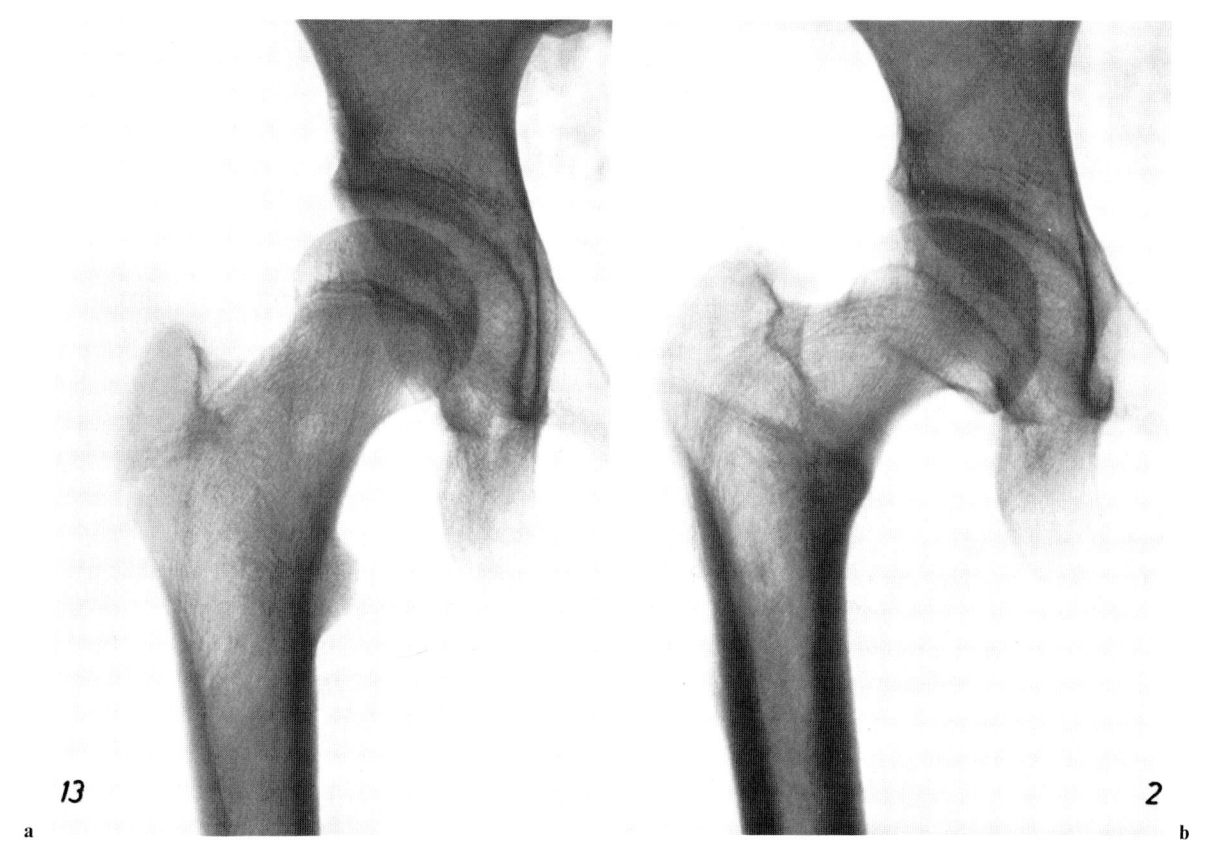

Fig. 36a, b. Change in the architecture of the cancellous bone following a varus osteotomy. **a** 13-year-old female patient before a varus osteotomy; **b** 2 years afterwards

A 13-year-old female patient presented with coxa valga and subluxation. The femoral neck was filled with cancellous trabeculae uniformly distributed (Fig. 36a). A varus osteotomy was carried out. Two years later, two bundles of trabeculae had developed in the femoral neck, surrounding a more translucent area (Fig. 36b). This represents the typical architecture in bone subjected to bending stress.

9.56   3.57   9.57

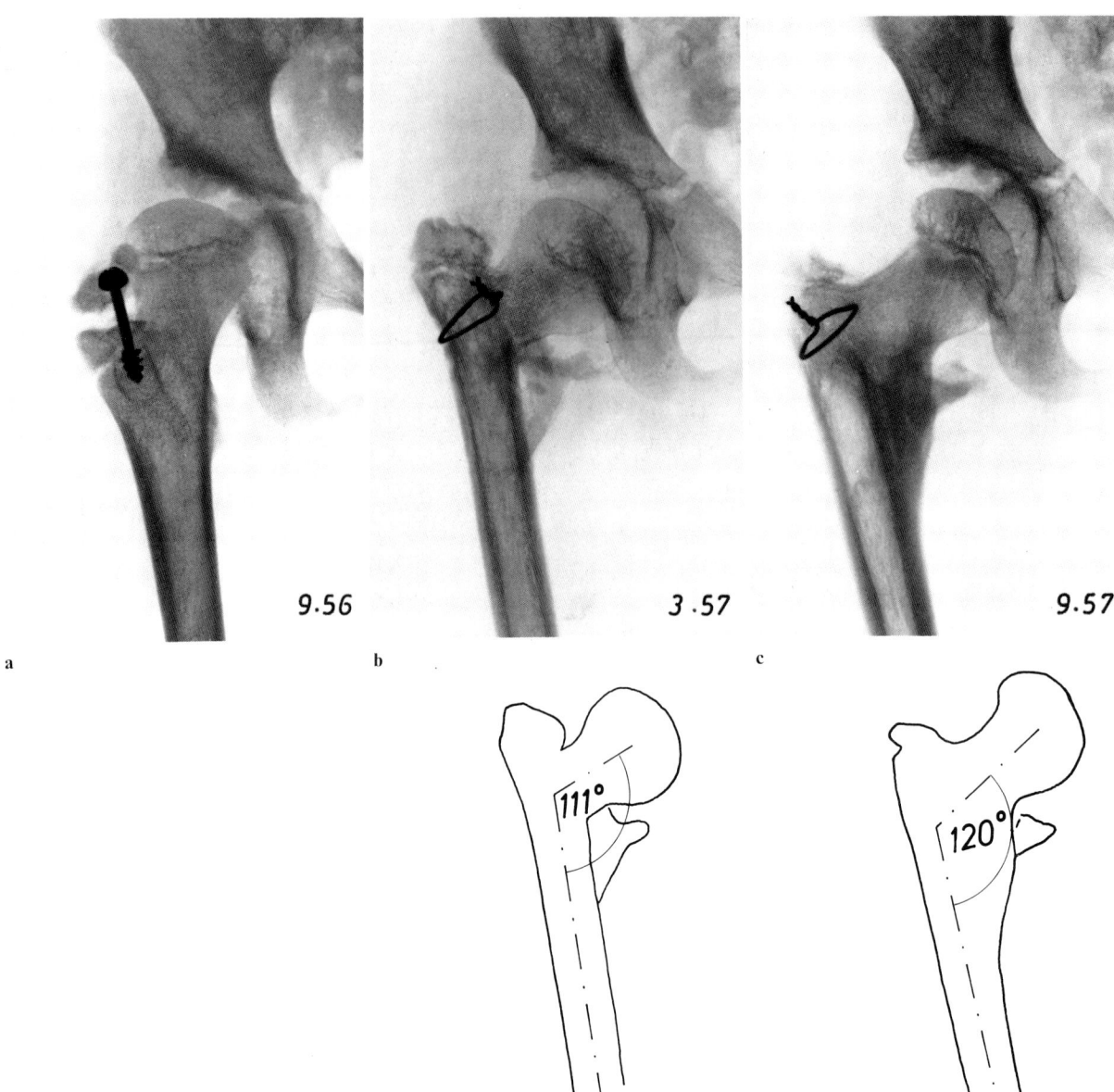

a   b   c

111°   120°

Fig. 37a–c

A 7-year-old female patient had undergone an open reduction of a congenitally dislocated hip (Fig. 37a): the structure of the femoral neck looked uniform. She underwent a varus osteotomy (Fig. 37b). Six months later two bundles of trabeculae surrounding a more translucent area were observed in the femoral neck (Fig. 37c). The Gothic arches were well visible a year afterwards (Fig. 37d). Uneven growth of the femoral neck transformed the coxa vara into coxa valga. Eleven years after the varus osteotomy, the femoral neck was again uniformly filled with trabeculae all directed vertically (Fig. 37e). A second varus osteotomy was carried out. At the 14-year follow-up the result remained excellent (Fig. 37f).

D. Conclusion

As Pauwels has shown, in coxa valga the compressive stresses in the hip are greater than in a comparable normal hip; the femoral neck is stressed moderately in pure compression; the shearing component is small or absent. In coxa vara, the articular compressive stresses are smaller than in a comparable normal hip; the femoral neck is subjected to more bending stress than is the case in a normal hip. This leads to significantly greater compressive and tensile stresses in the neck and a considerable shearing component. These differences in the stressing of the hip result in differences in the bony structure.

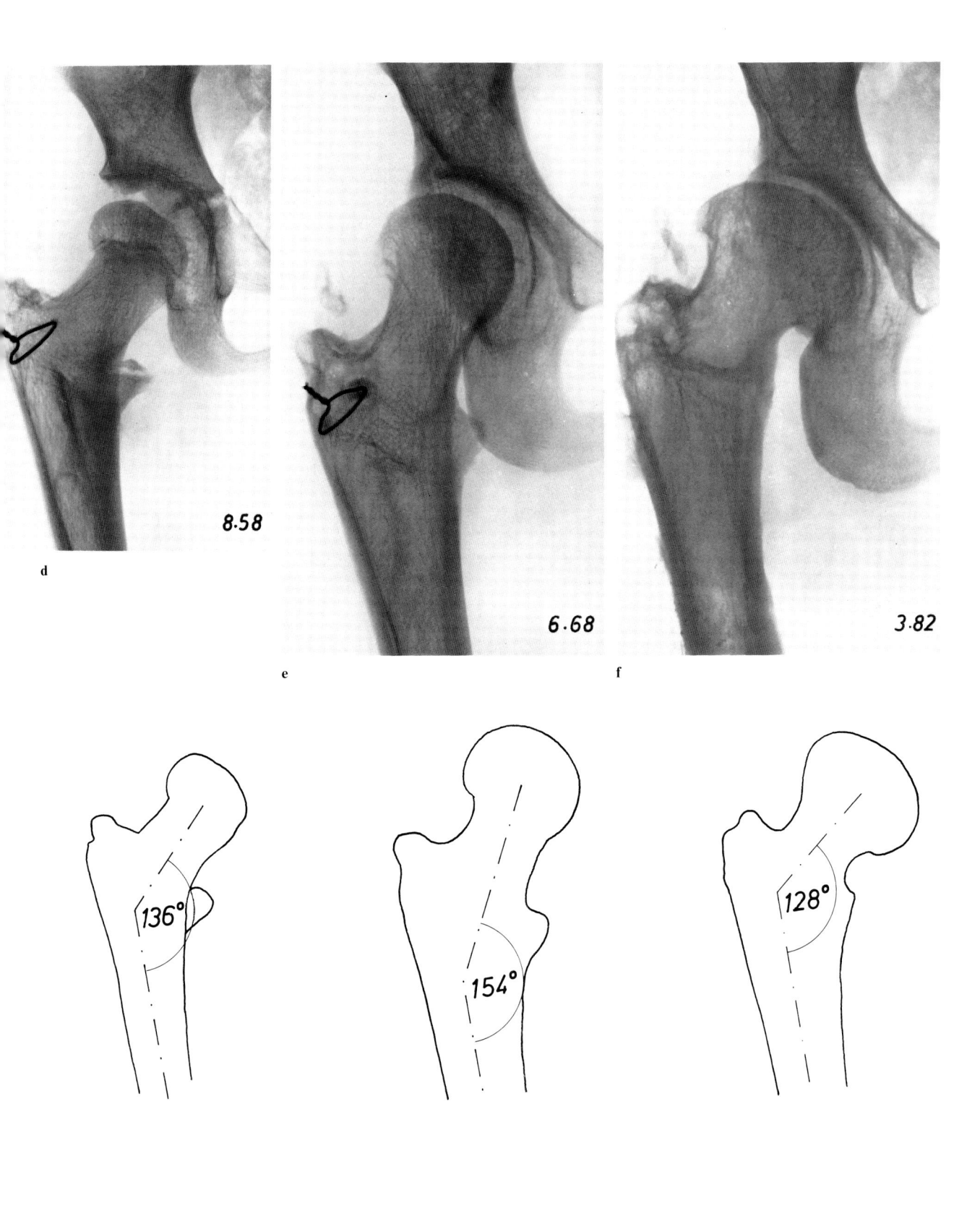

Fig. 37. a After open reduction of a congenital dislocation of the hip in a 7-year-old female patient. **b** After a varus intertrochanteric osteotomy. **c** Six months later. **d** Eighteen months after the osteotomy. **e** Eleven years after the osteotomy. **f** Fourteen years after a second varus osteotomy

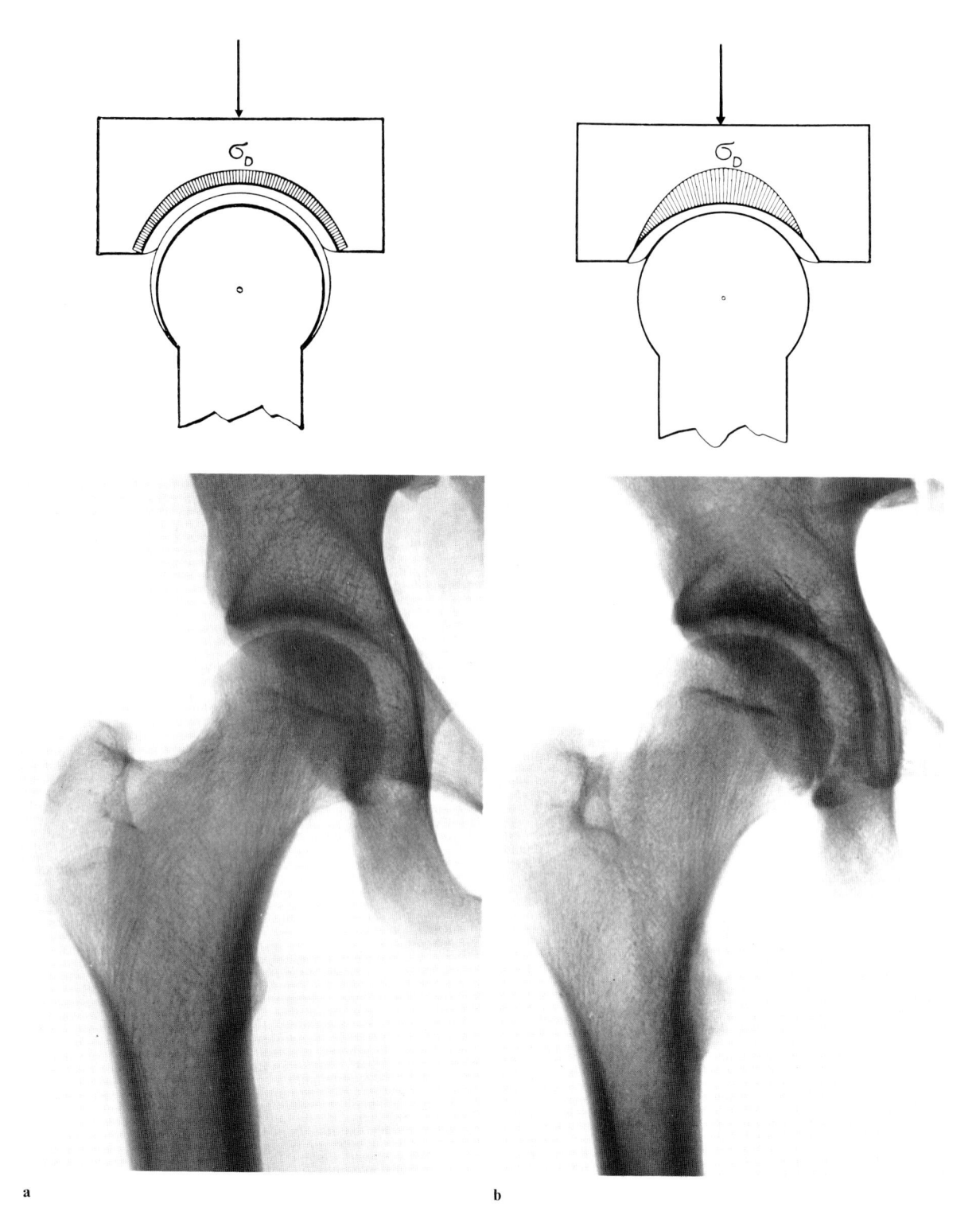

Fig. 38. a Distribution of the stresses in a model of a ball and socket joint with two interposed layers of shock-absorbing material (*top*). Normal hip with a subchondral sclerosis ("eyebrow") of uniform width throughout in the roof of the acetabulum (*bottom*). **b** Distribution of the stresses in the model of a ball and socket joint after removal of one layer of the interposed shock-absorbing material (*top*). Cup-shaped subchondral sclerosis as the first sign of primary osteoarthritis (*bottom*). σ_D, compressive stresses in the joint. (After PAUWELS 1961)

VIII. Significance of the Subchondral Sclerosis in the Acetabulum

A. Normal Hip Joint

According to PAUWELS (1973b), the quantity of bone depends on the magnitude of the stresses. He demonstrated this and enunciated a scientific law which KUMMER (1972, 1973) formulated mathematically, whereas WOLFF (1892) had only observed a change in the bony structure after an alteration in the stressing of the bone.

Subchondral sclerosis of even width throughout in the roof of the acetabulum of a normal hip corresponds to an even distribution of the compressive stresses over the weight-bearing surface of the joint (Figs. 25 and 38). Such an even distribution of the compressive stresses in a spherical joint requires:

1. The action of the transmitted force at the centre of the weight-bearing surface
2. The presence of cartilage
3. Probably a slight incongruence between the articulating surfaces in the non-loaded state

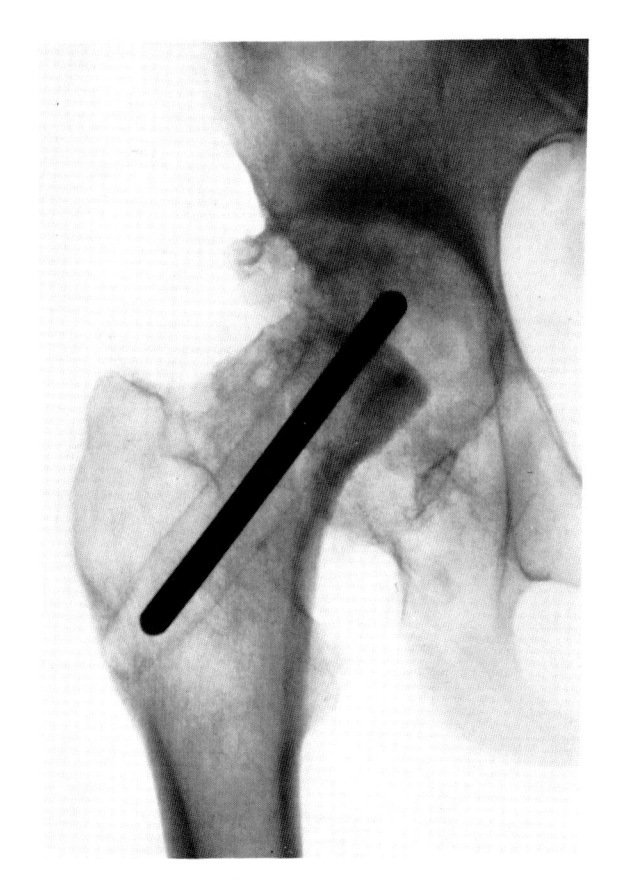

Fig. 39. Cup-shaped subchondral sclerosis in the roof of the acetabulum after prosthetic replacement of the femoral head

B. Primary Osteoarthritis

In a ball and socket joint of elastic and homogeneous material with negligible friction, when the load acts at the centre of the weight-bearing surface, even distribution of the compressive stresses can be achieved by interposing a sufficient layer of appropriate shock-absorbing material (Fig. 38a). Removing part of the layer of shock-absorbing material results in an uneven distribution of the stresses in the joint. The maximum stress coincides with the line of action of the central load and the stresses decrease progressively to zero symmetrically on both sides of the line of action of the load (Fig. 38b).

Similarly, in a normal hip the subchondral sclerosis is distributed evenly throughout in the roof of the socket (Fig. 38a). When cartilage or bone no longer distributes the stresses evenly in the joint, a cup-shaped subchondral sclerosis develops (Fig. 38b). This sclerosis indicates that the resultant force is still acting at the centre of the weight-bearing surface of the joint. The uneven distribution of the articular compressive stresses seems to result from a biological deficiency of the cartilage or from a stiffening of the bone rather than from a change in the acting forces. The cup-shaped subchondral sclerosis in the roof of the acetabulum constitutes the first sign of primary osteoarthritis. It can evolve towards a dense triangle either at the edge of the socket (subluxation) or in the depths of the socket (protrusio acetabuli). The same cup-shaped subchondral sclerosis develops in the roof of the socket after the femoral head has been replaced by a prosthesis and one layer of cartilage has thus been removed (Fig. 39).

Primary osteoarthritis seems to result from a failure of cartilage as biological material even when stressed normally. The underlying mechanisms seem to be metabolic impairment or loss of chondrocyte function and "may include death or injury to chondrocytes, defective chondrocyte replication or growth; inadequate or abnormal synthesis, secretion, maturation, or aggregation of proteoglycans; inadequate or abnormal synthesis, secretion, maturation, or cross linking of type II collagen; defective aggregation of collagen and proteoglycans" (GARDNER 1983). In osteoarthritis changes are observed in the proteoglycans and in the water content of cartilage.

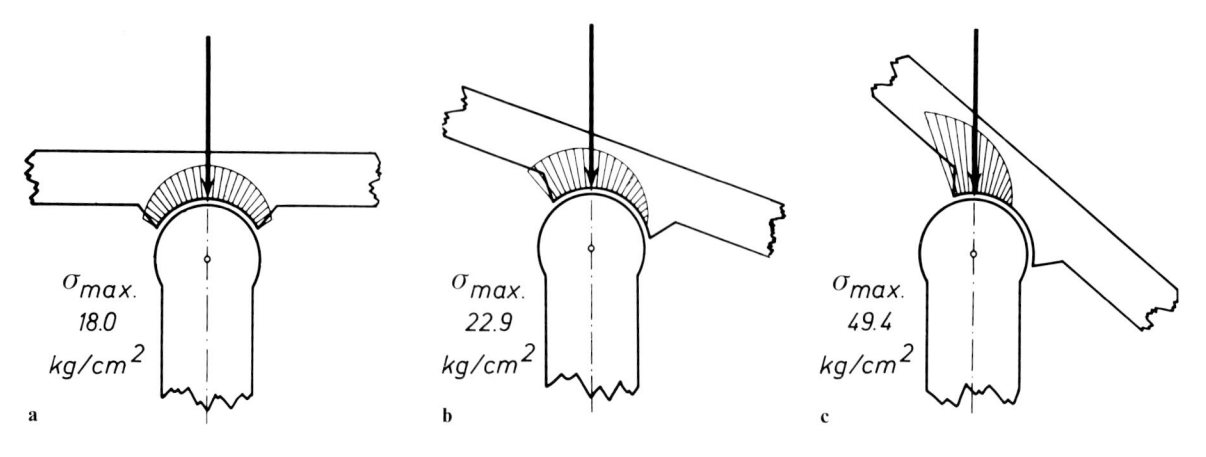

Fig. 40. a Central load. **b, c** Load acting off-centre. σ_{max}, maximum stress. (After Pauwels 1961)

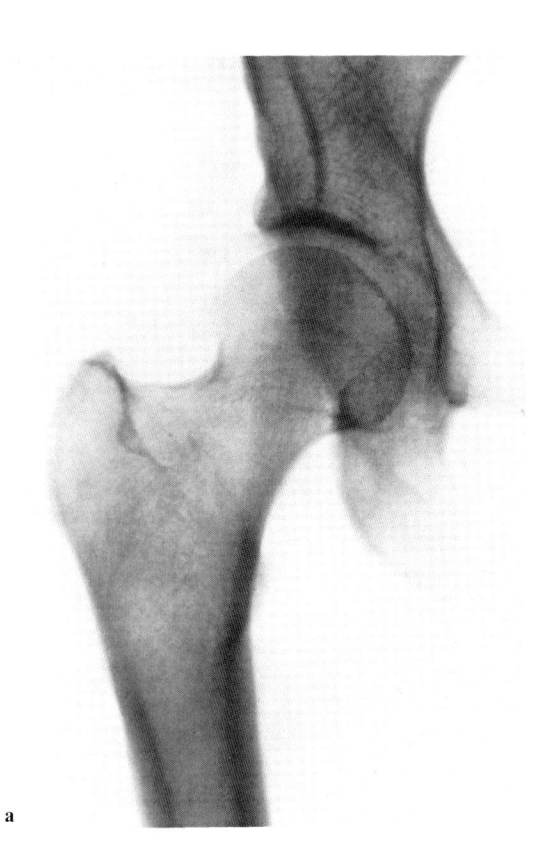

Fig. 41. a Subchondral sclerosis of uniform width throughout in a normal hip. **b** Dense triangle at the edge of the acetabulum in a subluxated hip. **c** Beyond the threshold of stress tolerance, cysts appear in the dense triangle

C. Osteoarthritis with Subluxation

In a ball and socket joint of elastic and homogeneous material with negligible friction, the compressive stresses are distributed symmetrically on both sides of the line of action of the load as long as the load acts at the centre of the articular weight-bearing surface (Fig. 40a). If the intersection of the articular surface by the line of action of the load is regarded as the pole, the weight-bearing surface obviously cannot extend beyond the equator (KUMMER 1968). In our example the whole contact surface is weight bearing.

If the line of action of the load is displaced towards the edge of the joint, the articular contact surface remains the same but only part of it is now weight bearing. The stress diagram is triangular with the maximum stress at the edge of the socket (Fig. 40b). The line of action of the load intersects the joint at about the junction of the lateral third and the medial two-thirds of the triangle. This results from the fact that the surfaces of the stress diagram on both sides of the line of action of the load must be equal. The closer the line of action of the load lies to the edge of the joint, the smaller the weight-bearing surface, although the contact surface remains unchanged. The smaller the weight-bearing surface, the greater the compressive stresses in the joint (Fig. 40c).

These are expressed by the triangular sclerosis at the edge of the acetabulum, called "PAUWELS' triangle" (Fig. 41b). This triangle appears similar to the stress diagram as long as the stresses are not increased beyond the tolerance threshold for the bone. Beyond this threshold cysts appear and bone is resorbed. This leads to remodelling of the socket (Fig. 41c).

The dense triangle at the edge of the acetabulum can be observed in congenital subluxation of the hip (Fig. 41b, c). It can also result from a lateral displacement of the resultant force R, the consequence of a progressive subluxation of the femoral head being pushed laterally by a medial osteophyte (Fig. 42). This was shown by PAUWELS (1973a). In these circumstances, the contact surface of the

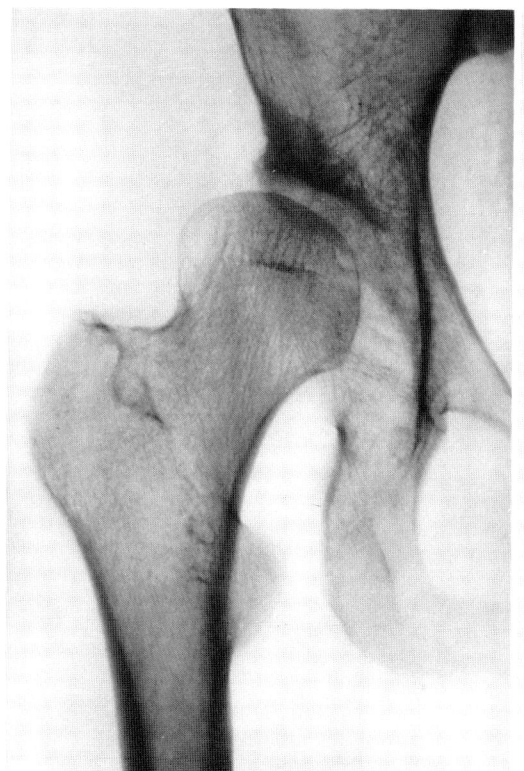

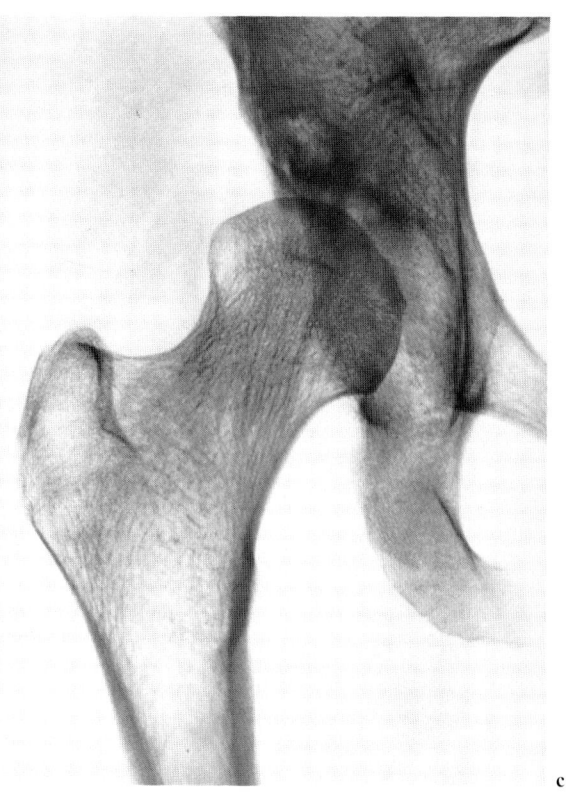

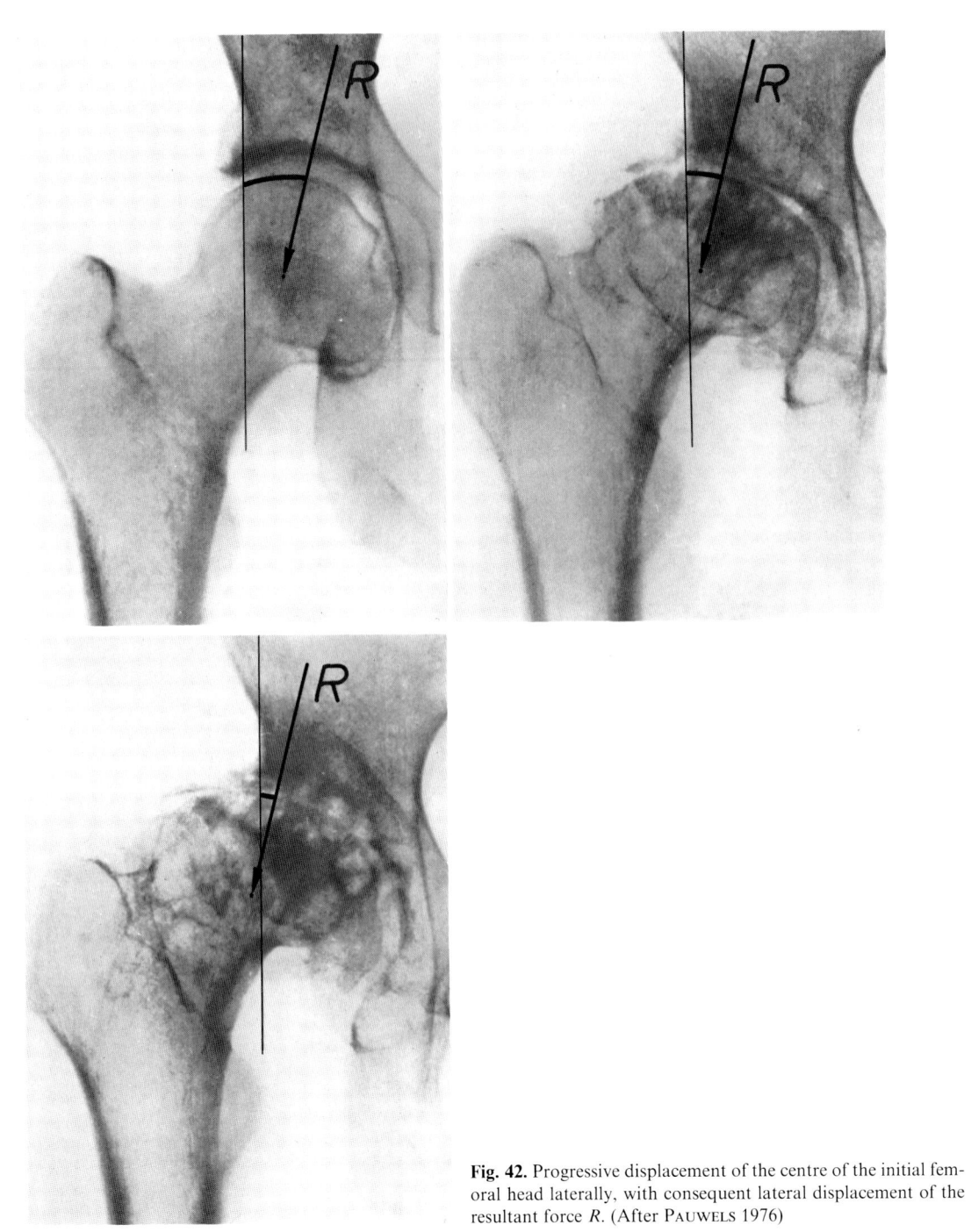

Fig. 42. Progressive displacement of the centre of the initial femoral head laterally, with consequent lateral displacement of the resultant force R. (After PAUWELS 1976)

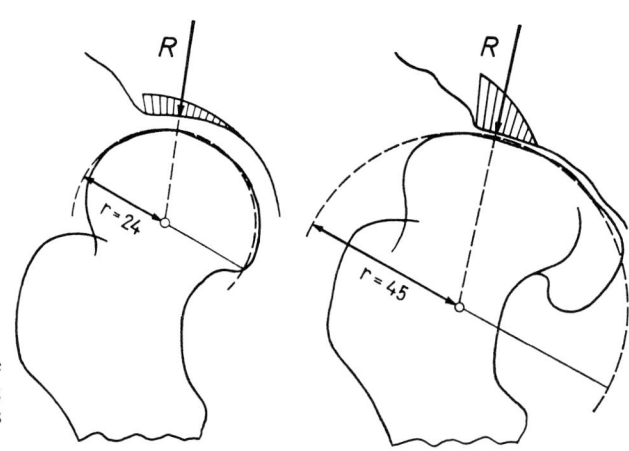

Fig. 43. Increase in the articular contact surface area; decrease in the weight-bearing area; increase in the stresses. r, radius; R, resultant of the forces acting on the hip. (After Pauwels 1976)

joint can increase considerably due to the remodelling, but the weight-bearing area progressively decreases and the articular compressive stresses thus increase (Fig. 43). This paradox results from the fact that the resultant force R continues to act at the initial centre of the femoral head, which is pushed further and further laterally. The medial osteophyte which develops on the medial aspect of the femoral head is at first made of cartilage and develops where there is moderate compression (Grasset 1960). It usually does not seem to bear weight significantly.

D. Osteoarthritis with Protrusio Acetabuli

In protrusio acetabuli the femoral head seems to be pushed medially. The transverse component Q of force R appears to be too great for the resistance of the tissues (Fig. 28). A triangular subchondral sclerosis develops in the depths of the acetabulum (Fig. 44). This suggests a displacement of R towards the medial edge of the facies lunata. If the stresses become sufficiently increased, cysts appear in the dense triangle (Fig. 217).

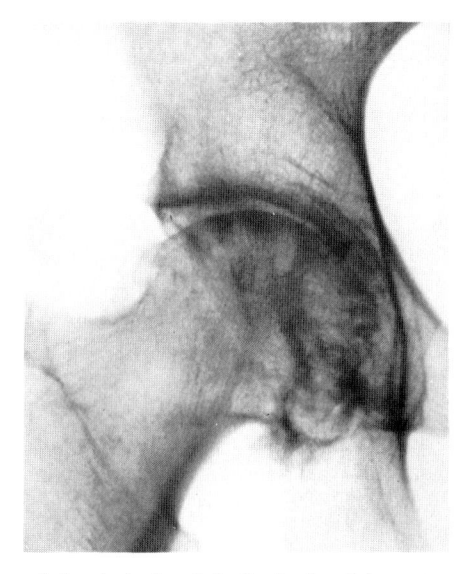

Fig. 44. Dense subchondral sclerosis in the depths of the acetabulum in protrusio acetabuli

E. Different Types of Osteoarthritis

Besides subluxating and protrusive osteoarthritis, there also exists a concentric type in which the joint space becomes narrowed everywhere and osteophytes developing from the acetabulum surround the femoral head, which is crowned by its own osteophytes. A dense triangle may or may not develop at the edge of the socket (Fig. 45).

Osteoarthritis can also be divided into hypertrophic and atrophic types. In hypertrophic types, remodelling is important and large osteophytes develop (Fig. 46a). These types appear to be most suited to biomechanical treatment: the osteophytes and the remodelling can often be put to use. In the atrophic types, the joint space disappears, abnormal sclerosis may or may not develop but there seem to be little remodelling and osteophytic reaction. The condition looks rather inflammatory even if the sedimentation rate and other tests for inflammation remain normal (Fig. 46b). As a rule, treatment is less satisfactory in these atrophic types.

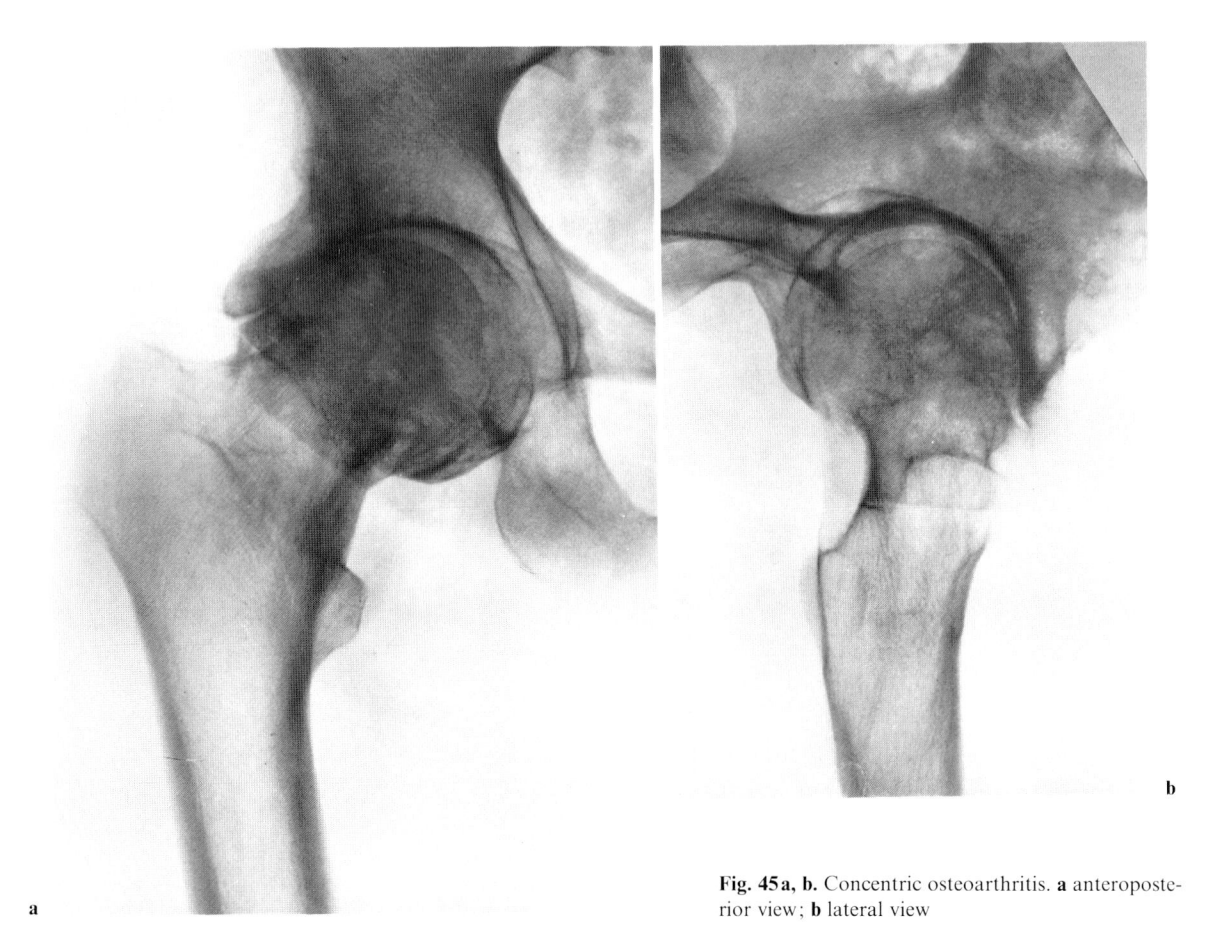

Fig. 45a, b. Concentric osteoarthritis. **a** anteroposterior view; **b** lateral view

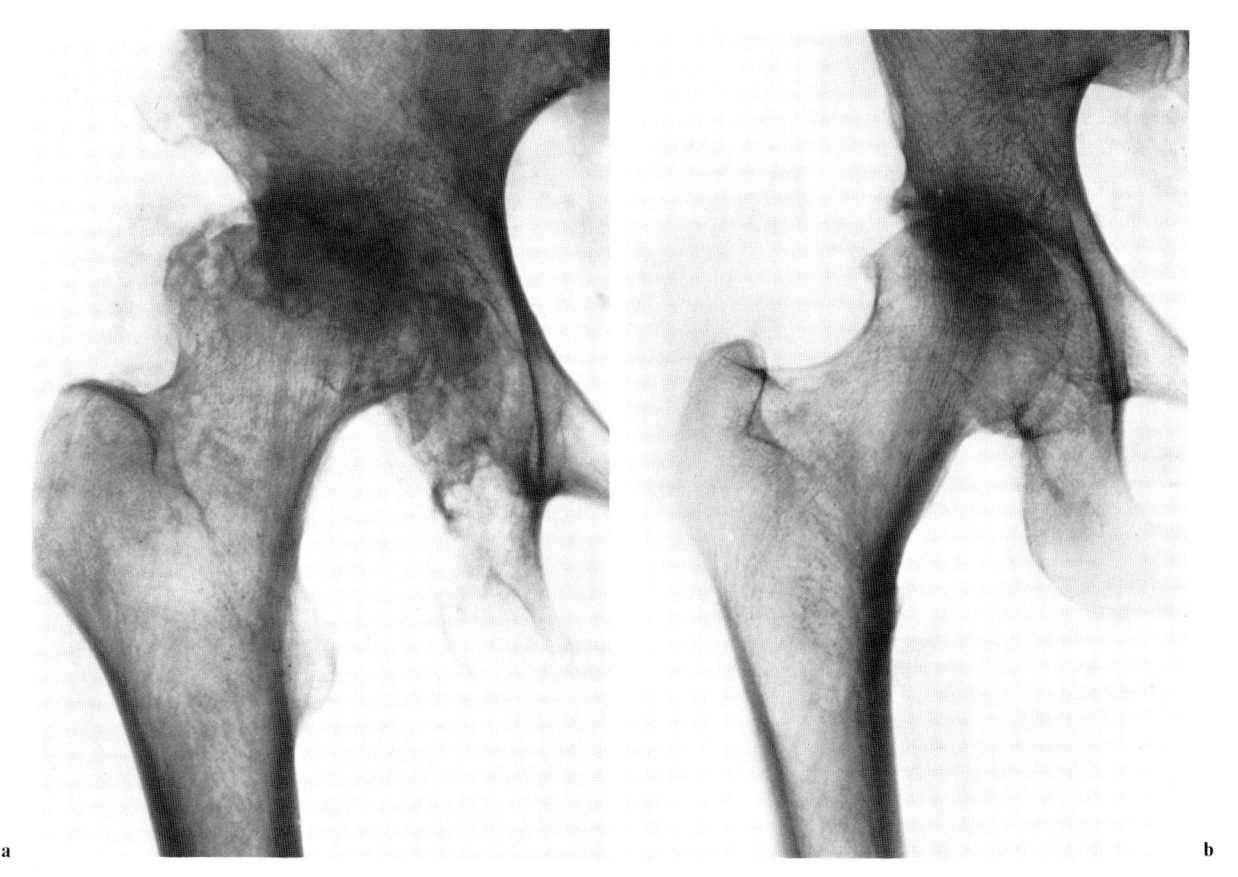

Fig. 46. a Hypertrophic osteoarthritis. **b** Atrophic osteoarthritis

Fig. 47a–c. Rapidly destructive osteoarthritis in a 66-year-old male patient

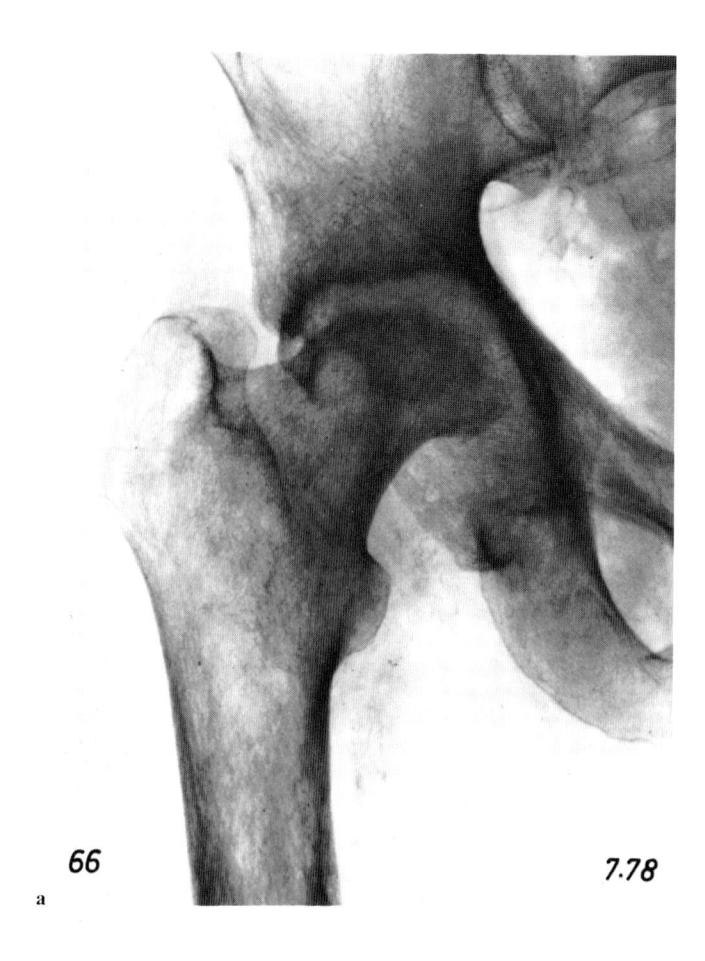

66

7.78

a

The rapidly destructive osteoarthritis of the hip represents an extreme example of this atrophic type. The femoral head and neck are resorbed in a few weeks or months without any clinical or laboratory sign of infection or even inflammatory reaction.

A 66-year-old male patient complained of severe pain in the hip (Fig. 47a). The range of movement was restricted. A biopsy was carried out at the same time as a hanging-hip procedure. The biopsy showed a thickened synovial membrane with congestive and oedematous areas. Other areas were fibrous, including small fragments of necrotic bone and cartilage. In some places the covering of synovial cells was hyperplastic. In the bony fragment the trabecular pattern bordering a necrotic area was interrupted by fibro-oedematous tissue infiltrated here and there by inflammatory cells, mostly mononuclear. The bony trabeculae appeared to have been considerably remodelled. Some segments were actually in the process of being resorbed. The pathologist reported a rapidly destructive osteoarthritis.

After the tenotomy, pain disappeared. At the 4-year follow-up (Fig. 47c) the hip remained pain-free and the range of movement had improved, but the femoral head had been resorbed completely.

8.79

1.83

b

c

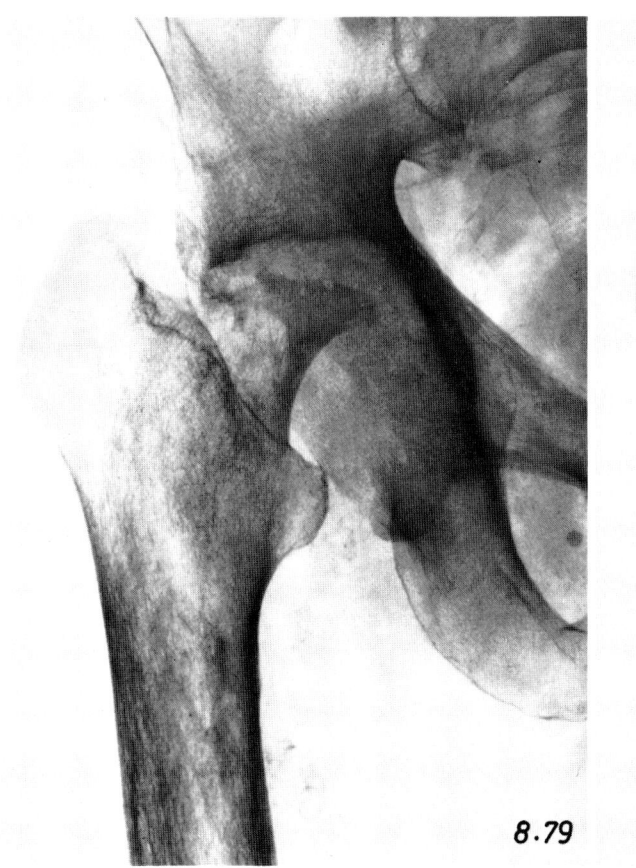

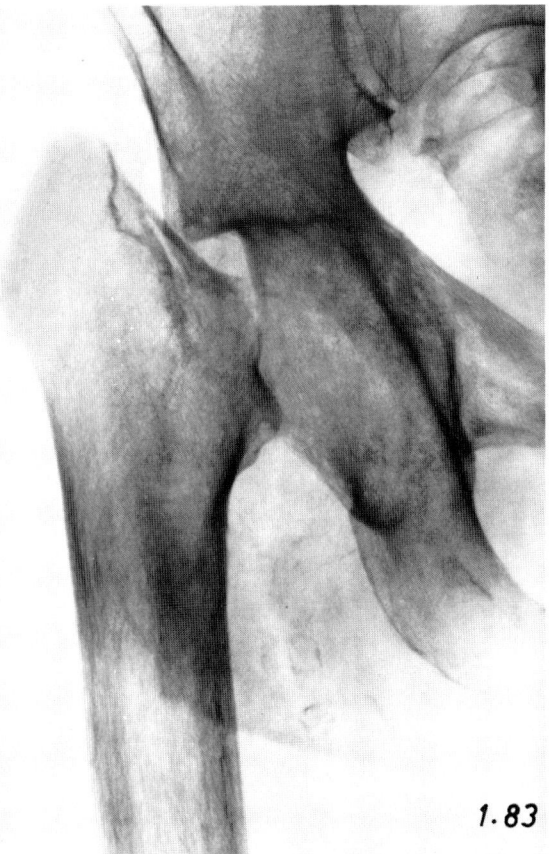

IX. Conclusion

During gait the hip is repeatedly subjected to a force which reaches more than four times body weight. This force is transmitted from the pelvis to the femur through weight-bearing surfaces which have been determined, and creates compressive stresses in the joint. In a normal joint these compressive stresses are distributed evenly over the weight-bearing surface of the articulation; this is due to the action of cartilage and probably to some slight incongruence of the joint surfaces when not loaded.

Osteoarthritis of the hip appears as the result of a disturbance of the balance which normally exists between the resistance of the tissues of the joint and their mechanical stressing. The tissue resistance depends on biological factors which are imperfectly understood. It can be lowered, and this seems to be the case in primary osteoarthritis. In the course of the evolution of the condition, destruction of cartilage and remodelling of bone will lead to incongruence of the joint surfaces and increase the mechanical stress. The mechanical stress may also be abnormally high initially, as in many dysplastic hips. In such hips the tissue resistance may also be congenitally low. Thus the two causes of disturbance of the physiological equilibrium probably often coexist. In any case, in osteoarthritis the articular compressive stresses seem to be too high for the tissue resistance.

Chapter II. Principles of a Biomechanical Treatment of Osteoarthritis of the Hip. Critical Analysis of Different Surgical Procedures. Instinctive Attempts to Relieve Stress in the Joint

Since in osteoarthritis the compressive stresses are too great for the resistance of the tissues, there are two sensible ways of dealing with this condition. One would consist of increasing the tissue resistance, the other of decreasing the compressive stresses in the joint.

I. Modifying the Biology of the Tissues

Several attempts have been made to modify the biology of the articular tissues and thereby to increase their resistance. Lumbar sympathectomy has been carried out in the hope of improving the blood supply to the affected hip (ROWNTREE and ADSON 1927; LERICHE and JUNG 1933). SCAGLIETTI (1964) ligated all the arteries which he could find about the femoral neck: the anterior and posterior circumflex arteries, the articular branch of the gluteal artery, and the obturator artery. He wanted to reduce hyperaemia, which he regarded as a factor aggravating the condition.

Drilling the femoral neck has been suggested by several authors (BOPPE 1936; HERBERT 1950; KIAER 1950), some with the idea of relieving venous stasis. Others have implanted a piece of muscle in a hole drilled in the femoral neck to improve blood supply (VENABLE and STUCK 1956; PALAZZI 1958). After carrying out as complete a curettage as possible of the femoral neck and head, CAMERA (1954) filled them with cancellous bone. NISSEN (1960) divided the femur by an intertrochanteric osteotomy without displacement. In order to be sure of preventing displacement, he implanted a nail and plate in the bone before its division.

A skin arthroplasty of the hip has been described (DELCHEF et al. 1959). The femoral head was dislocated, denuded of its osteophytes, covered by one or two layers of skin and replaced in the acetabulum. The skin was supposed to undergo metaplasia into cartilage. All these procedures fell into disrepute as a consequence of their unpredictable or short-lived results.

Recently, good results have been claimed following injection of extracts of cartilage into the affected joint. Improvements were observed mainly in cases in which the articular surfaces had remained congruent and in which there was no sign of overpressure. However, the follow-up is as yet short.

Even if the resistance of the tissues could be restored to normal, this would probably be insufficient in most cases, since the evolution of the condition often leads to an increase in the mechanical stressing of the joint. The only remaining alternative, therefore, is to decrease the compressive stresses in the joint if possible.

II. Reducing Joint Pressure

Most of the authors who have dealt with osteoarthritis of the hip with a mechanical goal in view have attempted either to decrease the load transmitted across the joint or to provide the femoral head with sufficient coverage. They have seemed to ignore the importance of a good congruence of the articular surfaces and of the weight-bearing area of the joint.

A. McMurray Osteotomy

McMURRAY (1935) described an oblique intertrochanteric osteotomy with proximal and medial dis-

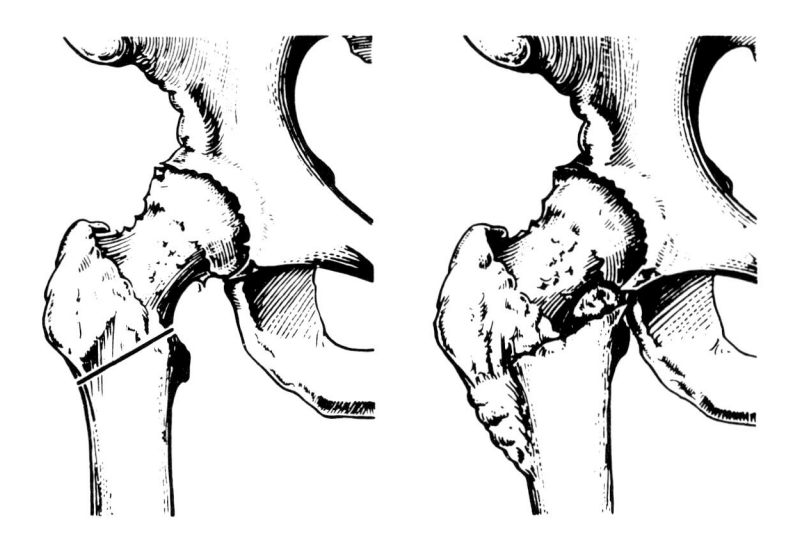

Fig. 48. McMurray osteotomy. (After McMurray 1939)

placement of the femoral shaft. The upper end of the shaft fragment, having been pushed below the lower border of the acetabulum (Fig. 48), was supposed to transmit part of the body weight directly from the pelvis to the femoral shaft, thus by-passing the affected hip.

Actually, the shaft fragment only rarely articulates with the pelvis, and when it does, the nearthrosis may be painful because of the concentration of the stresses over a very small weight-bearing surface. Medial displacement of the femoral shaft causes some valgus deformity of the knee (Fig. 49) but does not change the mechanical stressing of the hip joint. If an offset column supports a balance, this column will be subjected to bending stress below the angulation (Fig. 50a). If the axis of the lower part of the column is brought beneath the pivot of the balance, the column will then be subjected to compressive stress (Fig. 50b). Nothing will have changed in the joint with the balance whatever the shape of the column supporting it, whether it be offset or straight.

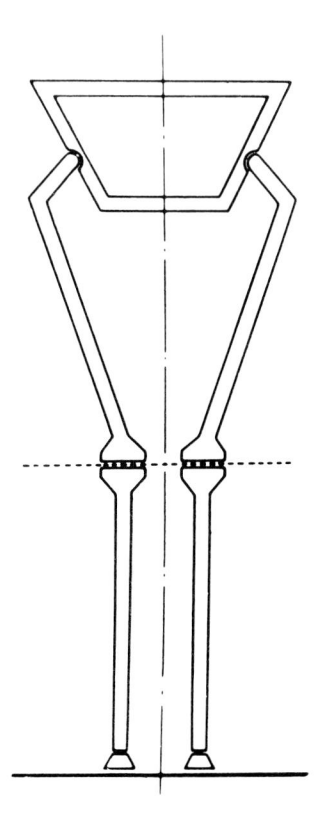

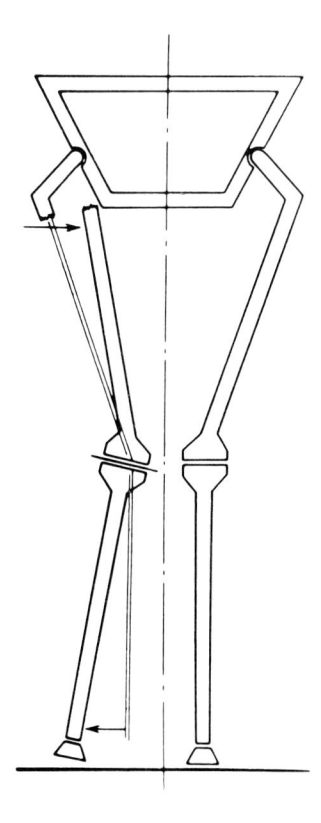

Fig. 49. Medial displacement of the upper extremity of the femoral shaft leads to a valgus deformity of the knee. (After Pauwels 1963a)

Fig. 50. a The balance lies off-centre in relation to the lower part of the offset column. **b** Displacing the lower part underneath the balance does not change the stresses in the pivot of the balance. *h*, lever arm of the force acting on the column (redrawn after PAUWELS)

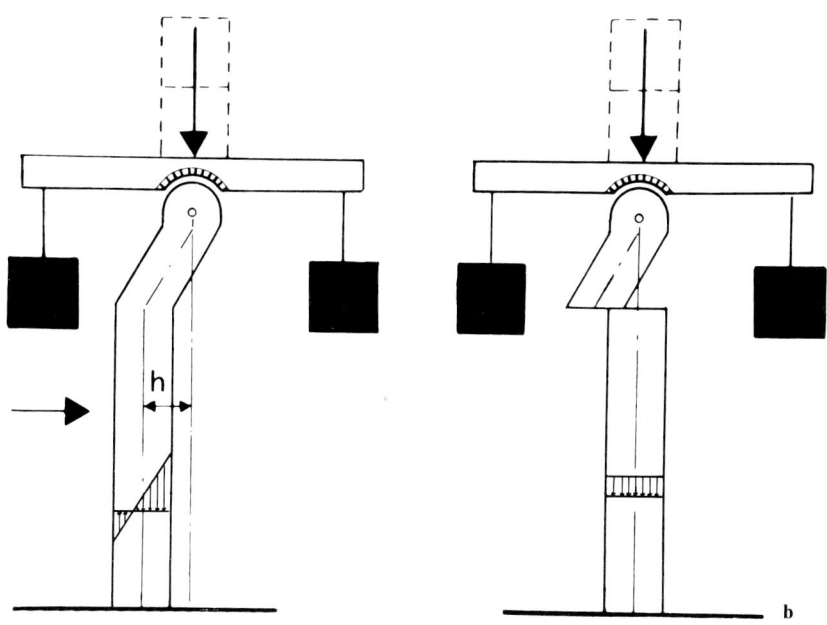

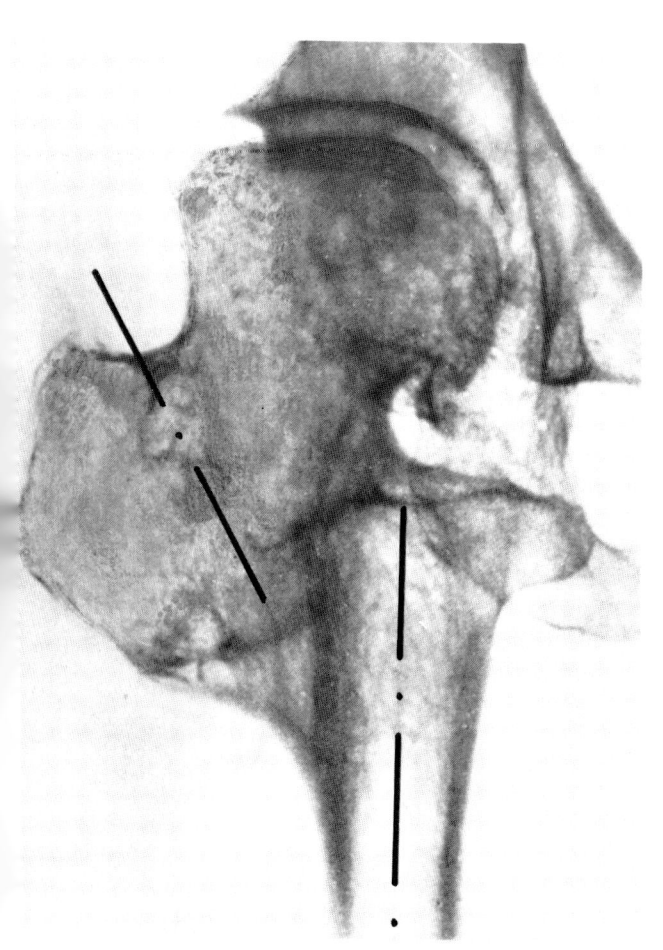

Fig. 51. Undesired rotation of the femoral head in a McMurray osteotomy. (After OSBORNE and FAHRNI 1950)

Similarly, displacing the femoral shaft medially does not modify the compressive stresses in the hip joint. In most of our valgus osteotomies, we actually displace the femoral shaft laterally in order to avoid a valgus deformity of the knee. This lateral displacement does not prevent the joint from healing (MAQUET 1966).

Actually, the McMURRAY osteotomy decreases the load acting on the hip by releasing two groups of muscles. Proximal displacement of the femoral shaft releases the iliopsoas and the adductor muscles. In some of his patients, McMURRAY (1939) observed a rotation of the femoral head as after a valgus osteotomy. Such a rotation of the femoral head may by chance improve the joint congruence and enlarge the articular weight-bearing surface (Fig. 51). Such an increase in the weight-bearing area of the articular surface was unforeseen and not desired by McMURRAY, who wrote: "The final position of the lower portion of the bone was left largely to chance", and "no effort is made to change the position of the upper fragment".

The good results sometimes observed after the McMURRAY osteotomy should be attributed either to the release of muscles or to an increase of the weight-bearing surface of the hip joint occurring by chance, unforeseen and undesired by McMURRAY. DOLIVEUX (1966) wrote a remarkable critical analysis of the McMURRAY osteotomy and of its developments and modifications, full of humour and well worth reading.

B. Multiple Tenotomy

Voss (1956) proposed carrying out tenotomy of the adductor and abductor muscles in order to decrease the load transmitted across the hip joint. This procedure fell into disrepute after it had been used for any kind of case of osteoarthritis. It did not succeed when the weight-bearing surface of the joint was significantly decreased. But it is still indicated in some circumstances: it is treated in more detail in Chap. III.

C. Shelf Operation

The shelf operations aim at covering the femoral head. The rationale behind them seems to be based on the idea that the hip is loaded vertically. This is erroneous, as was shown in Chap. I. The resultant force acting on the hip joint is normal to the weight-bearing surface and can be at a considerable angle from the vertical (Fig. 142). Improvement of a hip with severe osteoarthritis after a shelf operation is rarely observed. BERTRAND et al. (1964) have always noticed aggravation of the condition after this operation. They regard osteoarthritis as a contra-indication for the shelf operation.

The shelf operation provides, at best, a line of contact between the shelf and the femoral head, and more often only a point of contact. To increase the weight-bearing surface of the joint the shelf should have the same radius of curvature as the femoral head in every plane and be placed exactly in the prolongation of the articular surface of the socket. These two prerequisites are almost impossible to fulfill.

D. Pauwels' Approach to Osteoarthritis of the Hip

PAUWELS (1959, 1973a) wanted to decrease the joint pressure to bring it into line with the tissue resistance. The articular compressive stresses can be decreased either by reducing the load which creates them or by enlarging the surface area which transmits them. The example of the columns (PAUWELS 1963a) illustrates this. A vertical cylindrical column of homogeneous material supports a load of 200 kg which acts along the axis of the column (Fig. 52a). The cross section of the column is indicated below. The load of 200 kg evokes compressive stresses of 255 kg/cm^2 in the material of the column, as shown in the stress diagram. Reduction of the load to 100 kg lowers the compressive stresses in the material of the column to 127.5 kg/cm^2 (Fig. 52b). If the initial load of 200 kg is supported by a column with a diameter three times larger than that of the first column, the compressive stresses are only 28.3 kg/cm^2 (Fig. 52c). Because the diameter of the column is three times larger, the compressive stresses created by the same load become nine times smaller. The greatest reduction of compressive stresses will be attained by combining both possibilities, diminution of the load and enlargement of the weight-bearing surface. The compressive stresses, which were 255 kg/cm^2 in the first column, are then reduced to 14.1 kg/cm^2 (Fig. 52d).

The two PAUWELS operations, the varus intertrochanteric osteotomy (PAUWELS I) and the valgus intertrochanteric osteotomy combined with a tenotomy of the abductor, adductor and iliopsoas muscles (PAUWELS II), pursue the same aim. They enlarge the weight-bearing surface and they decrease the load transmitted across the joint. The lateral displacement of the greater trochanter combined with a tenotomy of the adductor and iliopsoas muscles (MAQUET 1976b) has exactly the same effects as the PAUWELS osteotomies. This procedure enlarges the weight-bearing surface of the joint and decreases the load supported.

E. Remarks on Bombelli's Concepts

Having carried out a large number of Pauwels osteotomies, BOMBELLI (1976) has tried to explain the results in his own way, and his explanation is very peculiar indeed. BOMBELLI regards the weight-bearing surface of the acetabulum of a normal hip joint as horizontal and nearly plane or only slightly concave. The resultant of the forces acting on the hip would form an angle of 16° with the vertical and 8° when pain in the joint causes the subject to limp. The acetabular surface would be in contact with the femoral head at one point which does not generally coincide with the intersection of the articular surface by the resultant force R. R is thus resolved into a component normal to the articular surface and a component tangential to the articular surface. When the inclination of the weight-bearing surface of the socket to the horizontal is greater than 16°, or 8° if limping, the tangential component would tend to push the femoral head outside the acetabulum, thus stretching capsule and ligaments. This stretching

Fig. 52. a Stresses in the cross section of a column supporting a load which acts along the axis of the column. **b** A smaller load creates smaller stresses. **c** Using a column with a larger cross section reduces the stresses considerably. **d** Combining both possibilities: decreasing the load and increasing the weight-bearing surface. *Below*: cross sections of the columns. (After Pauwels 1963a)

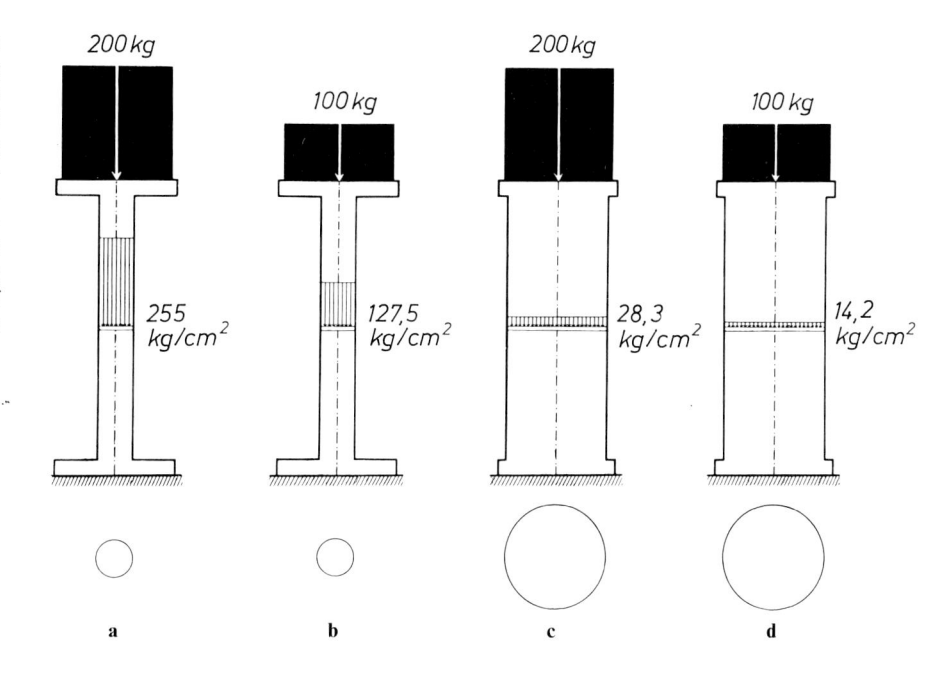

would promote the development of osteophytes. The beginning and evolution of osteoarthritis would depend essentially on the inclination of the roof of the acetabulum. A high-degree valgus osteotomy (30°–35°) would promote the formation of osteophytes, as does the tangential force tending to extrude the femoral head. These osteophytes, and particularly that developed at the edge of the acetabulum, would make the "plane" of the weight-bearing surface horizontal. Moreover, synovial fluid accumulating in the lateral gap between the joint surfaces after the valgus osteotomy would act as a pressure-distributing element. Simultaneously, it would also stretch the capsule.

The whole theory is based on a mechanical error and on disregard for the histological picture. First the acetabular articular surface is not, even approximately, plane. It is spherical and closely moulded over the femoral head. Any anatomical specimen demonstrates this. Contact is thus made by a surface and not a point, as assumed by Bombelli. Secondly, since friction in a joint is negligible [coefficient of friction = 0.002 according to Radin (1970), lower than the friction of a skate on ice] and since there is equilibrium, the resultant of the forces exerted on the hip must be normal to the weight-bearing surface of the joint[1]! If it is not normal to the weight-bearing surface there is no equilibrium. Indeed, most of the Bombelli's diagrams contradict a state of equilibrium. In other words, in circumstances such as those represented, the pelvis would rotate about the femur until equilibrium is achieved, that is to say until the resultant force has become normal to the weight-bearing surface. Thus the component tangential to the weight-bearing surface, which according to Bombelli provokes osteoarthritis, does not exist.

Thirdly, according to Bombelli, the formation of osteophytes results from stretching of the capsule and of the ligamentum teres. This means tension in these structures. Tension constitutes the stimulus for the formation of fibrous tissue. However, the osteophytes are made of cartilage before becoming ossified (Grasset 1960). The stimulus for the formation of cartilage is hydrostatic pressure, not tension (Pauwels 1965). In other words, the biological structure of osteophytes, and particularly of that developed over the medial aspect of the femoral head, completely contradicts the assumption of Bombelli. Carstens (1982) demonstrated this in a careful histological study related to the mechanical stressing of the osteophytes of osteoarthritic femoral heads.

From the X-rays presented by Bombelli himself to sustain his theory, it appears that, in most instances, the osteophytes did not develop further after a valgus osteotomy. The postoperative horizontal position of the roof of the acetabulum seems to be due to a projection of the X-rays different from that before the osteotomy, or simply to a rotation of the X-rays. Finally, the osteotomies carried out by Bombelli are Pauwels osteotomies.

---

[1] More exactly, the resultant R is at right angles to the plane tangential to the articular surface at the intersection of this articular surface and the line of action of force R.

III. Instinctive Attempts to Reduce the Stress on the Affected Hip

PAUWELS (1935) demonstrated how sideways limping works by shortening the lever arm h' of the force K exerted by the partial body mass. He also explained the action of a walking stick held in the hand opposite to the affected hip. Both limping and the use of a walking stick decrease the resultant force exerted on the hip joint, but both bring the line of action of this force closer to the vertical.

A. Limping

When the subject limps, the upper part of the body — the trunk, head and upper limbs — moves towards the affected leg at every single-support period involving this leg. The displacement of the upper part of the body is combined with a displacement of the pelvis and of the loaded leg in the opposite direction, which is necessary to maintain balance. At first glance, the limping individual seems to bring the whole body weight onto the affected leg. This might seem to increase the stress on the hip, but in fact the load exerted on this hip is decreased, as was shown by PAUWELS (1935).

PAUWELS made a film of an individual who limped because of a diseased but mobile right hip. He enlarged the successive pictures taken during the right single-support period and traced the outlines of the subject. Using the data of BRAUNE and FISCHER, he recorded the position of the centres of gravity of the different body segments and of the joints in the three-dimensional system of co-ordinates mentioned above (page 1).

The distance between the line of action of force K and the centre of the loaded femoral head is much shorter in the limping patient (Fig. 53) than in the normal individual (Fig. 2). The lever arm h of the muscular force M is unaltered. Therefore, force K can be counterbalanced by a smaller muscular force and the resultant force R is smaller. The line of action of force R passes through the intersection of forces K and M and through the centre of the femoral head. It is inclined at 8° to the perpendicular in PAUWELS' example, whereas it is inclined at 16° in the normal individual.

In the limping patient, at each phase of the right single-support period, the partial centre of gravity S_5 lies much closer to the perpendicular passing through the supporting foot than in the normal individual. This means that the forces of inertia are smaller when the subject is limping. These forces of inertia depend on the velocity of gait and the latter can vary during the evolution of the condition. PAUWELS calculated the forces of inertia assuming that the velocity was about one-third of that on which FISCHER based his calculation. He assumed the type of movement to be the same as during normal gait. He concluded that, under such conditions, the compressive force exerted on the hip of the individual weighing 58.7 kg attains only 100 kg when he limps, as opposed to 258 kg when he walks normally. The variations of this resultant force during the single-support period are also much slighter than in normal walking. The hammering of force R on the articular surface is thus considerably reduced. The line of action of the resultant force is less inclined from the vertical (8° vs. 16°).

Limping is usually observed in one of two sets of circumstances: it can result from a muscular weakness, or it can constitute an automatic reaction which tends to protect a deficient skeleton and, eventually, to lessen pain. If muscular power is diminished by paresis or paralysis and becomes insufficient to balance the eccentrically placed body weight, the individual must adopt an unnatural gait. During the single-support period on the weakened side he displaces his trunk towards that side. This tends to bring the centre of gravity above the loaded joint, requiring less muscular

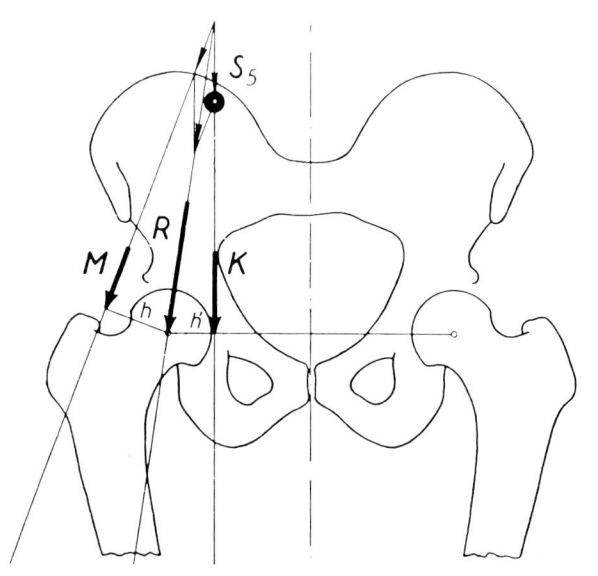

Fig. 53. Limping. S_5, centre of gravity of the part of the body supported by the right hip; K, force exerted by this part of the body; M, force exerted by the abductor muscles; R, resultant of forces K and M; h, lever arm of M; h', lever arm of K. (After PAUWELS 1935)

force to balance the force due to the body mass. By changing his gait the subject compensates for the insufficiency of his muscles. Such a limp must be regarded as a functional adaptation.

Limping can also be observed in the presence of normal muscular power. In this case, it is due to the tendency of the body to protect a painful bone or joint. The body tries to reduce the load exerted on the affected limb. A limp thus tends to be adopted by individuals with lesions of joints and bones of the lower limb. It progressively disappears as the diseased leg recovers strength. Its disappearance depends on the efficacy of treatment in restoring a normal mechanical equilibrium.

B. Using a Walking Stick

Many patients with a painful hip use a stick which they hold in the opposite hand. The use of a stick can prevent or reduce limping. It lessens the displacement of the upper part of the body toward the diseased side during the single-support period of gait.

The stick transmits a part of the body weight to the ground. Force C exerted on the stick by the hand acts with a lever arm f, which is the distance between the stick and the centre of the femoral head (Fig. 54). In Pauwels' example, $f = 30$ cm.

Fig. 54. a Using a walking stick. S_5, centre of gravity of the part of the body supported by the right hip; K, force exerted by this part of the body; h', lever arm of force K; M, force exerted by the abductor muscles; h, lever arm of force M; C, force exerted on the walking stick; f, lever arm of force C; F, resultant of forces K and C; s, lever arm of force F; R, resultant of forces F and M. R is the force actually transmitted across the hip joint (redrawn from PAUWELS 1935). **b** Using a walking stick increases the support area

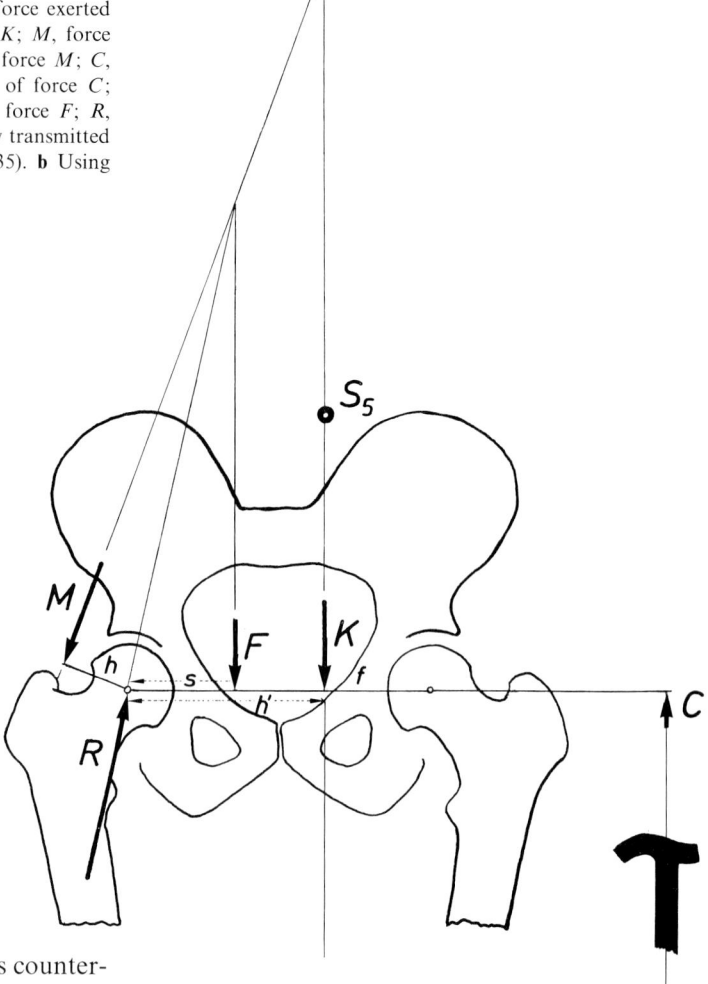

The moment Cf tends to rotate the pelvis counter-clockwise about the right femoral head in the diagram, whereas the moment Kh' of the force K exerted by the partial body weight ($K = 47.760$ kg and its lever arm $h' = 10.99$ cm) tends to rotate the pelvis clockwise. Both static forces C and K are vertical with opposite signs. Their resultant F is also vertical and $F = K - C$. The line of action of force F is at a distance s from the hip such that:

$$Fs = Kh' - Cf$$
$$s = \frac{Kh' - Cf}{K - C}$$

The force K, which normally tends to tilt the pelvis clockwise with the moment Kh', is now replaced by force F. The moment Fs is smaller because force F is less and it acts with a lever arm which is shorter than h'.

The stick allows the trunk to straighten without increasing the force acting on the hip. It thus becomes unnecessary to shift the trunk to the diseased side, i.e. to limp.

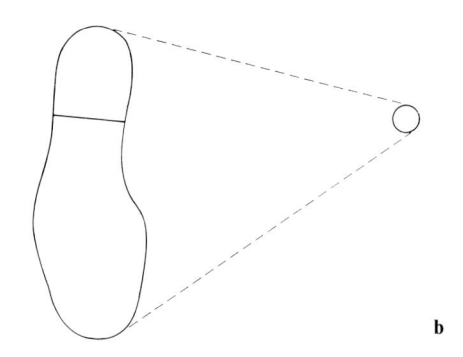

Fig. 55. The action of a walking stick can be compared with the use of a wheelbarrow. *C*, force exerted on the walking stick; *K*, force exerted by the part of the body supported by the hip; *R*, resultant of the forces *K* and *C*

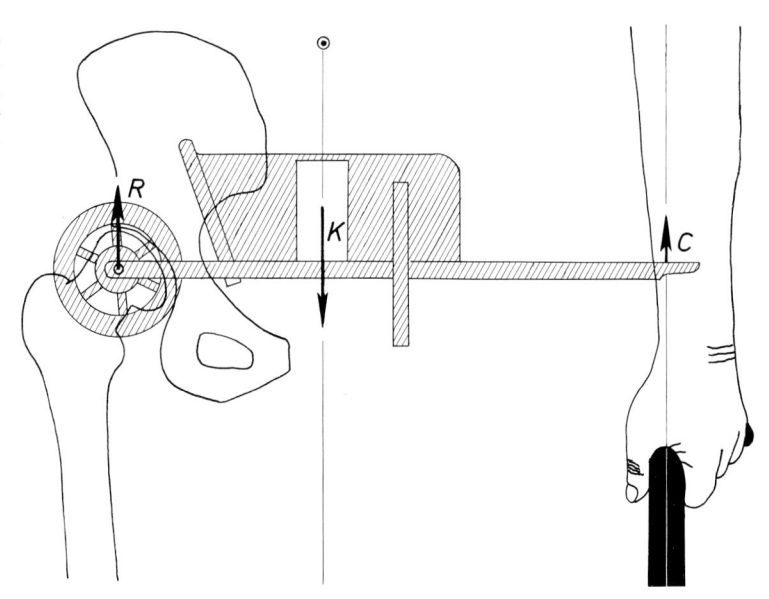

Force *K* is counterbalanced by *M*, the force exerted by the abductor muscles, acting with the lever arm h ($= 4$ cm):

$$M = \frac{Fs}{h} = \frac{Kh' - Cf}{h}$$

The hip supports the resultant *R* of forces *F* and *M*:

$$R = \sqrt{F^2 + M^2 + 2FM\cos(\widehat{FM})}$$

in which $\widehat{FM}$ is the acute angle formed by the lines of action of forces *M* and *F*. In this case $\widehat{FM} = 21°$.

The angle $(\widehat{RF})$ formed by the lines of action of *R* and *F* has also been calculated:

$$\sin(\widehat{RF}) = \frac{M}{R}\sin(\widehat{FM})$$

For a sufficient magnitude of force *C*, a muscular force *M* becomes unnecessary. Force *F* then becomes force *R*, which acts vertically on the hip (Fig. 54). The walking stick acts like the hands holding the handles of a wheelbarrow (Fig. 55). The axis of the wheel corresponds to the centre of the femoral head. The load in the wheelbarrow corresponds to the mass of the body minus the supporting leg (47.76 kg).

The values of the static forces and of the angle $(\widehat{RF})$ are presented in Table 7 for several forces exerted on the stick by the hand[2]. It appears that the use of a stick markedly reduces the load acting on the hip. Taking the forces of inertia into account would complicate the calculation without significantly altering the result because the patient with a stick moves slowly, thus reducing to a minimum the forces of inertia. These may, therefore, be disregarded.

The stick also enlarges the area of support. Normally, the latter roughly corresponds to the surface of the foot or shoe in contact with the ground. With a stick the area of support takes the shape of a large triangle with the tangent to the lateral edge of the foot or shoe on the ground as its base and the tip of the stick as its apex (Fig. 54b). Considerably enlarging the support, the stick obviously ensures better balance for the subject.

In summary, using a stick decreases the force transmitted across the hip but brings its line of action closer to the vertical. Furthermore, using a stick considerably enlarges the support of the subject and ensures a better equilibrium.

[2] For this calculation, we started from the data of phase 16 (subject of BRAUNE and FISCHER 1895; FISCHER 1899, 1900, 1901, 1903, 1904). The lever arm of *K* is 10.99 cm, that of *M* 4 cm.

Table 7. Using a walking stick

Force *C* exerted on the stick (kg)	Force *M* exerted by the abductor muscles (kg)	Force *R* exerted on the hip (kg)	Inclination of the line of action of force *R* to the vertical
0	131.221	176.640	15°26′
2	116.221	161.717	14°55′
5	93.721	139.363	13°57′
10	56.221	102.251	11°22′
15	18.721	65.282	5°52′
17.5	0	30.260	0°

IV. Conclusion

In dealing with osteoarthritis of the hip, various attempts have been made to restore a normal resistance to the tissues by modifying their biology, both by means of surgery and by means of drugs, usually to no avail. However, the patients affected by osteoarthritis of the hip try to diminish the load transmitted across the joint by limping and by using a walking stick. Both decrease the moment of the force eccentrically exerted by the mass of the body on the loaded hip. The stick acts by transmitting part of this force directly to the ground. The muscular force necessary for balancing the remaining part is, therefore, reduced and could eventually be completely eliminated. The resultant force acting on the hip is thus decreased. Limping shortens the lever arm of the force exerted by the mass of the body by shifting its centre of gravity towards the loaded hip. Consequently, equilibrium can be ensured by a smaller muscular force, and the compressive force acting on the hip is reduced.

The patient thus instinctively tends to decrease the stress on his affected hip joint. Different surgical procedures have been devised to the same end, the diminution of the load transmitted across the hip. They have been disappointing in many cases because the weight-bearing surface of the joint becomes smaller during the course of the condition. In order sufficiently to decrease the articular pressure, not only must the load supported be reduced but also the weight-transmitting surface of the joint must be enlarged. PAUWELS was the first to draw attention to this prerequisite. In Chap. III we shall deal in more detail with the hanging-hip procedure (VOSS-PAUWELS), the varus intertrochanteric osteotomy (PAUWELS I), the valgus intertrochanteric osteotomy combined with multiple tenotomy (PAUWELS II) and the lateral displacement of the greater trochanter combined with a tenotomy of the adductor and iliopsoas muscles (MAQUET). We shall also study the effect of shortening the opposite leg in certain cases (MAQUET). All these procedures are aimed at decreasing the articular pressure in the hip joint. Finally, we shall analyse the mechanical action of the SCHANZ osteotomy in old unreduced congenital dislocations.

Chapter III. Surgical Treatment of Osteoarthritis of the Hip

The rationale behind our surgical treatment of osteoarthritis of the hip is that of PAUWELS and consists of decreasing the load transmitted across the hip joint and above all of enlarging the weight-bearing surface of the articulation. The choice of the proper surgical procedure in each particular case is of decisive importance. Analysis of and tracings from appropriate X-rays are essential in making this choice.

I. X-rays

A. Before the Operation

Choice of operation and pre-operative planning are based on appropriate X-rays.

1. Overall Anteroposterior View of the Pelvis

The usual overall anteroposterior view of the pelvis with both hips and part of the femora provides information on the hips and on any adduction contracture or deformity which may be present (Fig. 56). In order to measure the deformity, a tangent to the iliac crests or to the ischial tuberosities is drawn. The longitudinal axis of each femoral shaft is also drawn. The angles formed by the pelvic line and the femoral axes medially and distally are measured. The smaller angle is subtracted from the larger and their difference is divided by two. The value thus obtained gives the degree of adduction contracture or deformity.

In the example in Fig. 56, the angle formed by the pelvic line and the right femoral shaft is 65°; that formed by the pelvic line and the left femoral shaft is 105°. The adduction contracture is:

$$\frac{105° - 65°}{2} = 20°.$$

2. Anteroposterior Views of the Affected Hip

The beam is centred on the femoral head and the leg is internally rotated as far as the condition allows. Three anteroposterior views of the affected hip are required:

1. One in neutral position between adduction and abduction
2. One in full abduction
3. One in full adduction

From the view in the neutral position the outlines of the joint and of the upper end of the femur will be traced and the pre-operative planning will be carried out. The two other views make it possible to decide which shadows belong to the femoral head and which to the pelvis. This is not always obvious from one view because of the superimposition of the different elements. The views in adduction and abduction also help to indicate the appropriate surgical procedure (Table 8). If the articular

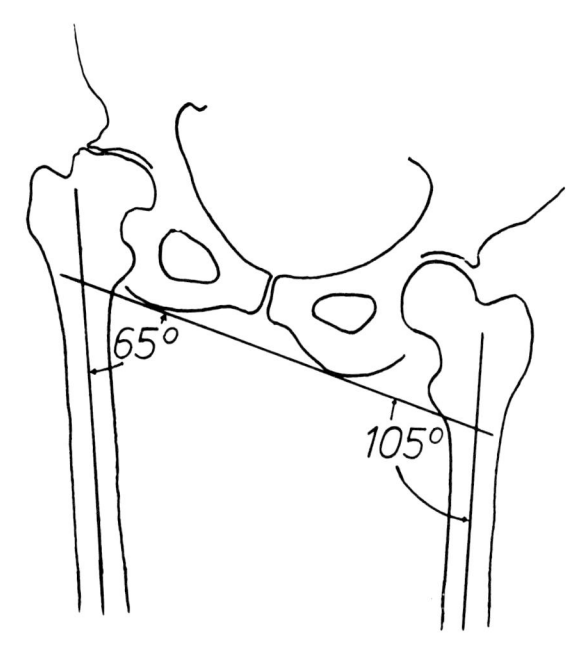

Fig. 56. Measurement of an adduction contracture or deformity

surfaces remain or become congruent in full abduction, a varus osteotomy may be considered (Fig. 57). If the congruence is poor in abduction and good in adduction, a valgus osteotomy should be considered (Fig. 58). If the articular surfaces are congruent in the three positions, one can choose between a hanging-hip operation, a varus osteotomy and a lateral displacement of the greater trochanter. The choice will be dictated by the shape of the subchondral sclerosis in the roof of the socket and by the level at which the greater trochanter lies. If there is a dense triangle at the edge of the acetabulum, the hanging-hip operation must be rejected. If there is a dense triangle at the edge of the acetabulum and there is coxa valga, a varus osteotomy should rather be carried out. If there is a dense triangle at the edge of the acetabulum and the greater trochanter is situated high, a lateral displacement of the greater trochanter should be chosen. A triangular subchondral sclerosis in the depths of the socket constitutes a sign of protrusive osteoarthritis. In such a case, a valgus osteotomy is generally indicated.

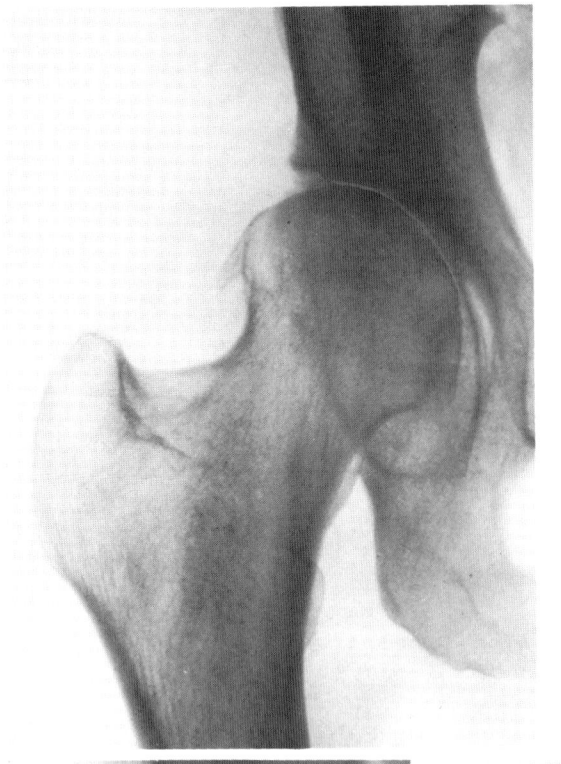

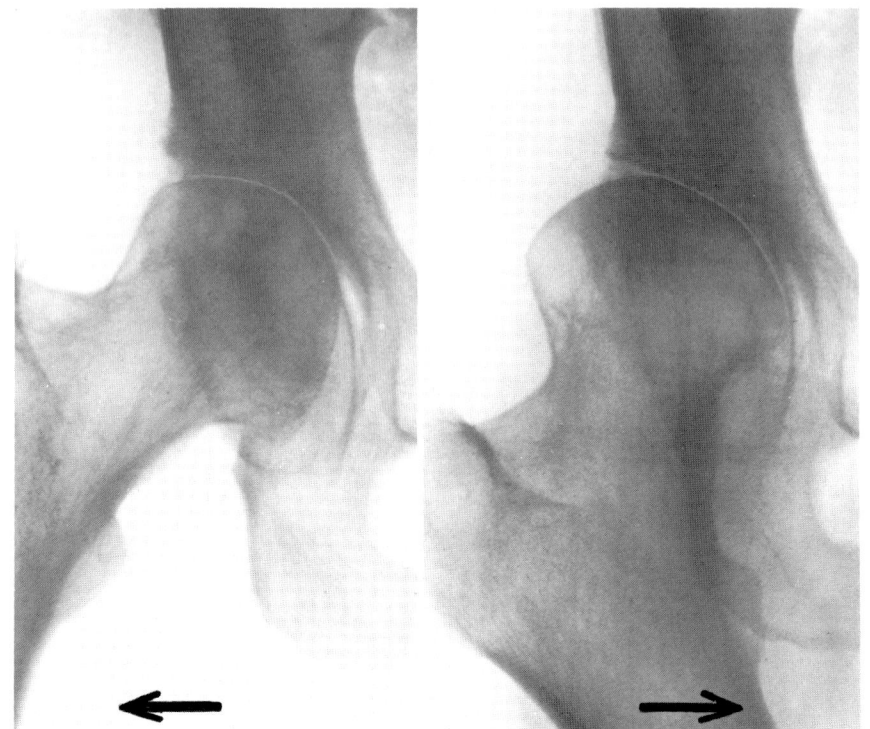

Fig. 57 a–c. Pre-operative X-rays. Congruence in abduction indicates a varus osteotomy. **a** Neutral position. **b** Full abduction. **c** Full adduction

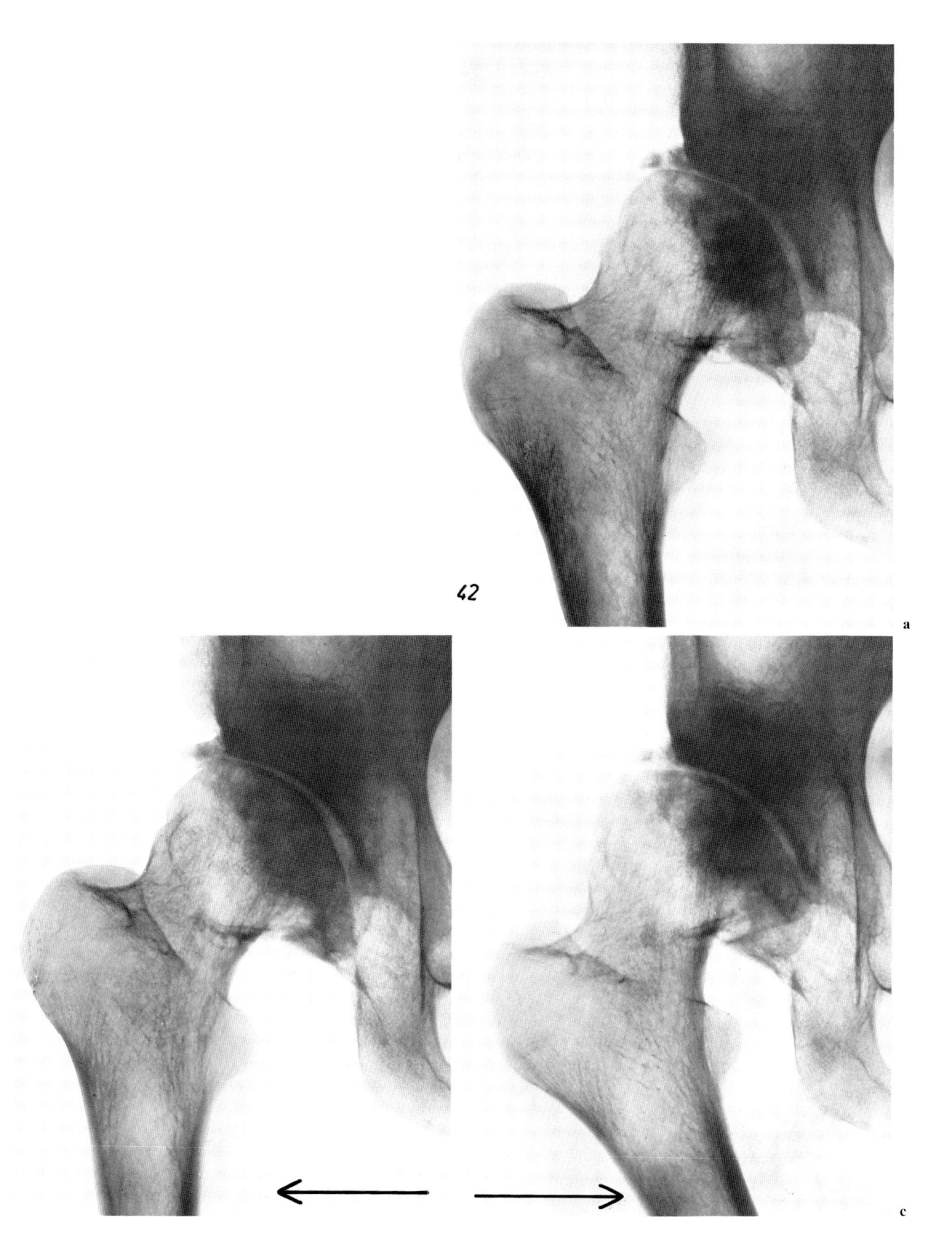

Fig. 58 a–c. Pre-operative X-rays. Incongruence in abduction and better congruence in adduction indicate a valgus osteotomy. **a** Neutral position. **b** Full abduction. **c** Full adduction

Table 8. Operative indications

	Congruence in all positions	Congruence only in abduction	Congruence only in adduction	No congruence
No dense triangle				
High greater trochanter	HH or LDGT	PI	PII	No osteotomy
Low greater trochanter	HH or PI	PI	PII	or tenotomy
Dense triangle at the edge of the acetabulum				
High greater trochanter	LDGT	PI	PII	
Low greater trochanter	PI	PI	PII	
Dense triangle in the depths of the acetabulum	PII		PII	

HH, hanging-hip procedure; LDGT, lateral displacement of the greater trochanter; PI, varus intertrochanteric osteotomy (Pauwels I); PII, valgus intertrochanteric osteotomy + tenotomy (Pauwels II)

When congruence or tendency to congruence occurs neither in the neutral position nor in abduction nor in adduction, the hip is not suitable for a joint-preserving operation at this stage (Fig. 59). One must choose another solution or await further evolution of the condition. In the course of the disease the edge of the acetabulum often collapses and the femoral head changes its shape in such a way that a valgus osteotomy becomes possible after some years.

3. Lateral View of the Femoral Neck and Three-quarter View

The lateral view of the femoral neck and the three-quarter view complement our information in the sagittal plane. At an early stage, when the joint is still spherical, they can help the surgeon to decide whether to carry out a derotation operation either to correct an exaggerated anteversion of the femoral neck or to improve the anterior coverage of the femoral head.

4. Anteroposterior View of the Lower Limbs

When there is a discrepancy in leg length and its correction is considered, a long X-ray showing the pelvis and the two legs is necessary in order to measure the difference in length precisely.

Fig. 59a–c. Congruence neither in abduction nor in adduction. This is not an indication for an osteotomy. **a** Neutral position. **b** Full abduction. **c** Full adduction

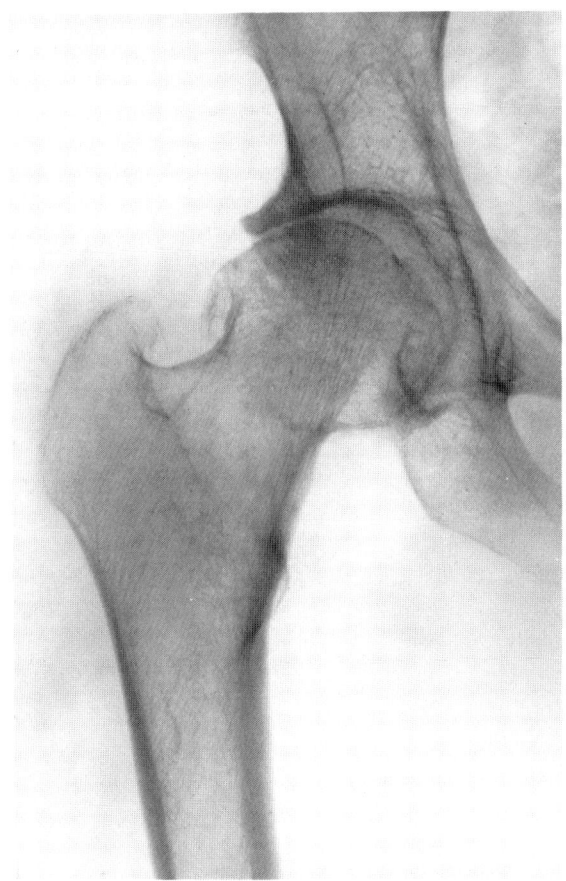

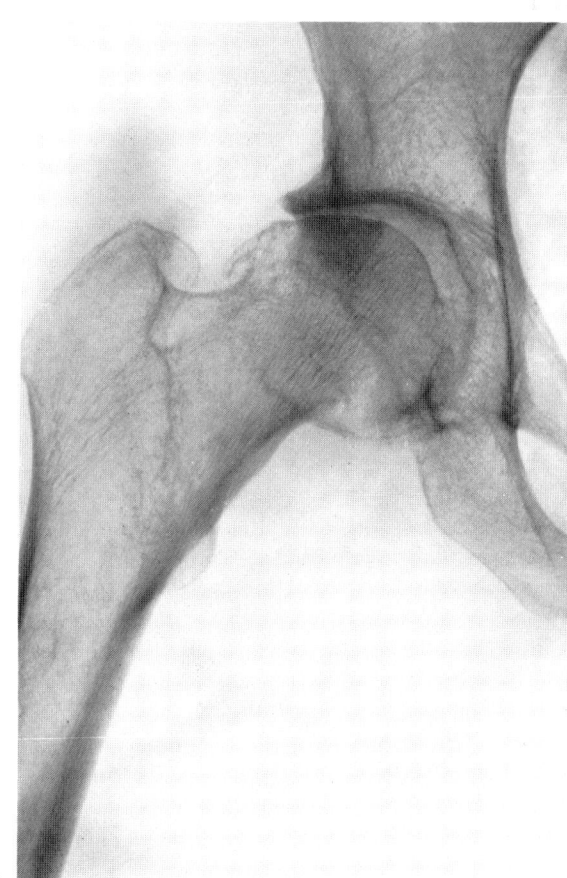

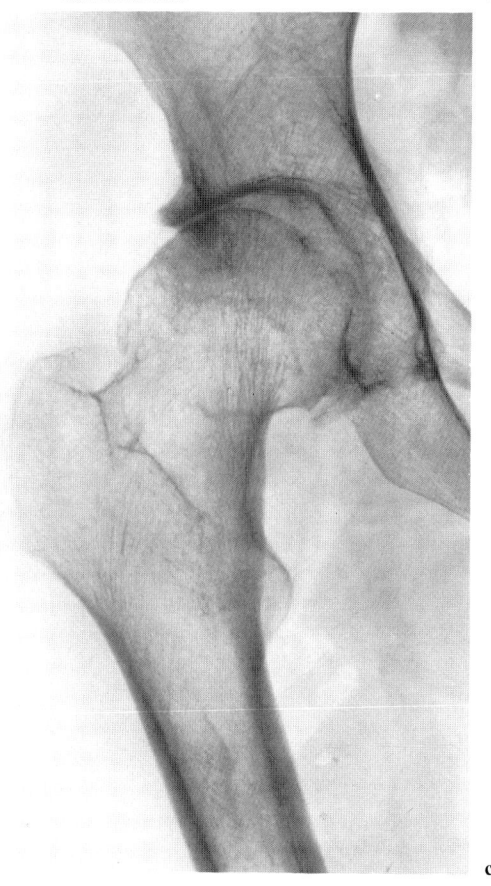

B. During the Operation

When the choice between a varus and a valgus osteotomy remains doubtful, X-rays must be taken in full abduction under anaesthesia after tenotomy of the adductor muscles. If they show good congruence a varus osteotomy is chosen. If not, a valgus osteotomy is preferred.

The articular surfaces looked congruent in abduction in the pre-operative X-ray of a 31-year-old female patient (Fig. 60a). Under anaesthesia, after the adductor muscles had been divided, full abduction became possible. In this position, the joint surfaces were incongruent (Fig. 60b). Therefore, a valgus osteotomy was carried out. At the 14-year follow-up the result remained excellent.

X-rays of the hip are taken on the operating table after the insertion of the KIRSCHNER wires which delineate the osteotomy (Fig. 61). They allow an exact measurement of the angles formed by the KIRSCHNER wires and by the wires with the axis of the femoral shaft.

C. After the Operation

In the postoperative follow-up, an anteroposterior view with the beam centred on the femoral head and a lateral view are regularly required. In the first weeks, attention is focused on the fixation of the fragments and on the bony union at the osteotomy site. Later, the evolution of the subchondral sclerosis and the joint space constitute the focal points of interest.

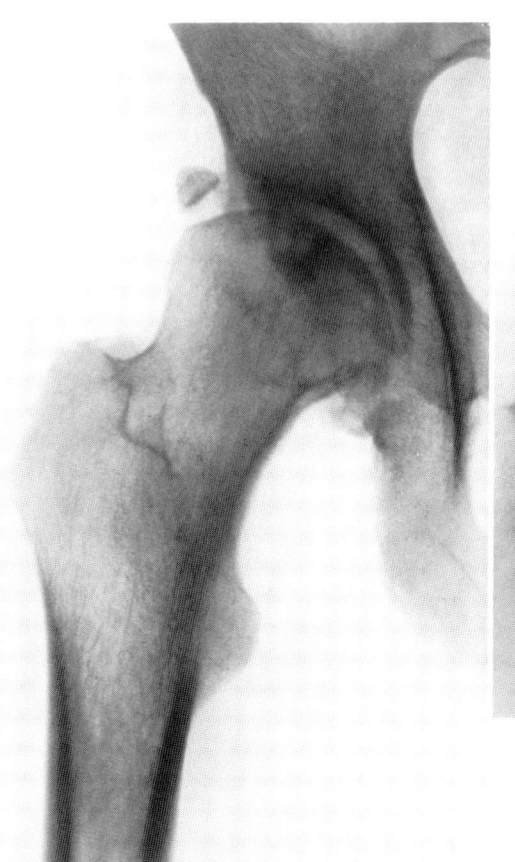

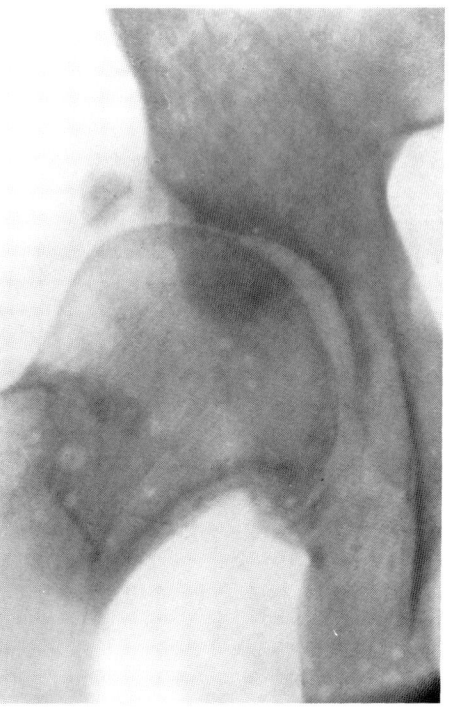

Fig. 60. a A pre-operative X-ray taken in abduction indicates a varus osteotomy. **b** A new X-ray taken under anaesthesia shows incongruence of the articular surfaces in abduction

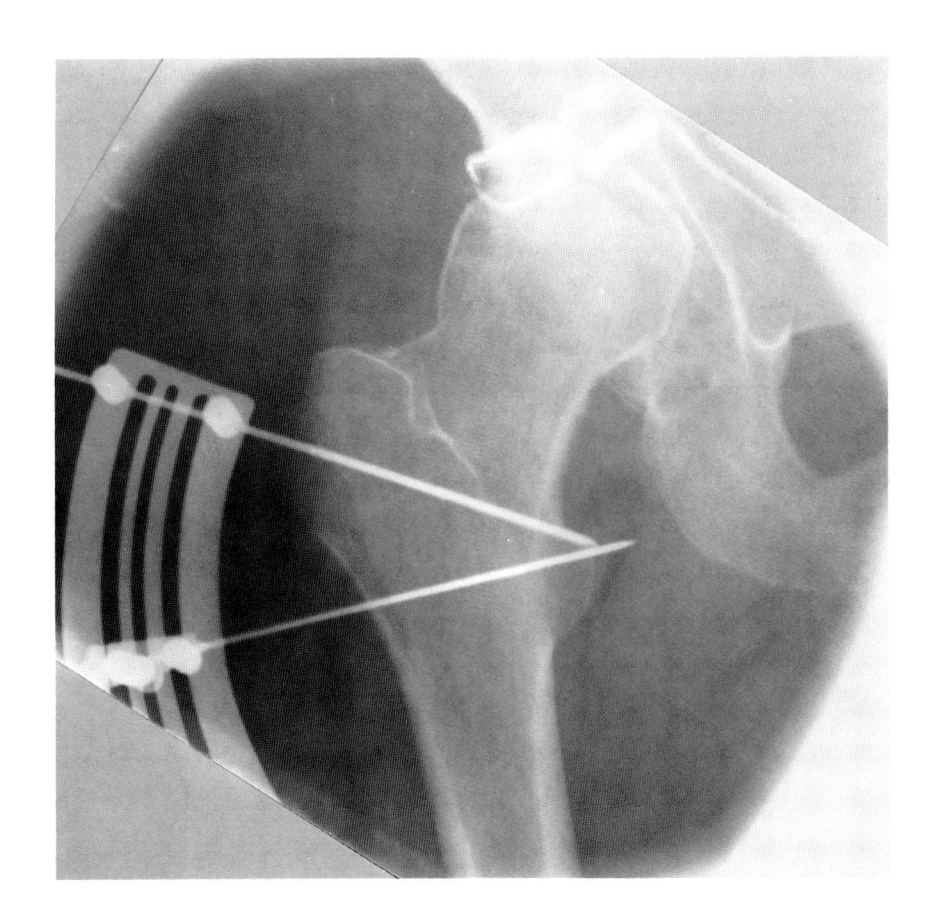

Fig. 61. X-ray taken during operation

II. Hanging-Hip Procedure

A. Rationale

In osteoarthritis the muscles spanning the hip are often permanently contracted. This limits the range of movement, increases the joint pressure and causes pain. Division of the main muscles spanning the joint, whether they are permanently contracted or not, decreases the force R transmitted across the articulation (Fig. 62). This division does not usually alter the weight-bearing surface of the joint.

Tenotomy of the adductor longus muscle, of the fascia lata and of the gluteus medius and minimus muscles was proposed by Voss (1956). Pauwels (1959) complemented the procedure by dividing the iliopsoas at its attachment to the lesser trochanter. Pauwels (1961) considered that the iliopsoas muscle, the direction of which is only a little oblique to the resultant force R, exerts nearly all of its force as compression acting on the hip joint. The other muscles develop a force more oblique to the line of action of the resultant force R. Only D, the component of this muscular force parallel to the resultant R, exerts a pure compression on the joint (Fig. 63).

B. Experimental Study

1. Material and Method

An experimental study was carried out by Radin et al. (1975) on 50 adult cats in which the proximal femoral epiphyses were closed; this was checked by means of pelvic X-rays. The animals were put under general anaesthesia. The right hip was approached through a posterolateral incision. The gluteus medius and minimus and the piriformis muscles were divided, the capsule incised and the femoral head dislocated. The cartilage from the weight-bearing areas of the socket and the femoral head was removed down to bleeding bone using a sharp curette. Twenty-one of the animals constituted the control group. In these the hip was reduced and the divided muscles were reattached. In the other cats, the hip was reduced but the divided muscles were not reattached before closure: moreover, the quadratus femoris and the iliopsoas muscles were divided at their femoral insertions and the adductor longus tendon was cut proximally. Three or four days after surgery, all the cats were transferred to a farm, where they lived in large pens and were allowed full activity. One animal (tenotomized) developed ischaemic necrosis of the hip and was not included.

2. Results

The results are summarized in Table 9. All the cats limped initially. The ones with the resutured muscles (controls) ceased to limp between the 3rd and 6th postoperative months. But the limp reappeared in this group by the 12th month and persisted in all but two animals to the 30th month. In the unsutured group, the limping disappeared between 6 and 12 months after surgery and was not observed in any of these animals subsequently.

The animals were killed at varying time intervals up to 30 months. At 1 and 2 months, the unsutured muscle attachments were flimsy fibrous bands. At 3 months, the iliopsoas and adductor attachments were firm and normal in appearance. By the 6th month, the external rotator and abductor muscles were firmly reattached. Their insertions were 0.5–1 cm smaller than normal. The muscle attachments in the sutured group appeared normal. In both groups the hip capsules were intact at the time of death, although they were never sutured. At up to 6 months the capsules in both groups were tense and contained a large amount of clear synovial fluid. After 6 months there was little or no effusion in the unsutured group, but there was a consistent significant effusion in the sutured group. This persisted throughout the remainder of the experimental study.

The articular surfaces fitted poorly in all animals until about the 12th month. The incongruence persisted in the sutured cats but the fitting of the surfaces markedly improved in the unsutured group. Osteophytes were consistently found in the sutured animals at the 24th month (Fig. 64). Most of the cats in this group had a limited range of movement and the articular capsule was thickened. Frank fibrous ankylosis was found in two sutured animals, one at 24 months and one at 30 months. The hip joints of the unsutured cats remained congruent and were free of osteophytes (Fig. 65).

Microscopically, fibrous tissue was present in the articular defects in all animals after only

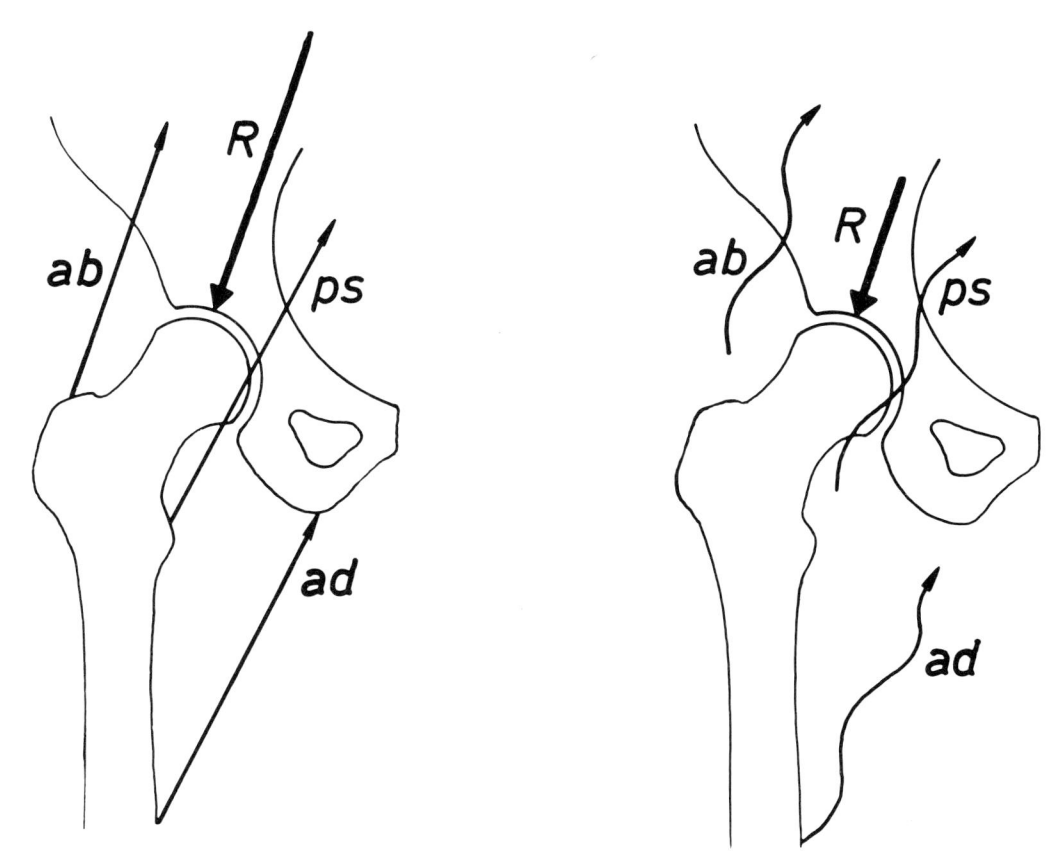

Fig. 62. The hanging-hip procedure decreases the overall force *R* transmitted across the joint. *ab*, abductor muscles; *ad*, adductor muscles; *ps*, iliopsoas muscle

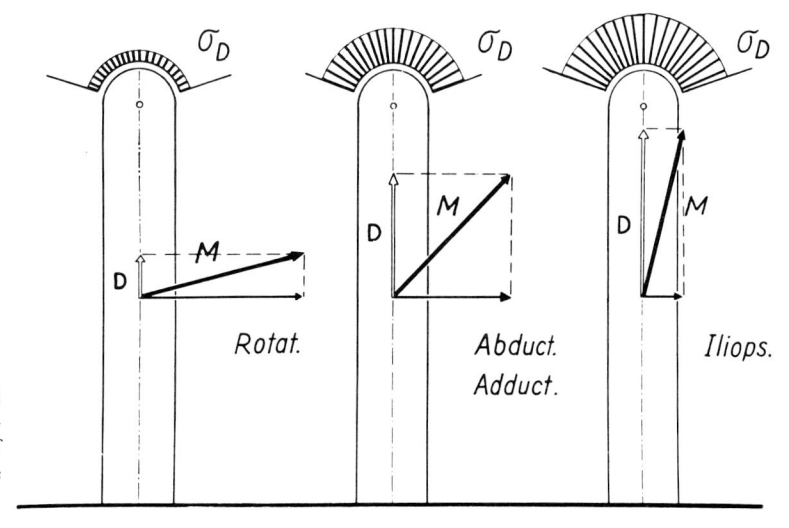

Fig. 63. Resolution of the force *M* exerted by different muscles into a component *D* parallel and a component normal to the line of action of the resultant force. σ_D compressive stresses in the joint. (After Pauwels 1961)

Table 9. Clinical evaluation of animals: average ratings (Radin et al. 1975)

Months postop.	No. of animals		Limp		Effusion		Lack of joint congruence		Hypertrophic changes	
	E	C	E	C	E	C	E	C	C	C
1	4	3	Mod	Mild	Mod	Mild	Severe	Mild	None	None
2	6	4	Mod	Mod	Mild	Mod	Severe	Severe	None	None
6	5	5	Mild	None	Mild	Mild	Mod	Severe	None	None
12	5	4	None	Mod	None	Mild	Mild	Severe	None	None
24	4	3	None	Mod	None	Mild	None	Severe	None	Mod
30	4	2	None	Mod	None	Mild	None	Severe	None	Mod
	28	21								

E, experimental; C, control

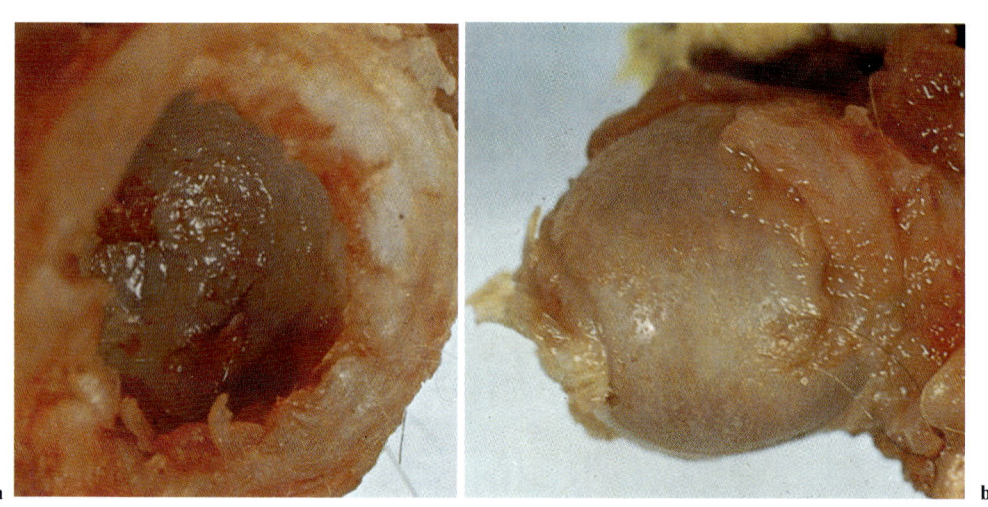

Fig. 64a, b. Hip joint of a control ("non-hanging-hip") animal at 24 months. Irregular joint with lips and spurs, eburnated bone. **a** socket; **b** femoral head. (Radin et al. 1975)

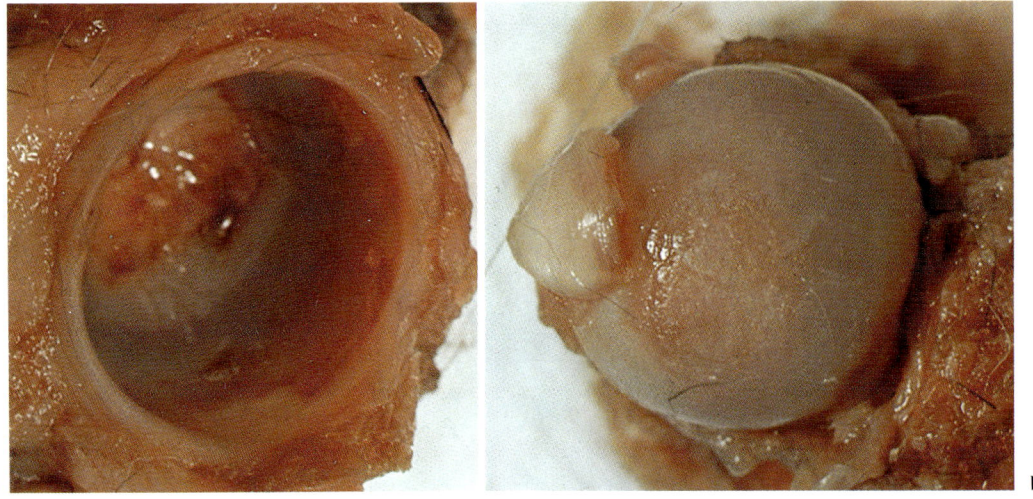

Fig. 65a, b. Hip joint of an animal from the experimental ("hanging-hip") group. Maintenance of joint congruence, absence of hypertrophic changes, re-formation of a smooth, glistening bearing surface on both sides of the joint. **a** socket; **b** femoral head. (Radin et al. 1975)

Fig. 66. Photomicrograph of the weight-bearing surface of the femoral head of an animal in the experimental (tenotomy) group 30 months after surgery (RADIN et al. 1975). Safranin-O and fast green staining, ×150

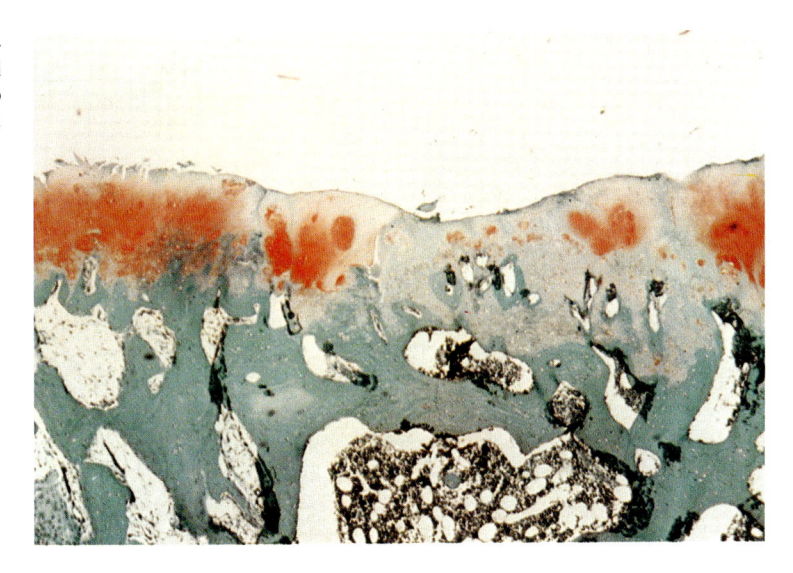

1 month, but was clearly more exuberant in the unsutured cats. After 1 year, histological sections through the weight-bearing portions of the heads and sockets of the unsutured group showed fibrocartilage (Fig. 66) and what appeared to represent remodelling of small foci of fibrocartilage into an intermediate stage, more hyaline than fibrous. This chondroid covering was not always continuous across the joint surfaces. More frequently it looked like an abundant layer of irregular cartilaginous-like tissue. The chondroid nature of this tissue was confirmed by safranin-O staining. Such staining quantitatively indicates the presence of proteoglycans. There was no indication that the small rim of cartilage left at the periphery of the joint in any way contributed to the healing.

The histological examination of the hips of the sutured animals after 1 year consistently showed eburnated bone (Fig. 67). This was in marked contrast to the unsutured animals, which consistently showed formation of an articulating surface.

3. Discussion

Hip joints experimentally denuded of their cartilage go on to progressive degeneration (KETTUNEN 1958). The findings in our sutured animals confirmed this. Similarly, osteoarthritic joints generally continue to degenerate. However, reconstitution of the joint space and regression of the abnormal subchondral sclerosis are observed after a proper

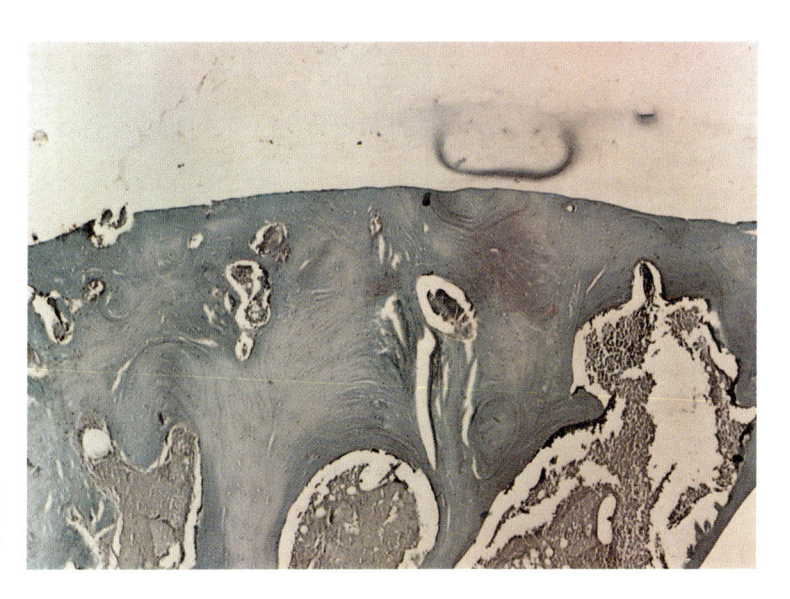

Fig. 67. Photomicrograph of the weight-bearing surface of the femoral head of an animal in the control group (with sutured muscles). (RADIN et al. 1975)

osteotomy close to the joint. Histological evidence exists to substantiate reconstitution of articular surfaces after such a procedure (NISSEN 1963; ENDLER 1972; BYERS 1974; FUJISAWA et al. 1976).

Attempts have been made to study cartilage degeneration by creating defects in the articular surfaces. Partial-thickness articular defects in adult animals do not heal. Small full-thickness defects in adult animals heal, usually with fibrocartilage. Extensive defects of articular cartilage on both sides of a joint, however, even those penetrating to the subchondral bone, were not healed in adult animals after several years, despite an attempt at initial healing by the cells. Healing apparently requires a source of cells existing in the base of the defect in the underlying bone.

Multiple tenotomy decreases the overall force and thus the compressive stresses across the hip joint. In these conditions of decreased articular pressure in which movement is maintained and the subchondral bone represents an obvious source of cells, chondroid tissue develops. This tissue is mostly fibrocartilage. Chondroid healing in our unsutured animals may have originated in hyaline remainders which persisted after curettage of the cartilage. However, it is significant that such healing was limited to the unsutured animals. After 1 year, none of the sutured cats demonstrated any cartilage or fibrocartilage in the weight-bearing areas.

The regenerated chondroid tissue observed in the unsutured animals does not always constitute a smooth fibrocartilaginous surface, but may be irregular and incomplete. It should be stressed, however, that by all clinical criteria it functioned well. If the animals had been observed for longer periods of time, later degeneration of this new cartilaginous tissue might have been apparent. It is also possible that further healing would have occurred.

This experiment suggests that the clinical improvement shown after multiple tenotomy has some biological basis. Damaged cartilage appears to be attempting to heal. Such cartilage healing seems to be made possible by decreasing the mechanical stress in the joint sufficiently.

C. Indications

We consider the hanging hip operation or multiple tenotomy to be indicated in hips with osteoarthritis, avascular necrosis or rheumatoid arthritis. The following conditions are required:

1. Good congruence of the joint surfaces in the neutral position as well as in adduction and in abduction of the limb.
2. No sign of lateral or medial concentration of the stresses in the joint as demonstrated by localized triangular sclerosis of the subchondral bone in the X-ray. The subchondral sclerosis should appear cup-shaped (Fig. 70) or should be distributed over the whole area in the roof of the socket (Fig. 74).

In these patients, the weight-bearing surface of the joint is not decreased by the pathological changes. The joint pressure can be reduced significantly by decreasing the overall force R transmitted across the hip.

A dense triangle at the edge of the acetabulum corresponding to a lateral displacement of R or a dense triangle in the depths of the acetabulum in protrusio acetabuli demonstrates a reduction of the weight-bearing surface of the joint with localized concentration of the compressive stresses in the joint. They jeopardize the results of the hanging-hip procedure and constitute a contra-indication.

However, we have carried out the operation in some hips despite such signs, as a temporary measure to relieve pain, because at that time the patients were not considered suitable candidates for other more extensive procedures. The patients knew that they would have to undergo another operation later, when the evolution of the condition had changed the shape of the hip sufficiently to make the joint suitable for a different procedure. The pre-operative range of movement is not taken into account, since experience shows that some patients with as little as 10° flexion, no adduction or abduction and no rotation can regain a nearly full range of movement postoperatively.

When the geometry of the joint allows a choice between the hanging-hip operation and another procedure, such as a varus osteotomy or a lateral displacement of the greater trochanter, the benignity of the hanging-hip procedure makes it the procedure of choice in old people.

D. Operative Procedure

The operation is carried out under general anaesthesia with tracheal intubation. The patient lies supine with the legs apart. Draping is such that only the medial aspect of the upper extremity of the thigh is visible. The surgeon stands at the level

Fig. 68. Positions of the patient (*1*), surgeon (*2*) and assistant (*3*) for the tenotomy of the adductor and iliopsoas muscles of the right hip

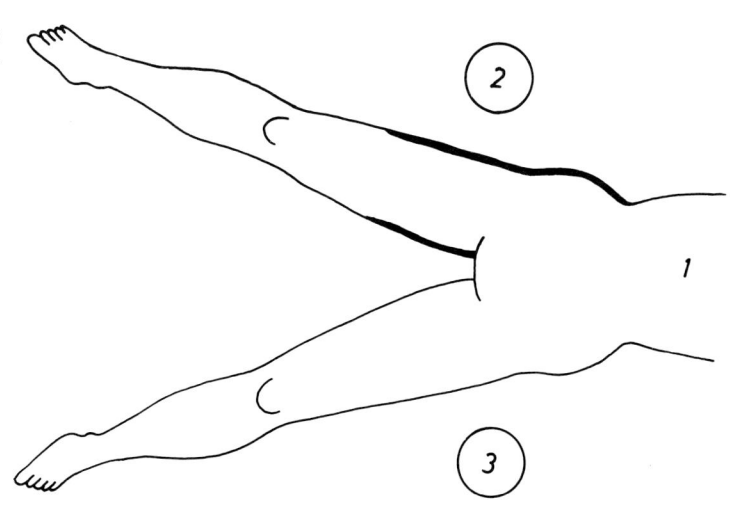

of the patient's groin on the side to be operated upon. The assistant stands opposite him (Fig. 68).

The skin is incised longitudinally for 5 cm as proximally as possible over the tendon of the adductor longus muscle, which is clearly felt. This tendon is divided transversely close to the pubic bone, as are the short adductor and gracilis muscles. The pectineus muscle is partially divided. The superficial branch of the obturator nerve and the accompanying vessels are seen between the pectineus and the adductor longus. The obturator vessels and the deep branch of the obturator nerve are encountered at a deeper level: they delineate the tenotomy in depth. The lesser trochanter is palpated with the left index finger. The tendon of the iliopsoas muscle is often found to be very taut. It is divided close to the lesser trochanter, using scissors.

There should be not bleeding during the whole procedure provided that the two mentioned groups of vessels are sought for and clearly seen. Only the skin is sutured.

The patient is then turned over and lies prone with a pillow beneath the chest in order to avoid stretching the brachial plexus. The leg to be operated on and the lower part of the trunk are prepared up to the waist and covered with stockinette, which is glued in position. The surgeon sits at the level of the patient's hip and the assistant stands at the level of the patient's knee on the same side of the table.

The skin incision is lateral and longitudinal, about 10 cm long, distal to the greater trochanter (Fig. 69). The fascia lata is divided by a cruciate incision longitudinally and transversely in the distal part of the incision. A muscle retractor is placed between the lesser trochanter and the femoral neck. The greater trochanter appears clearly. The tendons of the gluteus medius and gluteus minimus muscles are divided close to the greater trochanter until the scissors abut against the superior aspect of the neck of the femur.

Only the longitudinal cut in the fascia lata is sutured. The transverse cut relieves the tension of

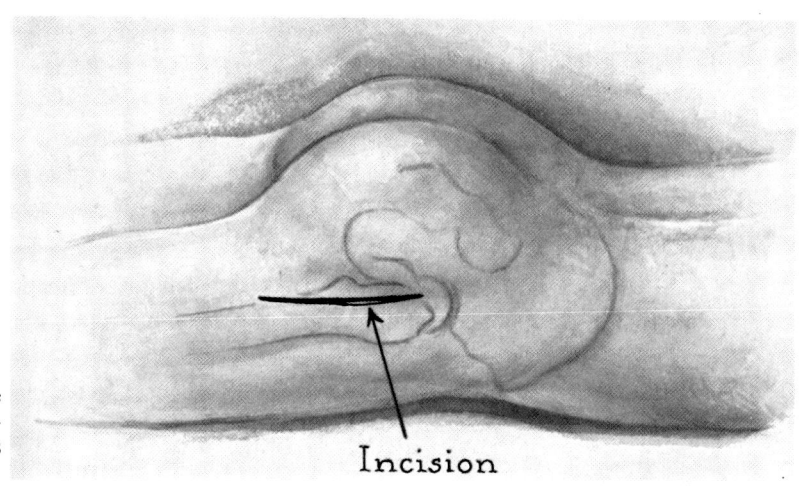

Fig. 69. Incision for the division of the fascia lata and the tenotomy of the gluteus medius and minimus. (After BANKS and LAUFMAN 1958)

the tensor fasciae latae. The subcutaneous fat and the skin are sutured using suction drainage. If carried out as described above, this part of the procedure should be practically bloodless.

E. Postoperative Care

The foot of the bed is elevated 20 cm and the patient is kept in a semi-recumbent position. Elderly patients lying supine in bed with the foot raised are apt to develop pulmonary oedema during the first hours after the operation. Sitting avoids this complication. Low molecular weight Dextran (Dextran 40) is infused for 3 days, starting at operation (one bottle a day). As soon as he awakes and then at 10-min intervals, the patient is asked to blow into a tube with its end under 20 cm of water. This represents our simple routine prophylaxis against thrombo-embolism. Whilst the patient lies in bed, 2-kg traction is put on the leg that was operated upon.

On the 2nd day after the operation, the patient is helped to stand and starts walking with the help of two crutches. Every day he walks further. He leaves the hospital after 12 days, the stitches having been removed. He is encouraged to use both his crutches for about 3 months and then one crutch for a further 3 months, in order to relieve joint pressure.

Except for walking, active exercises are forbidden. These would only strengthen the muscles and consequently increase joint pressure. This is the exact opposite of the goal of the hanging-hip procedure. Straight leg-raising must particularly be avoided. This exercise is very likely to damage the hip. During the 1st postoperative year night traction of 2 kg is recommended, with the foot of the bed elevated by 10–20 cm. The patients are seen at 3 months, 6 months and 1 year after surgery and then every year or two.

F. Postoperative Evolution

Relief of pain is usually immediate when the indication for a hanging-hip operation was correct. The range of movement increases progressively. In some patients the improvement is spectacular. The TRENDELENBURG sign often becomes negative after 6 months to 1 year postoperatively. In some patients it remains positive. Its disappearance seems unpredictable. Most of our patients abandoned their walking-sticks. The eldest patients

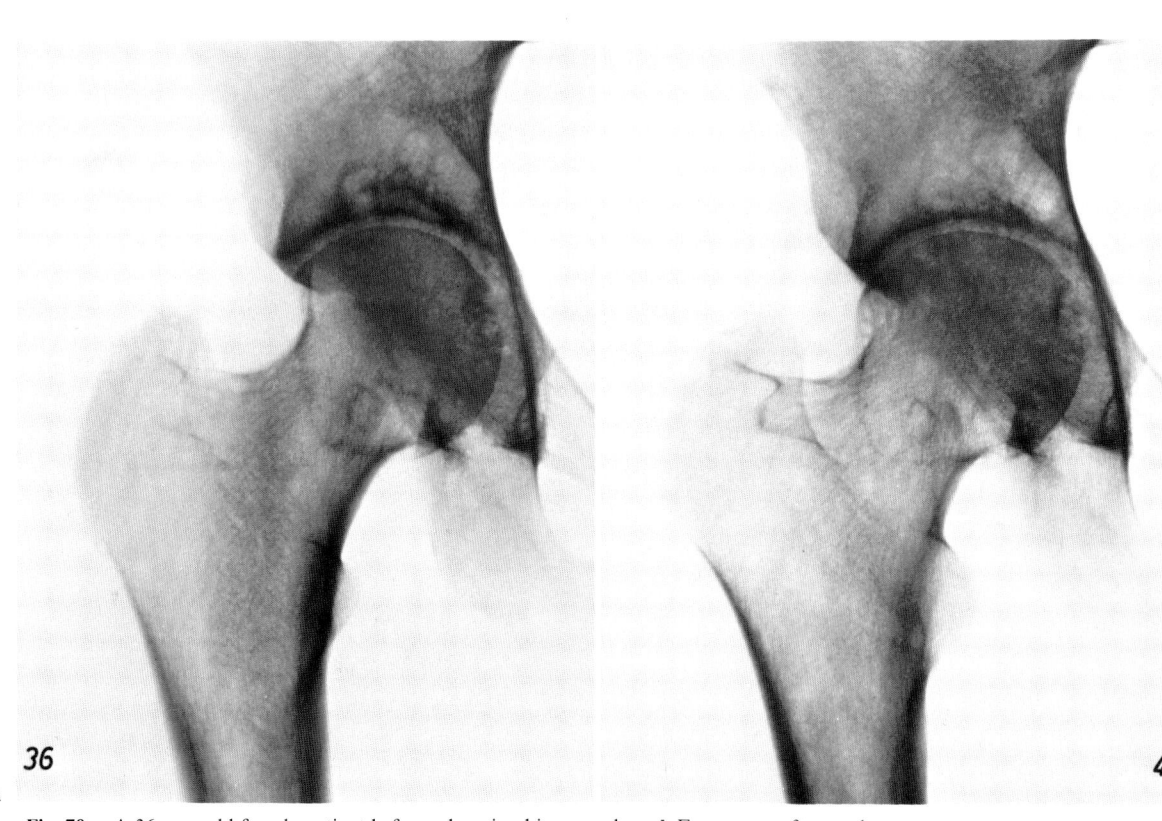

Fig. 70. a A 36-year-old female patient before a hanging-hip procedure. **b** Four years afterwards

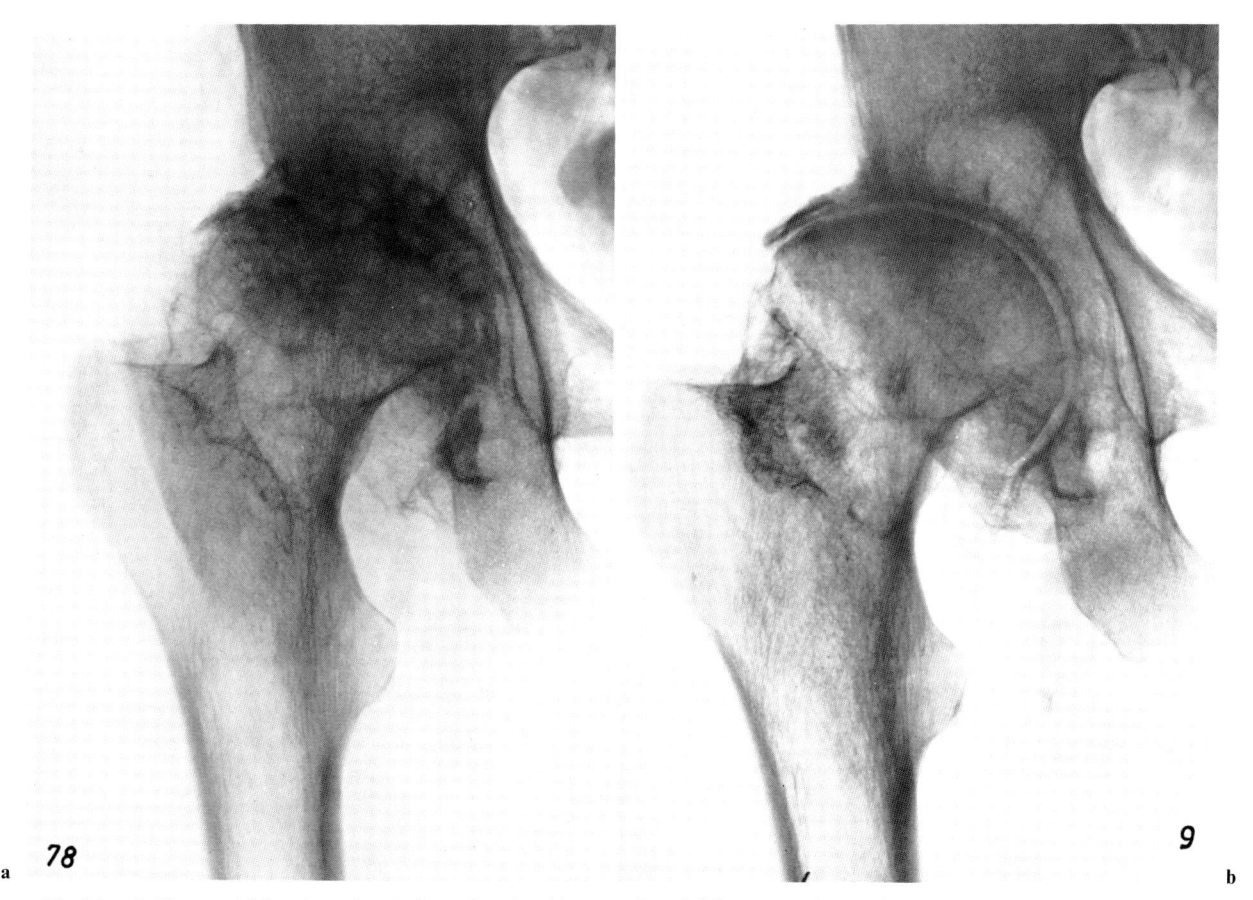

Fig. 71. a A 78-year-old female patient before a hanging-hip procedure. **b** Nine years afterwards

tend to continue to use one. We do not make any objection to its use since it further decreases the load exerted on the hip joint.

A 36-year-old female patient complained of pain day and night in her hip, the range of movement of which was restricted. A cup-shaped subchondral sclerosis with cysts in the roof of the acetabulum pointed to primary osteoarthritis (Fig. 70a). A tenotomy relieved pain completely. After a year the range of movement was once more complete. At the 4-year follow-up the clinical result remained excellent. The subchondral sclerosis had been replaced by a thin ribbon of even thickness throughout in the roof of the socket (Fig. 70b).

A 78-year-old female patient complained of a painful hip with considerable limitation of its range of movement (Table 10) and a severe limp. The X-ray (Fig. 71a) showed the joint space to have disappeared. There were a cup-shaped sclerosis and cysts in the roof of the socket. A hanging-hip procedure was carried out, and the pain disappeared immediately. At the 9-year follow-up, the hip remained pain-free. Its range of movement had improved considerably (Table 10) and the patient was not limping. The X-ray (Fig. 71b) showed a remarkable joint space to have developed. The subchondral sclerosis was thin and extended over a large area. The cysts had disappeared.

Table 10. Range of movement of the hip (Fig. 71)

	Before surgery	At the 9½-years follow-up	Gain
Flexion	75°	100°	35°
Extension	0°	10°	
Adduction	5°	35°	30°
Abduction	5°	5°	
Int. rotation	−5°	45°	95°
Ext. rotation	10°	55°	

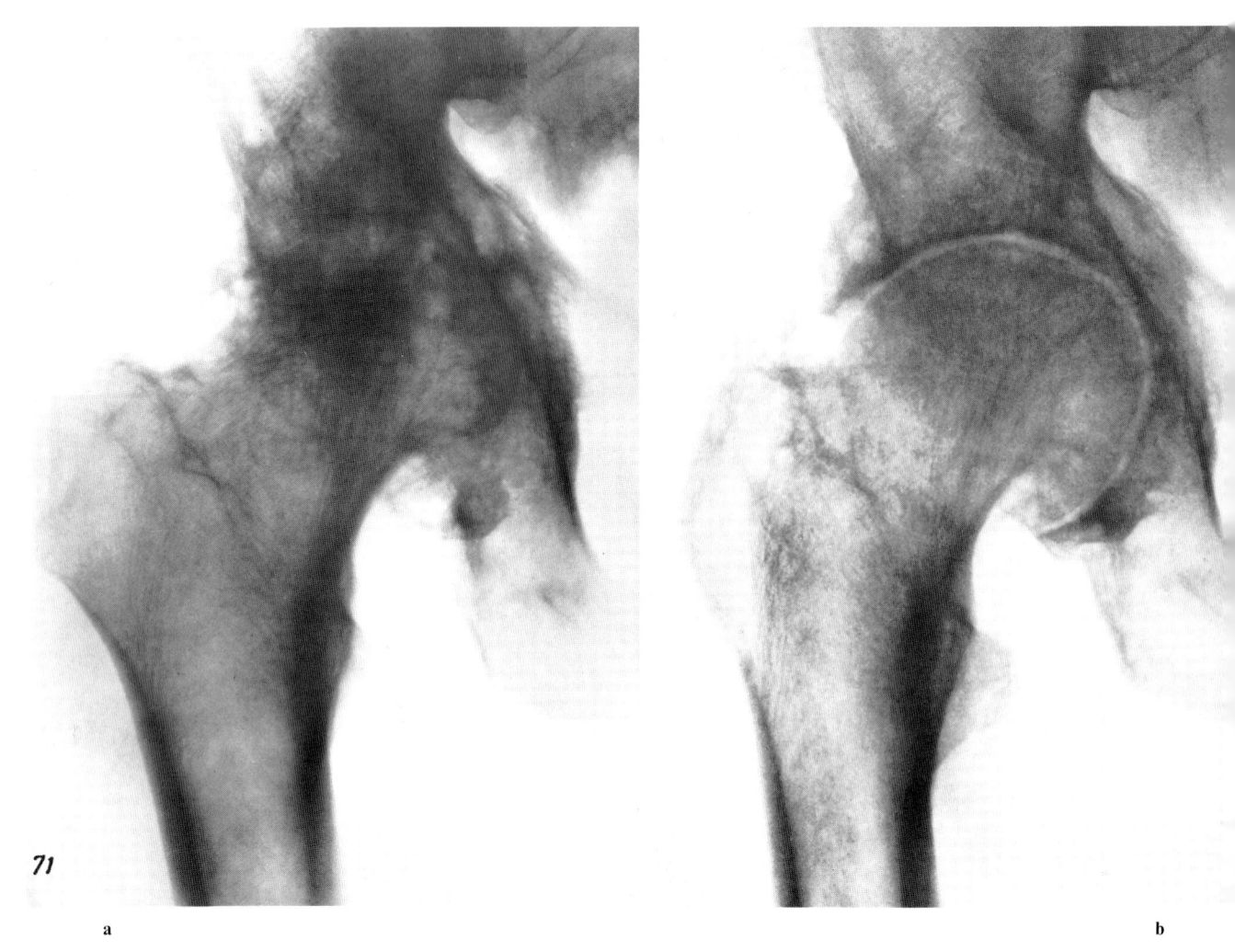

Fig. 72. a A 71-year-old male patient before a bilateral hanging-hip procedure. **b** Four years afterwards

The hanging-hip procedure can offer a simple solution to desperate problems in elderly patients. A 71-year-old male patient suffered rapid deterioration of both hips with severe pain and limitation of the range of movement (Figs. 72a and 73a). After a tenotomy carried out on both hips at the same session, he was free from pain. At the 4-year follow-up, the X-rays showed well-delineated joint spaces to have reappeared, and the other signs of osteoarthritis had regressed (Figs. 72b and 73b).

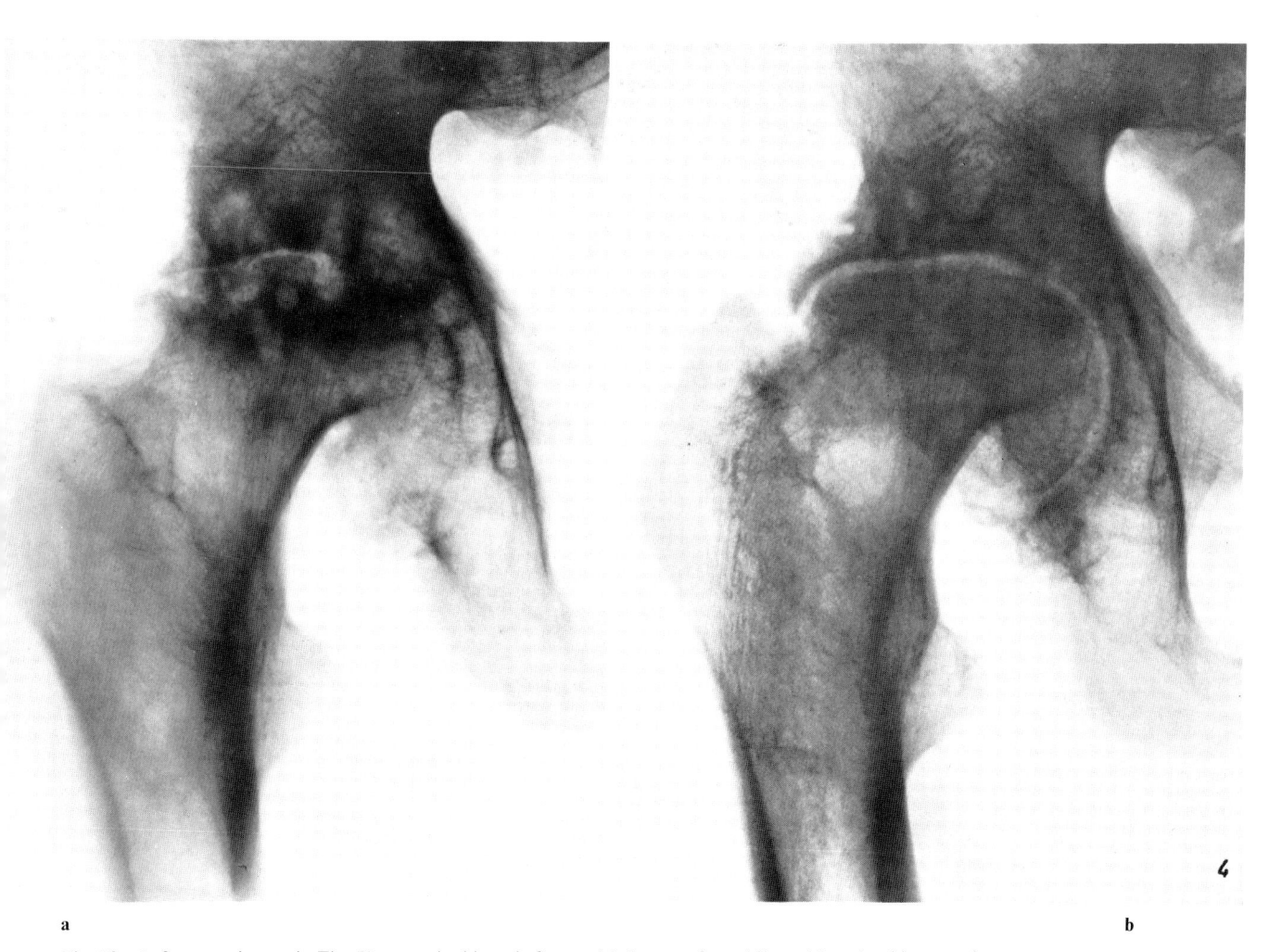

Fig. 73a, b. Same patient as in Fig. 72: opposite hip. **a** before and **b** 4 years after a bilateral hanging-hip procedure

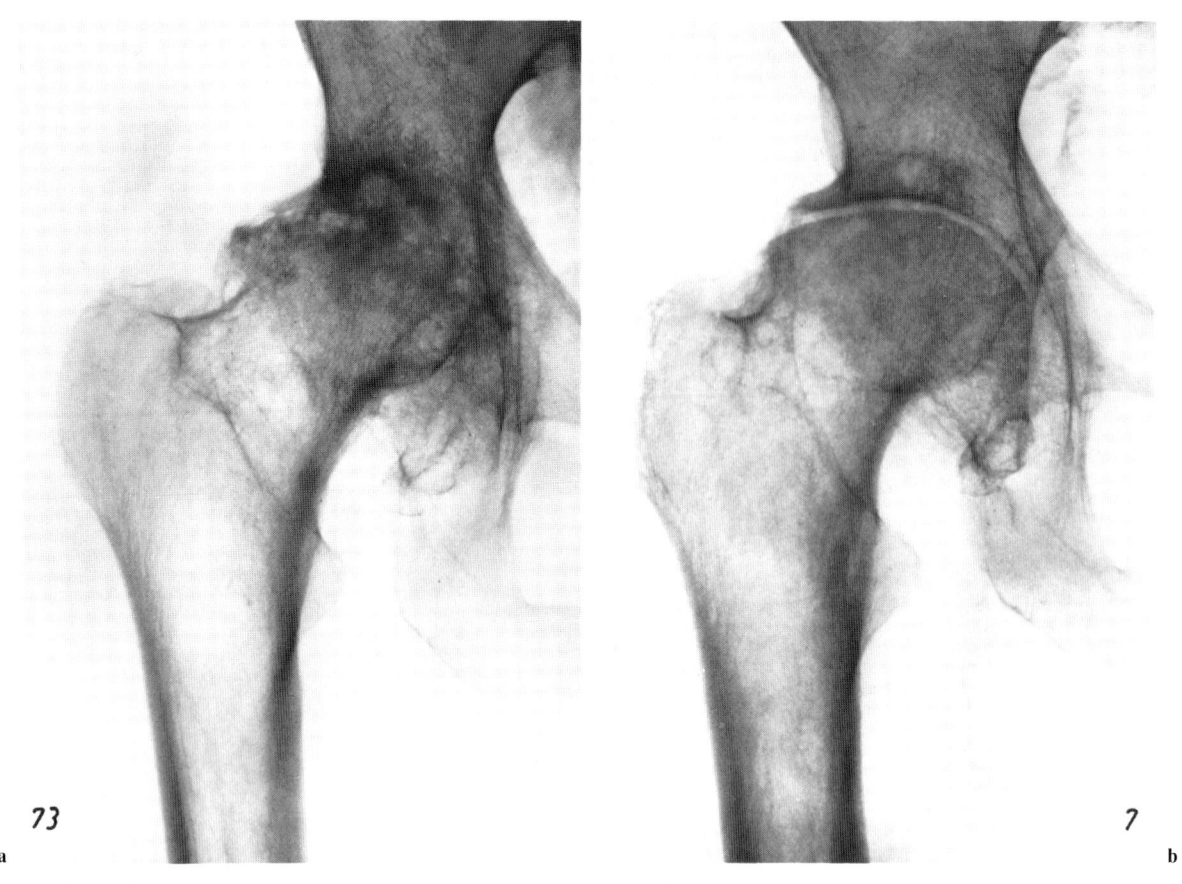

Fig. 74. a A 73-year-old female patient before a hanging-hip procedure. **b** Seven years afterwards

A 73-year-old female patient complained of severe pain in one hip, which was almost stiff (Table 11). She also suffered from diabetes, hyperuraemia and high blood pressure. X-rays revealed complete lack of joint space in the affected hip, a cup-shaped subchondral sclerosis with multiple cysts in the socket and in the femoral head (Fig. 74a). A hanging-hip procedure relieved the pain completely. At the 7-year follow-up the range of movement had increased considerably (Table 11). The patient walked with only a slight limp and the TRENDELENBURG sign had become negative. The signs of osteoarthritis had regressed and a large joint space had formed (Fig. 74b).

Table 11. Range of movement of the hip (Fig. 74)

	Before surgery	At the 7-year follow-up	Gain
Flexion	25°	85°	75°
Extension	−15°	0°	
Adduction	15°	25°	40°
Abduction	−15°	15°	
Int. rotation	−10°	10°	35°
Ext. rotation	10°	25°	

G. Incorrect Indications

Incongruence of the articular surfaces of the hip and a triangular subchondral sclerosis at the edge of the acetabulum (subluxation) or in its depths (protrusio) indicate that a reduction of the weight-bearing area of the joint has occurred. At this stage it is no longer sufficient to decrease the load transmitted across the hip. In these circumstances the hanging-hip procedure does not usually stop the evolution of the condition. It can, at best, be considered as an attempt to relieve pain temporarily.

A 64-year-old female patient presented with severe osteoarthritis of the hip with narrowing of the joint space, medial osteophyte of the head and triangular subchondral sclerosis at the edge of the acetabulum (Fig. 75a). Despite an extensive hanging-hip procedure, both the clinical condition and the X-ray appearance deteriorated. Four years later the dense triangle had increased in height and the subluxation had progressed (Fig. 75b). Such a failure must be attributed to a poor choice of procedure. With better knowledge of the biomechanics of the hip it could have been avoided. The hip had to be reoperated on. Enlarging the weight-bearing surface of the joint yielded an excellent clinical result, and this was confirmed by the X-ray evolution. The improvement remained unchanged at the 11-year follow-up (Fig. 75c).

H. Conclusion

The hanging-hip procedure thus appears to be an easy, simple and efficient way of treating osteoarthritis. However, if the joint surfaces are not congruent or if a triangular subchondral sclerosis substantiates reduction of the articular weight-bearing area, another solution must be sought for. Under those circumstances, the weight-bearing area of the joint must be increased by one of the following procedures.

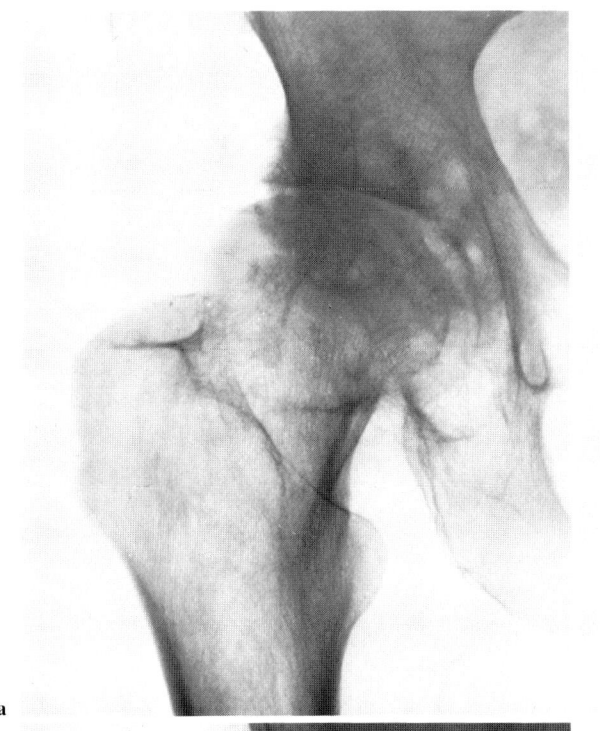

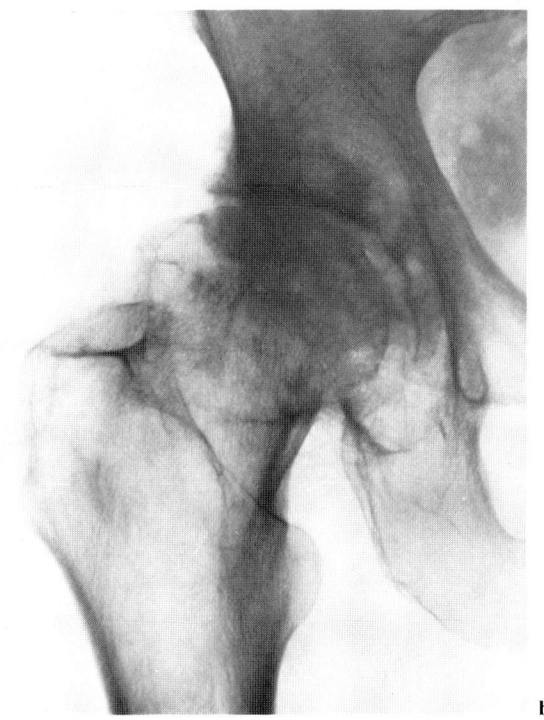

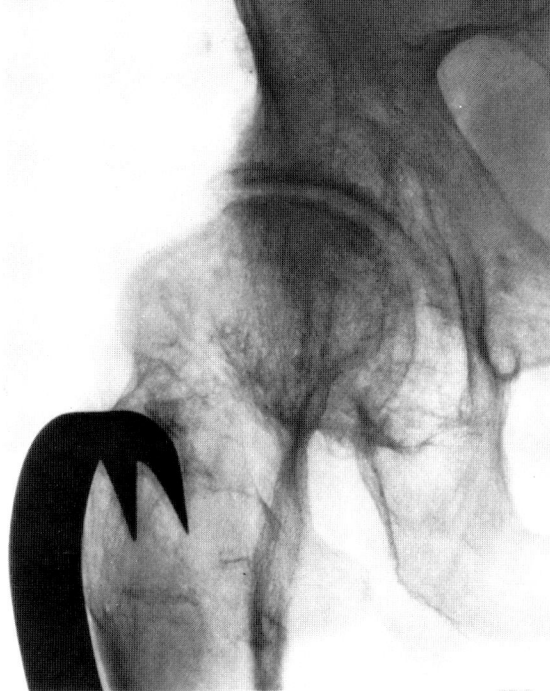

Fig. 75. a A 64-year-old female patient before a hanging-hip operation performed without the correct indications. **b** Four years afterwards: a valgus intertrochanteric osteotomy was then carried out. **c** Result at the 11-year follow-up

III. Varus Intertrochanteric Osteotomy (Pauwels I)

A. Rationale

The varus intertrochanteric osteotomy (PAUWELS 1959) lengthens the lever arm and changes the direction of the force M exerted by the abductor muscles (Fig. 76). Provided with a longer lever arm, the muscles carry out their work with less force. The change of direction of force M shifts the intersection of the two forces K and M downwards and thus displaces the resultant force R further into the socket (Fig. 28). This increases the weight-bearing area of the joint. It must be remembered that, in a congruent joint, the proportion of the contact surfaces which bears weight depends on the position of the resultant force R. A displacement of force R medially inside the acetabulum, therefore, increases the weight-bearing area even if the area of contact is not increased. Both decreasing force M and opening the angle formed by the lines of action of forces M and K reduce the resultant force R. The varus osteotomy must, therefore, result in a decrease in and an improved distribution of the compressive stresses in the joint.

The varus intertrochanteric osteotomy, although it decreases the resultant compressive force R and the reaction force R_1, actually (a) increases its transverse component Q, which pushes the femoral head into the acetabulum and (b) decreases its longitudinal component L, which pushes the femoral head upwards (Fig. 77). The varus osteotomy entails some shortening of the femur as a consequence of the closing of the neck-shaft angle. This shortens the distance between the origin and

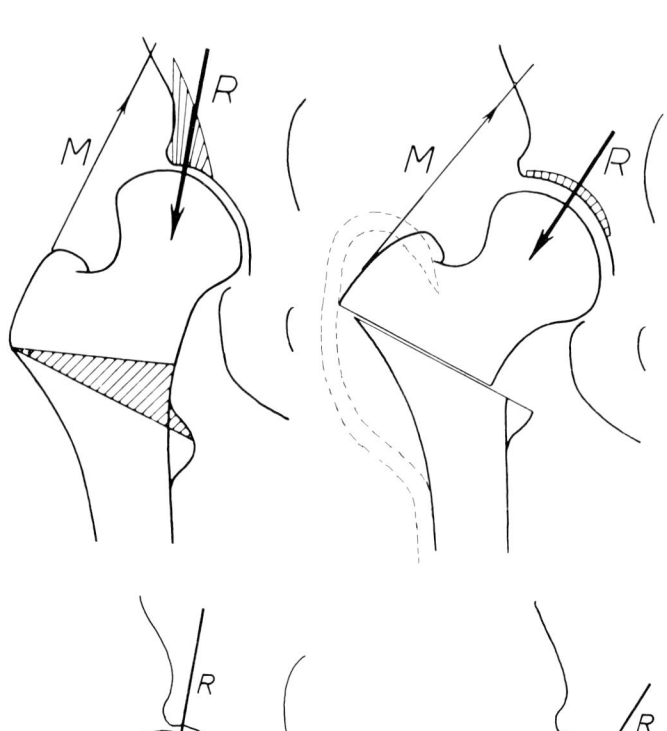

Fig. 76. Varus intertrochanteric osteotomy decreases the force R transmitted across the joint and enlarges the articular weight-bearing surface. M, force exerted by the abductor muscles. (Redrawn from PAUWELS 1959)

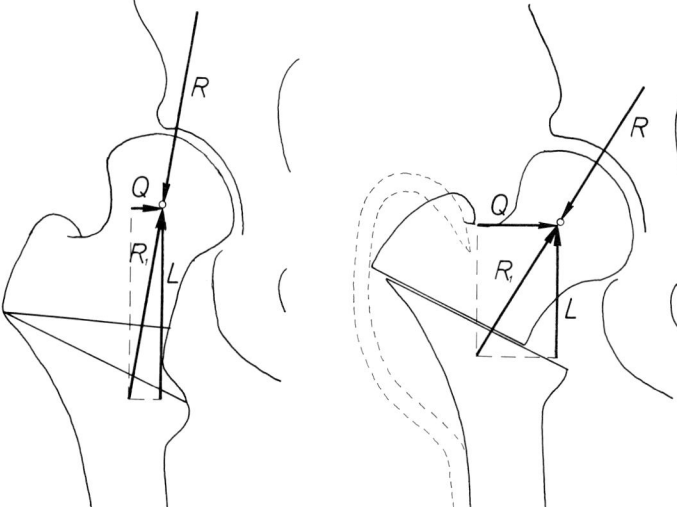

Fig. 77. Varus osteotomy increases the transverse component Q and decreases the longitudinal component L. R, resultant compressive force; R_1, reaction force

insertion of the muscles which span the hip and results in a relaxation of these muscles, thus further decreasing the resultant compressive force.

B. Indications

The essential prerequisite for the success of the procedure is good congruence of the articular surfaces when the leg is brought into full abduction pre-operatively (Fig. 78). If the femoral neck is long and the greater trochanter low, as in coxa valga subluxans, the varus osteotomy will lengthen the lever arm of force M significantly. If the greater trochanter is at its normal level or if the femoral neck is short, the varus osteotomy may not lengthen the lever arm of force M significantly. In this case the resultant force R is decreased only by opening the angle formed by the lines of action of forces K and M and the weight-bearing surface

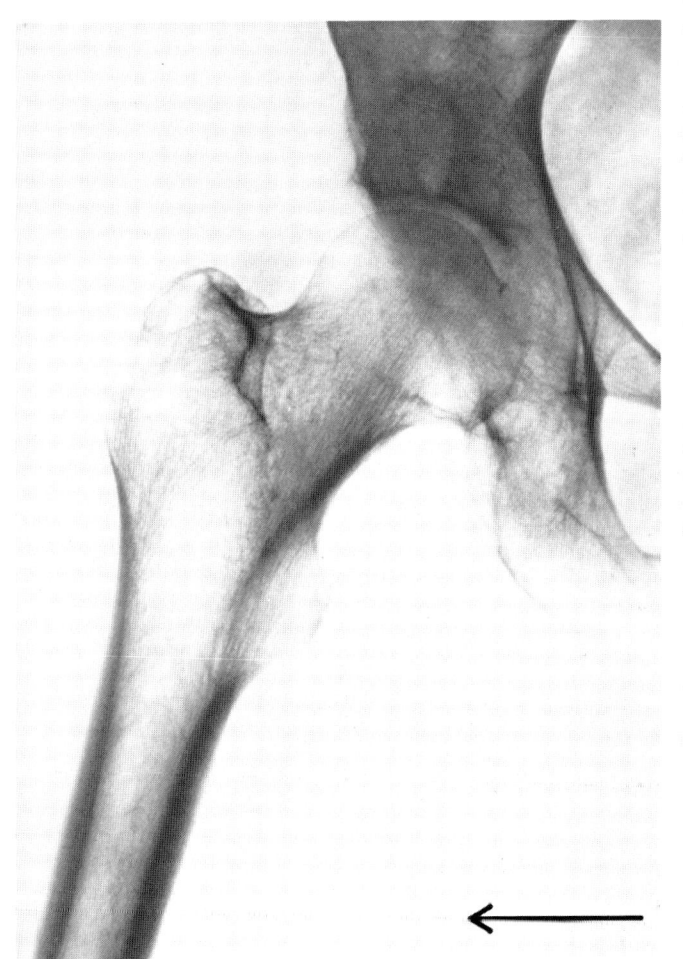

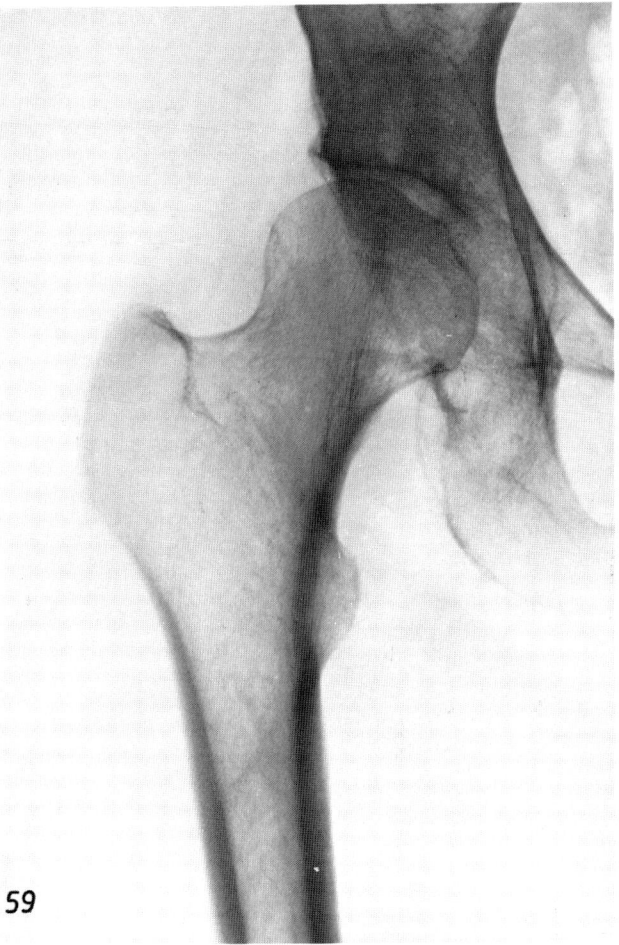

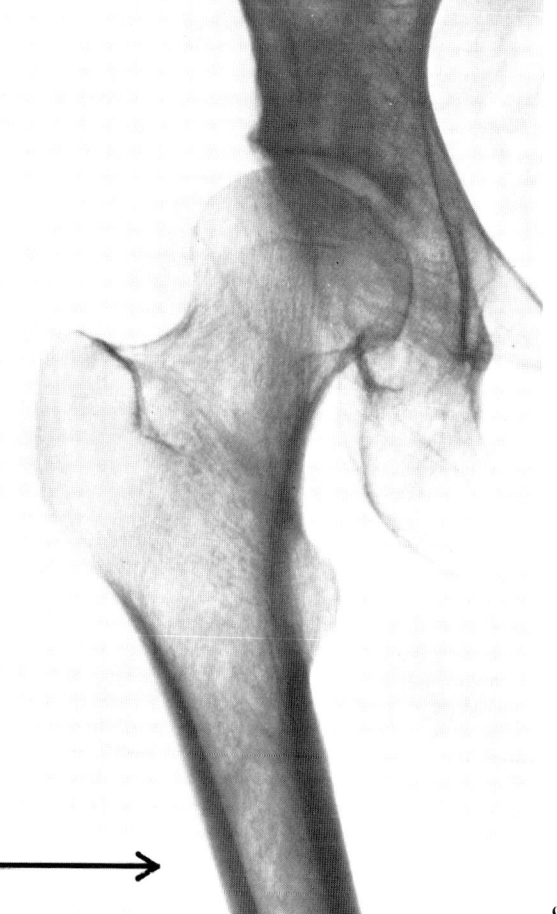

Fig. 78a–c. Congruence of the articular surfaces in abduction in a 59-year-old female patient. **a** neutral position; **b** full abduction; **c** full adduction

of the joint is enlarged by the change of direction of *R*. With a high greater trochanter or a short femoral neck and good congruence of the joint surfaces, it may be more efficient to displace the greater trochanter laterally (p. 134).

The best indications for a varus intertrochanteric osteotomy thus seem to be:

1. Osteoarthritis developing in coxa valga subluxans with congruent articular surfaces
2. Severe osteoarthritis with triangular subchondral sclerosis at the edge of the socket, provided that the articular surfaces are congruent in full abduction and that, in this position, the greater trochanter is not higher than the femoral head

In primary osteoarthritis with a cup-shaped subchondral sclerosis in the roof of the acetabulum, as long as the articular surfaces remain congruent in full abduction, a varus osteotomy may constitute an advantageous alternative to multiple tenotomy, mainly in younger patients (Fig. 104). The varus osteotomy presents the advantage of decreasing articular pressure by enlarging the weight bearing surface of the joint and by reducing the transmitted load, whereas the hanging-hip procedure only decreases the transmitted load. The varus osteotomy is, therefore, more efficient. The indications in children will be considered later (p. 260).

A varus osteotomy should not be carried out if, when the leg is fully abducted, the articular surfaces do not appear congruent in the X-ray. In these conditions, the procedure cannot enlarge and may even decrease the weight-bearing area of the hip and will therefore fail.

C. Pre-operative X-rays

Besides the overall X-ray showing the pelvis and both hips, the lateral view and the three-quarter view of the affected hip, three anteroposterior views are taken with the leg in internal rotation: one in the neutral position between adduction and abduction, one in full abduction and one in full adduction (Fig. 78).

The anteroposterior X-ray in abduction must show good congruence of the joint surfaces. However, only the drawing makes possible a definite decision as to the suitability of varus osteotomy and the degree of varus.

D. Pre-operative Planning

The equipment necessary for the tracing is: a viewing-box built in a table, tracing-paper, a hard pencil and a protractor. Using the anteroposterior X-ray of the hip in the neutral position, the contours of the acetabulum and of the upper end of the femur are carefully traced onto the left half of a transparent sheet. The axis of the femoral shaft is drawn (Fig. 79a). The transparent sheet is then folded along the middle, and the contour of the acetabulum is traced on the second half (Fig. 79b). This second half is detached and rotated over the first half — counter-clockwise for a right hip — until the articular surfaces of the acetabulum on the second half-sheet and the femoral head on the first are congruent, but with a joint space a little wider at the edge of the acetabulum. The greater trochanter should not be brought higher than the top of the femoral head. The angle formed by the edges of the two half-sheets is measured (Fig. 79c). The femoral head must be rotated in the socket by this angle if satisfactory congruence of the articular surfaces is to be achieved. The femoral neck and head are then traced on the second half-sheet (Fig. 79d). Coming back to the first half-sheet, two transverse lines are drawn from the innominate tubercle of the femur. The proximal one is drawn at right angles to the axis of the shaft. The distal one forms with the proximal an angle open medially (Fig. 79e). This angle is equal to the angle which has been measured between the edges of the two half-sheets. The distal transverse line is thus oblique medially and distally. Using the first half-sheet thus completed, the drawing is finished on the second half-sheet, giving the planned postoperative picture (Fig. 79f). The shaft of the femur must lie at the same distance from the pelvis as before the operation. This means that the distal fragment has to be displaced medially in relation to the proximal. Displacing the shaft fragment laterally in relation to the pelvis leads to a varus deformity of the knee. The contour of the compression-hook is drawn using a template so that the surgeon knows exactly where to position it and, if necessary, where to bend it. The two half-sheets will be displayed on a viewing-box during the surgical procedure (Fig. 79g). They show the size of the wedge to be resected, its position in the femur, the magnitude of the medial displacement of the distal fragment of the femur in relation to the proximal fragment and the position of the compression-hook.

If there is doubt about the choice between a varus and a valgus osteotomy, both procedures are planned. New X-rays in full abduction and in full adduction are taken after tenotomy of the adductor muscles, while the patient is under anaesthesia. The final decision is based on these X-rays (Fig. 60).

E. Instruments

The following instruments are required:

1. The usual instruments for soft tissues

2. Instruments for bone surgery
   a) Retractors (two)
   b) Periosteal elevator
   c) Lowman bone clamp
   d) Square awl
   e) Screwdriver
   f) Hammer
   g) Air-powered engine
   h) Screws 5 mm in diameter, 30–45 mm in length; appropriate drill and tap
   i) Kirschner wires 2 mm in diameter

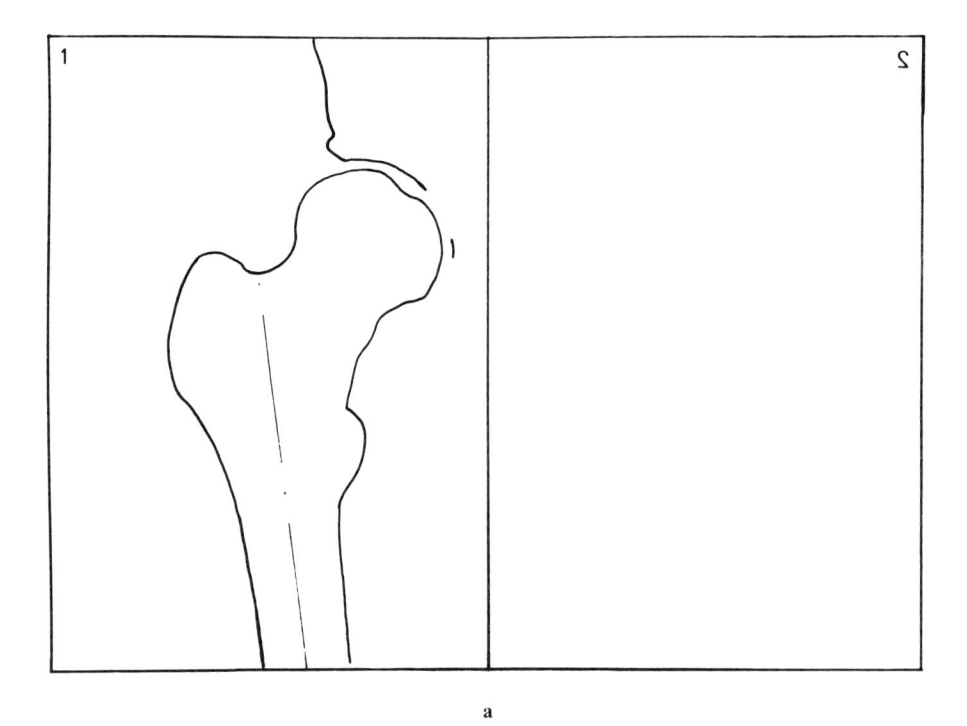

Fig. 79a–g. Pre-operative planning of a varus intertrochanteric osteotomy. *1, 2*, first and second half-sheets of tracing-paper

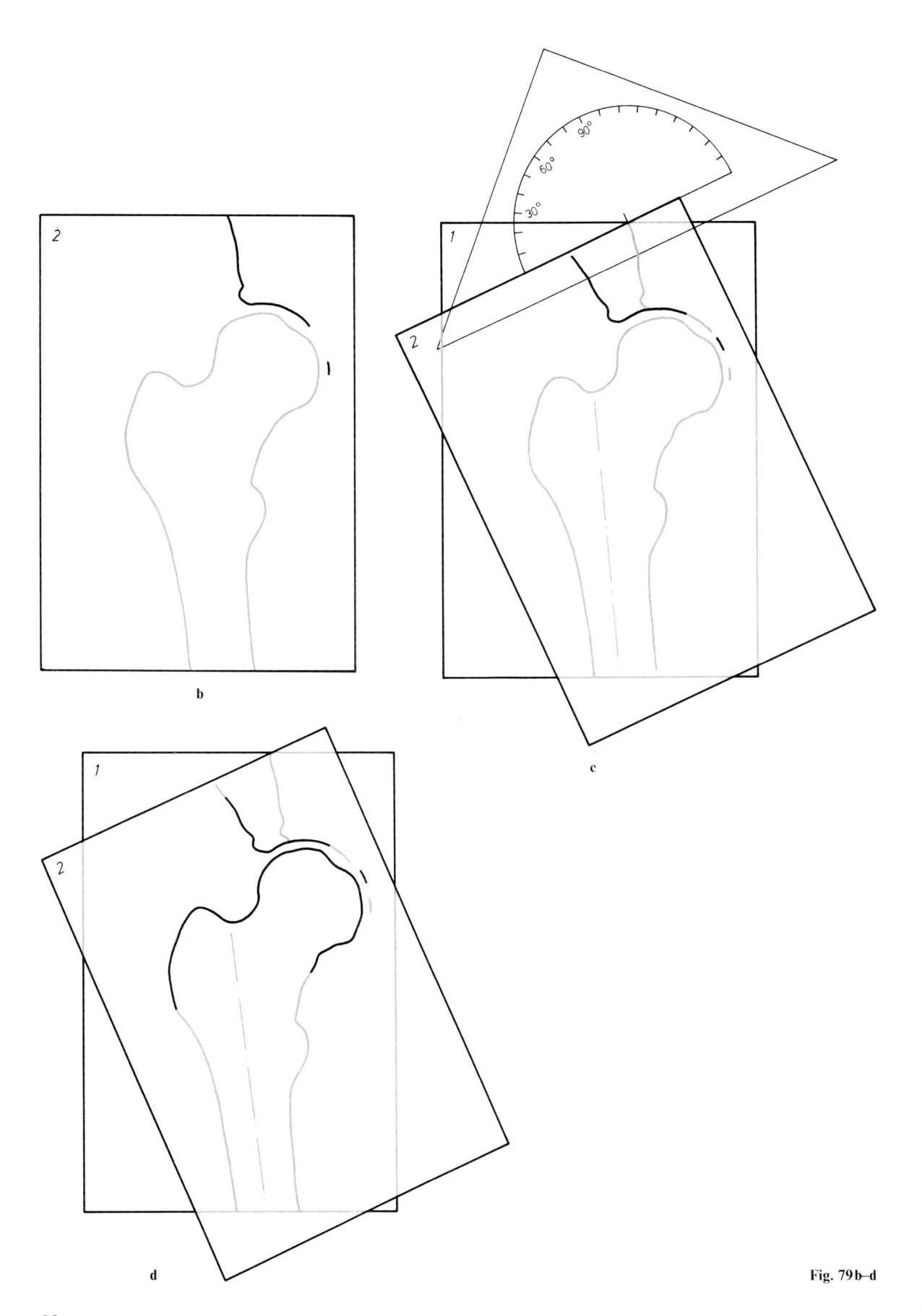

b

c

d

Fig. 79 b–d

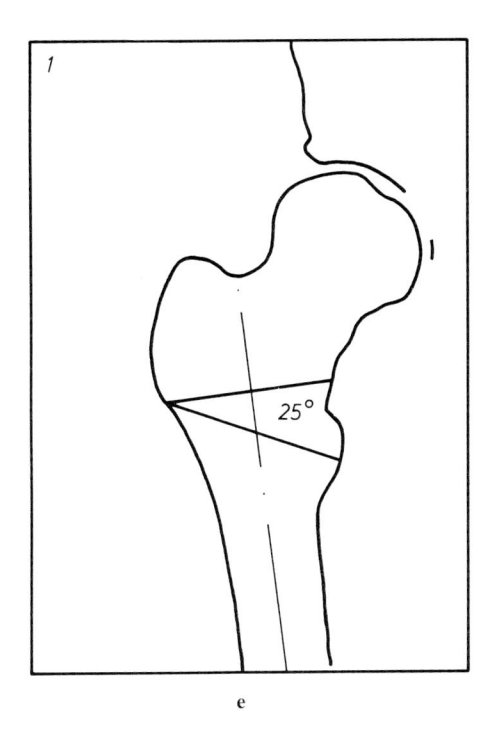

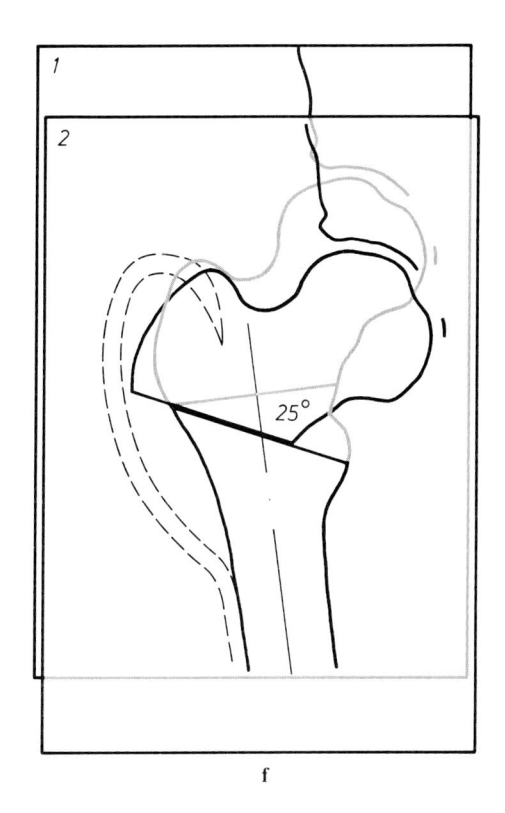

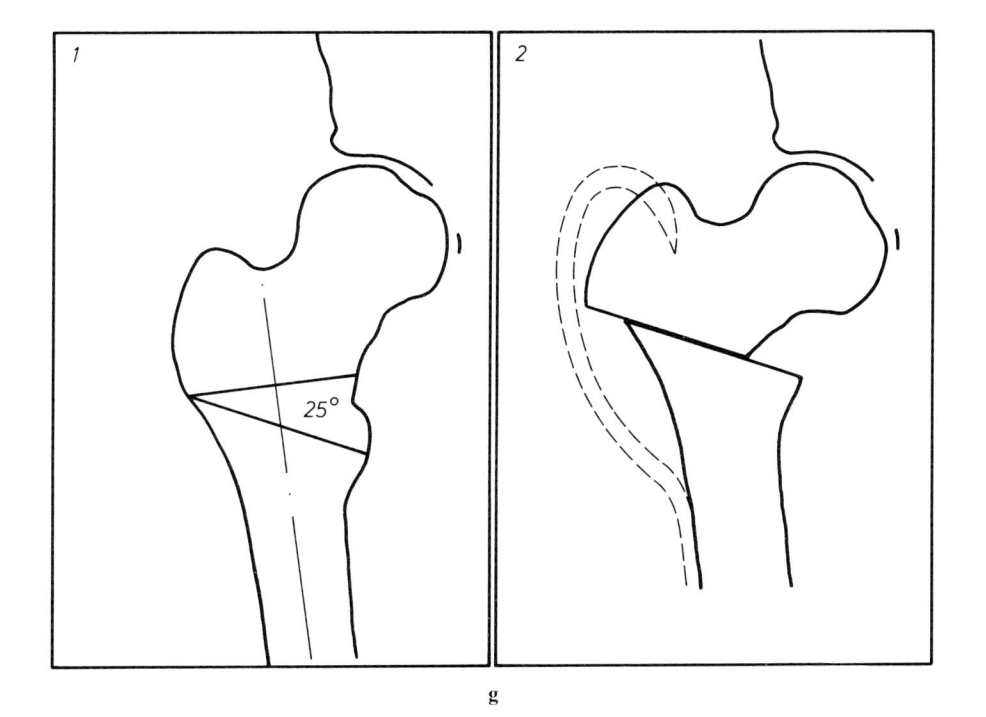

Fig. 79 e–g

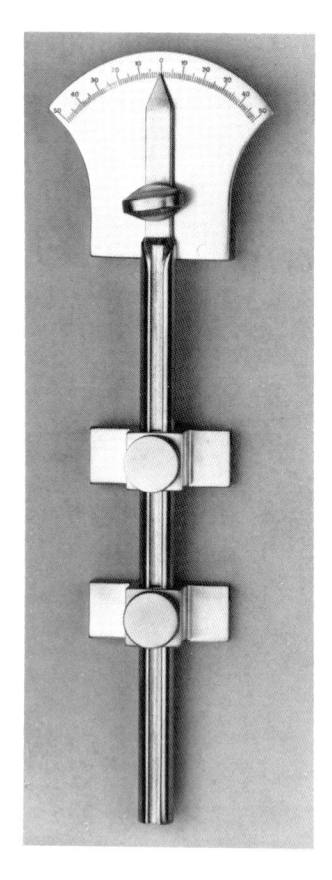

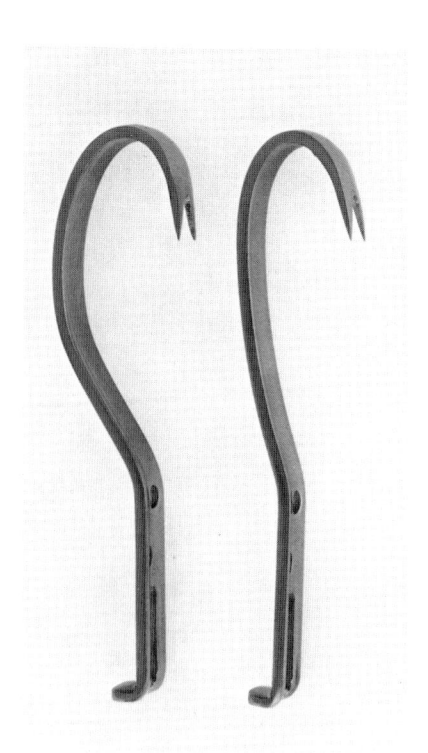

Fig. 82. Maquet compression-hooks *left* for varus osteotomy and *right* for valgus osteotomy

Fig. 80. Pin-insertion guide

3. Special instruments

a) Pin-insertion guide[1] (Fig. 80). This consists of a bar on which two mobile parts are mounted, and which ends as a pointer. One of the two mobile parts is engraved with a graduation in degrees and can rotate about an axis fixed in the bar. The other mobile part can glide along the bar and be fixed at any level. A KIRSCHNER wire is passed through a hole in each of the mobile parts. The two wires form an angle indicated by the pointer on the graduated scale. The gliding part allows modification of the distance between the wires without changing the angle which they form. The same instrument is used for osteotomy about the knee, but in that case STEINMANN pins are used, and these are passed through larger holes. The third mobile part shown in Fig. 80 is used for supraconolylar osteotomy of the femur.

b) A protractor[1] comprising a half-circle graduated in degrees, a fixed arm and a mobile arm with a pointer (Fig. 81). This is used to measure, on the X-rays taken during the operation, the angle formed by the KIRSCHNER wires which delineate the wedge to be resected.

c) A handsaw with disposable blades or an oscillating saw fitted to the engine.

d) MAQUET compression-hooks[1] (Fig. 82). These are made of stainless steel and comprise: two pointed prongs which are implanted into the

---

[1] Available from Joint Replacement Instrumentation, 104-112 Marylebone Lane, London W1.

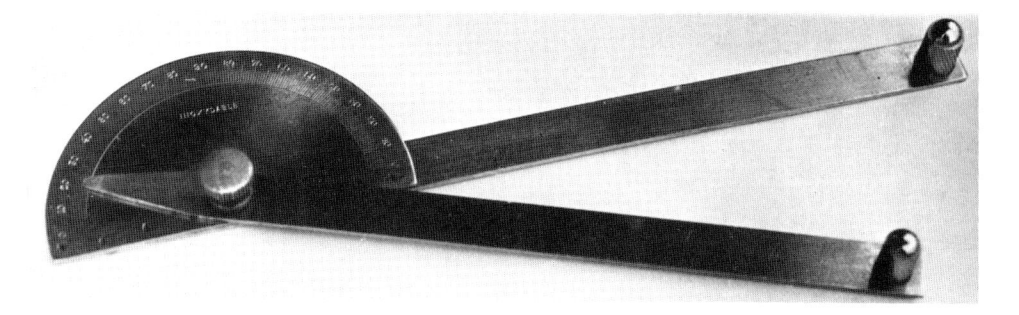

Fig. 81. Protractor

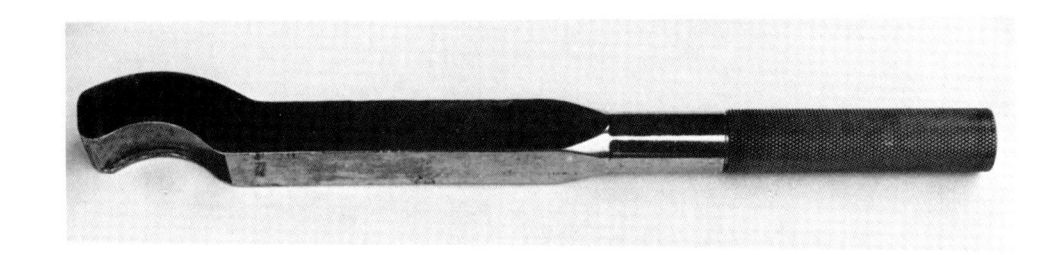

Fig. 83. Impacting-lever

greater trochanter and hinder its rotation; a bulging part placed lateral to the greater trochanter; a plate with two round holes and a slit for the screws; and a terminal abutment. There is a model for varus osteotomy and one for valgus osteotomy. In the former model the middle part bulges further laterally to allow for the medial displacement of the distal fragment of the bone in relation to the proximal. The hooks can be bent.

e) A plate-holder with an 11-mm wrench. It is used to hold and orientate the compression-hook and is one of the AO instruments (Association Suisse pour l'Etude de l'Ostéosynthèse).

f) An impacting-lever [2] (Fig. 83). Its curved end is applied over the proximal curve of the compression-hook and its other end is held in the left hand. Hammering on the middle part will make the prongs of the hook penetrate into the greater trochanter.

g) An eccentric disc [1] (Fig. 84) 24 mm in diameter. It has an eccentric 5.5-mm hole for a screw and two smaller holes for the prongs of the eccentric wrench. It is fixed in the bone over the compression-hook by means of a screw. The screw passes through the eccentric hole and the distal end of the slit in the compression-hook and penetrates the bone.

h) An eccentric wrench [2] (Fig. 84). This is a tube with a handle at one end and a disc with two prongs at the other end. The two prongs correspond exactly to the two small holes in the eccentric disc. Rotation of the wrench turns the eccentric disc about the screw fixed in the bone. When rotating, the eccentric disc pushes the compression-hook distally by acting against its terminal abutment (Fig. 85). When the screw arrives at the proximal end of the slit, the hook has been displaced distally by 17 mm.

---

[2] Available from J.R.I., 104-112 Marylebone Lane. London W1.

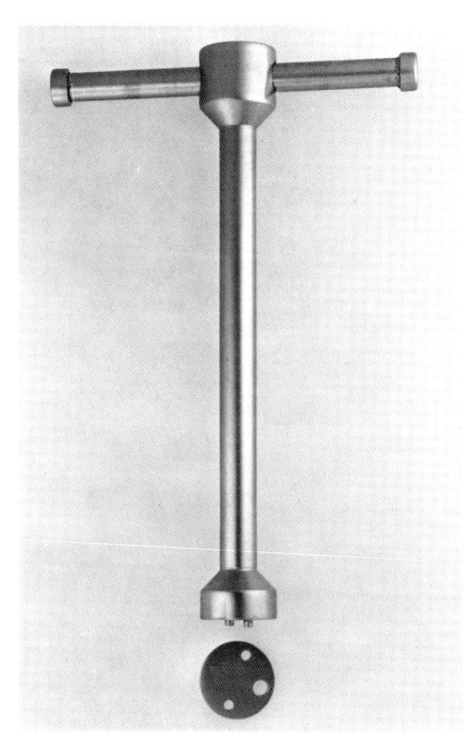

Fig. 84. Eccentric wrench and eccentric disc

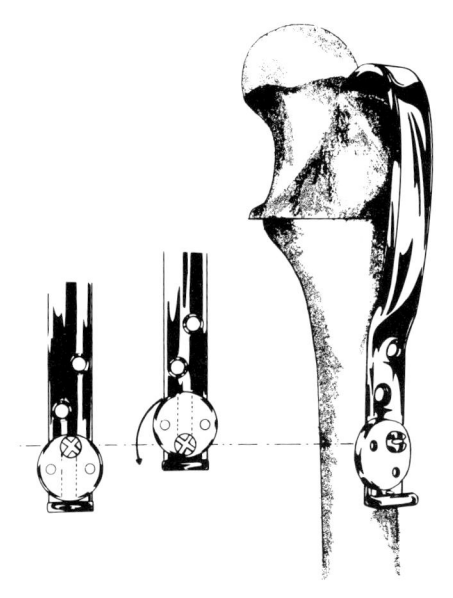

Fig. 85. How the eccentric disc works

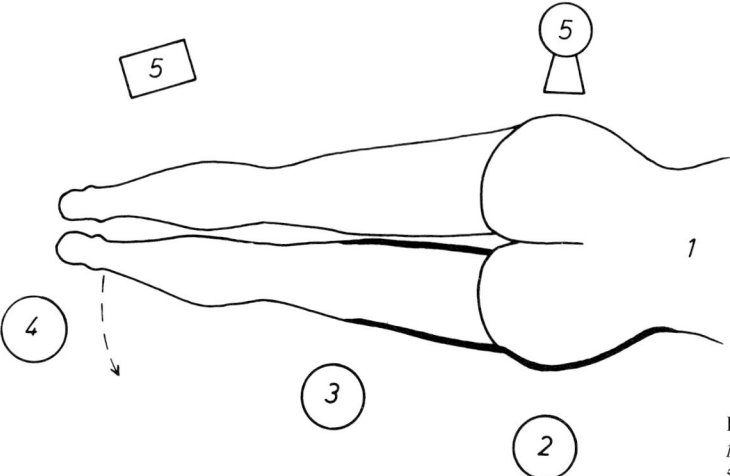

Fig. 86. Arrangement in the operating theatre.
1, patient; *2*, surgeon; *3, 4*, assistants;
5, X-ray apparatus and screen

F. Operative Procedure (Adults)

The patient is placed under general anaesthesia with tracheal intubation. The operation table must be transparent to X-rays. With the patient lying supine, the tendon of the adductor longus muscle is divided subcutaneously, close to the pubic bone. A more extensive tenotomy (p. 64) can be carried out if additional X-rays taken during full adduction and abduction under anaesthesia are necessary before the procedure can finally be chosen. Usually an extensive tenotomy is not needed, since all the muscles spanning the hip will be released by the shortening due to the varus osteotomy. The patient is then turned over and lies prone with a pillow beneath the chest to avoid stretching the brachial plexus.

1. Position

The lower limb to be operated on and the distal part of the trunk are prepared up to the waist and covered with stockinette, which is glued in place. The leg can thus be moved freely. The surgeon sits in front of the hip and the assistant stands at the level of the patient's knees (Fig. 86). A second assistant stands near the feet of the patient. The image-intensifier is positioned opposite the surgeon, at the same level; the screen must be clearly visible.

2. Approach

The skin incision is lateral and longitudinal, about 12–15 cm long, distal to the greater trochanter (Fig. 87). The fascia lata is incised longitudinally, further proximally than the skin incision, to give access to the greater trochanter. A retractor is passed behind the femur, distal to the lesser trochanter, through the gluteus maximus tendon (Fig. 88). The vastus lateralis is disinserted from the greater trochanter and the linea aspera. The first perforating artery and its accompanying veins are often encountered, and in this case they must be ligated and divided. The lateral aspect of the femur is cleared with the periosteal elevator. Only

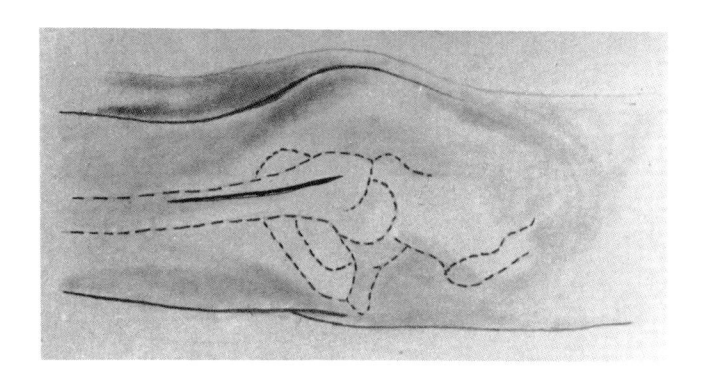

Fig. 87. Operative procedure: incision

in the intertrochanteric region are the anterior and posterior aspects cleared, just enough for the osteotomy.

3. Delineation of the Wedge to Be Resected

Using the air-powered drill, a KIRSCHNER wire is inserted from the innominate tubercle at right angles to the axis of the femoral shaft. A second KIRSCHNER wire is introduced using the pin-insertion guide. It forms with the former the desired angle, open medially, and should pass through the lesser trochanter (Fig. 89). An X-ray is taken and the angle is checked precisely, using the protractor.

4. Resection of the Wedge

The intertrochanteric wedge is cut with the handsaw, which is held parallel first to the proximal and then to the distal KIRSCHNER wire, under image-intensifier control (Fig. 90). The two cuts are begun. The proximal one is completed before the distal one, since it might be difficult to stabilize the proximal fragment during the second cut, whereas it is easy to hold the distal one with two retractors or a LOWMAN clamp.

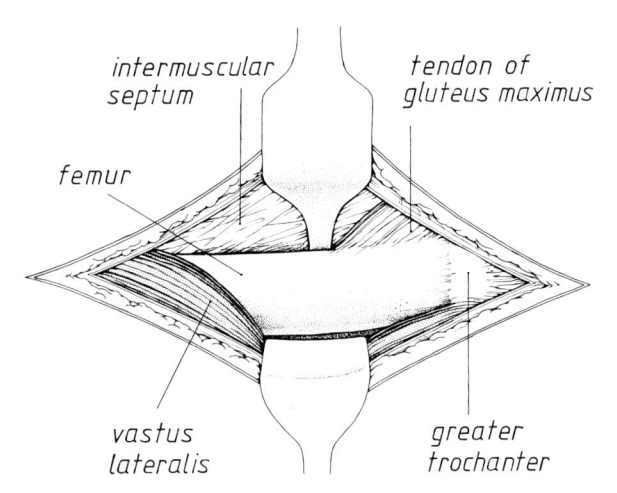

Fig. 88. Posterolateral approach to the upper end of the femoral diaphysis

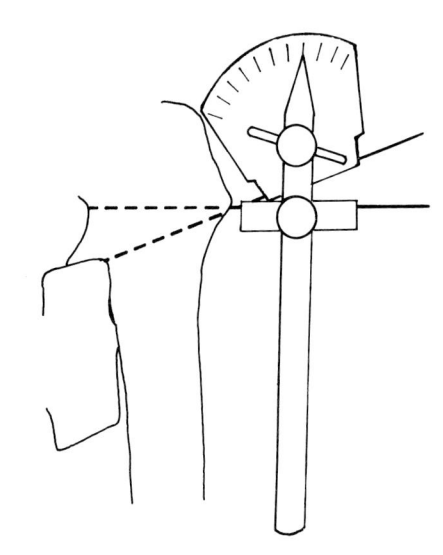

Fig. 89. Insertion of the KIRSCHNER wires using the pin-insertion guide

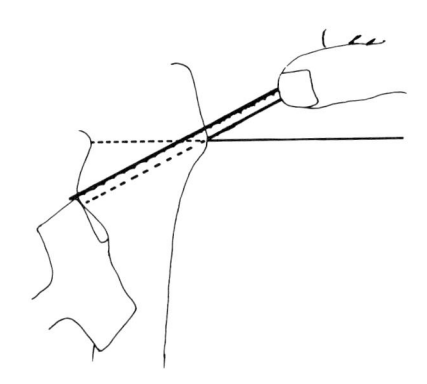

Fig. 90. Removal of an intertrochanteric wedge

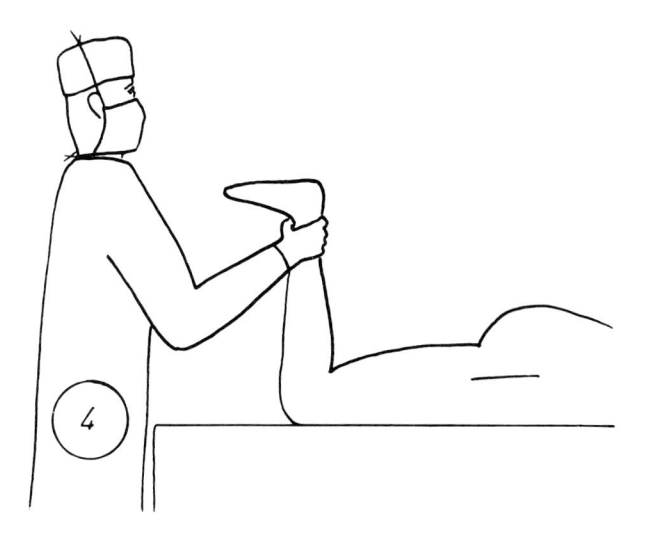

Fig. 91. An assistant ensures proper rotation of the leg

5. Derotation

If a derotation is necessary, the proximal cut is carried out completely, the leg is derotated, and only then is the distal cut carried out. After the wedge has been removed, the knee is flexed by the second assistant, who uses both hands to keep the lower leg vertical (Fig. 91). The thigh is pushed proximally. Sometimes, the square awl must be used as a lever to coapt the two osteotomy cuts.

6. Positioning the Compression-hook

The distal fragment is pushed medially using the LOWMAN clamp. The compression-hook held in the plate-holder is placed laterally, taking hold in the greater trochanter, exactly as represented in the pre-operative plan. It is held against the shaft by the LOWMAN clamp (Fig. 92). A KIRSCHNER wire is introduced from behind, between the lateral cortex of the distal fragment and the proximal fragment. This KIRSCHNER wire will prevent the lateral cortex from penetrating the cancellous bone of the greater trochanter. The prongs of the hook are lightly hammered into the greater trochanter using the impacting-lever (Fig. 93). Then a hole is drilled in the femur, through the distal end of the slit in the compression-hook. The hole is tapped. A screw is passed through the eccentric disc and through the slit and screwed into the bone (Fig. 94). A 180° rotation of the wrench will rotate

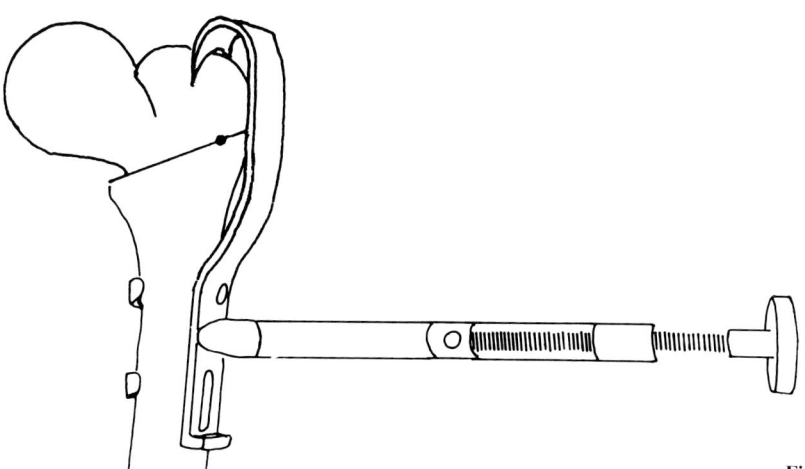

Fig. 92. Positioning the compression-hook

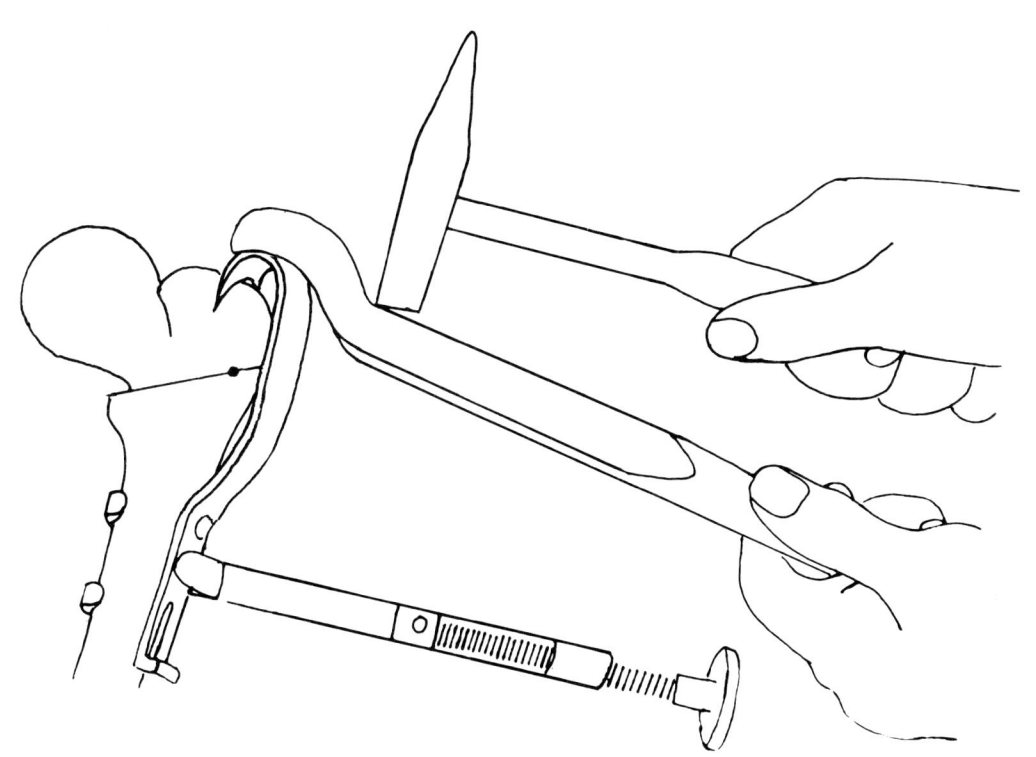

Fig. 93. Hammering in the compression-hook

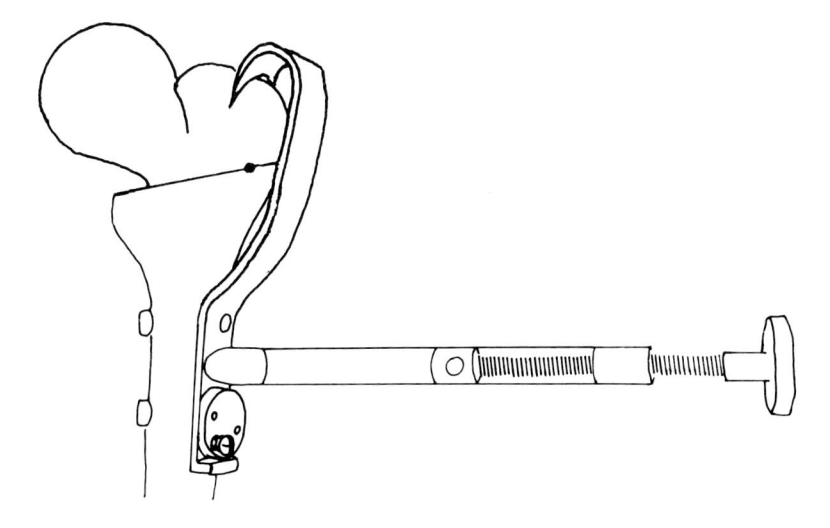

Fig. 94. Positioning the eccentric disc

Fig. 95. Compression of the fragments

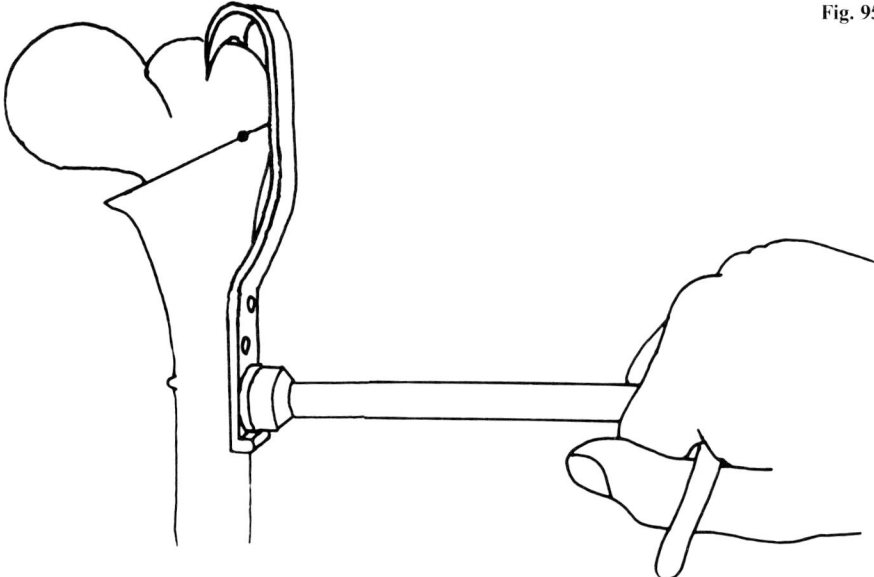

the eccentric disc about the screw and thus displace the compression-hook distally by 17 mm (Fig. 95). This makes the prongs of the hook penetrate further into the greater trochanter and compresses the fragments. If the penetration of the prongs and the compression between the fragments seem to be insufficient, the manoeuvre with the disc can be repeated after a new hole has been drilled at the distal end of the slit in the hook.

The second assistant rotates the leg internally and externally so that the surgeon can check the stability of the arrangement. The compression-hook is then fixed to the femur with two screws passed through its circular holes. The eccentric disc is removed and another screw replaces the one which has served as a pivot and which is usually bent (Fig. 96). If there remains any doubt as to the stability of the fixation of the fragments, two or three KIRSCHNER wires can be introduced through the latter in a cross-like fashion, in order to hinder any rotation.

7. Suture

The vastus lateralis is reattached to the greater trochanter by means of an absorbable suture. The fascia lata, the subcutaneous fat and the skin are sutured using suction drainage. The total loss of blood is very little (often less than 100 ml).

8. Using the Resected Wedge

Shortening resulting from the varus osteotomy can be minimized by removing a wedge the angle of which is half the necessary size. This wedge is then rotated by 180° and reinserted between the two fragments. For example, in order to carry out a 50° varus osteotomy, a wedge of 25° with its base medial is removed. It is reinserted between the fragments with its base now lateral (Fig. 97). This procedure has given us excellent results in children. In adults it entails a significant risk of non-union or at least of delayed union and is not recommended.

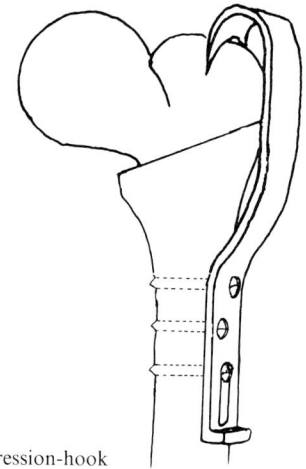

Fig. 96. Fixation of the compression-hook

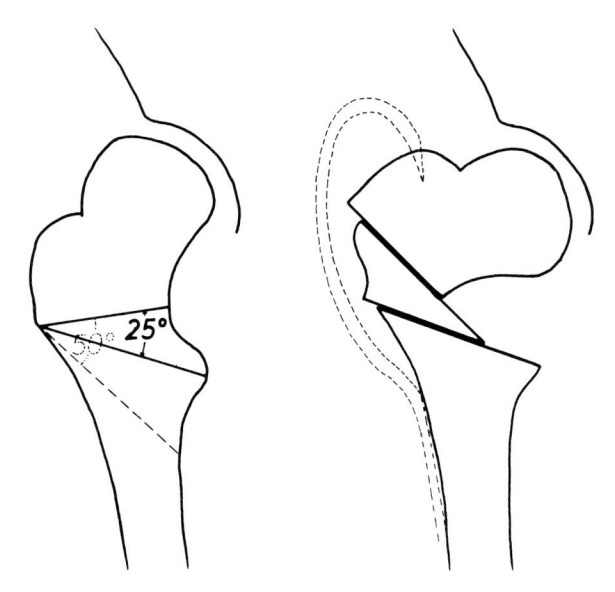

Fig. 97. Reinserting the removed wedge after rotating it (not recommended in adults)

G. Postoperative Care

As after all our operations, the foot of the bed is elevated by 20 cm and the semi-recumbent patient is asked to blow into a tube with its end 20 cm under water. Low-molecular-weight Dextran is infused for 3 days. The patient is encouraged to move immediately. The suction drainage is removed on the 2nd day, and the patient is then helped to get up and starts walking with two crutches. If there was still a good joint space before the operation, the crutches are discarded as soon as the patient feels able to walk without them. If there was no joint space, it is recommended that the two crutches be retained for 6 months and that one crutch then be used for another 6 months. This one crutch is held in the hand opposite to the hip that was operated upon. During the first 6 months the patient puts about 15%–20% of his weight on the affected limb when he walks with his crutches. Active exercise should be avoided, and the patient kept away from the physiotherapist. Active exercise tends to strengthen the muscles and increases joint pressure, which is exactly the opposite of what is desired.

The implant is usually removed after 1 year, sometimes earlier, sometimes not at all. The removal is carried out under general anaesthesia, using two short incisions along the initial scar, one for the screws and the other at the top of the hook to pull it out. A special tool is used for hammering out the hook through the proximal incision (Fig. 98).

No night traction is used following this procedure.

H. Postoperative Evolution

Relief of pain is usually immediate, and the hip joint remains pain-free provided that the operation has decreased the joint pressure. This supposes that the operation was correctly indicated. In most patients, the range of movement improves in the course of the postoperative months or even years. In some, a temporary limitation of flexion may occur despite improvement in adduction and abduction and in rotation. This limitation of flexion usually lasts only a few months. Limping progressively disappears; the younger the patient, the sooner this happens. The TRENDELENBURG sign soon becomes negative, often long before limping has completely disappeared.

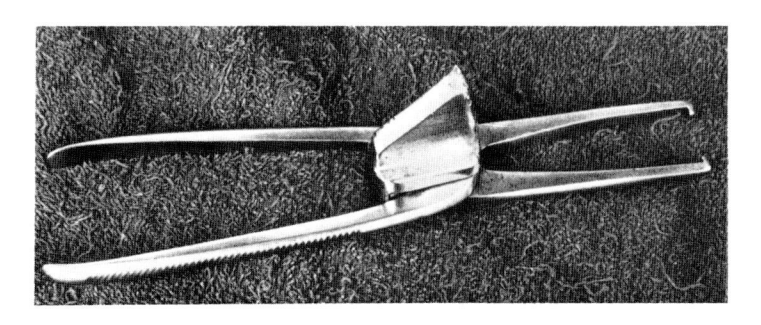

Fig. 98. Hook-extractor

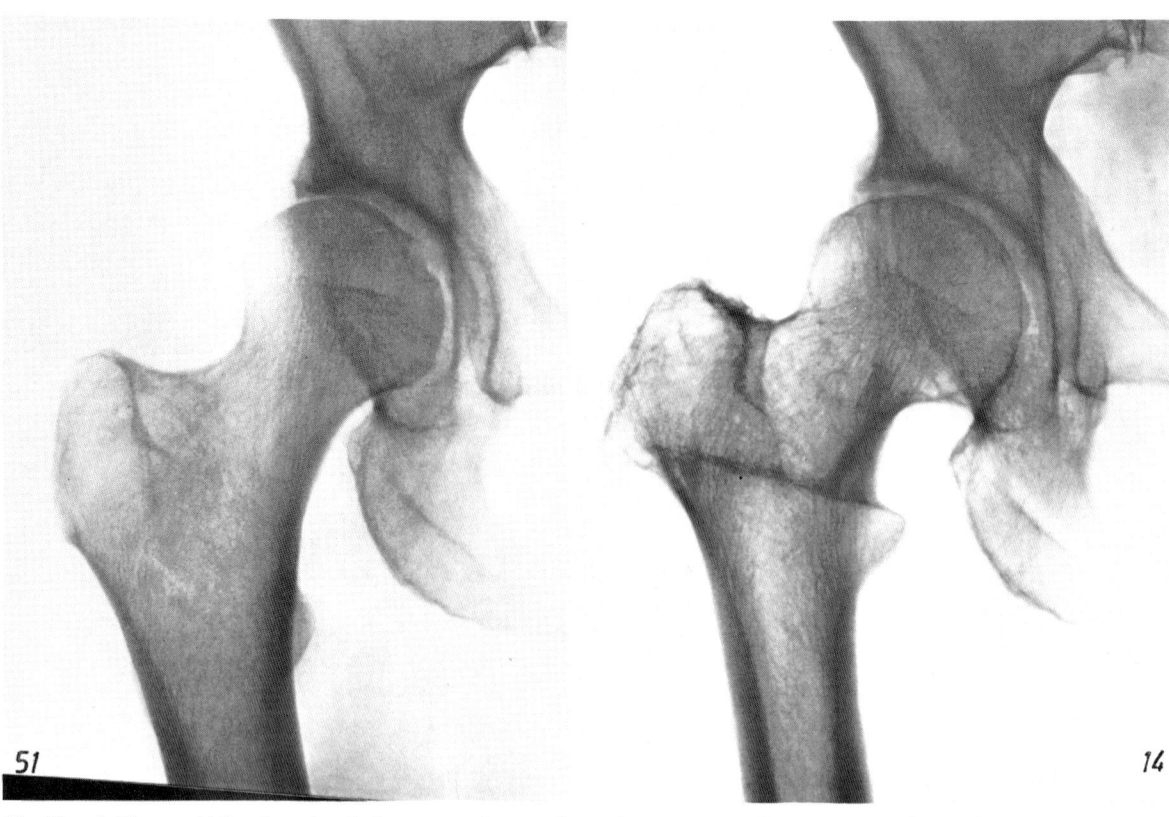

Fig. 99. a A 55-year-old female patient before a varus intertrochanteric osteotomy. **b** Fourteen years afterwards

In the X-rays, the lateral triangle of subchondral sclerosis is replaced by a thin ribbon of dense bone, the normal "sourcil" (PAUWELS). This indicates an even distribution of the compressive stresses in the joint. The cysts slowly disappear and a wide joint space develops (Fig. 99; Table 12).

Tightening the hook may provoke some medial separation between the fragments. When this occurs, the patient is asked to walk with his full weight on the leg from the very first. Only after the osteotomy surfaces have become parallel is the patient advised to put only partial weight on it.

In a 59-year-old patient with severe osteoarthritis of the hip (Fig. 100a), the X-ray of the joint with the leg in abduction showed good congruence of the articular surfaces (Fig. 78). Therefore, a valgus osteotomy was planned (Fig. 79). In the X-ray taken on the 5th day after the operation, the fragments were separated medially (Fig. 100b). The patient was told to put her full weight on the leg. In the X-ray taken on the 12th postoperative day, the contact between the fragments looked ideal (Fig. 100c). The patient then continued to put only part of her weight on the affected limb. At the 8-year follow-up the clinical result was excellent (Table 13). In the X-ray the signs of osteoarthritis had disappeared (Fig. 100d).

Table 12. Range of movement of the hip (Fig. 99)

	Before surgery	At the 14-year follow-up	Gain
Flexion	90°	140°	55°
Extension	−5°	0°	
Adduction	5°	40°	70°
Abduction	15°	50°	
Int. rotation	5°	45°	85°
Ext. rotation	5°	50°	

Table 13. Range of movement of the hip (Fig. 100)

	Before surgery	At the 8-year follow-up	Gain
Flexion	85°	90°	10°
Extension	5°	10°	
Adduction	10°	40°	35°
Abduction	20°	25°	
Int. rotation	10°	0°	50°
Ext. rotation	5°	65°	

Fig. 100. a Painful hip of a 59-year-old female patient before surgery. **b** Five days after a varus intertrochanteric osteotomy. **c** Twelve days after surgery. **c** Eight-year follow-up

Op.+5d

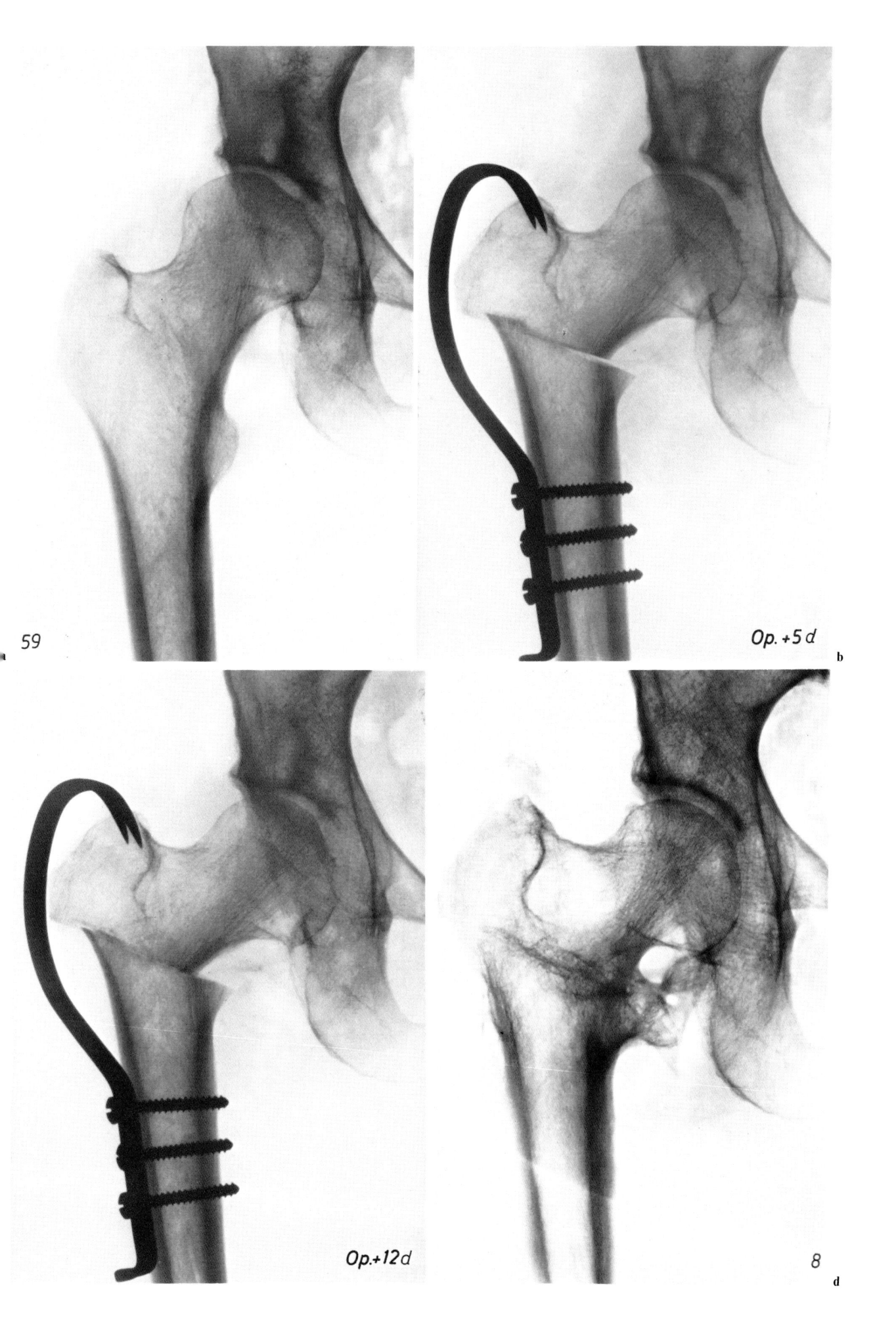

Op.+12d

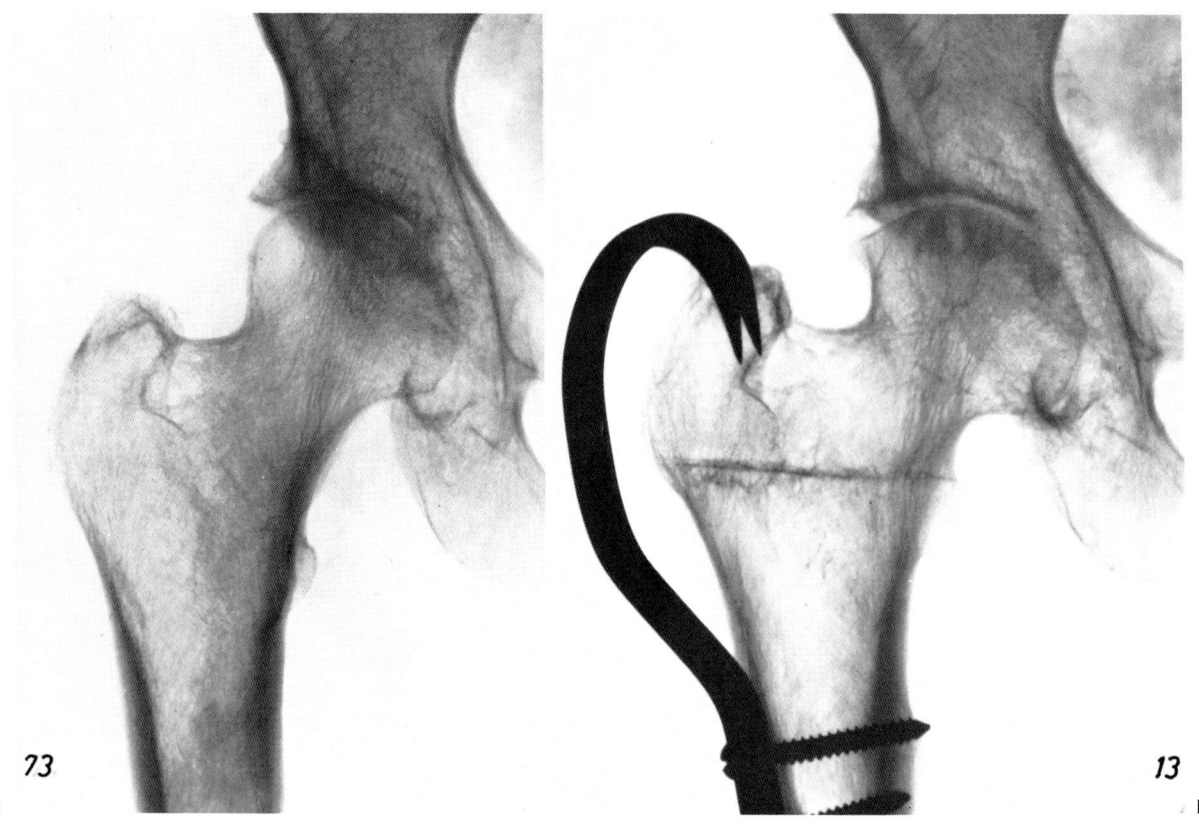

Fig. 101. a A 74-year-old female patient before a varus intertrochanteric osteotomy. **b** Thirteen years afterwards

There seems to be no age limit to healing. A 74-year-old female patient with a painful hip, limited range of movement and severe limp showed narrowing of the joint space and a sclerotic triangle at the edge of the acetabulum (Fig. 101a). After a varus intertrochanteric osteotomy, the pain was relieved and the range of movement became normal again (Table 14). In the X-ray, the dense triangle was replaced by a subchondral sclerosis of even width throughout and a wide joint space had reappeared. The result remained excellent at the 13-year follow-up (Fig. 101b).

This patient provided us with the opportunity of comparing progress following an osteotomy with that after a total replacement. When she was 77, her other hip was replaced elsewhere by a total prosthesis with cement (Fig. 102a). We would have carried out a valgus osteotomy (Fig. 102b) (see p. 102), but the patient took the fashionable option. The X-ray picture looked satisfactory 1 year after the total replacement (Fig. 102c), although the patient continued to refer to her osteotomized hip as her "good hip". Nine years after the total replacement, far-reaching resorption of bone around the prosthesis was certainly jeopardizing the future of this hip. Even the femoral cortex was reduced to about 50% of its initial width (Fig. 102d). Compare this with the osteotomy side!

Table 14. Range of movement of the hip (Fig. 101)

	Before surgery	At the 13-year follow-up	Gain
Flexion	70°	95°	30°
Extension	0°	5°	
Adduction	40°	55°	10°
Abduction	30°	25°	
Int. rotation	40°	15°	45°
Ext. rotation	50°	30°	

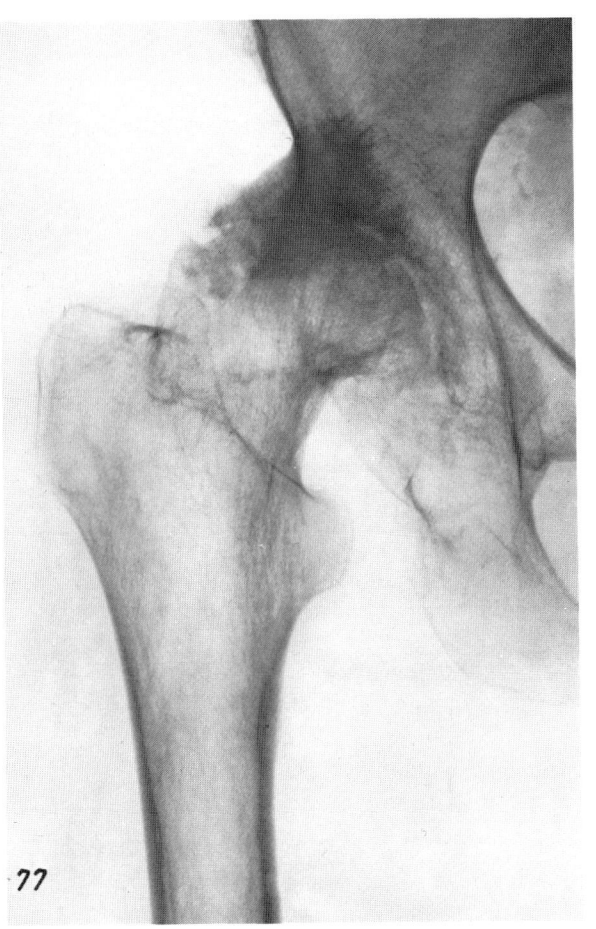

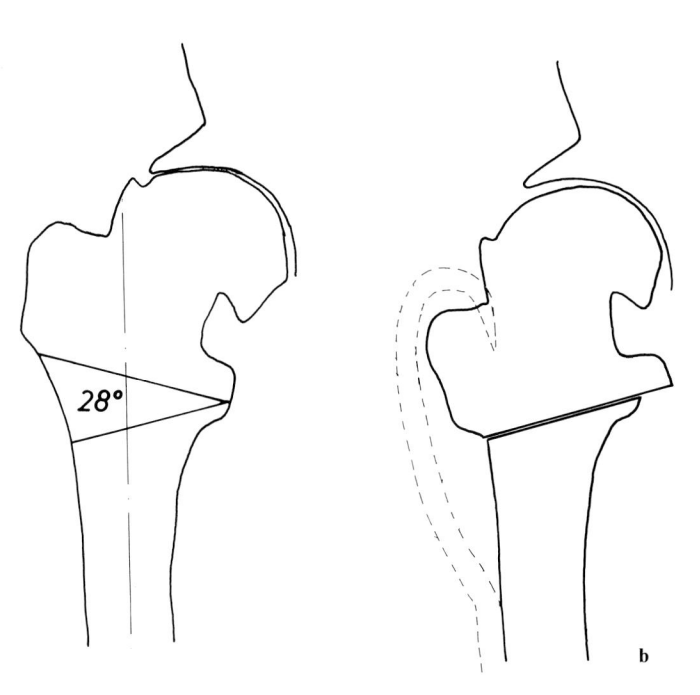

Fig. 102a–d. Same patient as in Fig. 101: opposite hip. **a** A total replacement arthroplasty was carried out when she was 77. **b** A valgus intertrochanteric osteotomy should have been carried out. **c** One year after replacement. **d** Nine years after replacement

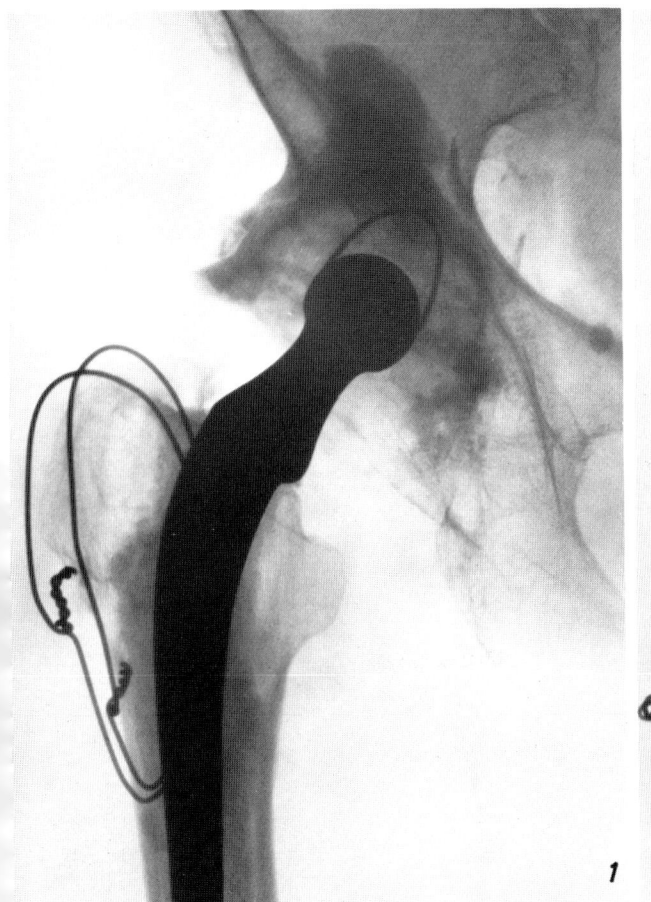

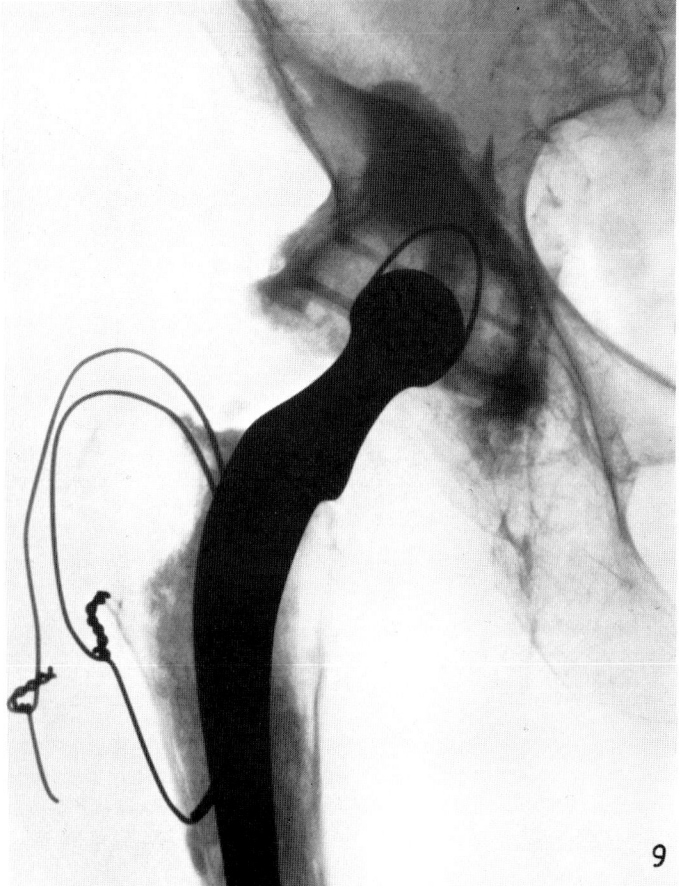

Another 71-year-old female patient had osteoarthritis of the hip with a sclerotic triangle at the edge of the socket, abnormal sclerosis and huge cysts in the femoral head (Fig. 103a). At the 5-year follow-up, the subchondral sclerosis had become uniform throughout, the joint space was wider and the cysts had dramatically regressed (Fig. 103b). Here again healing took place despite the age of the patient.

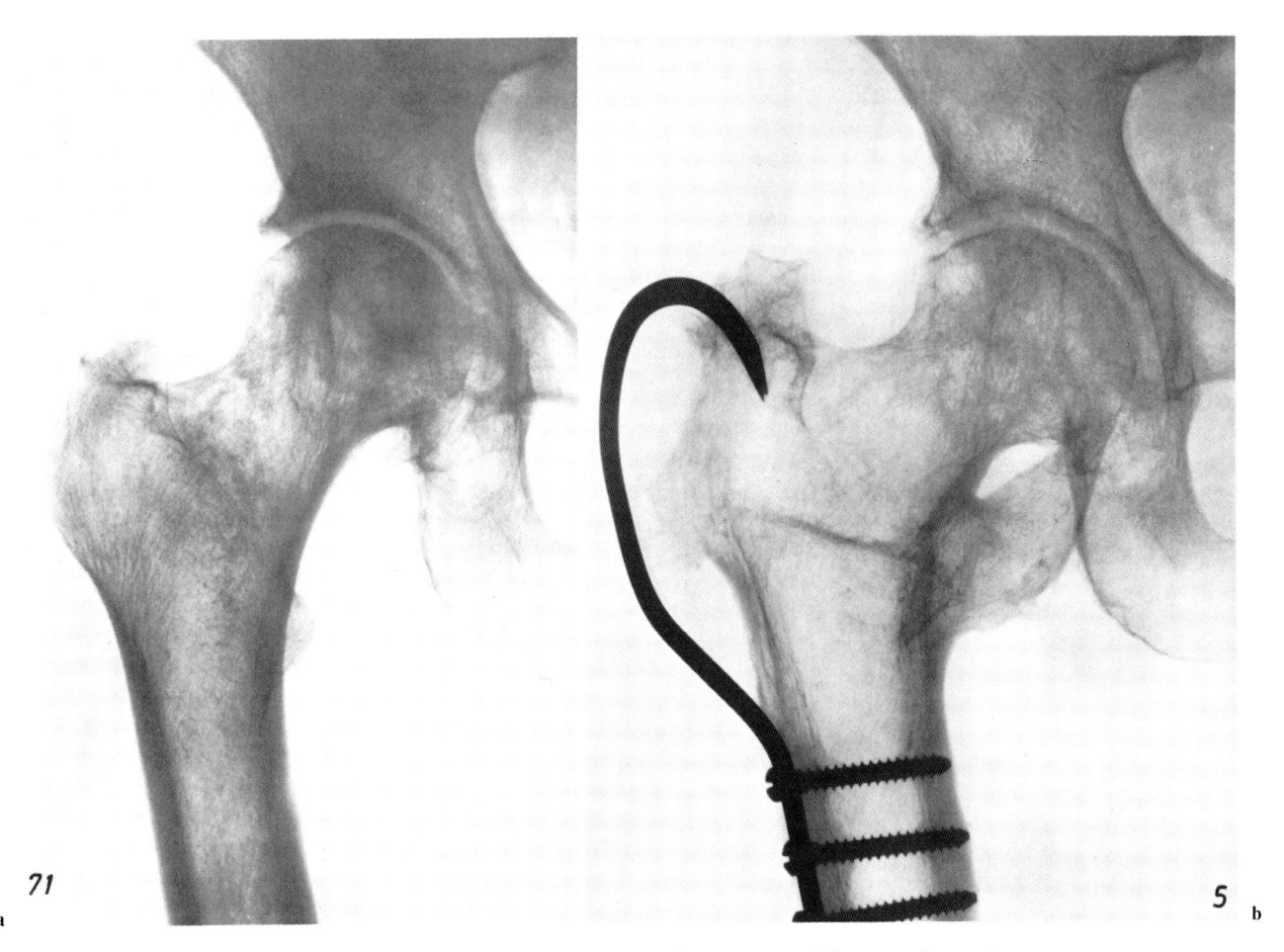

Fig. 103. a A 71-year-old female patient before a varus intertrochanteric osteotomy. b Five years afterwards

53

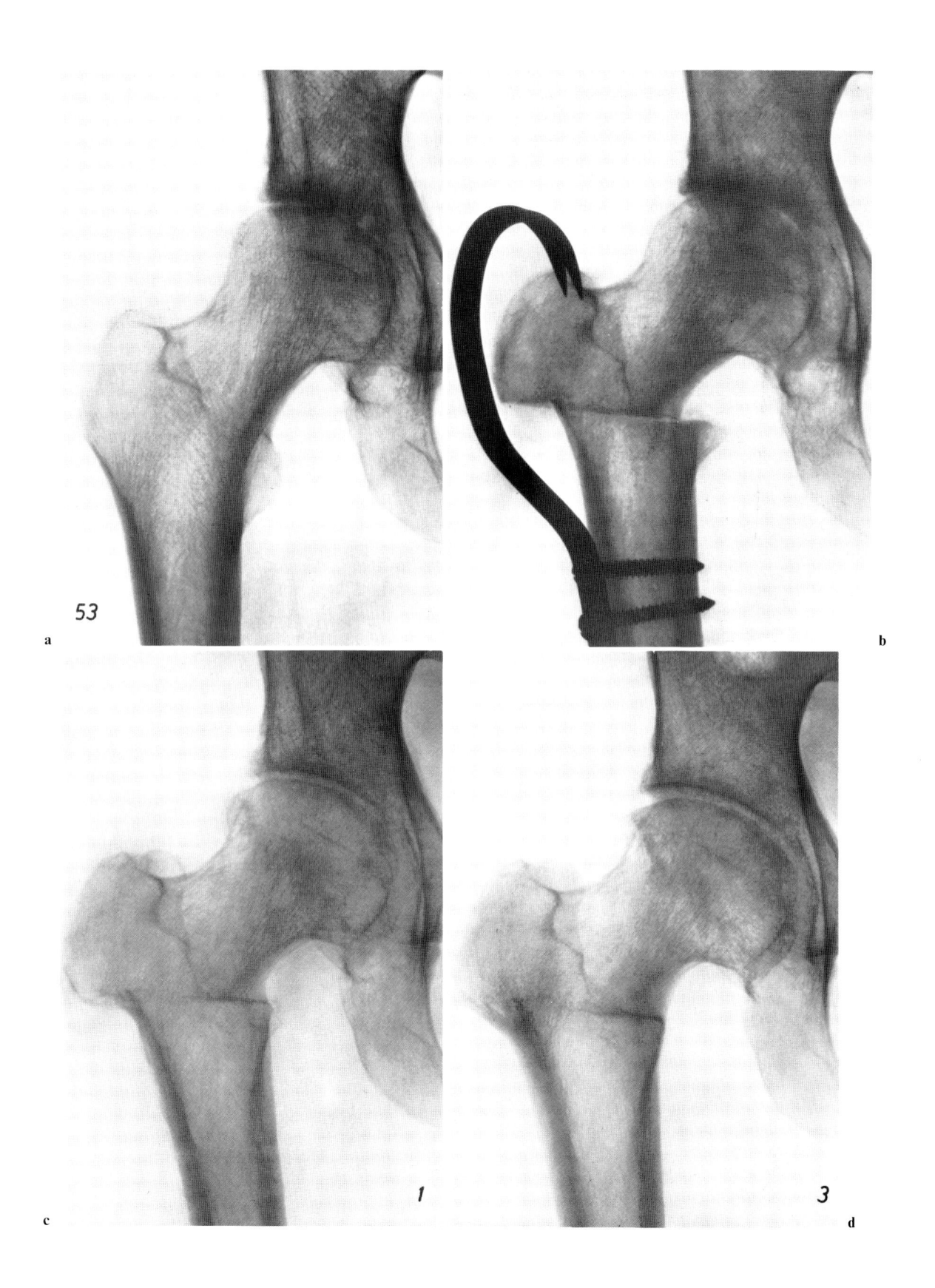

a

b

c   *1*

d   *3*

96

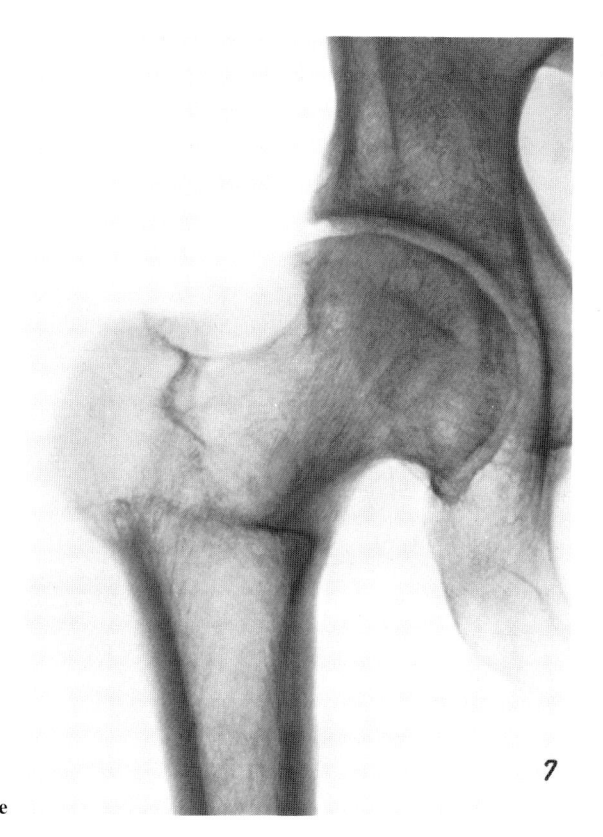

Fig. 104. a A 53-year-old female patient before a varus intertrochanteric osteotomy. **b** Immediately afterwards. **c** One year, **d** 3 years and **e** 7 years after the operation

Some authors have claimed that the procedure replaces in the socket a part of the femoral head from which the cartilage has been worn by another part on which it has been preserved. This may be true in some rare instances, but most often a joint space develops only progressively after the operation. A 53-year-old female patient presented with a painful hip with no joint space and a cup-shaped sclerosis in the roof of the acetabulum (Fig. 104a). This appeared as primary osteoarthritis resulting from a biological tissue defect. A varus osteotomy was carried out. Immediately afterwards, no joint space could be seen in the X-ray (Fig. 104b), but one year later a joint space had reappeared (Fig. 104c). Two more years later, it looked wider (Fig. 104d). Seven years after the osteotomy it seemed to have attained its definitive and normal width and the subchondral sclerosis was of even width throughout (Fig. 104e).

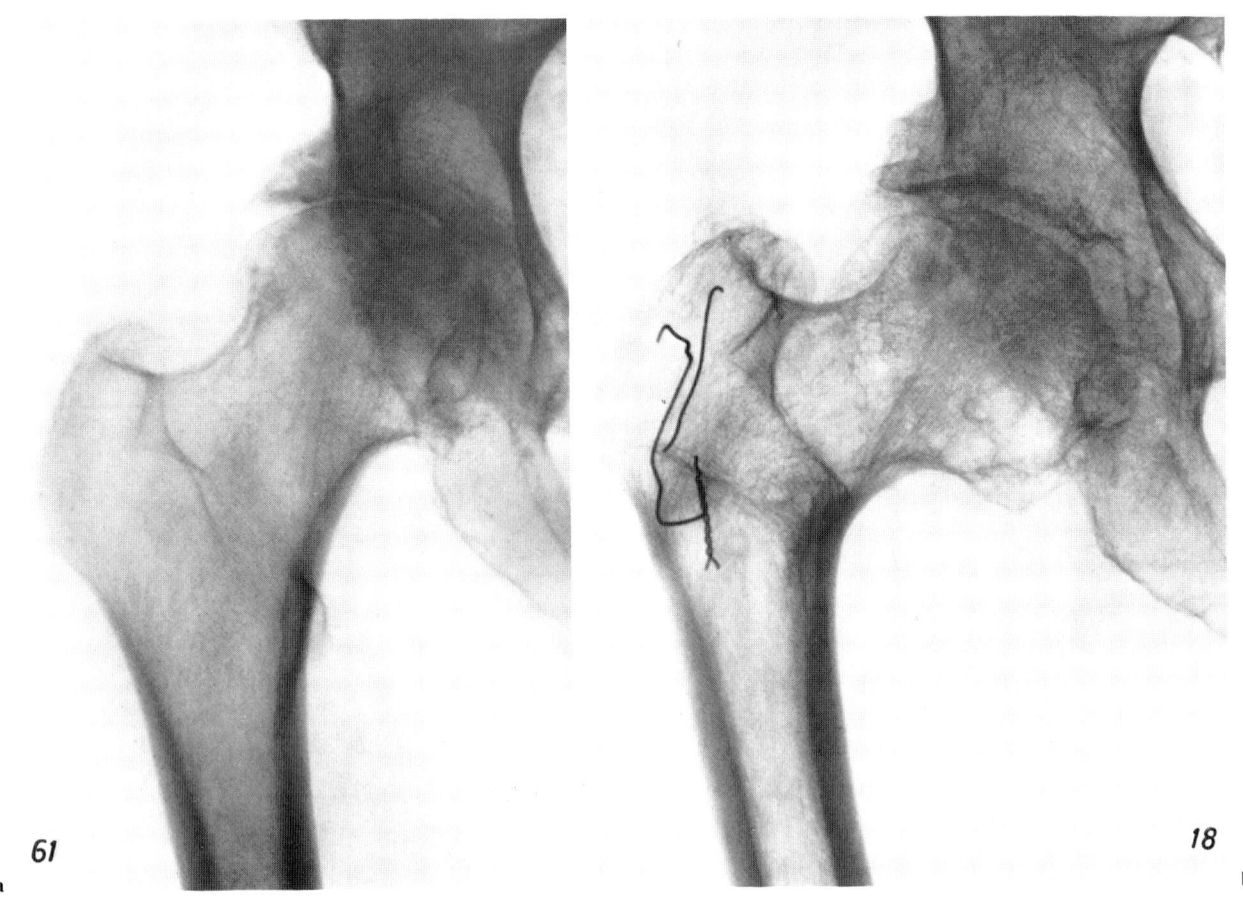

Fig. 105. a A 62-year-old female patient before a varus intertrochanteric osteotomy on the right hip. **b** 18 years afterwards

As shown earlier by PAUWELS, the results seem to be lasting. A female patient underwent the operation on one side at the age of 62 and on the other at the age of 63 (Figs. 105a and 106a). Over a follow-up period of 18 years and 17 years respectively (Figs. 105b and 106b), the clinical result remained excellent (Tables 15 and 16).

Table 15. Range of movement of the hip (Fig. 105)

	Before surgery	At the 18-year follow-up	Gain
Flexion	40°	85°	65°
Extension	−10°	10°	
Adduction	15°	40°	45°
Abduction	0°	20°	
Int. rotation	0°	25°	45°
Ext. rotation	0°	20°	

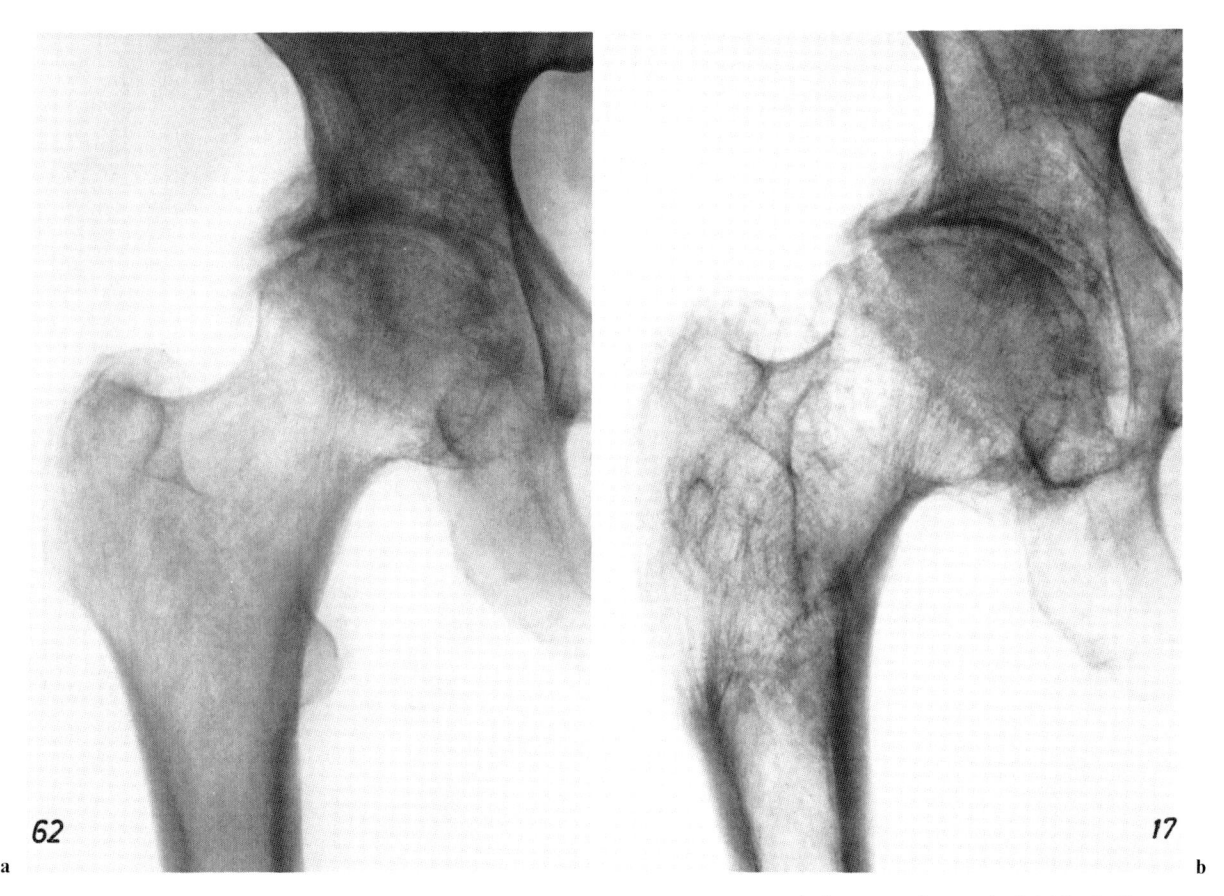

Fig. 106a, b. Same patient as in Fig. 105: opposite hip. Age at operation: 62 years. **a** before operation on the left hip; **b** 17 years after the operation

Table 16. Range of Movement of the hip (Fig. 106)

	Before surgery	At the 17-year follow-up	Gain
Flexion	50°	60°	20°
Extension	0°	10°	
Adduction	20°	30°	5°
Abduction	25°	20°	
Int. rotation	5°	0°	35°
Ext. rotation	5°	45°	

Fig. 107. A varus intertrochanteric osteotomy may not enlarge the weight-bearing surface of the joint and in this case should not be carried out

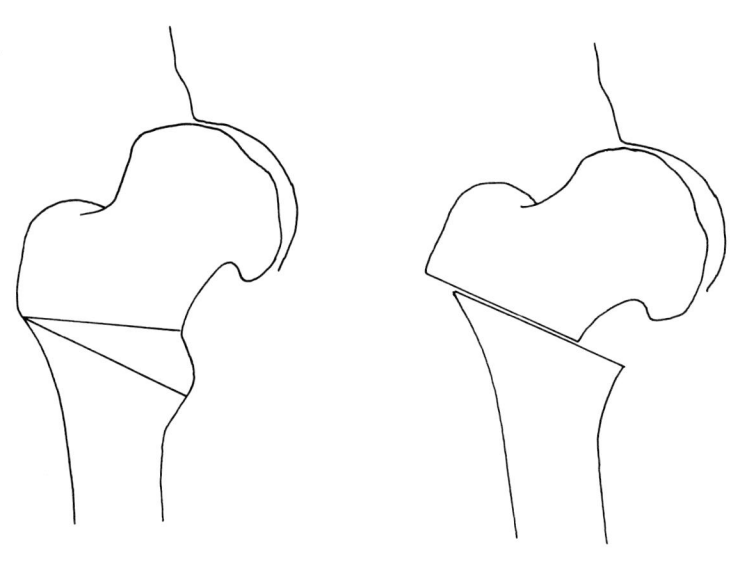

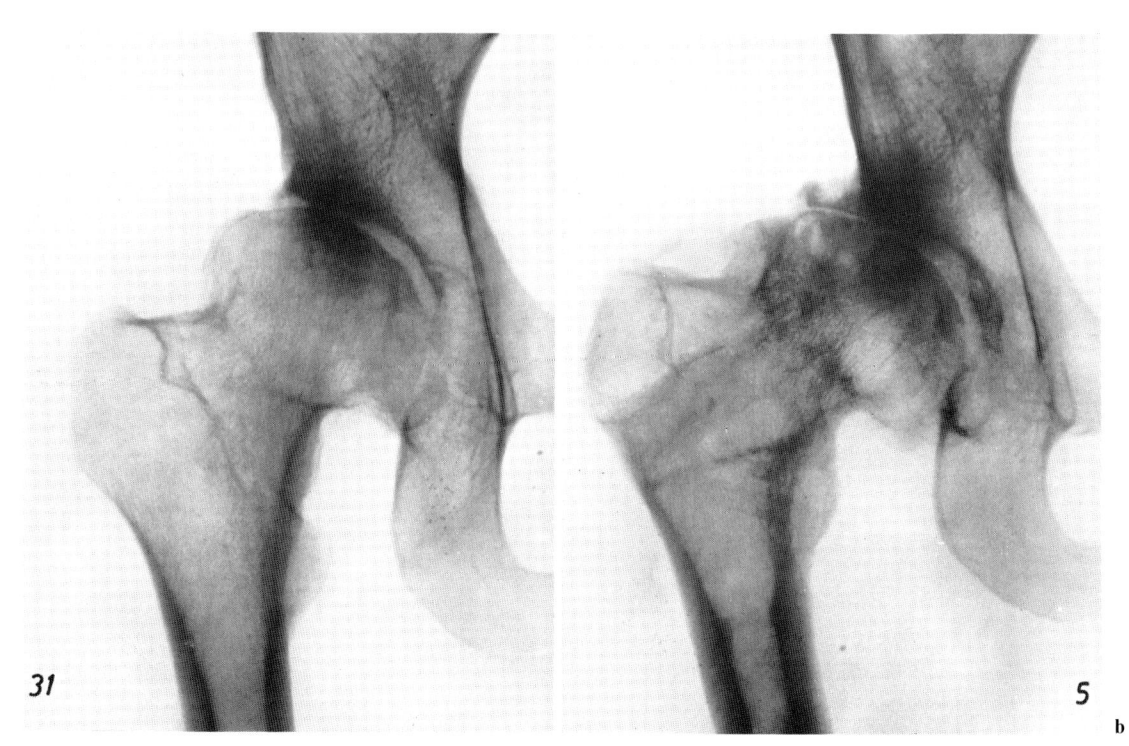

Fig. 108. a A 31-year-old female patient before a varus intertrochanteric osteotomy. **b** Five years afterwards: the operation decreased the weight-bearing surface of the joint

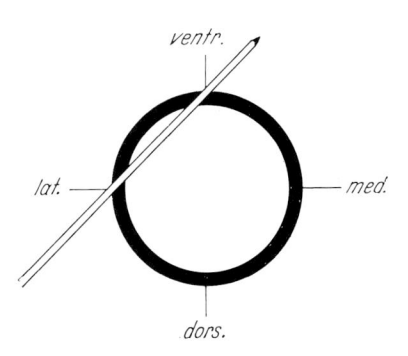

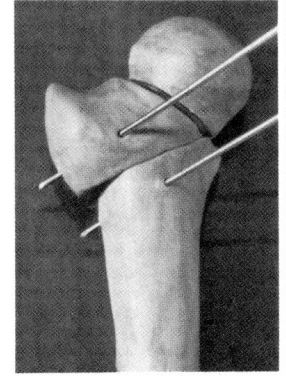

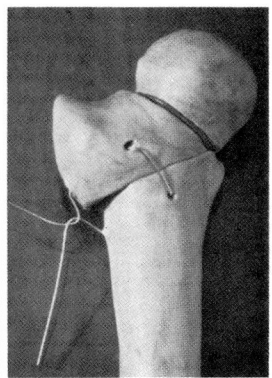

Fig. 109. Varus intertrochanteric osteotomy in a child. (After PAUWELS 1966)

I. Incorrect Indications

If varus osteotomy does not ensure congruence of the joint surfaces (Fig. 107) it may fail to change or may even decrease the articular weight-bearing area. This usually results in failure. A 31-year-old female patient with severe osteoarthritis of the hip (Fig. 108a) underwent a varus osteotomy elsewhere. Because of the deformity of the articular components, this could not ensure congruence of the joint surfaces. It probably decreased the weight-bearing area of the joint. Consequently, the clinical symptoms became worse and so did the X-ray picture (Fig. 108b). The sclerotic triangle at the edge of the acetabulum had increased at the 5-year follow-up.

Such failures demonstrate the essential contribution of the mechanical factors to the evolution of the condition and they must be attributed not to the method but to the poor choice of procedure by the surgeon. In these cases it often proves possible to enlarge the weight-bearing area of the joint by turning the femoral head the other way, that is by carrying out a proper valgus osteotomy.

J. Procedure in Children

Except in some spastic children, no tenotomy is required as a rule. The patient lies prone. The approach is posterolateral, as in the adult, but the incision is much shorter, giving access to the osteotomy site. A wedge is marked and resected as described above. Beforehand, two holes are drilled from the lateral aspect of the femur to its anterior aspect (Fig. 109), one on each side of the osteotomy site. A steel wire is passed through these holes, and when the fragments are in contact a long nail is introduced from the upper aspect of the neck through the femoral shaft. The steel wire is then tightened and secured. It will work as a double tension band, anterior and lateral, since at this level the resultant force acts posteriorly and medially.

K. Conclusion

Varus intertrochanteric osteotomy constitutes a very efficient means of decreasing joint pressure as long as the joint surfaces of the hip remain or become congruent in abduction. The reduction and better distribution of joint pressure can be read in the X-ray: the dense triangle at the edge of the acetabulum is replaced by a subchondral sclerosis of uniform width throughout.

IV. Valgus Intertrochanteric Osteotomy and Tenotomy (Pauwels II)

A. Rationale

The procedure consists of removing an intertrochanteric wedge with a lateral base (Fig. 110). By rotating the femoral head in the socket it takes advantage of the osteophyte developed on the medial aspect of the head. This osteophyte, which has evolved in an area of low pressure (GRASSET 1960), is incorporated in the weight-bearing area, which is thereby increased. The osteotomy is combined with a tenotomy of the abductor, adductor and iliopsoas muscles. The tenotomy reduces the transmitted load. The procedure results in a considerable diminution and an even distribution of the compressive stresses in the joint.

It has been objected that the valgus osteotomy shortens the lever arm of the abductor muscles and may displace the resultant force R towards the edge of the socket. This would obviously be true if the osteotomy were carried out on a normal hip. But when the hip is grossly deformed, the line of action of the resultant force R continues to pass through the centre of the original femoral head. Therefore, even if the contact surface of the joint has been considerably increased by the medial osteophyte and the remodelling of the articulation, the weight-bearing area of the joint can become much reduced (Figs. 42 and 43). This has been documented by PAUWELS (1973a, 1976). After an appropriate valgus intertrochanteric osteotomy, the line of action of the resultant force R passes through the centre of curvature of the femoral head remodelled by its medial osteophyte. This centre of curvature usually lies more medially than the centre of the original femoral head. Consequently, (a) the lever arm of the abductor muscles, far from being shortened, may be considerably lengthened; (b) at the same time, the lever arm of the force K exerted by the partial body mass is shortened; and (c) the line of action of the resultant force R is brought further medially into the acetabulum thus enlarging the weight-bearing area of the joint. This can be observed by comparing the pre-operative and postoperative X-rays of a female patient operated on at the age of 53 years (Figs. 111 and 169).

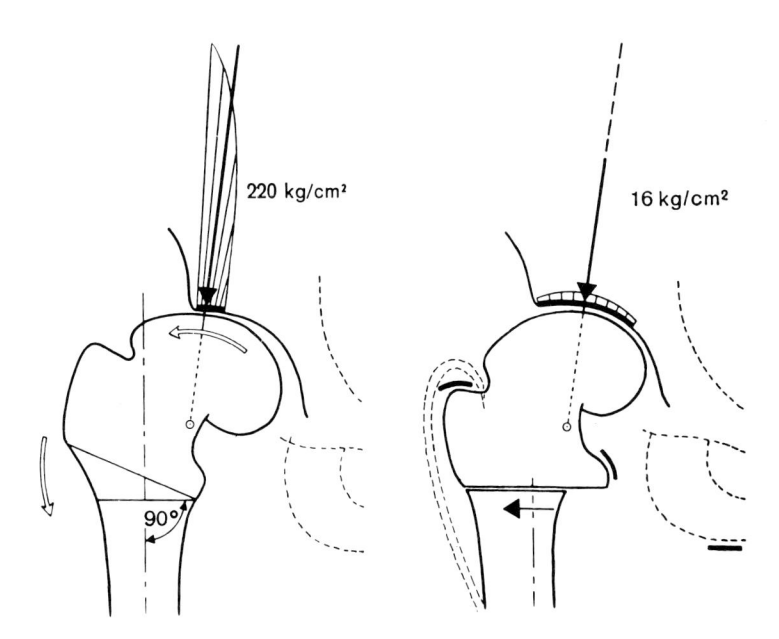

Fig. 110. The valgus intertrochanteric osteotomy takes advantage of the osteophyte developed over the medial aspect of the femoral head. Combined with a tenotomy of the abductor, adductor and iliopsoas muscles, it decreases the load transmitted across the hip and enlarges the weight-bearing surface of the joint (Pauwels II). (Redrawn after PAUWELS 1976)

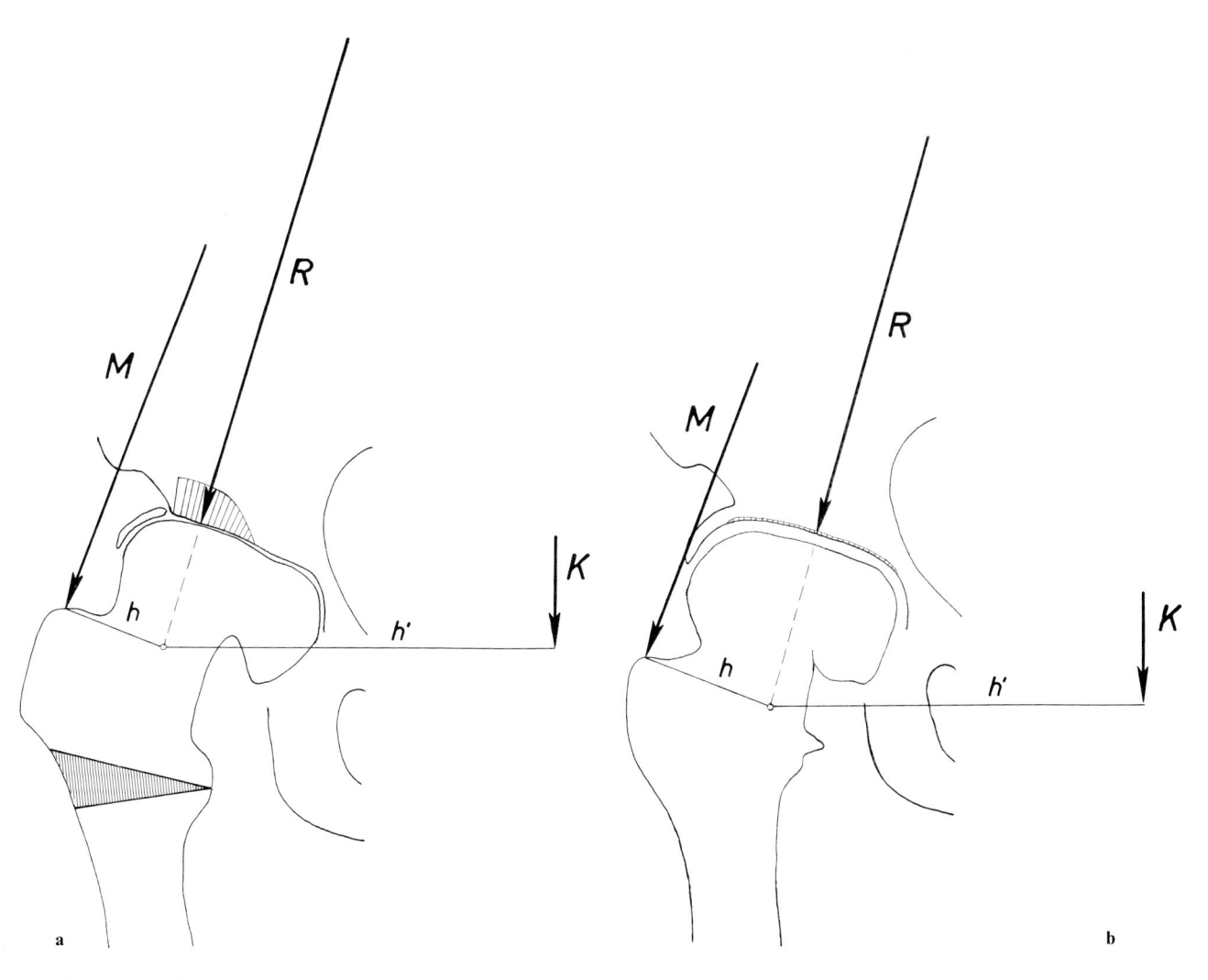

Fig. 111. a Before and **b** 2 years after a valgus osteotomy. The lever arms h and h' of the forces M exerted by the abductor muscles and K exerted by the part of the body supported by the hip are changed advantageously by the operation. R, resultant of M and K (see Fig. 169e and g)

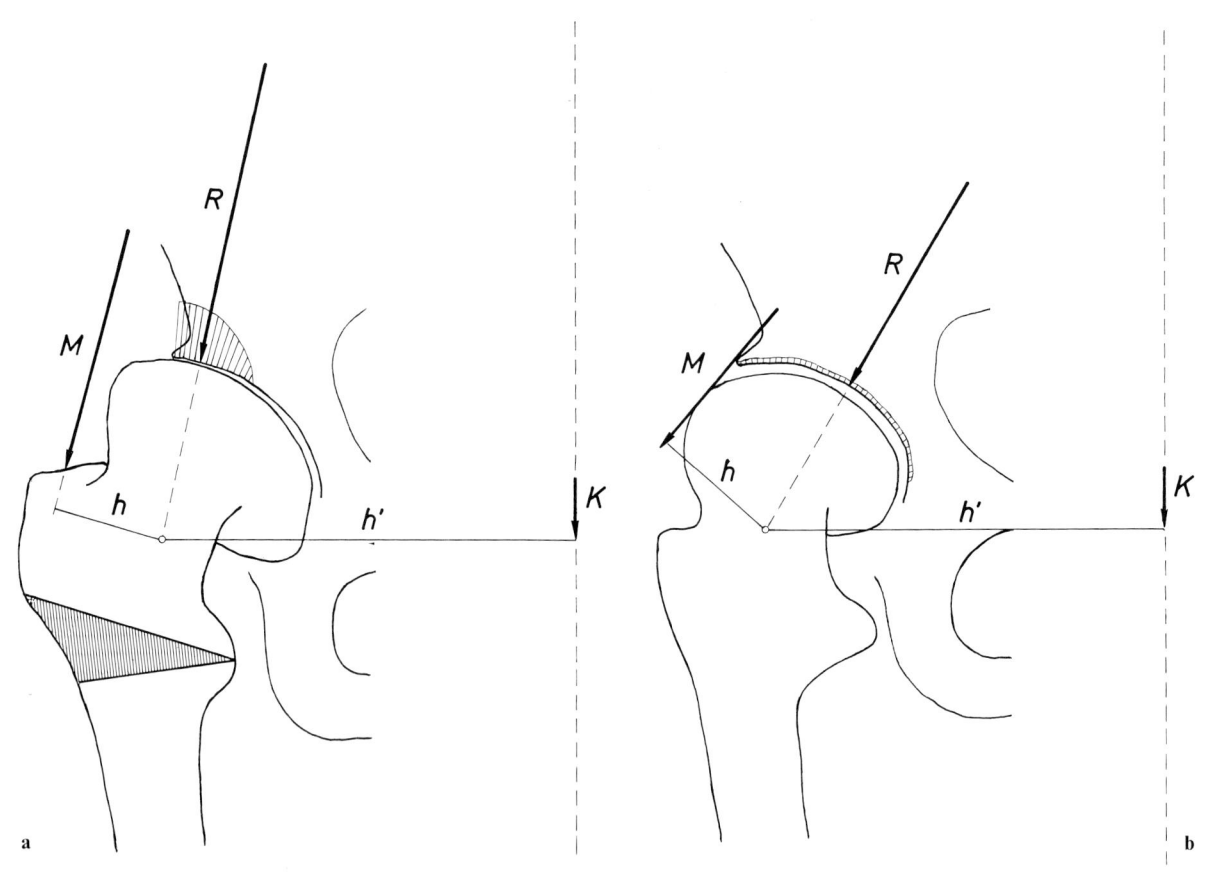

Fig. 112. a Before and **b** 10 years after a valgus osteotomy. The abductor muscles are pushed laterally by the femoral head bulging out of the socket. This lengthens the lever arm *h* of the force *M* exerted by the abductor muscles. *K*, force exerted by the part of the body supported by the hip; *h'*, lever arm of *K*; *R*, resultant of forces *M* and *K* (see Fig. 113)

The abductor muscles may also be pushed laterally by the lateral aspect of the femoral head, which remains bulging out of the socket after a valgus osteotomy. The femoral head then acts as a fulcrum, lengthening the lever arm of the muscles and changing their direction (Fig. 112). Consequently, the resultant force *R* is decreased and displaced medially into the acetabulum. This results in a decrease in and a better distribution of the articular compressive stresses.

This is confirmed by the evolution in a 48-year-old female patient who had severe osteoarthritis of one hip (Fig. 113a). A valgus intertrochanteric osteotomy was planned (Fig. 112) and carried out. At the 10-year follow-up the clinical result remained excellent (Table 17). In the X-ray the signs of osteoarthritis had regressed dramatically (Fig. 113b).

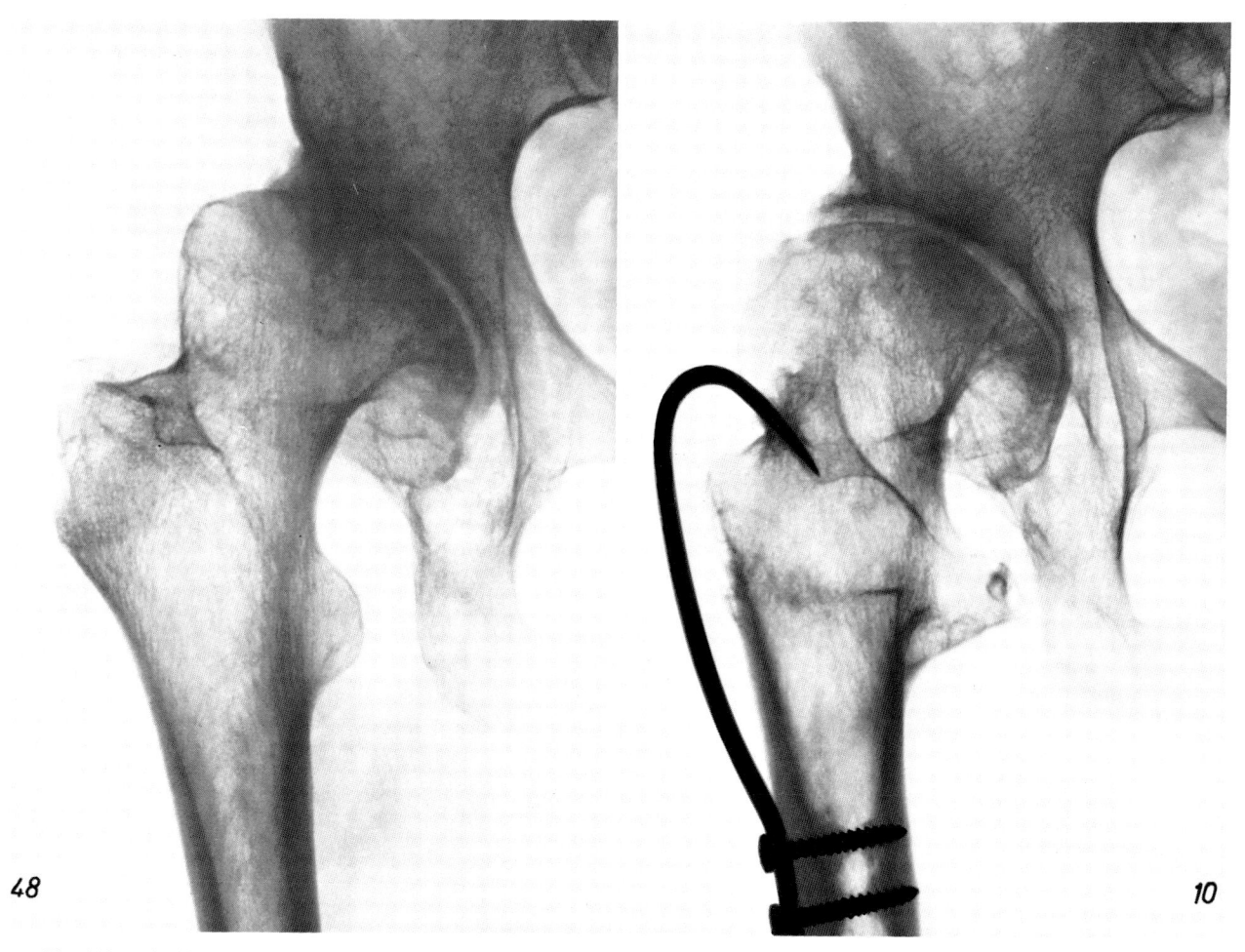

Fig. 113. a A 48-year-old female patient before a valgus intertrochanteric osteotomy combined with a tenotomy. **b** Ten years afterwards. The same hip is represented in Fig. 112

Table 17. Range of movement of the hip (Fig. 113)

	Before surgery	At the 10-year follow-up	Gain
Flexion	60°	95°	35°
Extension	10°	10°	
Adduction	10°	30°	65°
Abduction	−5°	40°	
Int. rotation	−5°	30°	35°
Ext. rotation	20°	20°	

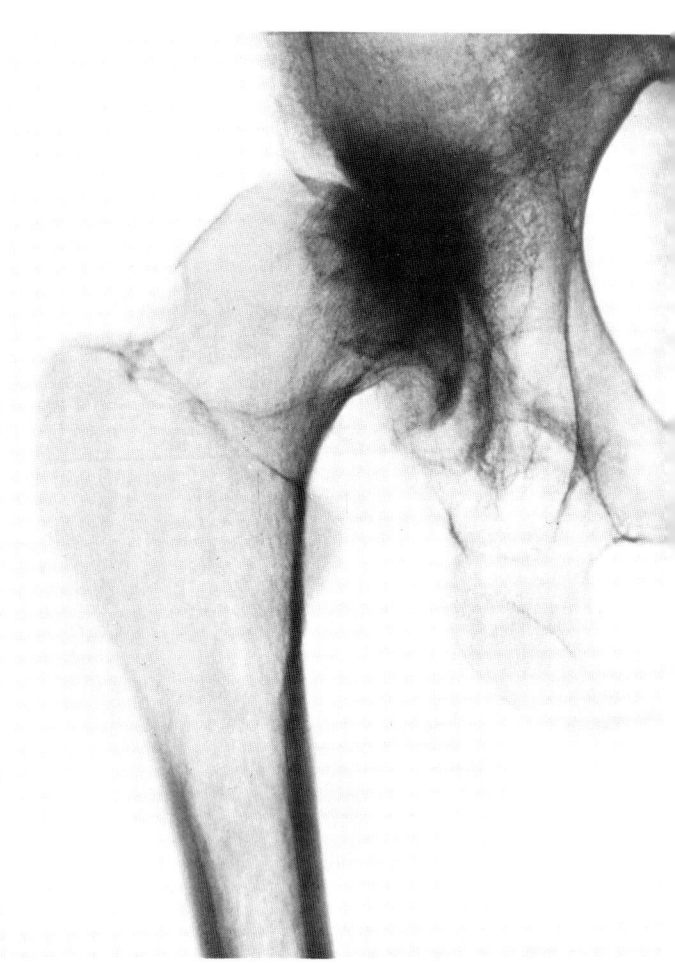

Fig. 114. a Neutral position. **b** No congruence in abduction.
c Tendency to a better congruence in adduction

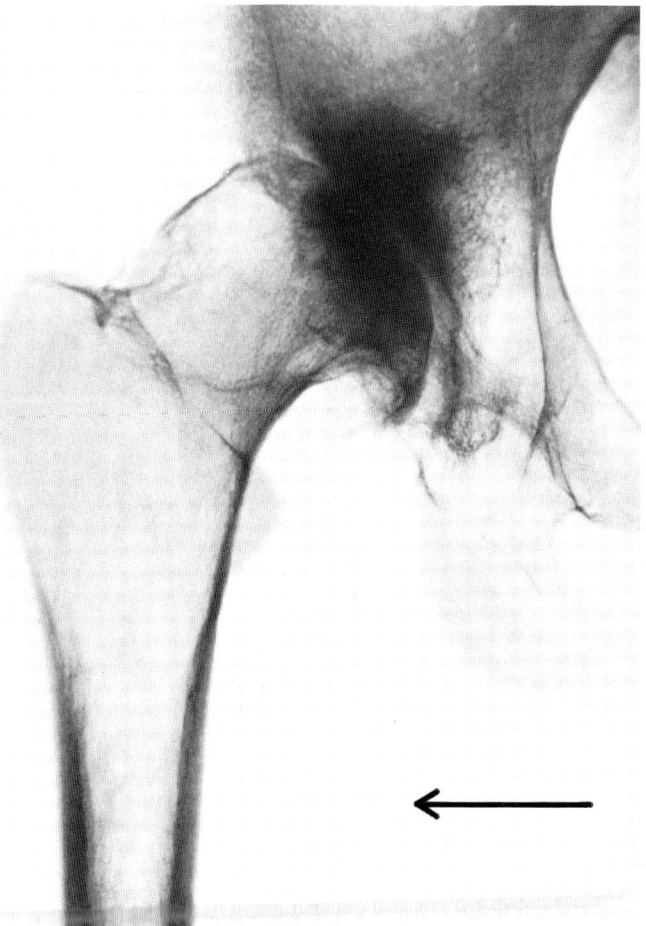

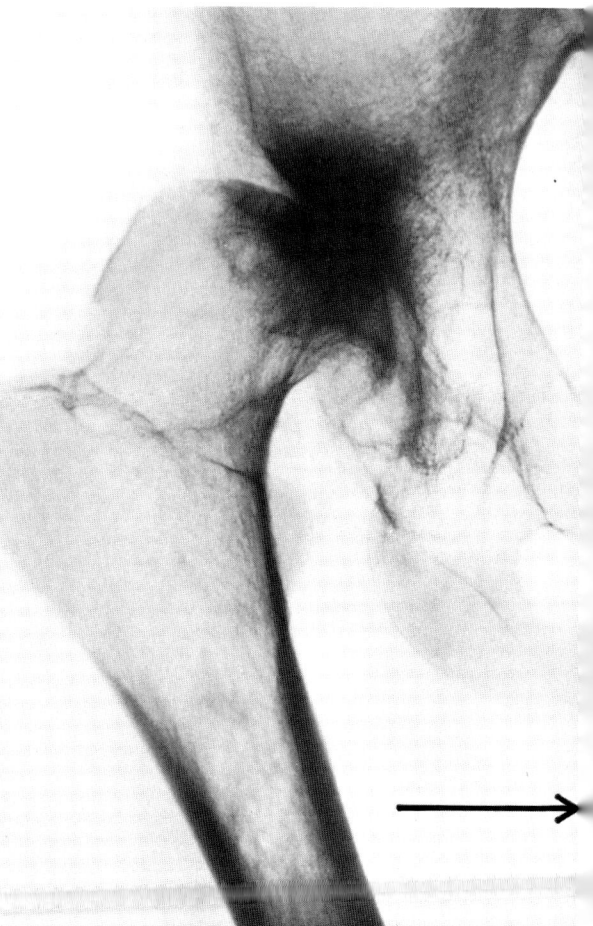

B. Indications

A hip suitable for a valgus osteotomy should present incongruent joint surfaces in abduction and congruence or tendency to congruence in adduction (Fig. 114). This occurs when the acetabulum is flattened by resorption of its lateral edge and the femoral head by resorption of its top and by apposition of a large osteophyte on its medial aspect. As shown by PAUWELS (1973), the radius of curvature of the articular pieces can be considerably increased by the deformation. The bigger the femoral head the better. Another indication for a valgus osteotomy is the hip with protrusio acetabuli and a sclerotic triangle in the medial aspect of the roof of the socket (see Chapter IV).

A small, round-shaped femoral head with congruent joint surfaces in abduction as well as in adduction and with no protrusio contra-indicates a valgus osteotomy. In such circumstances either a varus osteotomy or a lateral displacement of the greater trochanter should be considered.

C. Pre-operative Planning

The pre-operative planning follows the same guide-lines as for the varus osteotomy (p. 78). The contours of the acetabulum and of the upper extremity of the femur are traced on the left half of a sheet of tracing-paper from the anteroposterior X-ray in neutral position. The axis of the femoral shaft is drawn (Fig. 115a). The right half of the sheet is folded over the left and the contour of the acetabulum is traced on the right half from the left half-sheet (Fig. 115b). The sheet is cut in half and the second half-sheet is rotated over the first until the contour of the socket in the second and that of the femoral head in the first are congruent. The two contours should diverge a little laterally. The angle formed by the edges of the two half-sheets is measured with a protractor (Fig. 115c). The upper extremity of the femur is then traced on the second half-sheet of transparent paper (Fig. 115d). The angle which has been measured between the edges of the sheets is now drawn on the first half-sheet in order to delineate the wedge to be removed (Fig. 115e). It represents the angle by which the femoral head must be turned in the socket to ensure good congruence of the articular surfaces. The distal arm of this angle is at right angles to the axis of the shaft and is situated at the level of the tip of the lesser trochanter. The proximal arm of the angle is oblique upward and outward. The angle necessary to ensure congruence may be much larger than the possible clinical adduction of the hip. The apex of the wedge to be resected usually lies at the tip of the lesser trochanter and the upper side of the wedge passes through the innominate tubercle. To prevent the upper cut from being too high in the greater trochanter, that is, above the innominate tubercle, the apex of the wedge may be placed less deeply along the distal cut (Fig. 116).

From the first half-sheet, the tracing of the second half-sheet is completed. The contour of the

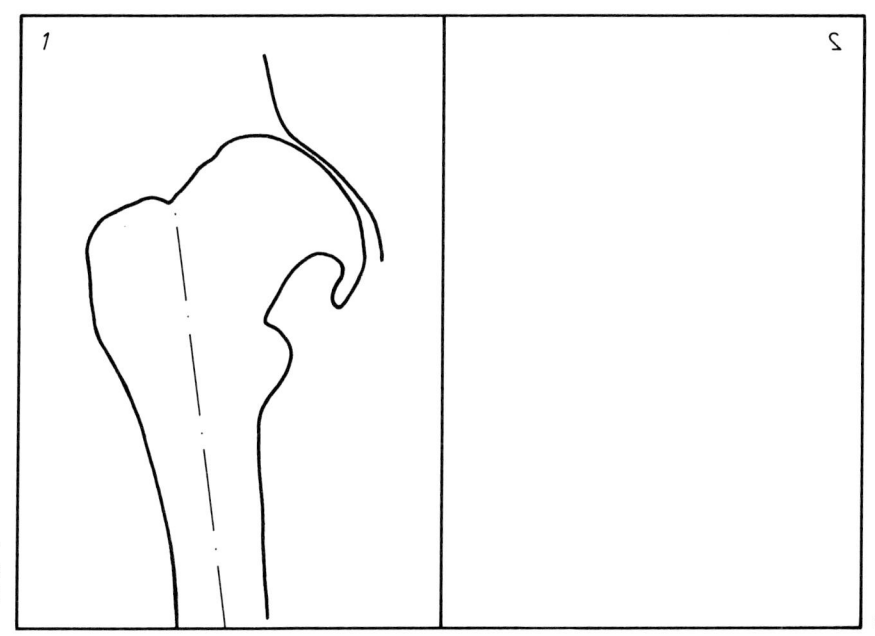

Fig. 115a–g. Pre-operative planning of a valgus intertrochanteric osteotomy. *1, 2*, first and second half-sheets of tracing-paper

Fig. 115b–d

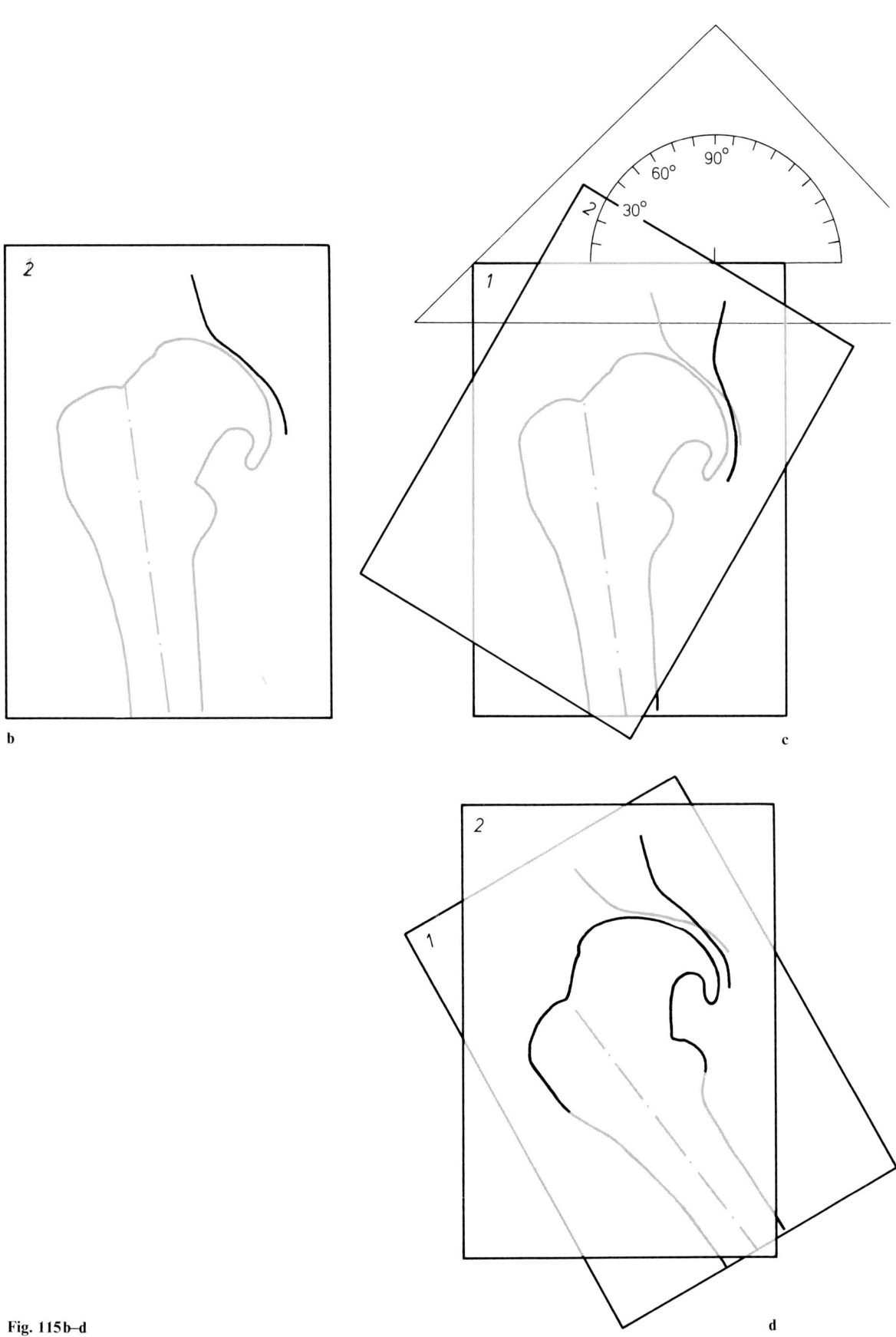

compression-hook is drawn using a template (Fig. 115f). The femoral shaft should lie at the same distance from the pelvis as before the operation. This means a lateral displacement of the distal fragment in relation to the proximal fragment. Displacing the distal fragment medially leads to a valgus deformity of the knee. The two half-sheets are displayed on a viewing-box in the operating-theatre (Fig. 115g). They show the wedge to be resected, its level and the place where the compression-hook must take hold in the greater trochanter or in the upper part of the femoral neck.

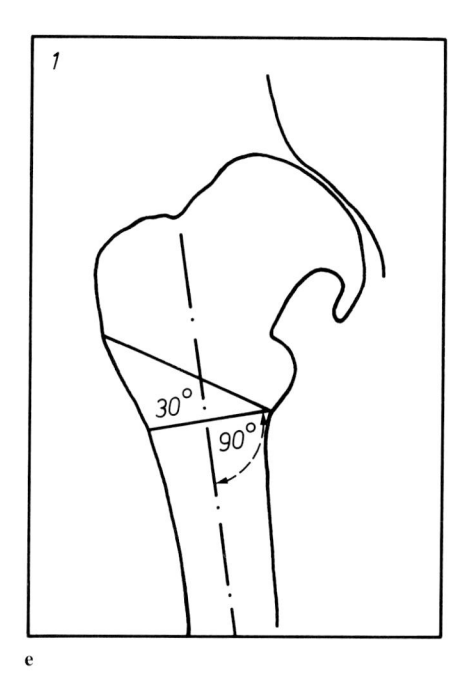

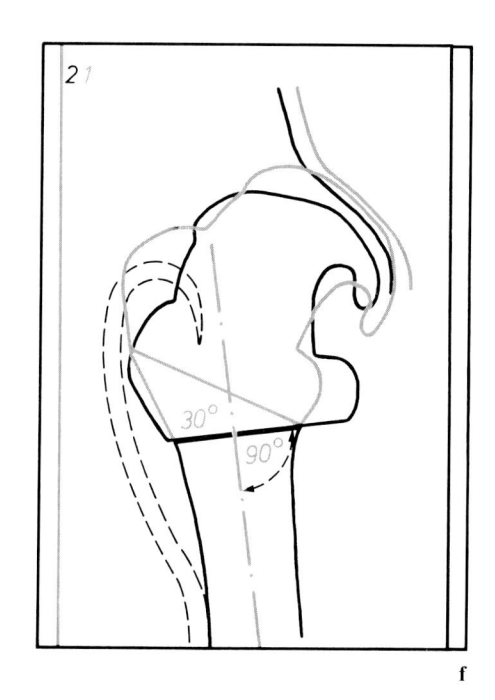

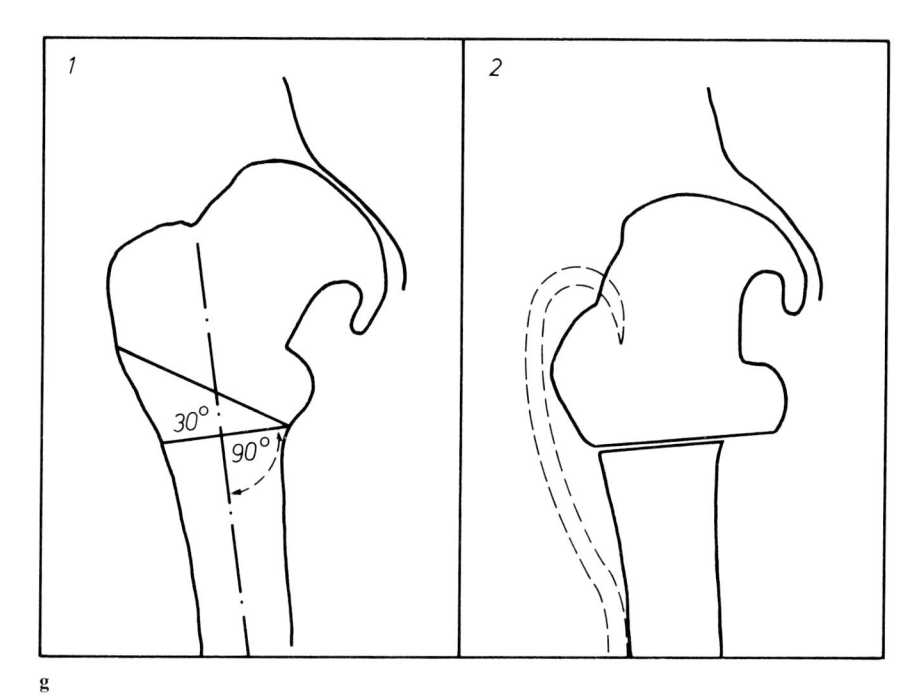

Fig. 115e–g

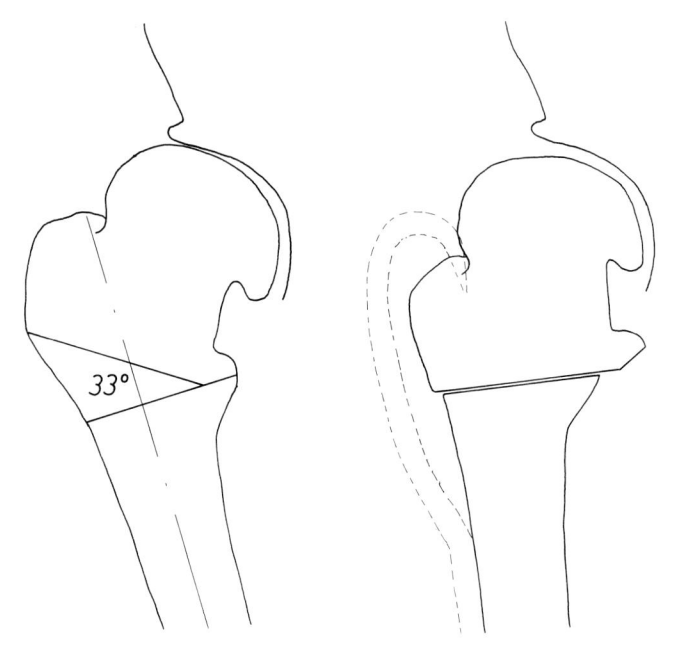

Fig. 116. Enough of the greater trochanter must be retained to provide the stressing-hook with a good hold

If there is any doubt about the adequacy of the indication, both a varus and a valgus osteotomy are planned. In the present instance (Fig. 117a) the diagram demonstrates that a varus osteotomy would reduce the weight-bearing surface of the joint (Fig. 117b). A valgus osteotomy will ensure congruence and enlarge the weight-bearing surface (Fig. 117c).

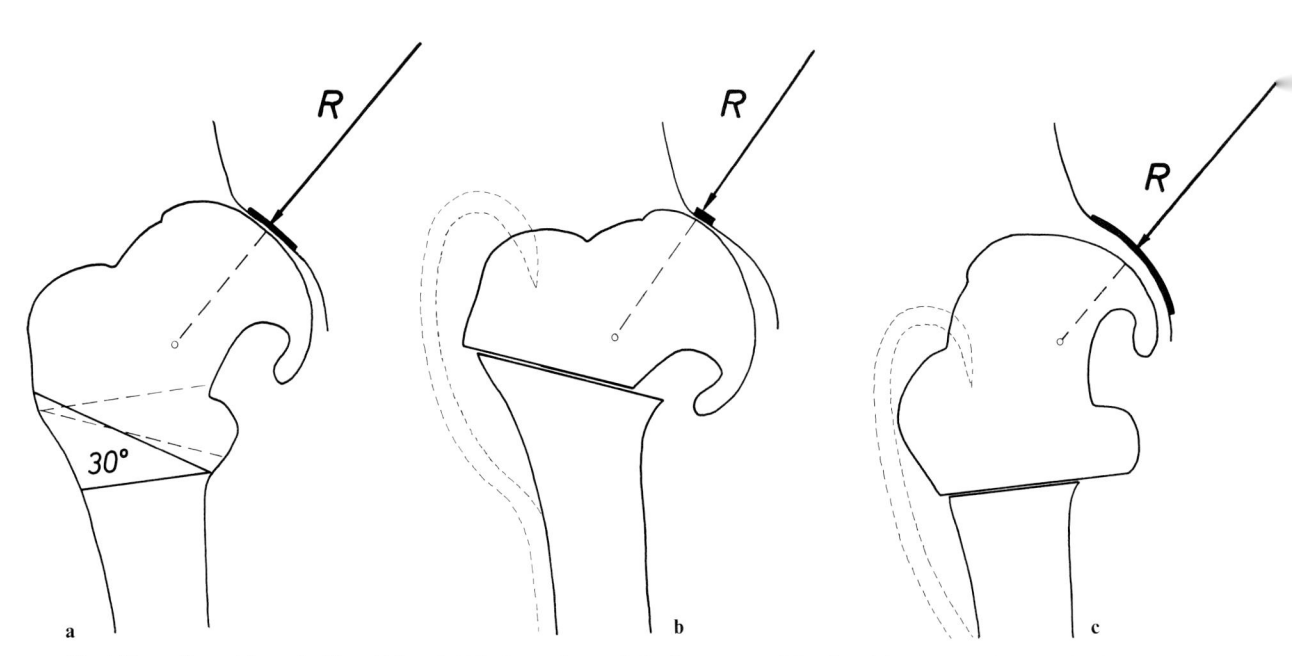

Fig. 117a–c. Same hip as in Figs. 114 and 115. *R*, resultant of the force exerted by the abductor muscles and the force exerted by the part of the body supported by the hip. **b** A varus osteotomy would decrease the weight-bearing area of the joint. **c** A valgus osteotomy will increase the weight-bearing area

D. Operative Procedure

1. Standard Procedure

The instruments are the same as for the varus osteotomy (p. 79). The operating-table must be transparent to X-rays. For tenotomy of the adductor and iliopsoas muscles, the patient lies supine. The operation is carried out exactly as described on p. 68. The patient is then turned over and the leg and lower trunk are prepared from foot to waist.

For valgus osteotomy and tenotomy of the abductor muscles, the patient lies prone. The approach is similar to that described for the varus osteotomy (p. 84). The lateral aspect of the upper end of the femur and the greater trochanter are clearly exposed.

a) Delineating the Wedge to Be Resected

A KIRSCHNER wire is inserted at right angles to the axis of the femoral shaft at the level of the lesser trochanter. Using the pin-insertion guide set at the necessary angle of correction, a second KIRSCHNER wire is inserted from the innominate tubercle of the femur, thus forming with the first the angle indicated in the pre-operative plan (Fig. 118). The second wire is oblique medially and distally. The apex of the wedge should lie at the tip of the lesser trochanter. If this brings the upper cut too high in the greater trochanter, i.e. above the innominate tubercle, the apex of the wedge will be chosen at a point somewhere across the lower cut. This must be carefully planned pre-operatively. An X-ray is taken to measure the angle formed by the KIRSCHNER wires (Fig. 61).

b) Tenotomy of the Abductor Muscles

Whilst the X-ray is being developed, the trochanteric insertions of the gluteus medius and minimus muscles are divided close to the greater trochanter, using scissors (Fig. 119).

c) Resection of the Wedge

The intertrochanteric wedge is cut with a handsaw maintained parallel successively to the proximal and to the distal KIRSCHNER wires (Fig. 120).

d) Derotation

When the wedge has been removed, the leg is put in abduction in such a way that the osteotomy surfaces are brought into contact and made parallel. The second assistant flexes the knee of the patient at right angles and holds the lower leg vertical (Fig. 91). This ensures an automatic derotation. If the two osteotomy surfaces do not fit, the square awl is used as a lever to bring them into close contact.

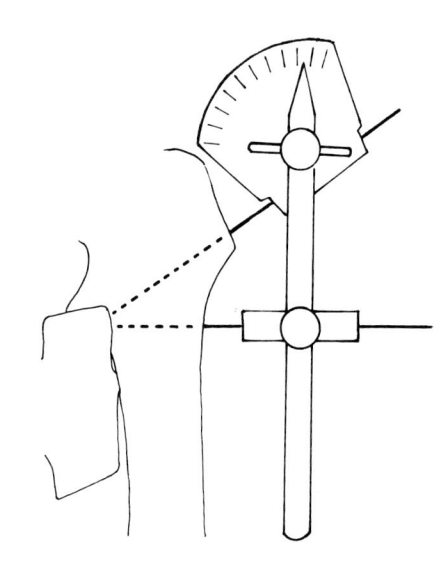

Fig. 118. Insertion of KIRSCHNER wires delineating the wedge to be resected

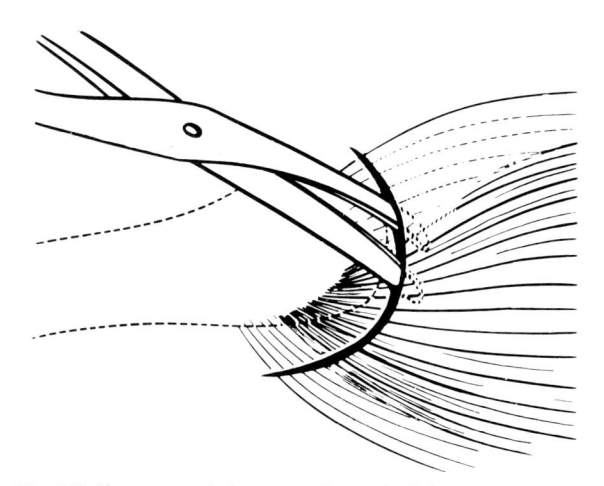

Fig. 119. Tenotomy of gluteus medius and minimus

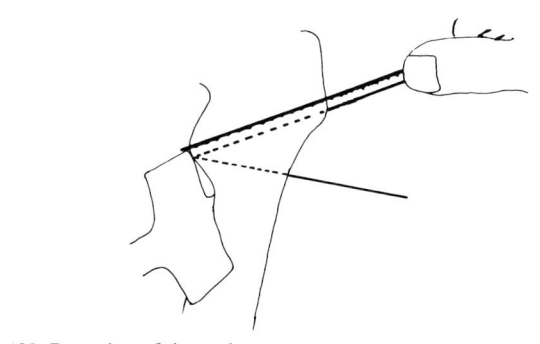

Fig. 120. Resection of the wedge

Fig. 121. Positioning of the compression-hook

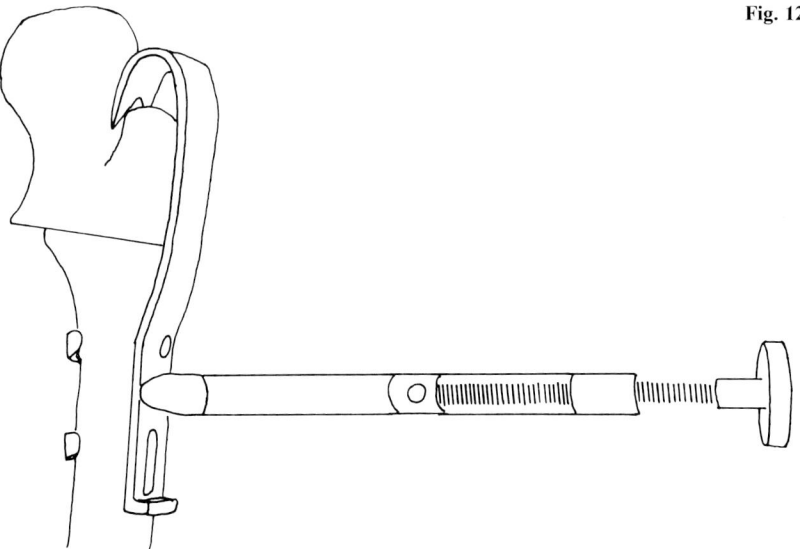

e) Fixing the Fragments

The compression-hook held in the plate-holder is placed with its prongs in the greater trochanter or medial to it, according to the pre-operative plan. The plate is applied over the lateral aspect of the femoral shaft and held by a LOWMAN clamp (Fig. 121). The prongs of the hook are lightly hammered into the greater trochanter using the impacting-lever (Fig. 122). A hole is drilled and tapped in the femur, through the distal end of the slot in the plate. The pivot screw passed through the eccentric disc is introduced into this hole (Fig. 123). The limb is then brought back from abduction into a neutral position, the second assistant maintaining the lower leg vertical. The eccent-

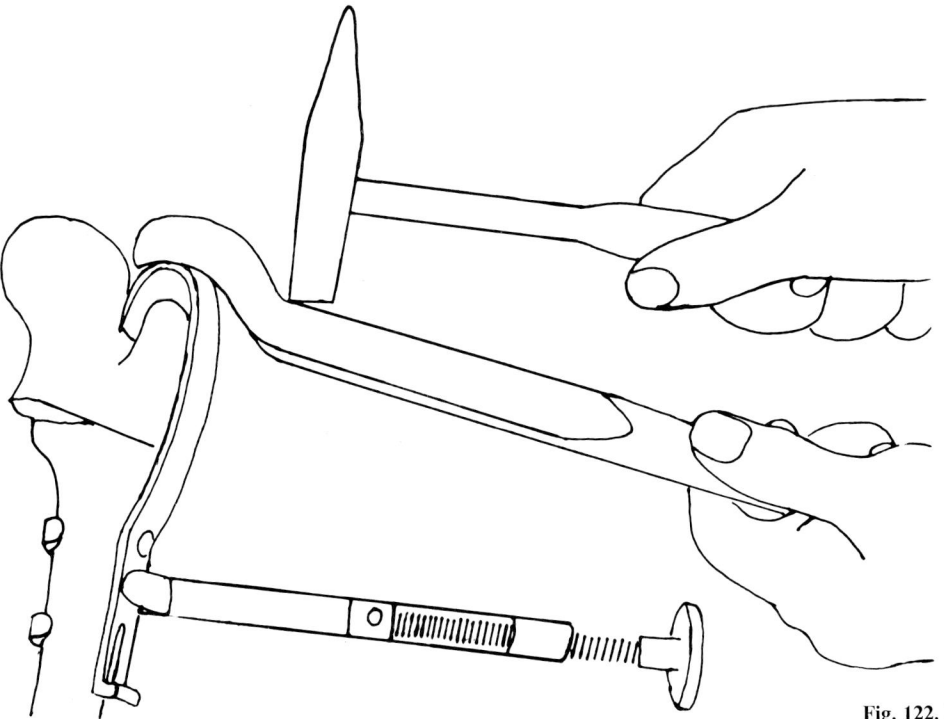

Fig. 122. Hammering in the hook

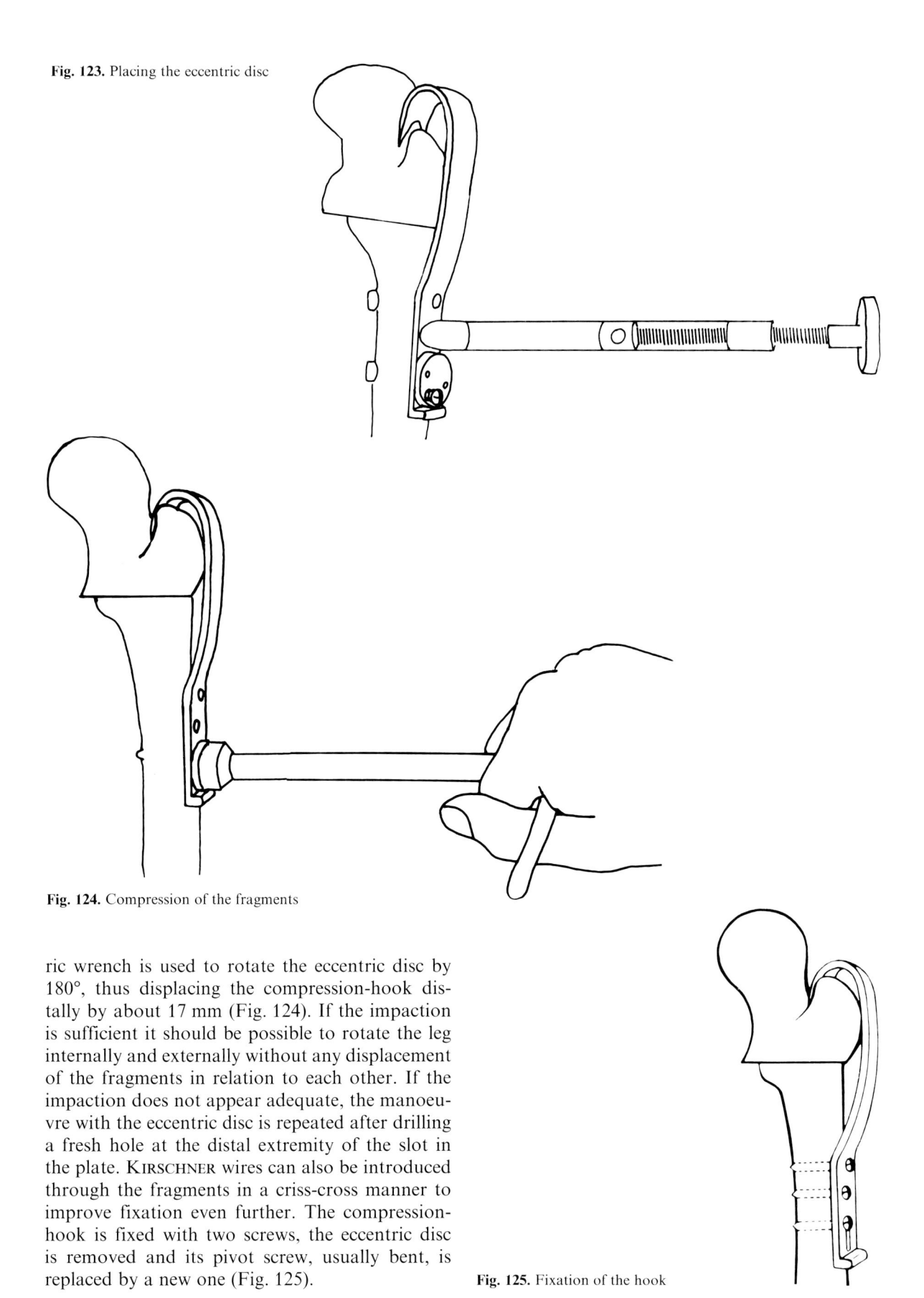

Fig. 123. Placing the eccentric disc

Fig. 124. Compression of the fragments

Fig. 125. Fixation of the hook

ric wrench is used to rotate the eccentric disc by 180°, thus displacing the compression-hook distally by about 17 mm (Fig. 124). If the impaction is sufficient it should be possible to rotate the leg internally and externally without any displacement of the fragments in relation to each other. If the impaction does not appear adequate, the manoeuvre with the eccentric disc is repeated after drilling a fresh hole at the distal extremity of the slot in the plate. KIRSCHNER wires can also be introduced through the fragments in a criss-cross manner to improve fixation even further. The compression-hook is fixed with two screws, the eccentric disc is removed and its pivot screw, usually bent, is replaced by a new one (Fig. 125).

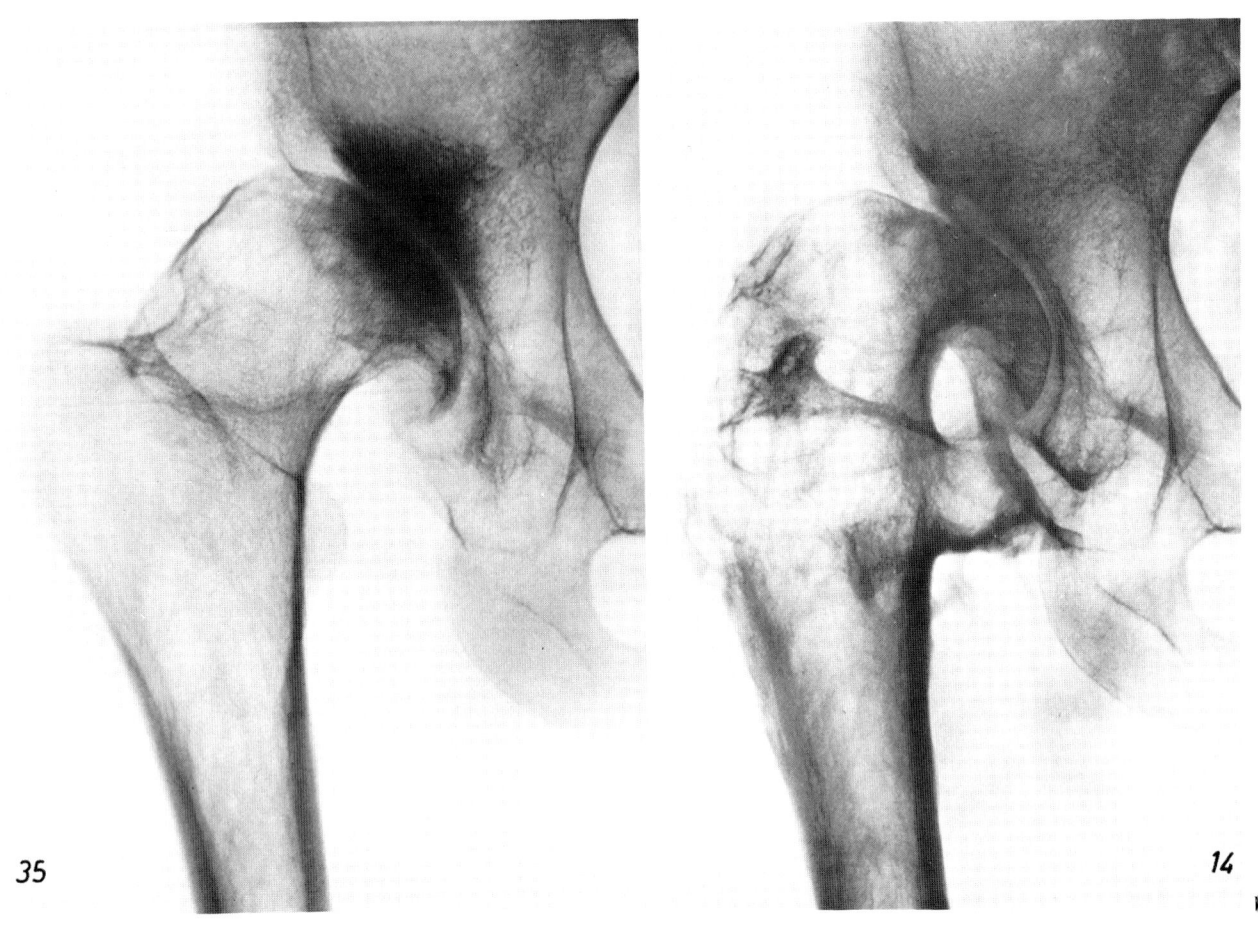

Fig. 126. a A 35-year-old female patient before a valgus intertrochanteric osteotomy and tenotomy. **b** 14 years afterwards

f) Suture

The vastus lateralis is reattached to the greater trochanter and the different layers of tissues are sutured over suction drainage.

The X-rays used to illustrate the planning of a Pauwels II operation (Fig. 115) were those of the hip of a 35-year-old female patient (Figs. 114 and 126a). One year after the procedure had been carried out the result was excellent and remained so at the 14-year follow-up: no pain, improvement of the range of movement and no limitation on walking. The X-rays show development of a wide joint space and regression of the subchondral sclerosis in the roof of the acetabulum (Fig. 126b).

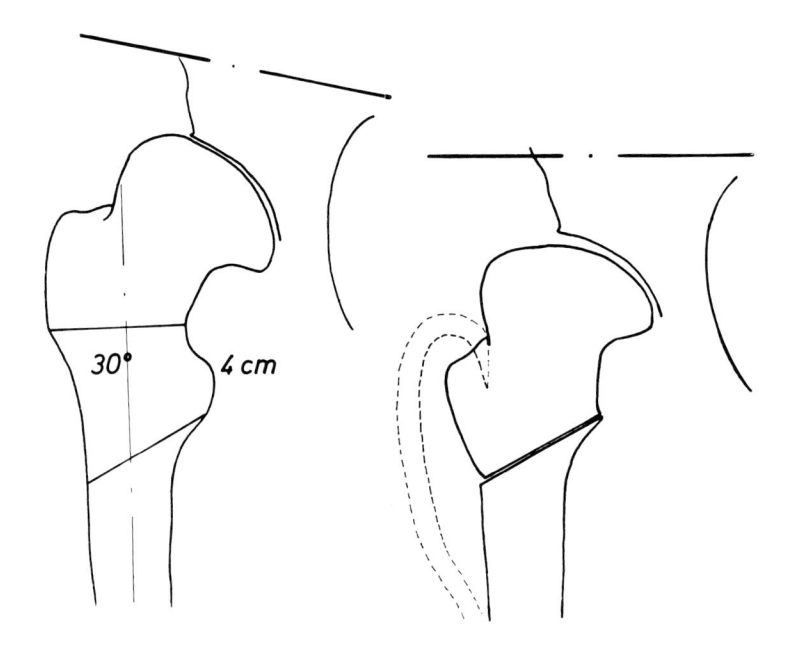

Fig. 127. Special bone section used when a shortening is combined with valgus osteotomy

2. Valgus Osteotomy Combined with a Shortening of the Leg

A valgus osteotomy may have to be combined with a shortening of the femur. In this case the tilt of the pelvis towards the shortened side must be taken into account and the degree of valgus increased accordingly. A 1-cm shortening roughly entails a 2°30′ tilting of the pelvis about the opposite hip.

Shortening by several centimetres necessitates removal of the lesser trochanter and the medial support which it provides for the proximal fragment. In these circumstances, in order to avoid medial tilting of this fragment, the upper cut is made normal to the axis of the femoral shaft and the distal cut oblique medially and proximally. In this way the osteotomy surfaces fit better and the medial support is provided by the medial cortex of the distal fragment (Fig. 127).

If a derotation is necessary it should be carried out after the first cut before inserting the distal KIRSCHNER wire and carrying out the distal cut.

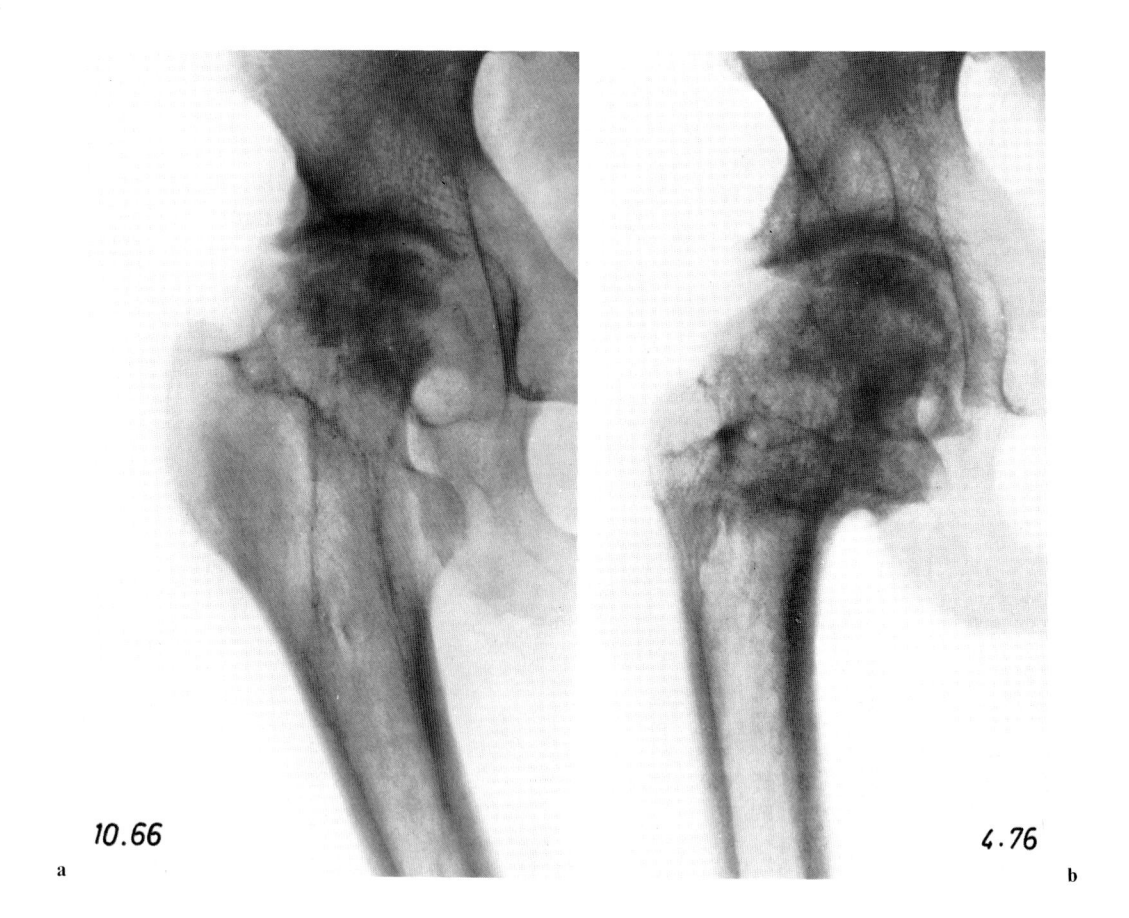

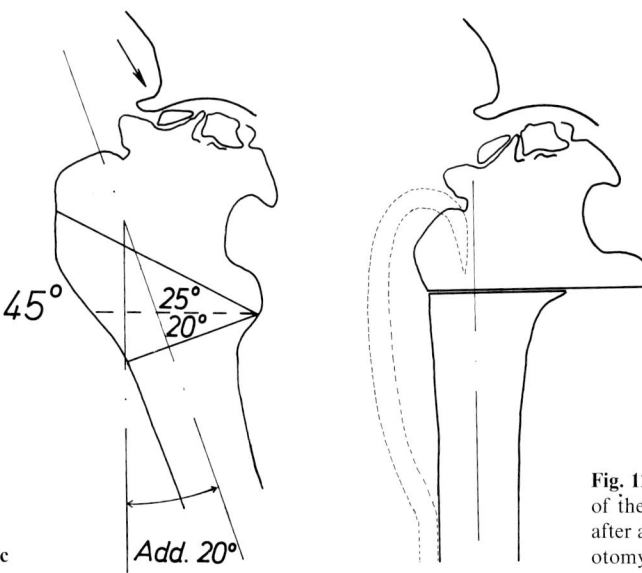

Fig. 128. a A 43-year-old female patient with avascular necrosis of the femoral head and adduction contracture. **b** Nine years after a valgus intertrochanteric osteotomy combined with a tenotomy. **c** Pre-operative planning. *Add.*, adduction

3. Correction of a Flexion Contracture

A flexion contracture persisting after tenotomy of the iliopsoas muscle probably results from osteoarthritic deformation of the bones and should be corrected at osteotomy level. To this end the wedge to be removed must be wider posteriorly than anteriorly. The angle of correction in the sagittal plane (= the degree of flexion contracture) can be marked in the bone by two KIRSCHNER wires introduced from behind forward, one on each side of the osteotomy. The distal wire must be normal to the axis of the femoral shaft. The saw blade is held parallel to the direction of these KIRSCHNER wires.

4. Correction of an Adduction Contracture or Deformity

If there is an adduction contracture or an adduction deformity, the angle of this adduction must be added to the measured angle (Fig. 56). Otherwise, the articular surfaces would be congruent only when the limb is in its deformed position. We have described above (p. 57) how to measure the deformity.

A 43-year-old female patient complained of a painful hip with a post-traumatic avascular necrosis of the femoral head (Fig. 128a). The leg was held in adduction (Fig. 56). The angles formed by the ischial line and the femoral axes were 65° on the adducted side and 105° on the opposite side. The adduction contracture thus attained $\frac{105°-65°}{2}=20°$. A 25° wedge had to be resected to ensure congruence of the articular surfaces. The 20° corresponding to the adduction contracture were added to the 25°. Finally, a wedge of 45° was resected (Fig. 128c). At the 9-year follow-up the result remained good (Fig. 128b).

5. Too Much Valgum

It usually seems better to make a little too much valgum than too little. If the degree of valgum is insufficient, the articular pressure remains concentrated at the edge of the socket. If the valgum is too great, overpressure may develop in a restricted area within the acetabulum. Resorption of tissue will take place with flattening of the head and socket, and this forcefully leads to an increase in the weight-bearing surface of the joint.

A 45-year-old male patient (Fig. 129a) underwent a 35° valgus osteotomy combined with a tenotomy. One year after the operation a gap appeared between the edge of the socket and the femoral head. Articular pressure seemed to be concentrated further medially (Fig. 129b). There the subchondral sclerosis had increased. At the 2-year follow-up the subchondral sclerosis had become uniform throughout and the joint space was delineated by congruent articular surfaces (Fig. 129c).

E. Postoperative Care

Postoperative care is the same as that following varus intertrochanteric osteotomy (p. 89). The suction drainage is removed on the 2nd day, the stitches on the 12th day just before the patient is discharged. The patient stands up from the 2nd day. He uses two crutches for 6 months, but from the beginning he puts 15%–20% of his body weight on the affected limb when he walks. This can be controlled by means of a scale. Otherwise, a rough but practical way of evaluating pressure is to make the patient walk over one's hand laid flat on the floor: one should feel the pressure without experiencing pain. After the 6th month only one crutch is used, held in the hand opposite to the affected hip.

Night traction of 2 kg on the limb operated upon is recommended after the 1st month and until the end of the 1st year. No active exercises should be done. It is often difficult to restrain the physiotherapists from imposing such exercises.

Rarely, valgus intertrochanteric osteotomy is considered when a wide joint space is still present. When this is the case, the crutches may be discarded as soon as the patient feels able to walk without them.

Again the compression-hook is removed after 1 year, using two short incisions and the appropriate tool.

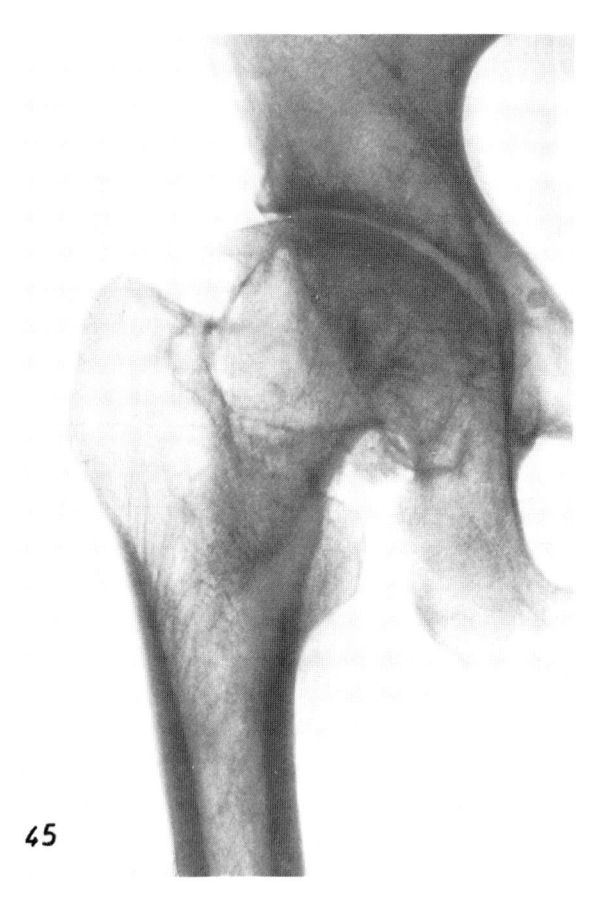

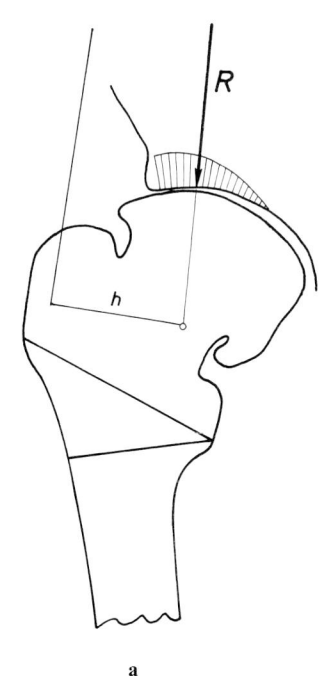

Fig. 129. a A 45-year-old male patient before a Pauwels II. **b** One year and **c** 2 years afterwards. *R*, resultant of the forces *M* exerted by the abductor muscles and *K* exerted by the part of the body supported by the hip; *h*, lever arm of *M*

1 2

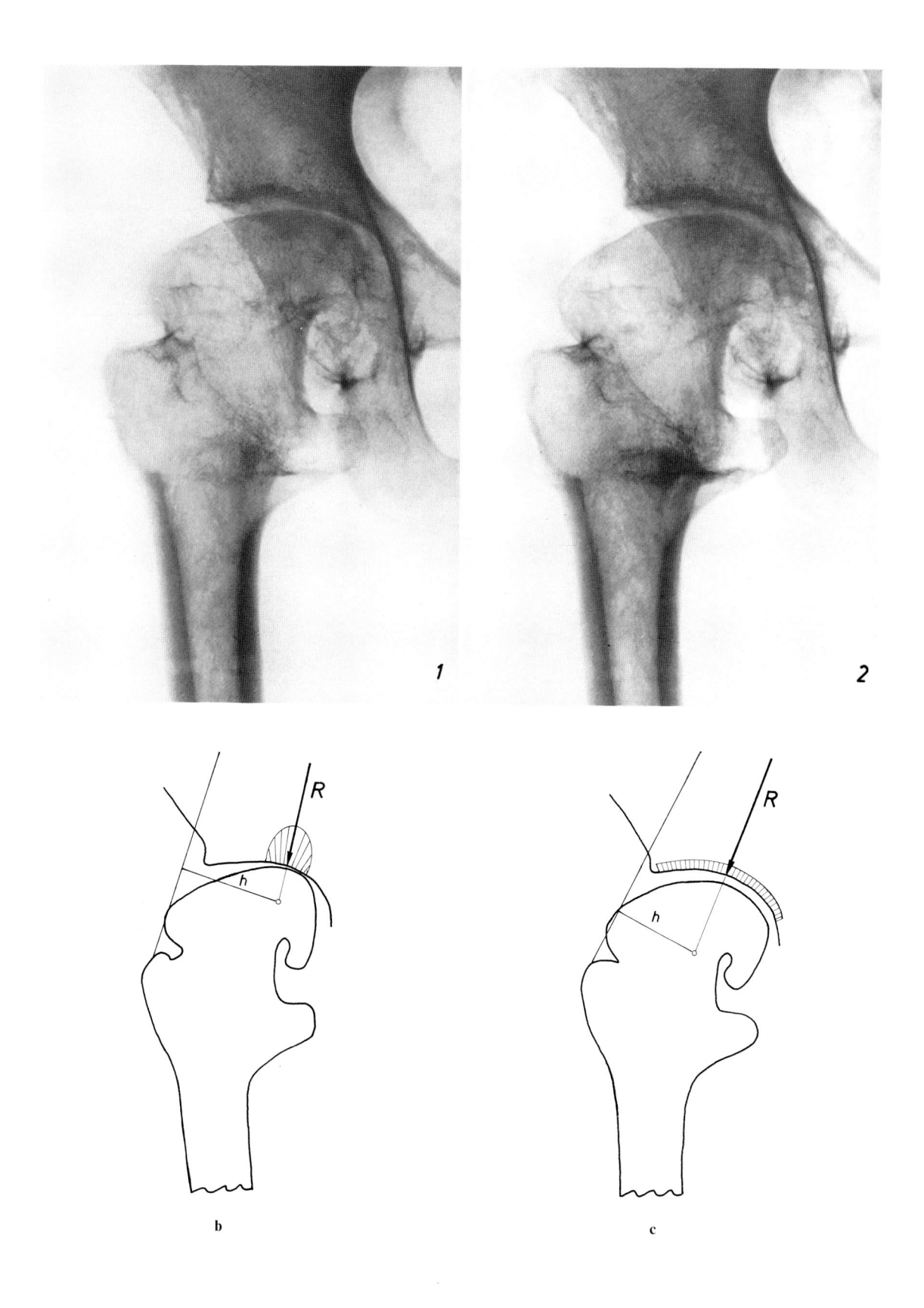

b c

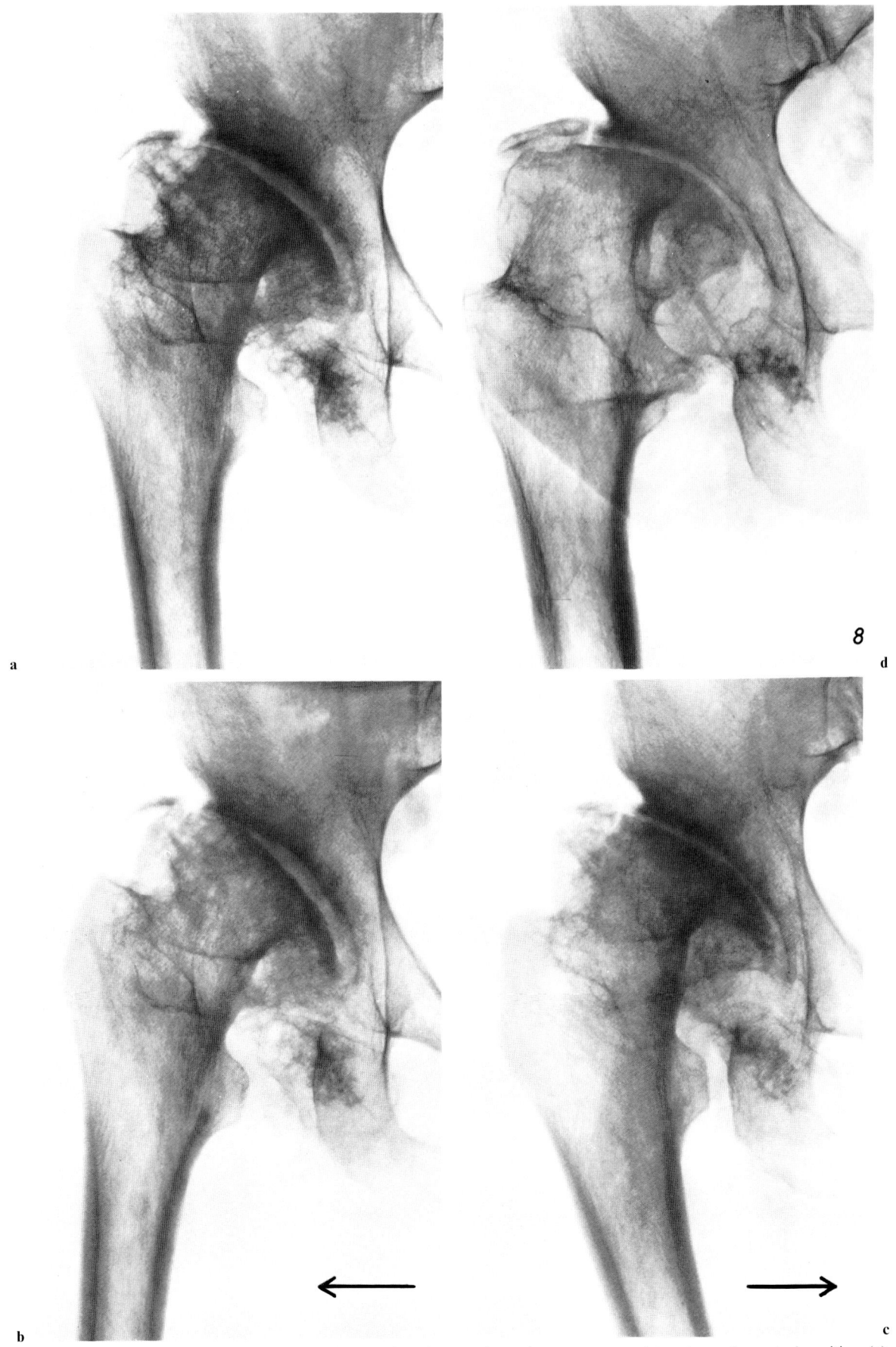

Fig. 130. a–c A 55-year-old female patient before a valgus intertrochanteric osteotomy and tenotomy, in neutral position (**a**), in full abduction (**b**) and in full adduction (**c**). **d** Eight years afterwards

F. Postoperative Evolution

Pain usually disappears immediately after surgery. Some flexion may be lost temporarily but is recovered during the 1st postoperative year. Very often the range of movement dramatically increases in the following years. Most patients no longer limp after 1 or 2 years. Some, mainly in the older group, continue to limp somewhat. X-rays show progressive development of a joint space during the first postoperative year. The subchondral sclerosis in the roof of the acetabulum may resolve much more slowly.

During the first postoperative months the X-ray picture may be alarming, suggesting septic arthritis, although this is not supported by clinical symptoms. This tremendous reaction of the articular bone actually constitutes a favourable omen for the future. It seems that metabolic changes take place as a result of the reduced joint pressure.

A 55-year-old female patient complained of a painful hip with limping and progressive limitation of the range of movement (Table 18). The X-ray showed severe osteoarthritis in a subluxated hip with a dense triangle at the edge of the acetabulum (Fig. 130a). Incongruence was worse in abduction (Fig. 130b). Adduction improved congruence (Fig. 130c). A 20° valgus osteotomy was planned (Fig. 131) and carried out. This operation altered and displaced the centre of rotation of the joint (Fig. 131). The extruded part of the femoral head pushed the abductor muscles laterally and changed their direction. This resulted in a lengthening of the lever arm h of the force M exerted by the abductor muscles, and in a diminution and a medial displacement of the resultant force R into the socket. The area of the weight-bearing surface of the joint was thus increased. Consequently, the articular compressive stresses were considerably reduced and became evenly distributed. At the 8-year follow-up the hip was pain-free and the range of movement had improved (Table 18). The subchondral sclerosis confirmed the decrease in and better distribution of joint pressure (Fig. 130d). A wide joint space pointed to the formation of fibrocartilage in the joint.

Table 18. Range of movement of the hip (Fig. 130)

	Before surgery	At the 8-year follow-up	Gain
Flexion	90°	95°	5°
Extension	0°	0°	
Adduction	25°	45°	45°
Abduction	10°	35°	
Int. rotation	0°	5°	20°
Ext. rotation	10°	25°	

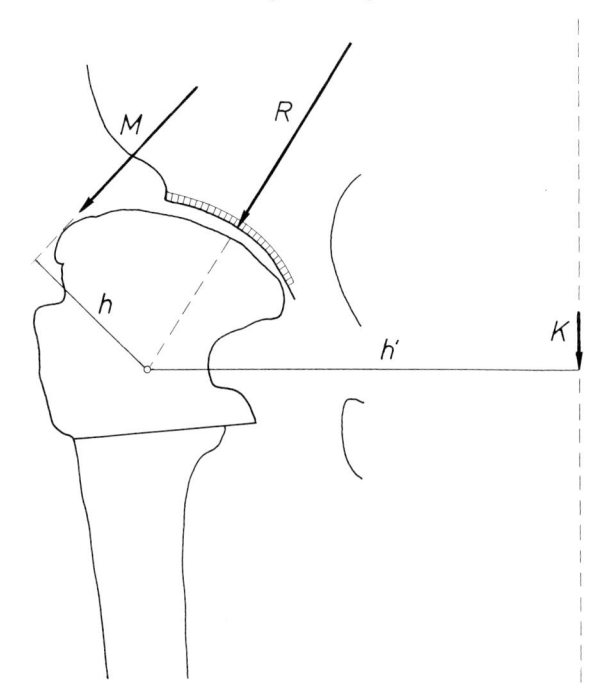

Fig. 131. Planning of the operation on the hip shown in Fig. 130. M, force exerted by the abductor muscles; K, force exerted by the part of the body supported by the hip; R, resultant of M and K; h, lever arm of M; h', lever arm of K

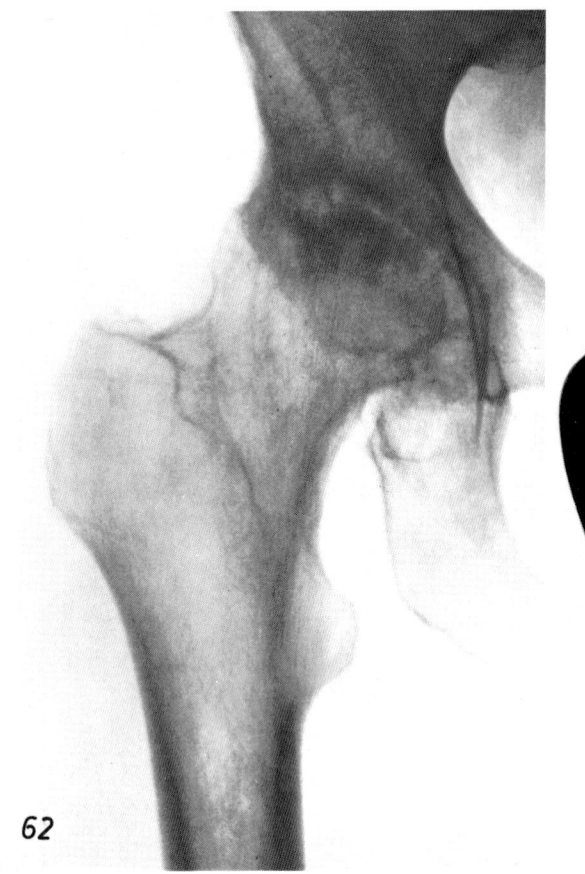

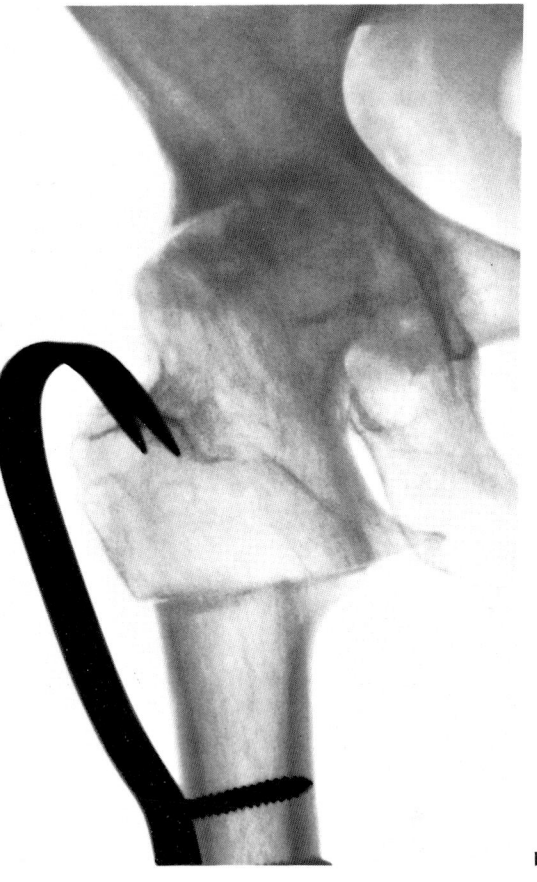

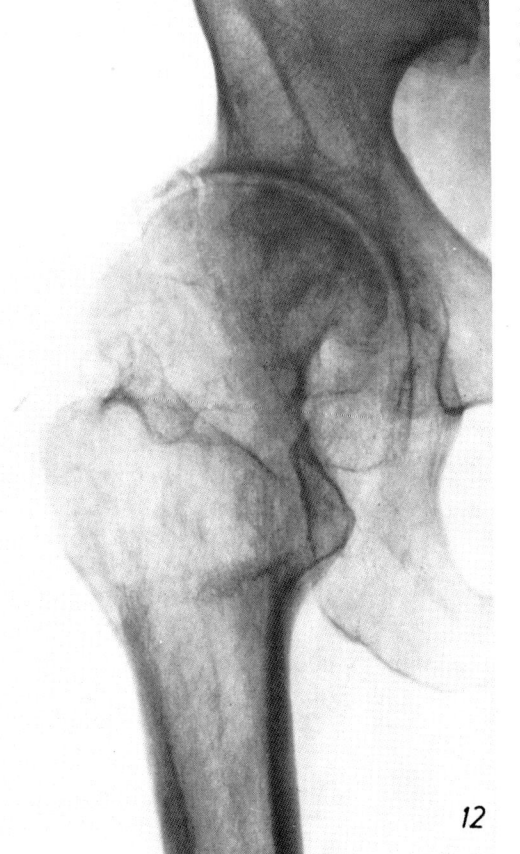

Fig. 132a–e. A 62-year-old female patient **a** before and **b** immediately after a Pauwels II. **c** One year, **d** 2 years and **e** 12 years later

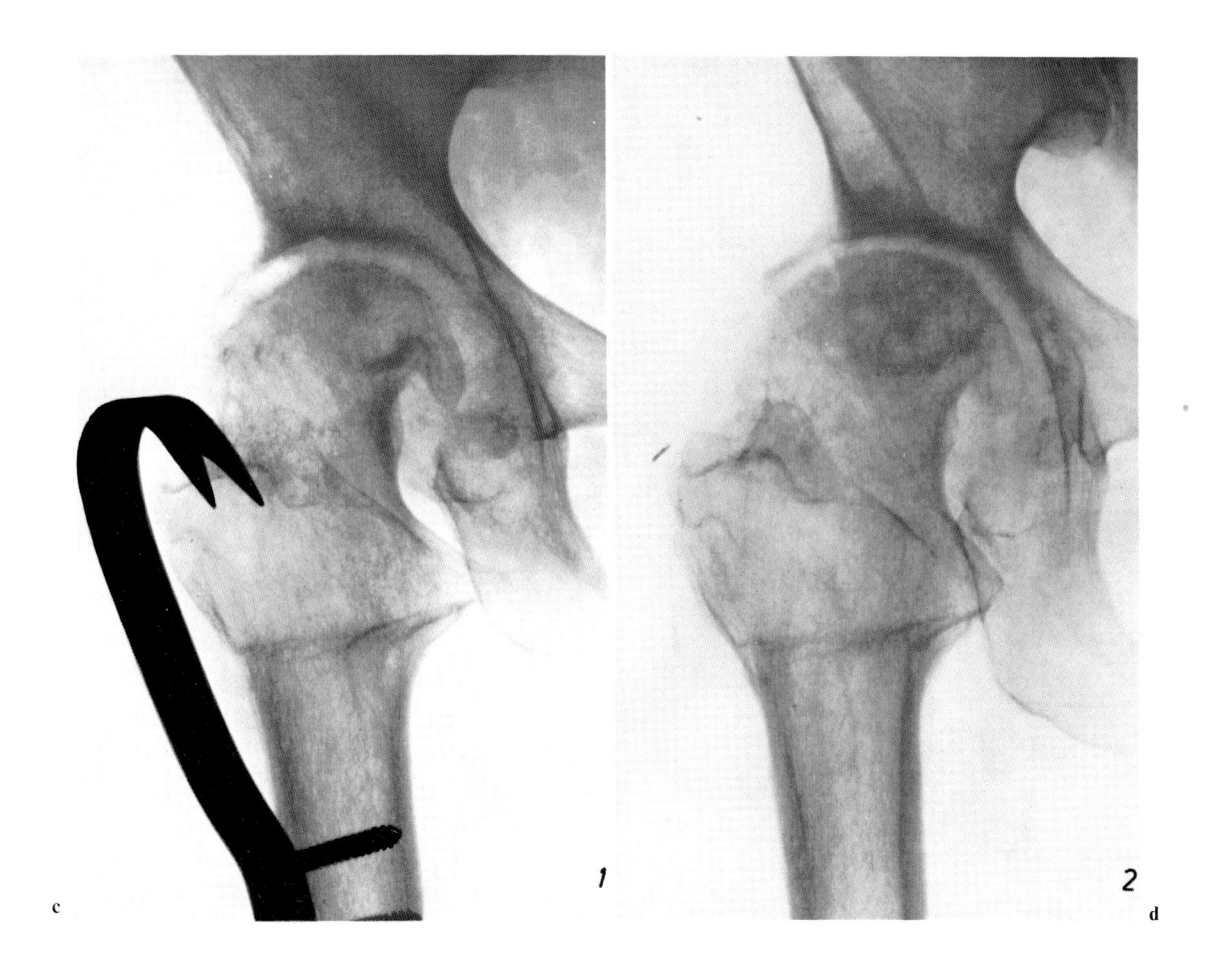

A 62-year-old female patient underwent a valgus osteotomy for severe osteoarthritis (Fig. 132a). Immediately after the operation, no joint space appeared in the X-ray (Fig. 132b). One year later, a wide joint space had developed but a dense triangle persisted at the edge of the socket (Fig. 132c). At the 2-year follow-up, the joint space appeared a little narrower and the dense triangle persisted (Fig. 132d). At the 12-year follow-up, the joint space was a little narrower still but the subchondral sclerosis in the roof of the acetabulum presented an even width over the weight-bearing area of the joint (Fig. 132e).

When there is overpressure, the dense triangle seems to appear much more quickly than it disappears when the joint pressure is again evenly distributed over a large weight-bearing surface. Bone remodels quickly to ensure its strength, more slowly to ensure its lightness. It is surprising how severely deteriorated hips can regenerate after a valgus osteotomy.

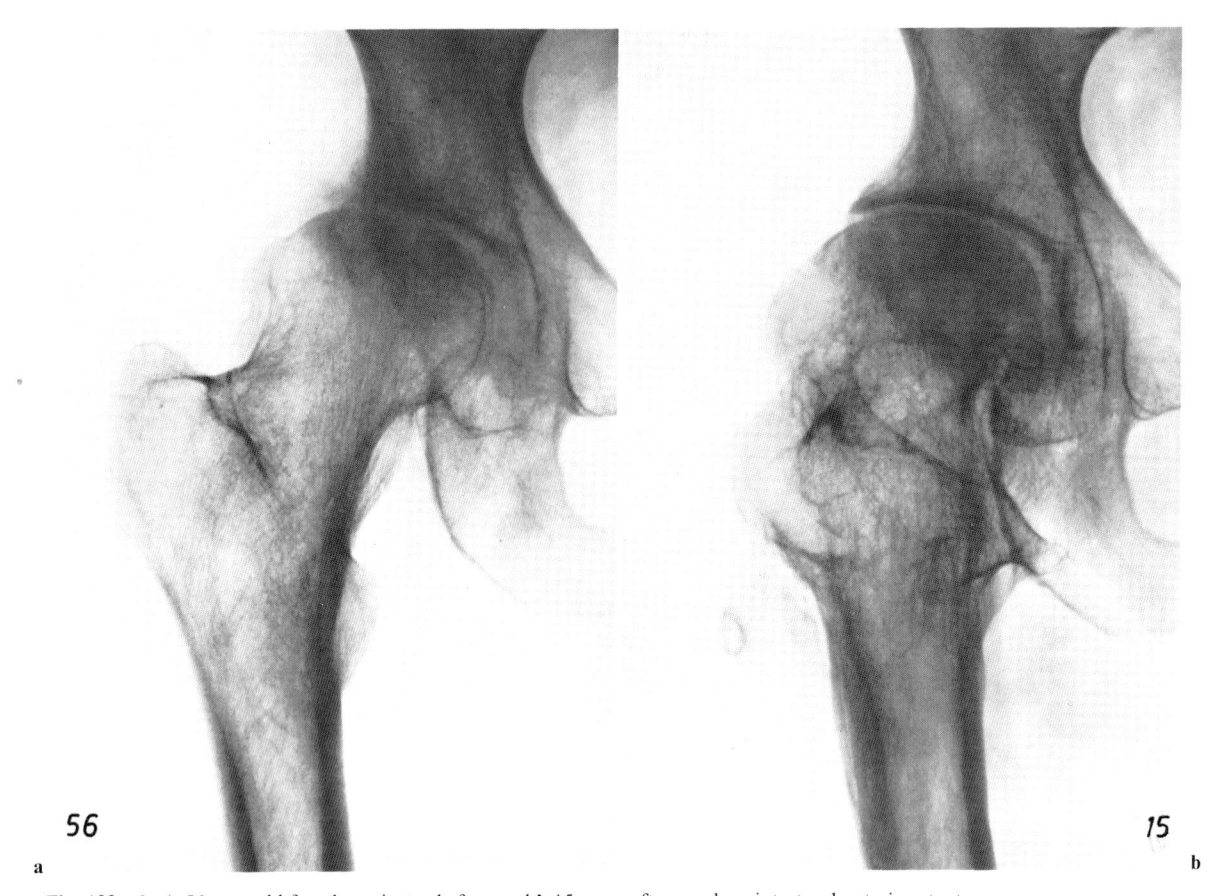

Fig. 133a, b. A 56-year-old female patient **a** before and **b** 15 years after a valgus intertrochanteric osteotomy

A 56-year-old female patient with severe osteoarthritis of both hips (Figs. 133a and 134a) underwent valgus intertrochanteric osteotomy, first of the right hip and then, 1 year later, of the left hip. Fifteen years later, the two hips appeared remarkably well remodelled. The dense triangle in the roof of the acetabulum had been replaced by a subchondral sclerosis of even thickness throughout, delineating a wide joint space (Figs. 133b and 134b).

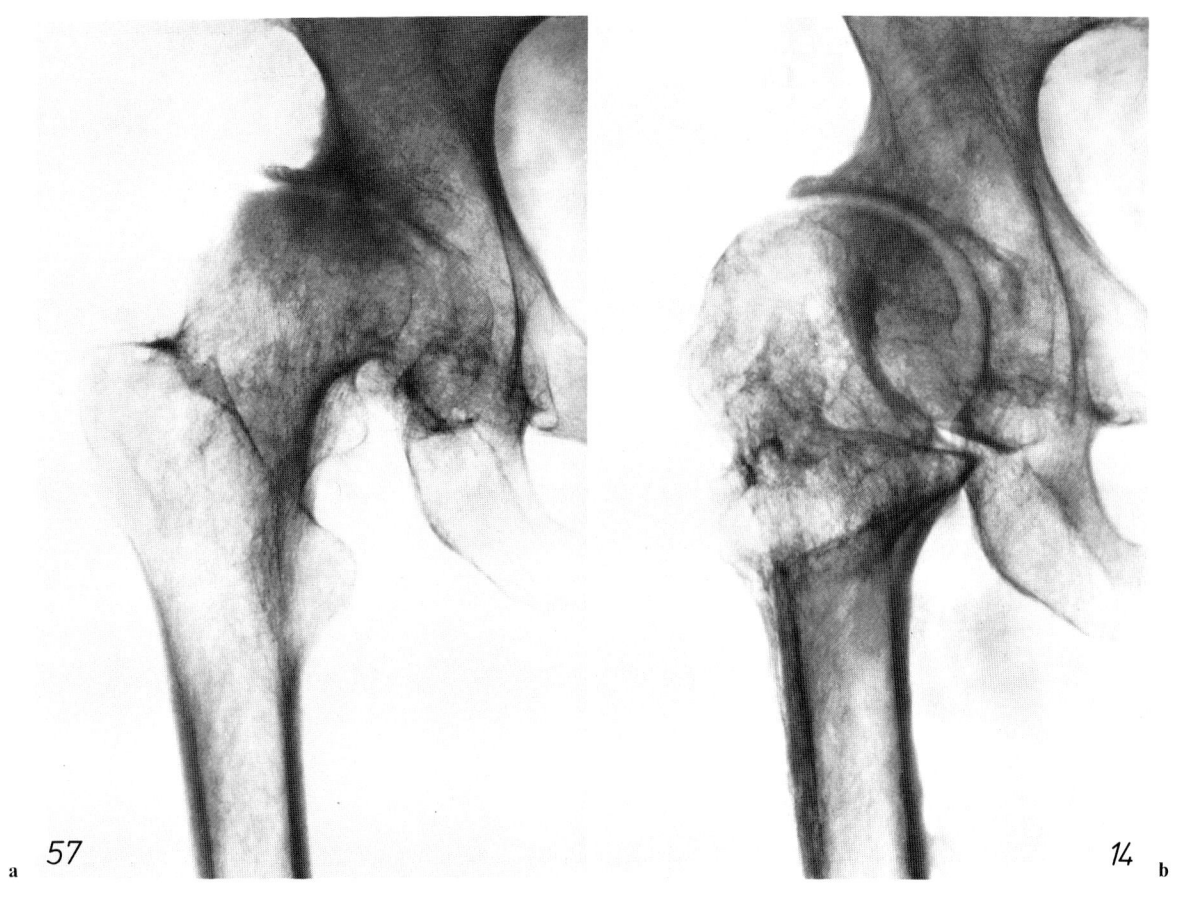

Fig. 134a, b. Same patient as in Fig. 133: opposite hip. Age at operation: 57 years. **a** before and **b** 14 years after a valgus intertrochanteric osteotomy

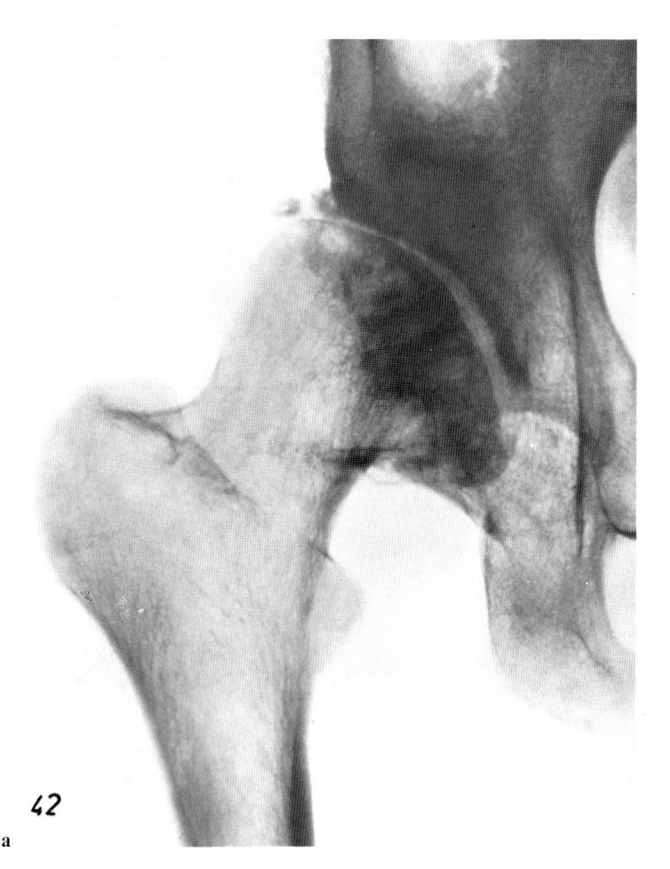

Fig. 135. a A 42-year-old female patient before a Pauwels II. **b** 19 years afterwards. **c** Pre-operative planning. Same hip as in Fig. 58

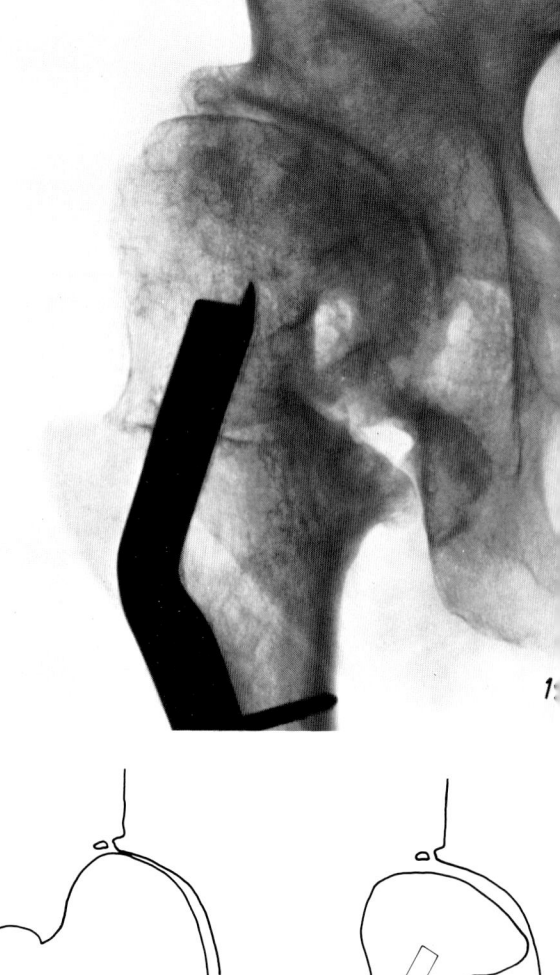

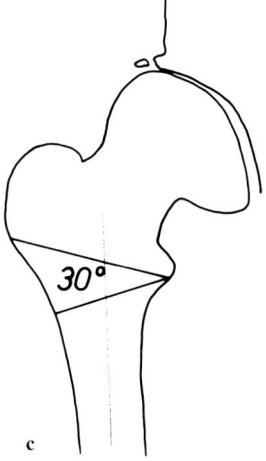

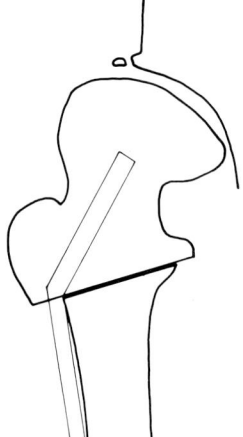

A 42-year-old female patient complained of severe and persistent pain in the hip (Fig. 135a). Abduction worsened the incongruence of the articular surfaces and adduction improved congruence (Fig. 58). The pre-operative plan showed that a 30° wedge would have to be resected (Fig. 135c). Nineteen years after a valgus osteotomy combined with a tenotomy, the clinical result remained excellent. In the X-rays the joint space was wide and a thin ribbon of dense bone of uniform width throughout had replaced the dense triangle in the roof of the acetabulum (Fig. 135b).

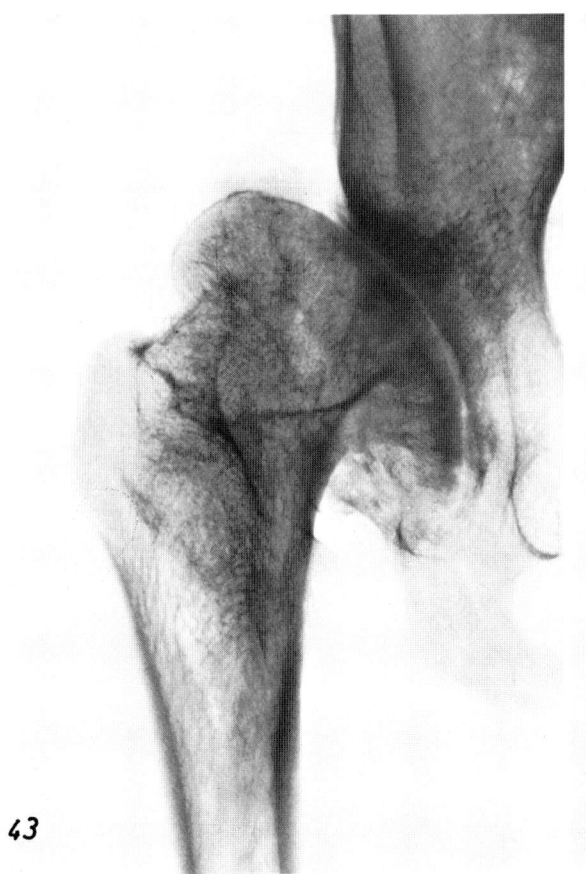

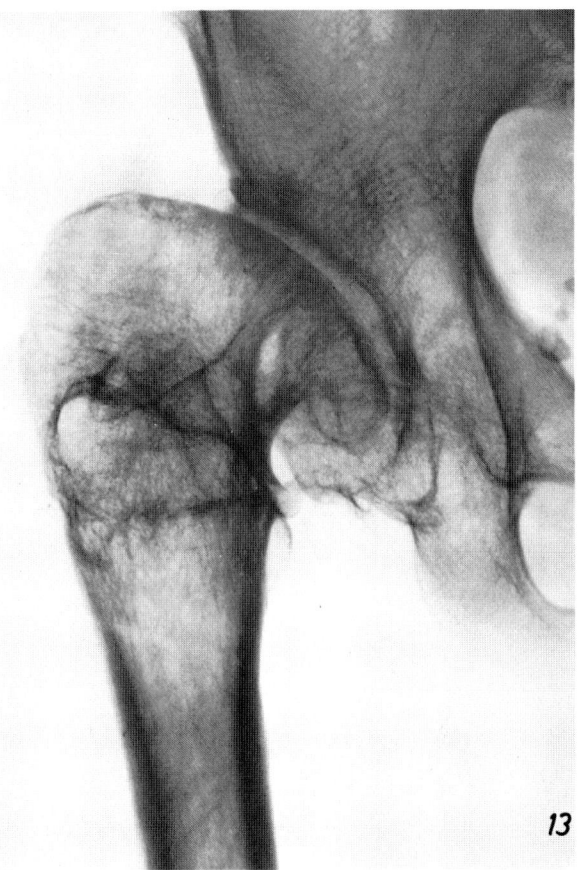

Fig. 136. a A 43-year-old female patient before a Pauwels II.
b 13 years afterwards

As a rule the largest femoral heads provide the best indications for a valgus osteotomy. In a 43-year-old female patient with an osteoarthritic hip which was flattened and increased in volume (Fig. 136a), a valgus osteotomy was carried out taking advantage of the medial osteophyte of the femoral head. Thirteen years later, the clinical result remained excellent (Table 19). The extruded head had pushed the abductor muscles laterally, lengthening their lever arm. The subchondral sclerosis pointed to an even distribution of the joint stresses over a large weight-bearing surface. A wide joint space had reappeared (Fig. 136b)

Table 19. Range of movement of the hip (Fig. 136)

	Before surgery	At the 13-year follow-up	Gain
Flexion	60°	90°	40°
Extension	−5°	5°	
Adduction	20°	45°	35°
Abduction	0°	10°	
Int. rotation	−5°	5°	30°
Ext. rotation	15°	30°	

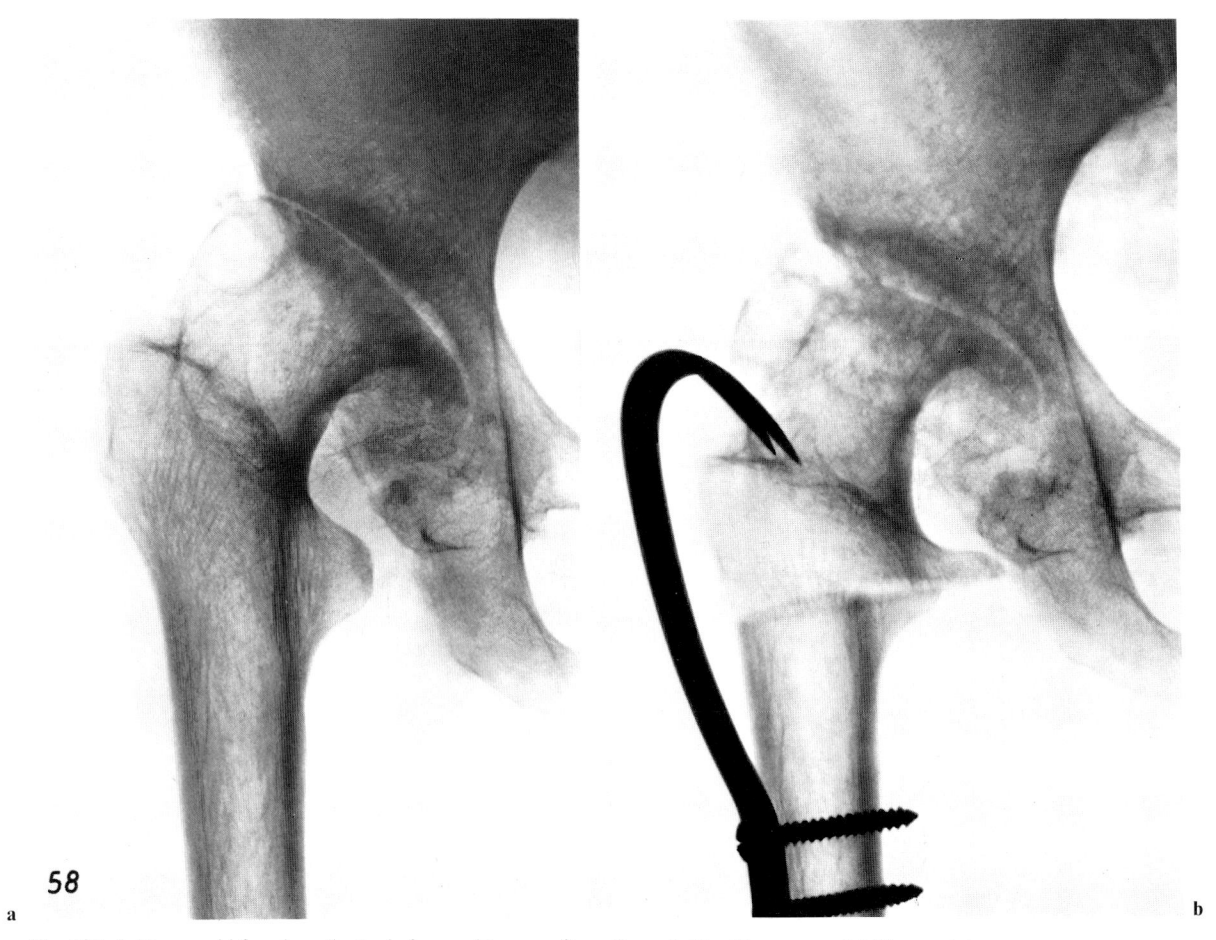

Fig. 137. A 58-year-old female patient **a** before and **b** soon after a Pauwels II. **c** One year and **d** 10 years later

In a 58-year-old female patient the femoral head was considerably widenend by a medial osteophyte, whereas the acetabulum was shallow (Fig. 137a). One year after a Pauwels II operation the result looked extremely good (Fig. 137c). Ten years after surgery the joint space remained wide (Fig. 137d) and the clinical result was still excellent.

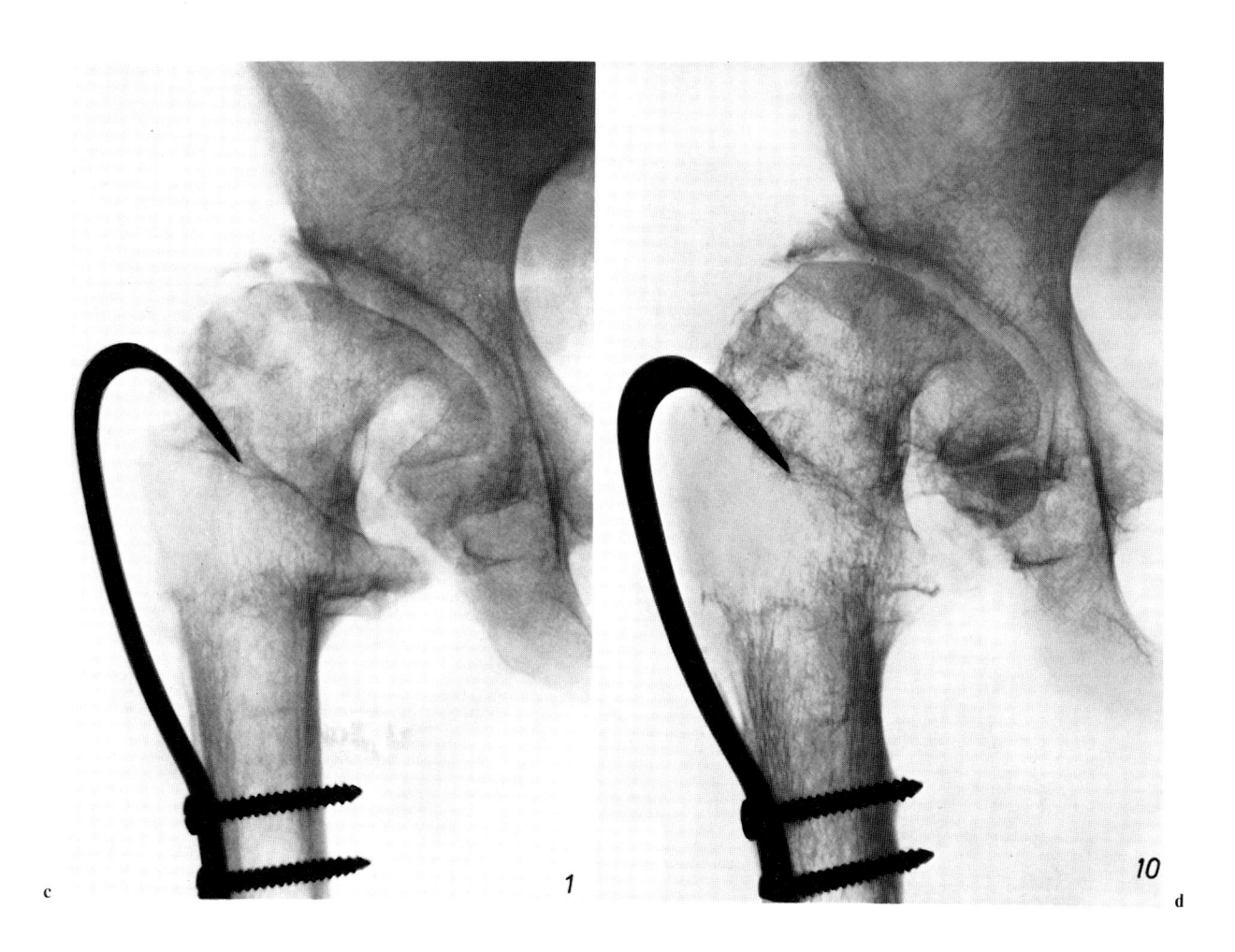

G. Reducing the Compressive Stresses in the Joint Rather than Restoring Normal Anatomical Shape

Whereas varus intertrochanteric osteotomy usually tends to restore anatomy to normal by replacing the femoral head in the acetabulum, valgus intertrochanteric osteotomy very often rotates part of the femoral head outside the socket and further increases a large neck-shaft angle. This results from the PAUWELS approach to the problem of osteoarthritis. This aims at decreasing the compressive stresses in the joint in order to make them tolerable for the tissues. In many cases a decrease in the articular compressive stresses can only be achieved by distorting anatomy further.

37

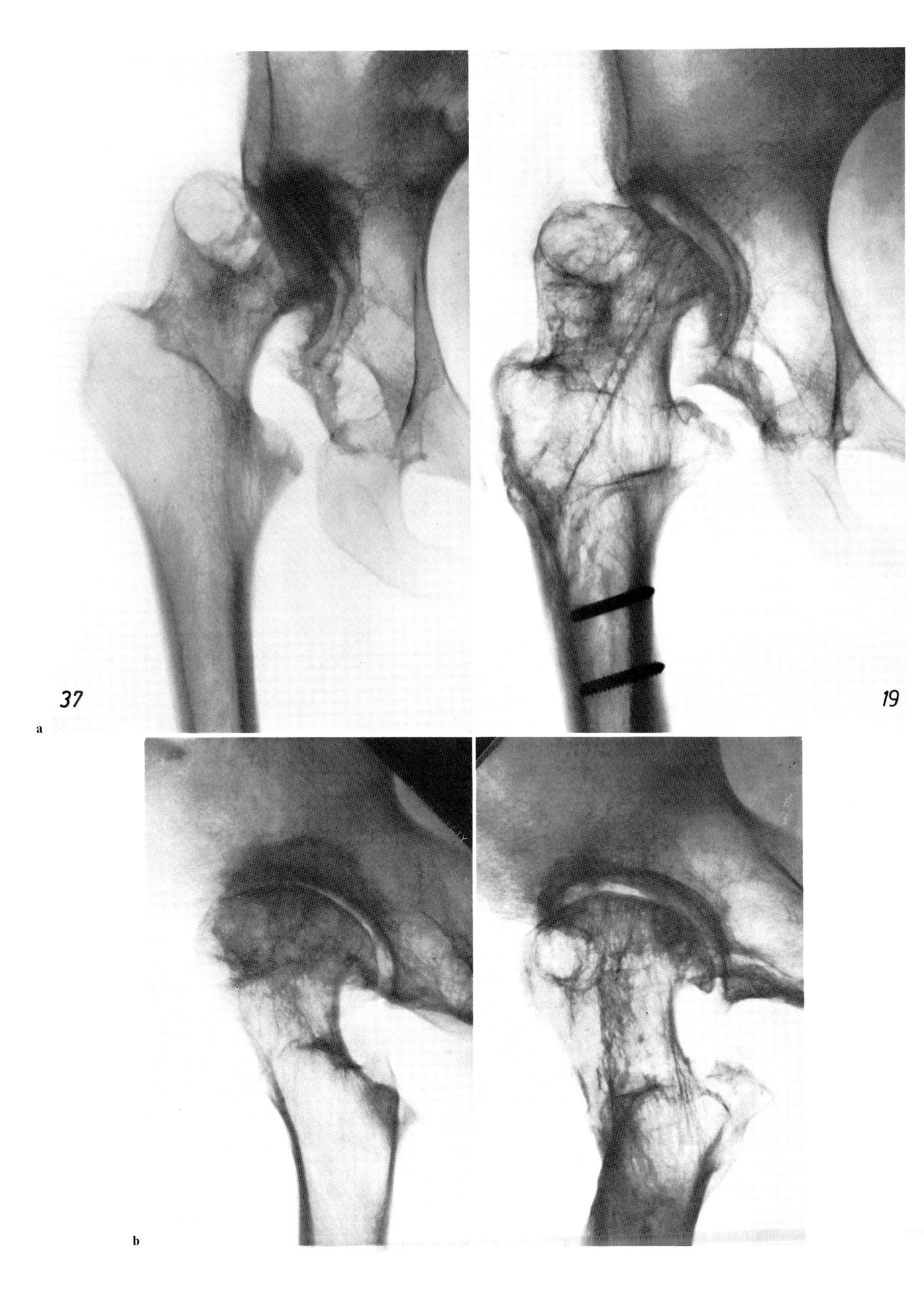

19

a

b

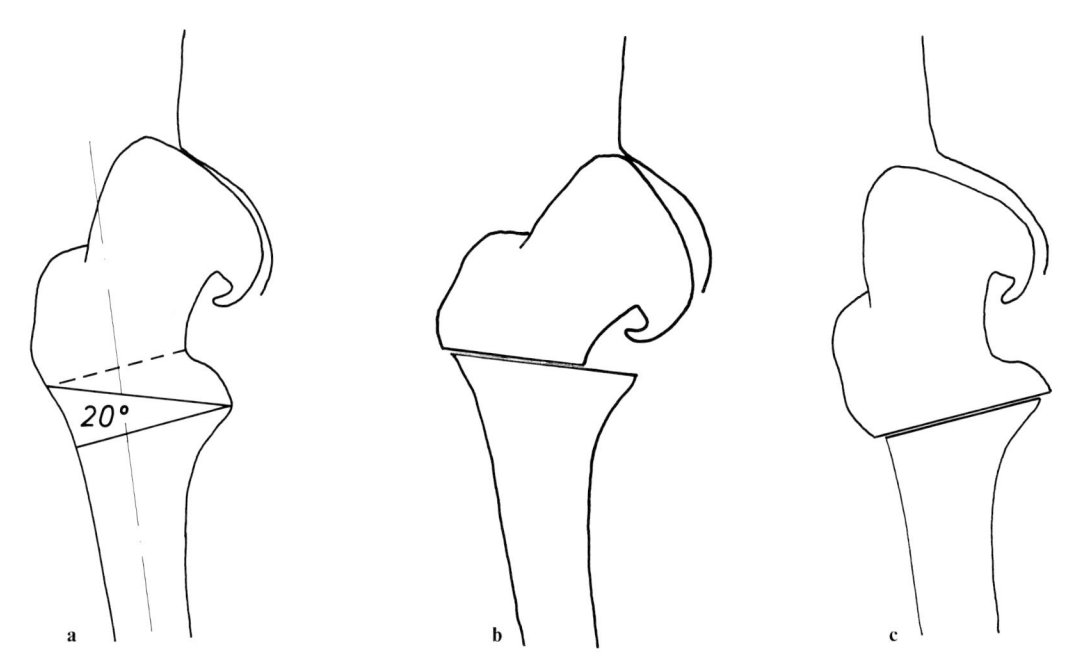

Fig. 139a–c. Pre-operative planning. A varus osteotomy would have decreased the weight-bearing surface of the joint. **a** Planning of a varus and of a valgus osteotomy. **b** Varus osteotomy. **c** Valgus osteotomy

A 37-year-old female patient developed severe osteoarthritis in a subluxated dysplastic hip, with coxa valga and a shallow acetabulum. A dense triangle at the edge of the latter demonstrated the increase and concentration of the stresses in that part of the joint (Fig. 138a). A varus osteotomy would have tended to restore normal anatomical shape but would certainly not have ensured congruence of the articular surfaces (Fig. 139b). It would therefore not have enlarged the weight-bearing area of the joint. To achieve this, a valgus osteotomy appeared to be necessary (Fig. 139c). The valgus osteotomy increased the deformity of the upper end of the femur as well as the subluxation. However, it was carried out with a multiple tenotomy and did indeed considerably reduce the compressive stresses in the joint (Fig. 140), as shown by the regression of the dense triangle at the edge of the socket and its progressive replacement by a subchondral sclerosis of uniform width throughout (Fig. 138b). At the 19-year follow-up the clinical result remained excellent.

Fig. 140. Predicted change in the distribution of the stresses after a Pauwels II. *R*, resultant force exerted on the hip. Same hip as in Figs. 138 and 139

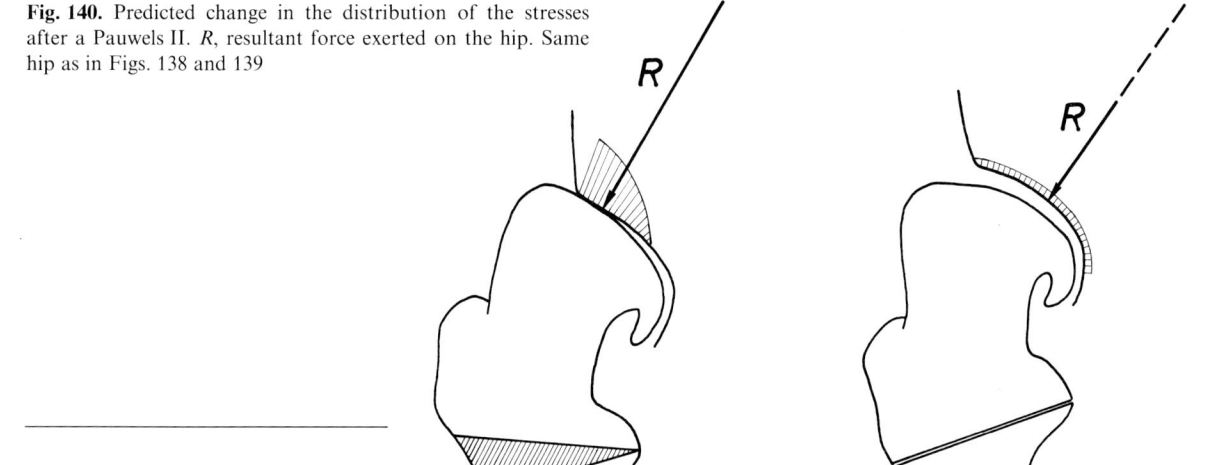

Fig. 138. a A 37-year-old female patient before a Pauwels II. **b** 19 years afterwards. *Top*, anteroposterior view; *bottom*, lateral view

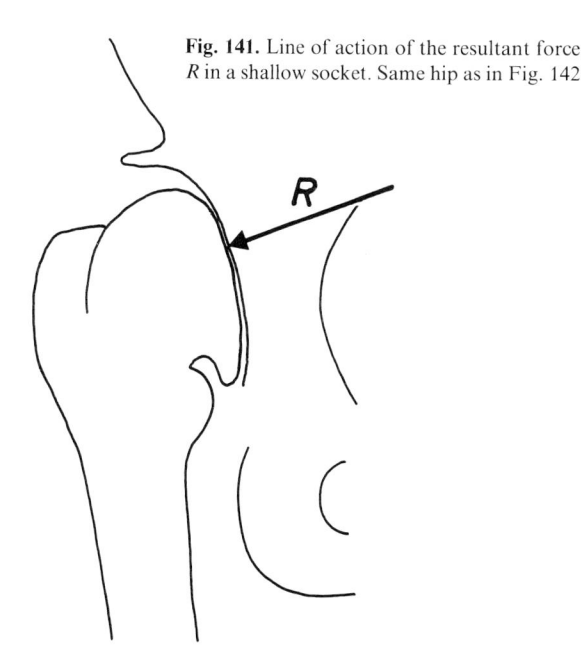

Fig. 141. Line of action of the resultant force R in a shallow socket. Same hip as in Fig. 142

The socket can be very shallow and nearly vertical in direction. If the femoral head has not become completely dislocated, this confirms the fact that the resultant force R acts at right angles to the articular surfaces (Fig. 141), since the coefficient of friction of a joint is very low, lower than that of skates on ice. This contradicts not only the concept of a vertical load acting on the femoral head, but also that of the importance of coverage of the femoral head in the classic sense, as by a shelf operation.

In a 50-year-old female patient (Fig. 142a) with such a shallow acetabulum, a valgus osteotomy was carried out. It enlarged the weight-bearing area of the joint and gave a good result (Fig. 142b) which was still obvious at the 13-year follow-up. Coverage of the femoral head as it is usually understood is irrelevant. What is important is the area of the weight-bearing surface of the joint.

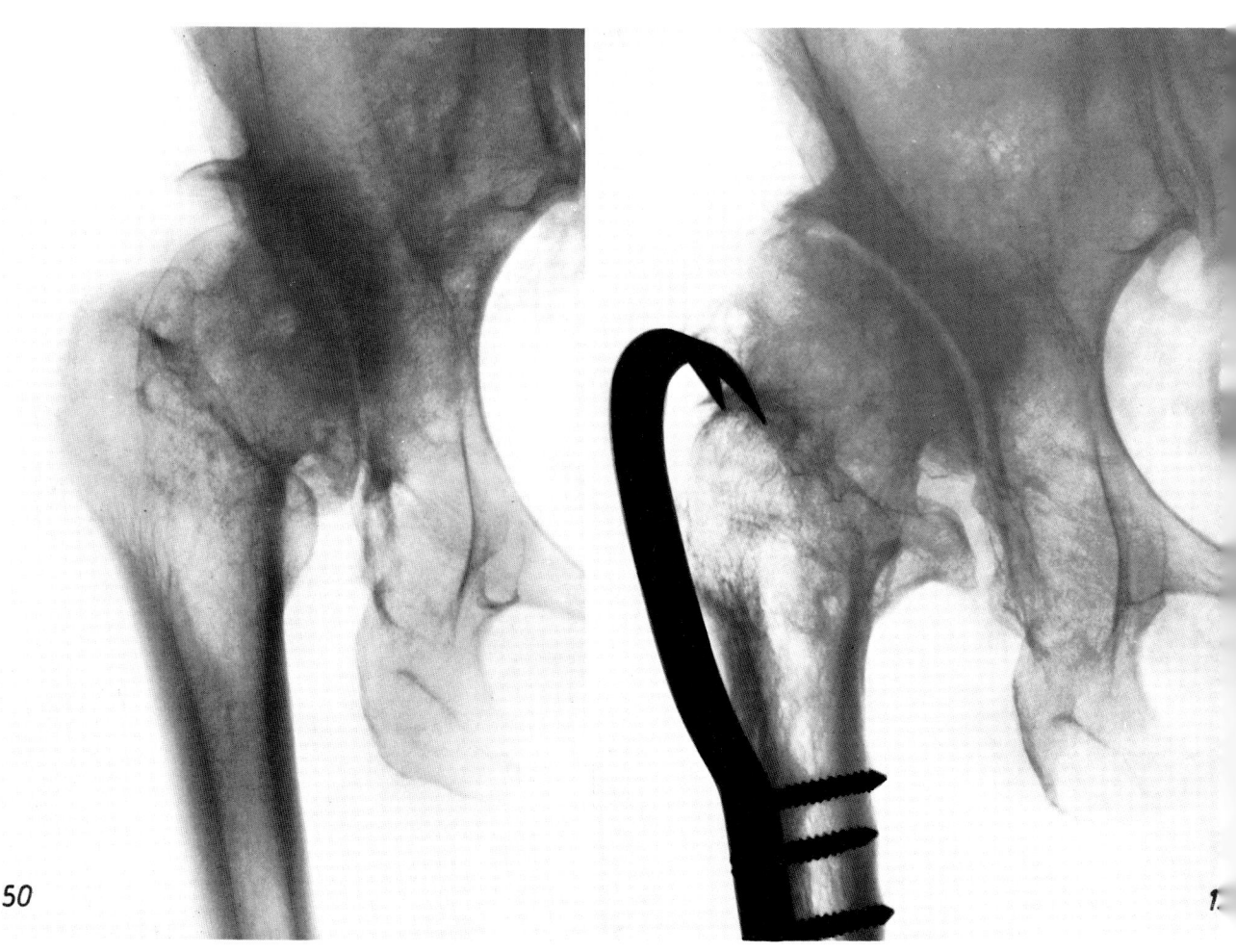

Fig. 142. a A 50-year-old female patient before a Pauwels II carried out despite the shallowness of the socket. **b** Thirteen years afterwards

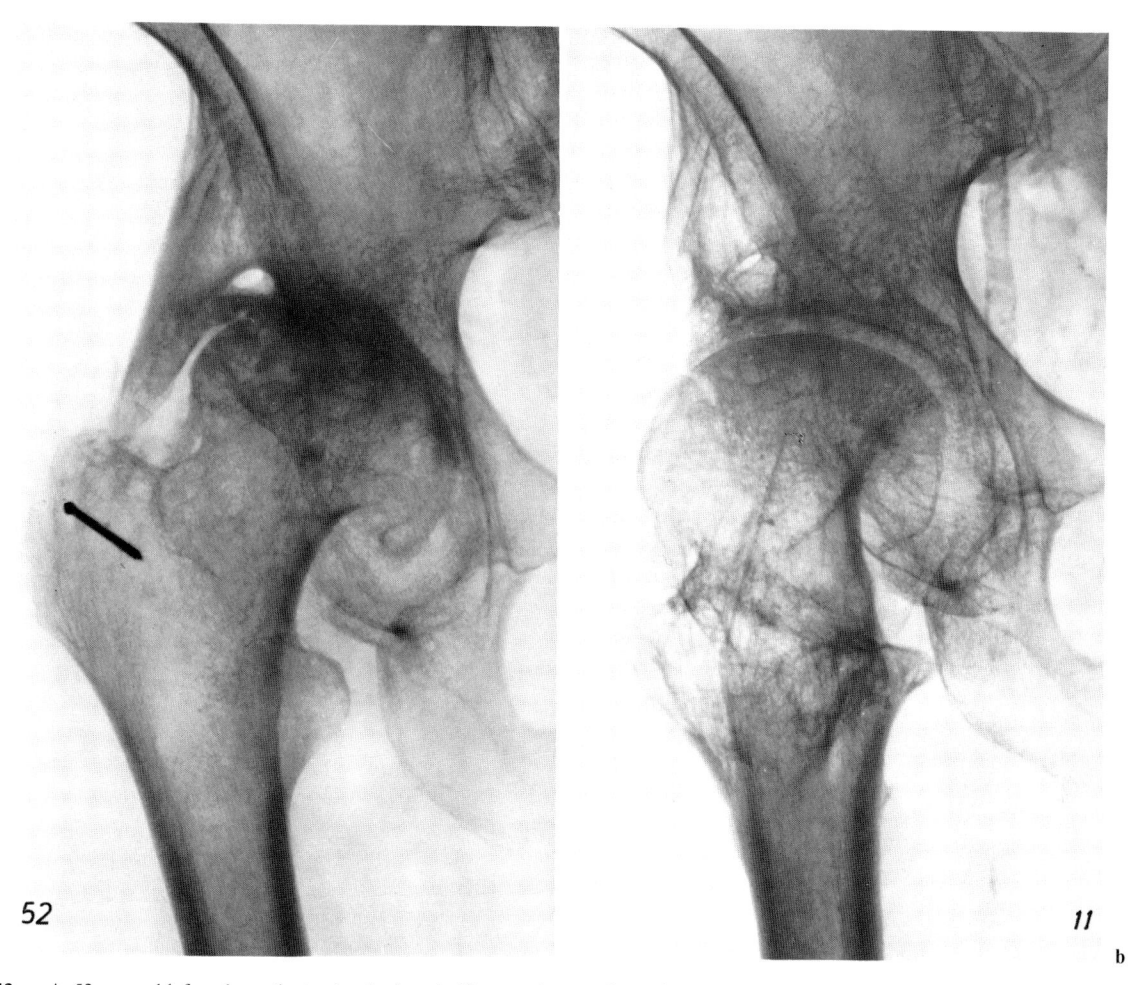

Fig. 143. a A 52-year-old female patient who had a shelf operation performed 11 years previously. **b** Eleven years later, after a valgus intertrochanteric osteotomy combined with a tenotomy and the removal of part of the shelf

A 52-year-old female patient had undergone a shelf operation 11 years previously. Despite the generous coverage of the femoral head thus provided, symptoms persisted and the hip deteriorated further. When we saw her, a sclerotic triangle at the edge of the socket indicated an increase in and concentration of the articular stresses; the joint space had disappeared (Fig. 143a). We removed most of the shelf and carried out a valgus osteotomy combined with a tenotomy, thus further uncovering the femoral head and opening the neck-shaft angle. Although the operation distorted the anatomy to some degree, it enlarged the weight-bearing surface of the joint and decreased the articular compressive stresses. This is confirmed by the result, which remained excellent at the 11-year follow-up (Fig. 143b): a subchondral sclerosis of even thickness throughout underlined the roof of the acetabulum and a wide joint space had reappeared.

H. Conclusion

The valgus intertrochanteric osteotomy is aimed at enlarging the weight-bearing area of the hip joint when the joint is grossly deformed. Diminution of the force transmitted across the joint is additionally achieved by a tenotomy of the abductor, adductor and iliopsoas muscles. The principle is exactly that of a varus osteotomy, but it is carried out differently and the indications are quite different.

V. Lateral Displacement of the Greater Trochanter

A. Rationale

The line of action of the resultant force R passes through the intersection of the lines of action of the forces K exerted by the partial body mass and M exerted by the abductor muscles and through the centre of the femoral head (Fig. 144a). The magnitude of force R depends on the magnitude of the forces K and M and on the angle formed by their lines of action. Opening this angle reduces R.

The resultant force R is transmitted across the weight-bearing surface of the joint. The weight-bearing area depends on the position of R in the joint. The articular compressive stresses (kg/cm^2) depend on the extent of the weight-bearing area of the joint and on the magnitude and position of force R. As a rule, the more medially the line of action of R intersects the acetabulum, the larger is the weight-bearing surface area and the less the joint pressure.

Laterally displacing the greater trochanter provides the abductor muscles with a better leverage (Fig. 144b). These muscles can then carry out their work with a smaller force (M). Lateral displacement of the greater trochanter also changes the direction of force M and lowers its point of intersection with the line of action of force K. This opens the angle formed by the lines of action of the forces K and M and displaces R medially into the socket. The resultant force R is decreased by the diminution of force M and by the opening of the angle formed by the lines of action of forces K and M. Displaced medially into the acetabulum, it is also distributed over a larger weight-bearing

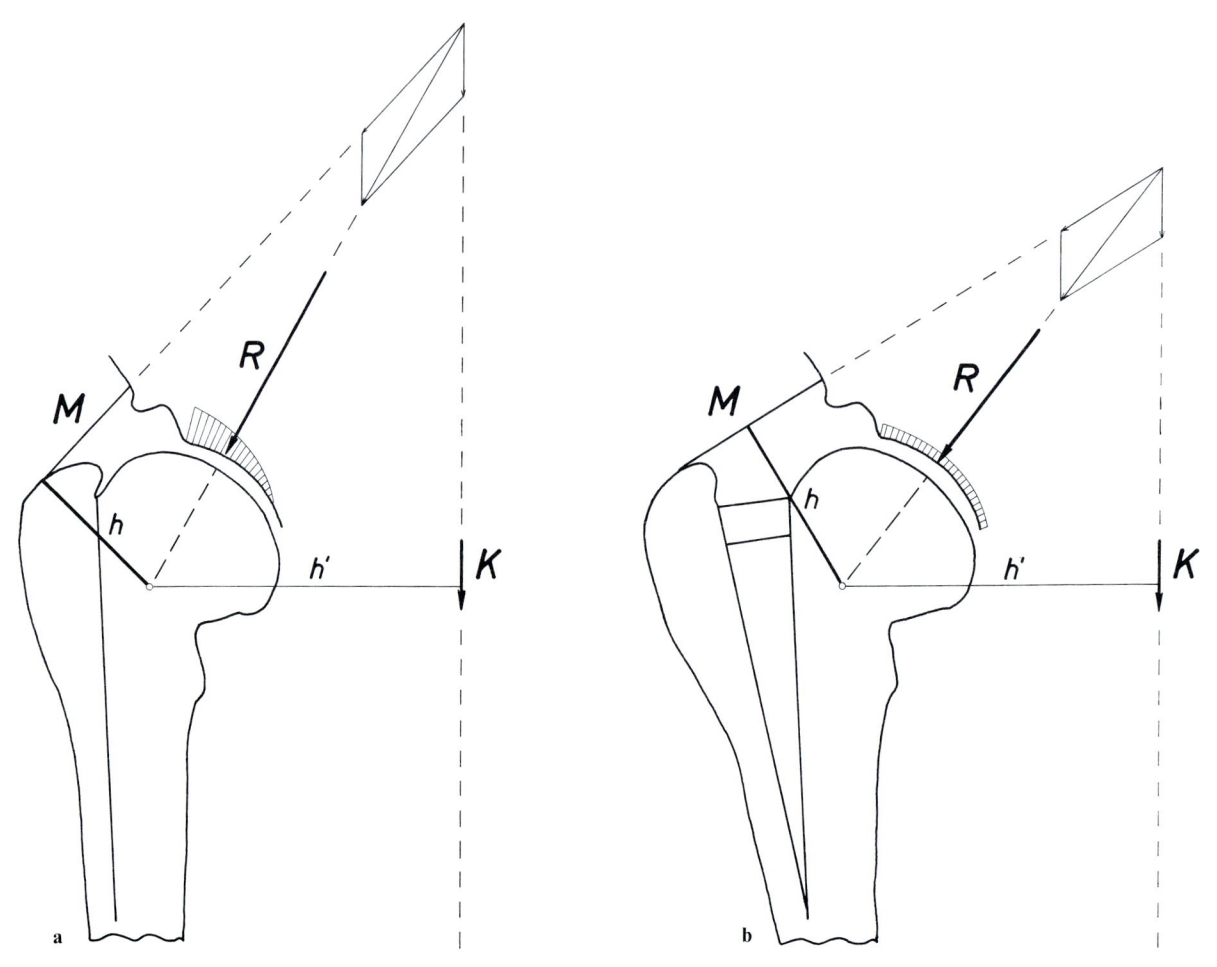

Fig. 144a, b. Lateral displacement of the greater trochanter decreases the force transmitted across the hip and enlarges the weight-bearing surface of the joint. K, force exerted by that part of the body supported by the hip; h', lever arm of force K; M, force exerted by the abductor muscles; h, lever arm of force M; R, resultant of forces K and M. **a** Before operation; **b** after operation

surface than previously. This results in a considerable diminution of the articular compressive stresses, which become more evenly distributed.

A tenotomy of the adductor and iliopsoas muscles is always additionally carried out. It further decreases the force transmitted across the hip joint. Lateral displacement of the greater trochanter combined with a tenotomy of the adductor and iliopsoas muscles reduces the compressive stresses in the hip joint exactly as the varus osteotomy does, by lengthening the lever arm of the abductor muscles, by releasing other muscles and by displacing the resultant force medially into the acetabulum. Both procedures thus decrease the load transmitted across the joint and enlarge the weight-bearing area of the latter.

A distal displacement of the greater trochanter, such as has been suggested in order to tighten the abductor muscles after a total hip replacement, can increase joint pressure (Fig. 145). Distal displacement of the greater trochanter shortens the lever arm h of the force M exerted by the abductor muscles and brings the line of action of this force closer to the vertical. This closes the angle formed by the lines of action of the forces M and K. Shortening the lever arm of the force M exerted by the abductor muscles and closing the angle formed by the lines of action of forces M and K both increase the resultant force R. Moreover, the intersection of the lines of action of forces M and K is displaced upwards. Therefore, R is brought closer to the edge of the acetabulum, thus reducing the weight-bearing part of the joint surface. Increasing the resultant force R and decreasing the weight-bearing area of the joint both increase joint pressure.

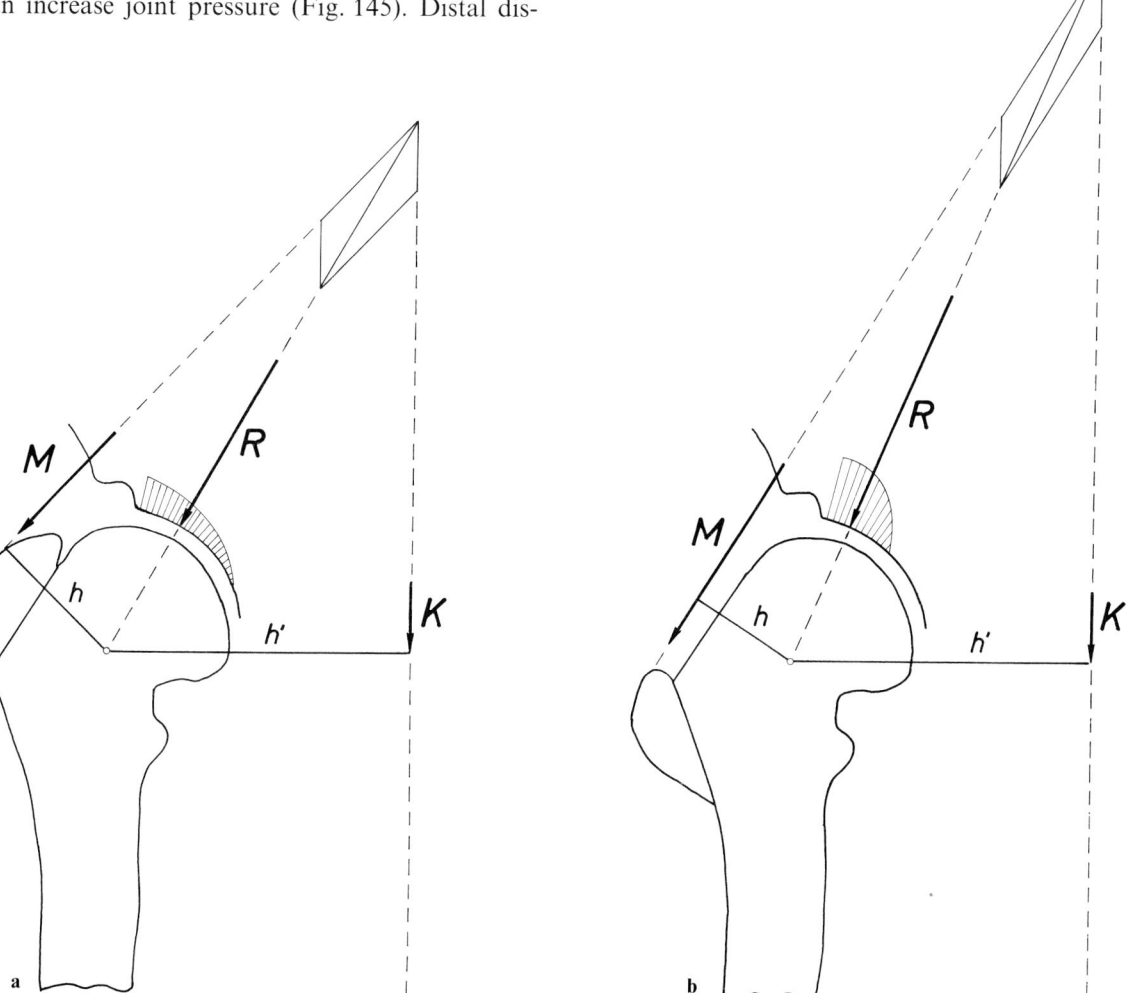

Fig. 145a, b. Displacing the greater trochanter distally may increase the articular compressive stresses in the hip joint by increasing R and reducing the weight-bearing joint surface. K, force exerted by that part of the body supported by the hip; h', lever arm of K; M, force exerted by the abductor muscles; h, lever arm of M; R, resultant of K and M. **a** Before operation; **b** after operation

B. Indications

The indications for lateral displacement of the greater trochanter include:

1. Osteoarthritis or avascular necrosis of the femoral head with congruent joint contours in all positions of the hip, when a proper varus intertrochanteric osteotomy would result in the greater trochanter lying higher than the centre of the femoral head. In patients with incongruent articular surfaces, a lateral displacement of the greater trochanter should not be carried out. A triangular sclerosis at the edge of the socket does not constitute a contra-indication, as long as the joint surfaces are congruent, since the procedure is also aimed at enlarging the weight-bearing area of the joint. This is in contrast to the hanging-hip operation, for which a triangular sclerosis is a contra-indication.

A 56-year-old female patient showed severe osteoarthritis of the hip with narrowing of the joint space and a triangular subchondral sclerosis at the edge of the acetabulum (Fig. 146a). The weight-bearing area of the joint was thus decreased. A 2.5-cm lateral displacement of the greater trochanter was carried out and combined with a tenotomy of the adductor and iliopsoas muscles. At the 6-year follow-up the hip remained pain-free; the full range of movement had been recovered and the patient was not limping. In the X-ray, the dense triangle at the edge of the acetabulum was replaced by a subchondral sclerosis of even width throughout. A wide joint space had reappeared (Fig. 146b).

When the joint surfaces are congruent and there is no sclerotic triangle at the edge of the acetabulum, if the greater trochanter is high, one may choose between a hanging-hip procedure and a lateral displacement of the greater trochanter. A

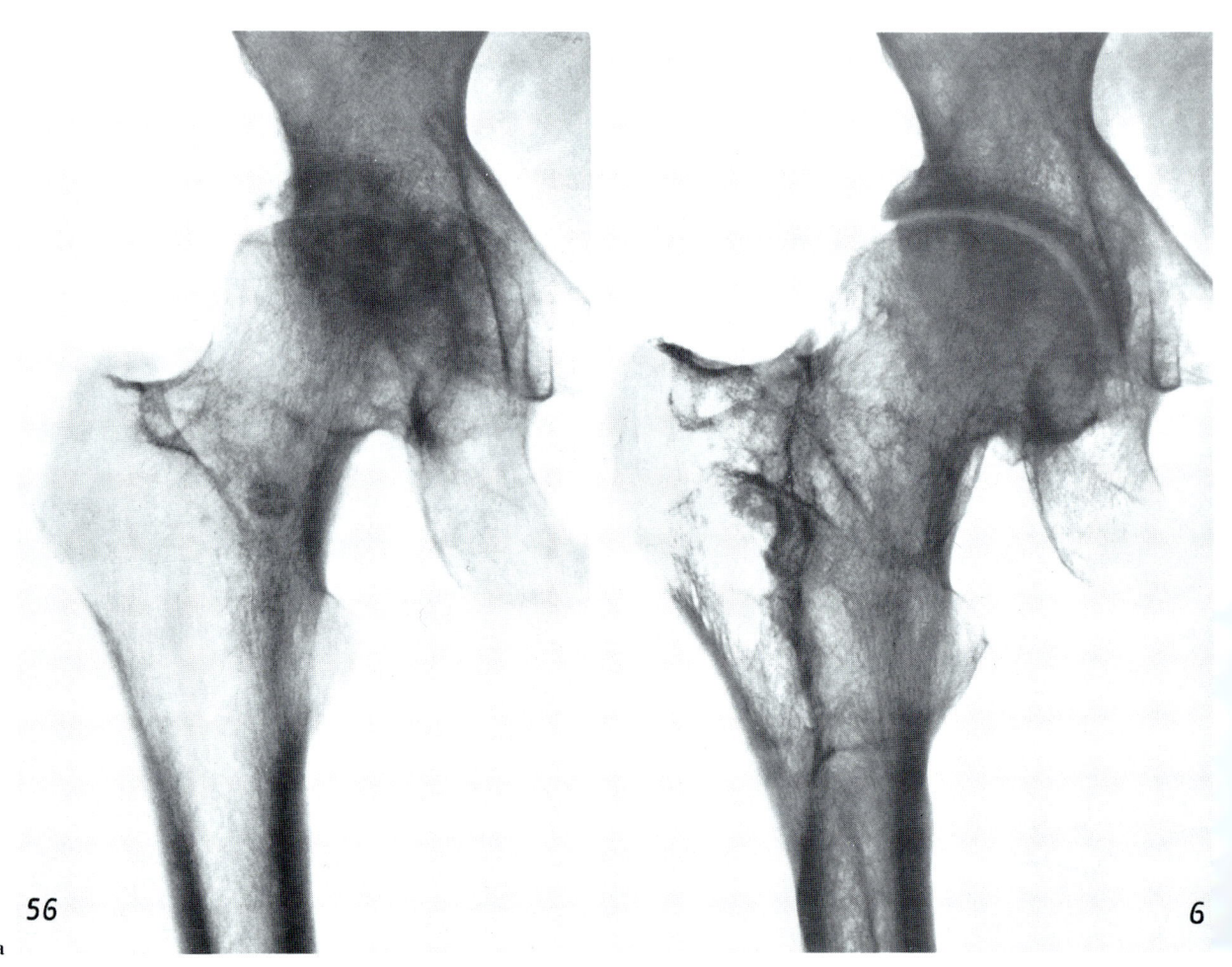

Fig. 146. a A 56-year-old female patient before lateral displacement of the greater trochanter. **b** Six years afterwards

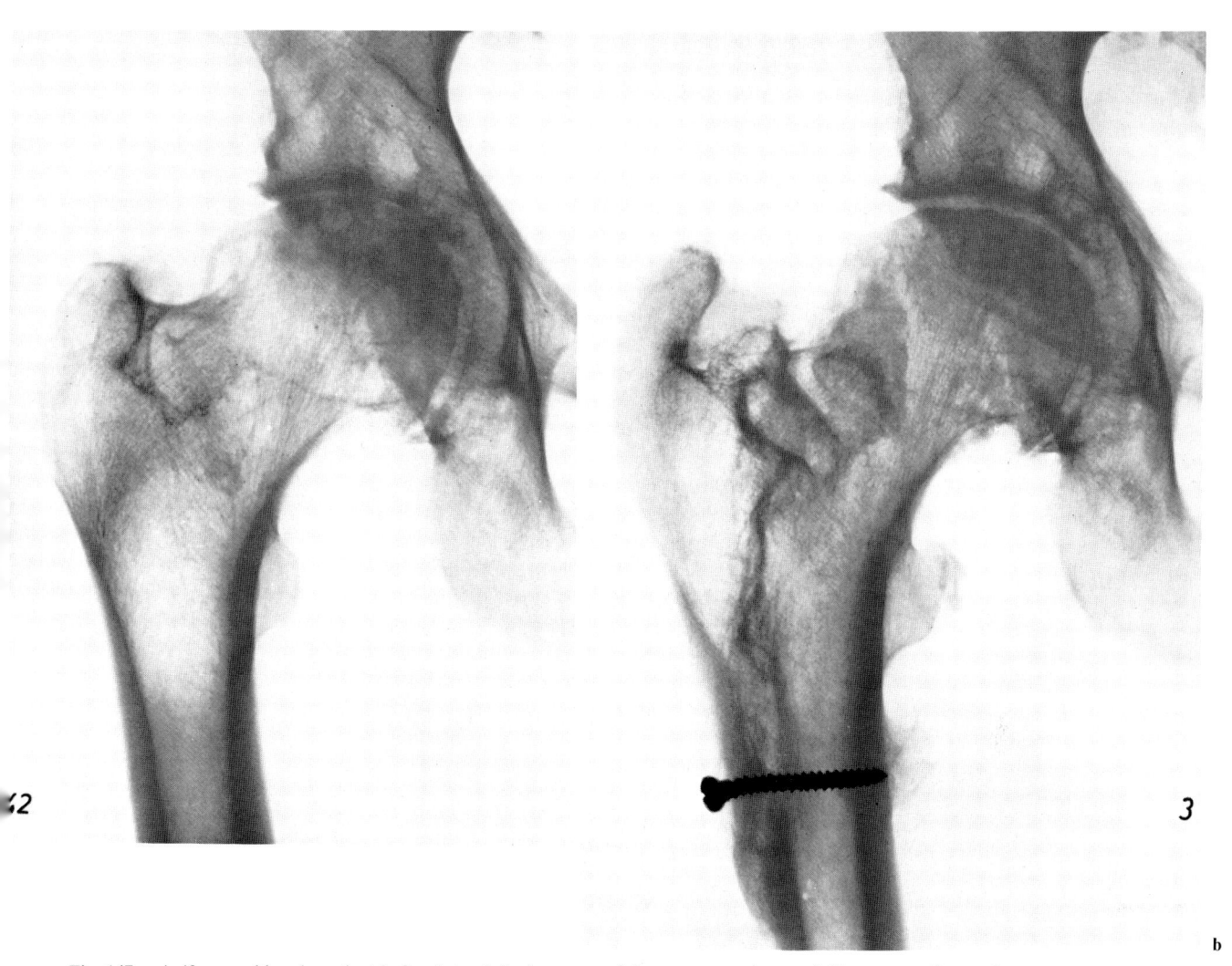

Fig. 147. a A 42-year-old male patient before lateral displacement of the greater trochanter. b Four years afterwards

lateral displacement of the greater trochanter is usually preferable in younger patients, since the procedure has a more significant mechanical effect than the hanging-hip operation.

A 42-year-old male patient had a hanging-hip operation for osteoarthritis ten years previously with a good result. He complained of pain in the opposite hip, which showed signs of osteoarthritis without reduction of the weight-bearing area, since there was no dense triangle at the edge of the acetabulum (Fig. 147a). A 2.5-cm lateral displacement of the greater trochanter was carried out on the painful side. At the 4-year follow-up the hip remained pain-free; the patient had recovered the full range of movement and was not limping. A wide joint space had reappeared (Fig. 147b). The patient was employed as a lorry driver.

2. Hips in which a varus or a valgus osteotomy has been carried out for osteoarthritis, ensuring good congruence of the articular surfaces and resulting in an enlarged weight-bearing area but which have either a short femoral neck or pronounced coxa valga with a short lever arm of the abductor muscles.

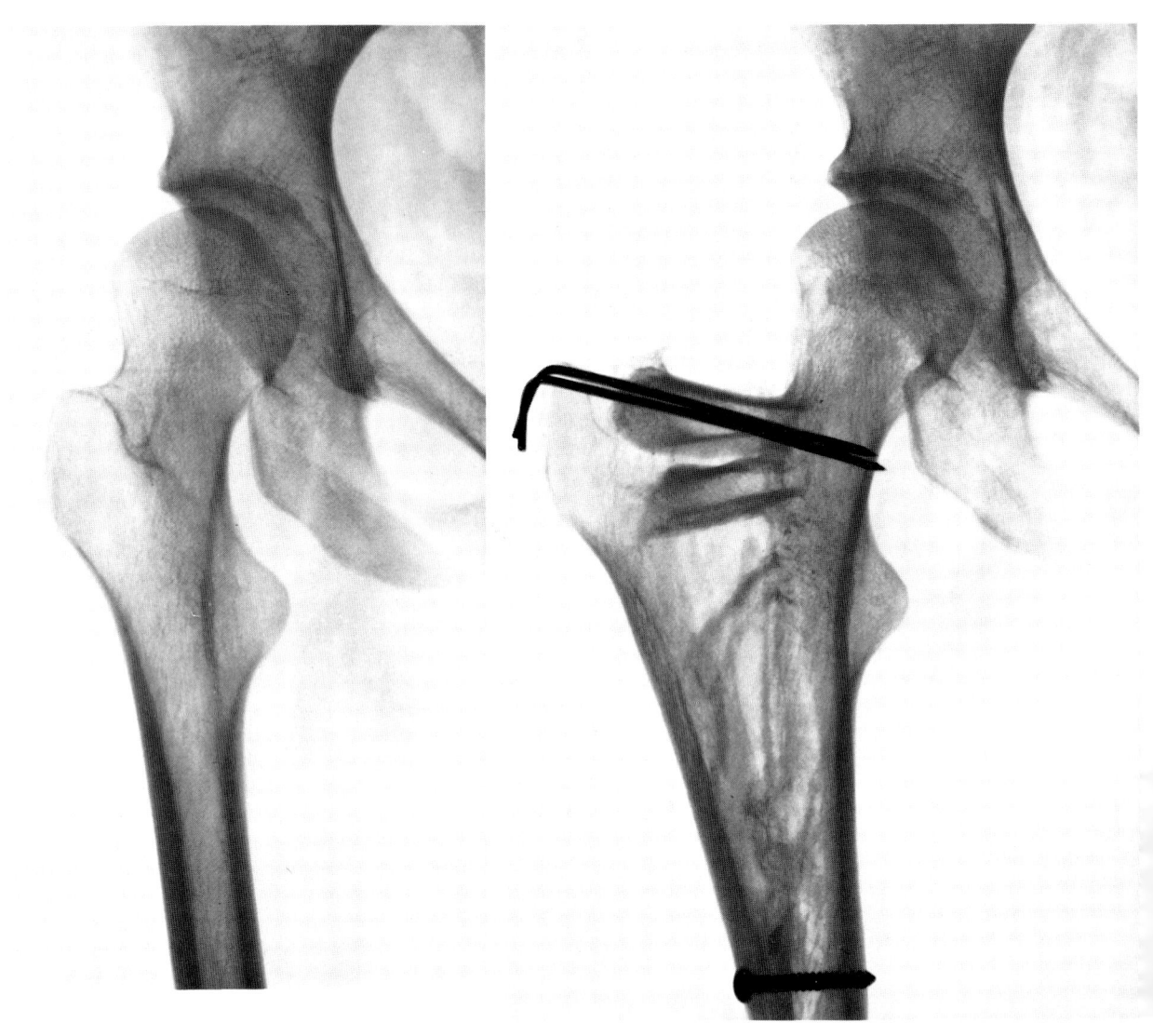

Fig. 148. a A 26-year-old female patient with a post-poliomyelitis limp before lateral displacement of the greater trochanter. **b** Two years afterwards

3. Limping due to weakness of the abductor muscles, for instance after poliomyelitis. In such cases the aim is to improve the leverage of the abductor muscles. A 26-year-old female patient limped badly after poliomyelitis, as a result of the weakness of the abductor muscles (Fig. 148a). The greater trochanter was displaced laterally by nearly 5 cm (Fig. 148b). At the 2-year follow-up the limping had disappeared. When lying on the opposite side, the patient could raise the leg in abduction. Provided with a much longer lever arm, the abductor muscles were now able to carry out their work.

Except in the case of the last indication (3.), the prerequisites for a lateral displacement of the greater trochanter can be summarized as follows:

1. Subluxating or concentric osteoarthritis; aseptic necrosis of the femoral head
2. Congruent joint surfaces
3. High location of the greater trochanter

Fig. 149. Pre-operative planning for the procedure carried out on the hip shown in Fig. 146

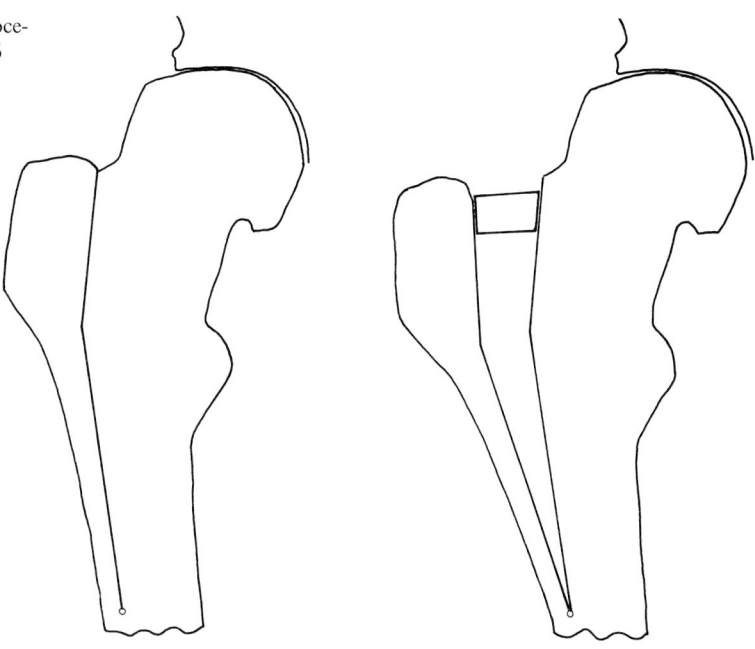

C. Pre-operative Planning

The contours of the socket and of the upper end of the femur are traced on a half-sheet of transparent paper (Fig. 149). A longitudinal line is drawn from the junction of the greater trochanter and the femoral neck to a point 12–15 cm distally, positioned at the junction of the lateral quarter and the medial three-quarters of the cross section of the femur. The sheet is then folded. The hip and that part of the femur medial to the longitudinal line are traced from the first onto the second half-sheet. The two half-sheets are then separated and the second is rotated over the first about the distal end of the longitudinal line (clockwise for a right hip) until the greater trochanter of the first half-sheet appears 2.5–3 cm or more, as desired, lateral to the remainder of the femur on the second half-sheet. The greater trochanter and the lateral part of the upper femur are then traced from the first onto the second half-sheet.

When there is a choice to be made between a lateral displacement of the greater trochanter and a varus osteotomy it is often useful to execute the drawings for both operations and to represent the forces as in Fig. 153. The mechanical action of the two procedures thus becomes evident and the better solution can be chosen.

D. Operative Procedure

The usual instruments for soft tissues and the instruments for bone surgery listed on p. 79 are used, with the addition of one special instrument, the MAQUET bone-spreader[3] (Fig. 150). This instrument derives from the LOWMAN bone clamp. It presents two longitudinal parts, one sliding in the other under the action of a screw. A flat piece of metal is fixed at 90° at the extremity of the supporting longitudinal part. Another flat piece of metal is articulated about an axle at the extremity of the sliding longitudinal part. The two flat pieces of metal brought together are inserted in the gap between the two fragments of bone. By sliding the mobile longitudinal part, its flat piece of metal is brought away from that fixed on the other longitudinal part and can pivot about its axle, according to the inclination of the elevated bone fragment.

The operation is carried out on a table transparent to X-rays, using general anaesthesia and tracheal intubation.

1. The patient lies supine. A full-thickness graft is taken from the lateral aspect of the ilium beneath the iliac crest. Its size is at least 4 cm × 2 cm, preferably more. The crest is preserved for cosmetic reasons. The aponeurosis, subcutaneous fat and skin are sutured using suction drainage.

2. A tenotomy of the adductor and iliopsoas muscles is carried out as described above (p. 68).

3. The patient is turned over on the abdomen with a pillow beneath the chest. The lateral incision extends from the greater trochanter about 15 cm distally. The fascia lata is incised along its fibers. The vastus lateralis is detached from the base of the greater trochanter and along the linea aspera, sufficiently to show the posterolateral aspect of the femur for a width of about 1 cm. The bone is cleared as far as the upper and medial junction between greater trochanter and femoral neck. A 2-mm hole is drilled from behind forwards at the distal end of the incision, 7–10 mm from the lateral border of the femoral shaft. The osteotomy is then begun with a rotating or an oscillating saw, from this distal hole proximally to the junction of the greater trochanter and the upper aspect of the femoral neck. The osteotomy is completed with a thin chisel. The limb is then brought into full abduction. The lateral flap of bone and the greater trochanter are separated from the main part of the femur using the special spreader. The iliac graft is then tailored to the proper size and inserted on edge, in the gap, medial to the greater trochanter, as proximally as possible. The femoral flap nearly always breaks at its distal attachment. It is fixed with a cortical screw, as far distally as possible. The graft is squeezed by the pressure of the bony flap. This may be sufficient to hold it. If not, two KIRSCHNER wires can be drilled transversely through the greater trochanter and graft and into the femoral neck. The different tissue layers are carefully sutured with drainage but without suction. The blood loss may be greater than in a varus or valgus osteotomy.

E. Postoperative Care

The postoperative care is the same as after the varus or valgus osteotomy.

The patient may move in bed immediately. Two days after surgery, he is helped to stand up, and on the third day he starts walking with two crutches. If the condition was severe, he is advised to use his crutches for about 6 months, putting only part of his weight (15%–20% of body weight) on the affected limb. He then uses one crutch for another 6 months in order to relieve the pressure

---
[3] Available from J.R.I., 104–112 Marylebone Lane, London W1.

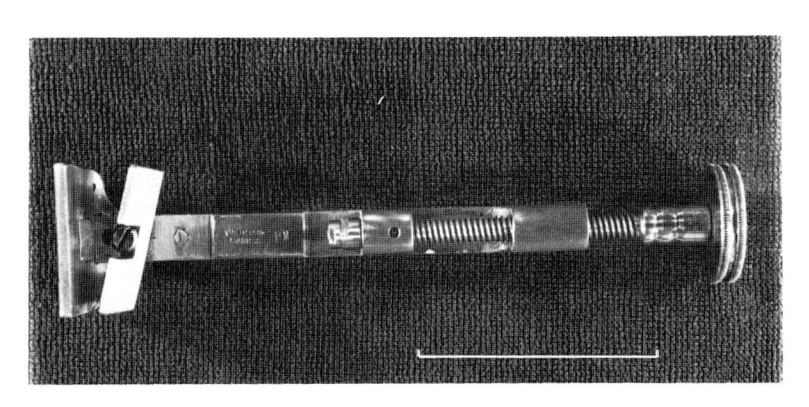

Fig. 150. Maquet bone-spreader

on the joint during the process of remodelling. All active exercises except walking are avoided. Strengthening of the muscles would increase joint pressure, which is just the opposite of the aim of the operation.

F. Postoperative Evolution

The postoperative evolution compares favourably with that of the varus or valgus intertrochanteric osteotomy. The pain disappears immediately. The range of movement usually improves, often dramatically. The patient limps for a shorter period of time and feels stable on the operated leg sooner than after an intertrochanteric osteotomy. The X-ray evolution is essentially similar.

The procedure was carried out in a 54-year-old female patient with primary osteoarthritis of the hip (Fig. 151a). The cup-shaped subchondral sclerosis in the roof of the acetabulum pointed to a normal position of the line of action of the resultant force R. The joint space was completely obliterated and cysts were visible in the femoral head and in the socket. One year after a considerable lateral displacement of the greater trochanter, the hip remained pain-free with a full range of movement, and the patient no longer limped. In the X-ray, a subchondral sclerosis of uniform width throughout appeared in the roof of the acetabulum and a clearly delineated joint space had developed (Fig. 151b).

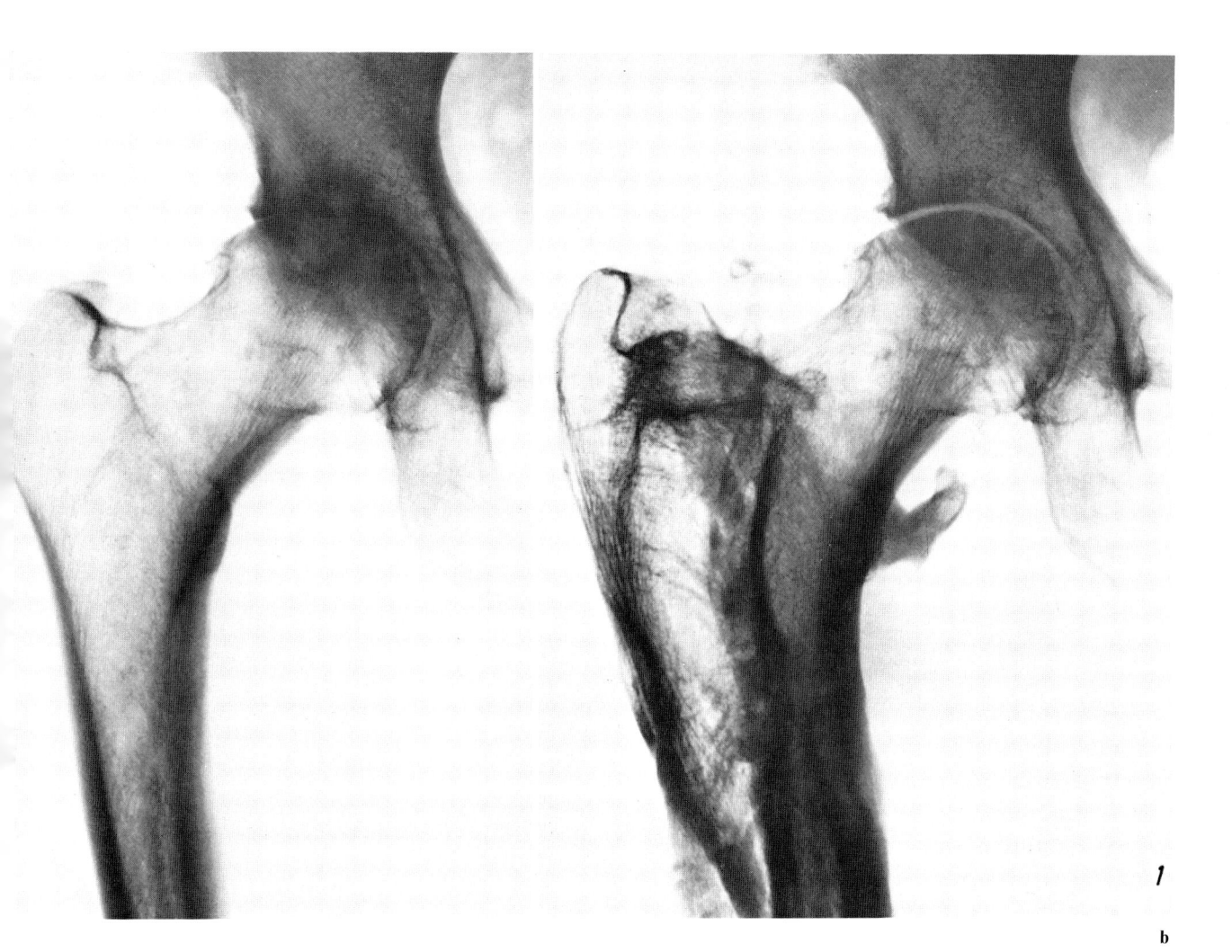

Fig. 151. a A 54-year-old female patient before lateral displacement of the greater trochanter. **b** One year afterwards

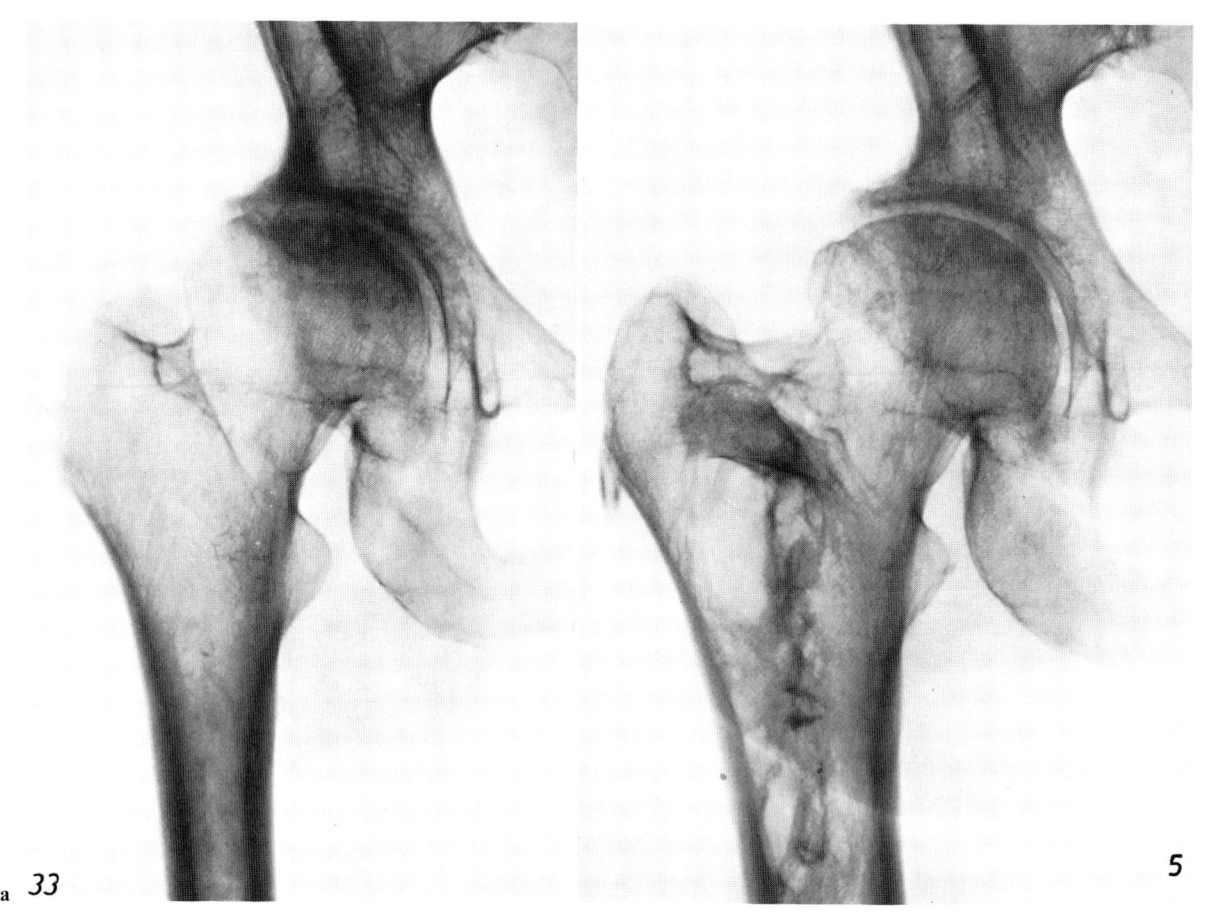

Fig. 152. a A 33-year-old female patient before lateral displacement of the greater trochanter. **b** Five years afterwards

The same procedure was carried out in a 33-year-old female patient with an avascular necrosis of the femoral head (Fig. 152a). In this instance the mechanical effect of the lateral displacement of the greater trochanter was calculated and compared with that of a varus intertrochanteric osteotomy (Fig. 153). Because of the shortness of the femoral neck and the position of the greater trochanter, a varus intertrochanteric osteotomy would hardly have lengthened the leverarm h of the force M exerted by the abductor muscles (Fig. 153a). Changing the direction of M would somewhat have decreased the resultant force R and would have brought it further into the acetabulum. However, a 2-cm lateral displacement of the greater trochanter appeared to be mechanically more efficient in decreasing R and in enlarging the weight-bearing area of the joint (Fig. 153b). Five years after the lateral displacement of the greater trochanter, the clinical result remained excellent: no pain, full range of movement (Table 20), normal gait and unrestricted walking capacity. In the X-ray, the dense triangle in the roof of the acetabulum had been replaced by a thin ribbon of dense bone of the same width throughout, delineating a wide joint space (Fig. 152b).

Table 20. Range of movement of the hip (Fig. 152)

	Before surgery	At the 5-year follow-up	Gain
Flexion	90°	115°	30°
Extension	5°	10°	
Adduction	5°	45°	75°
Abduction	25°	60°	
Int. rotation	5°	70°	115°
Ext. rotation	0°	50°	

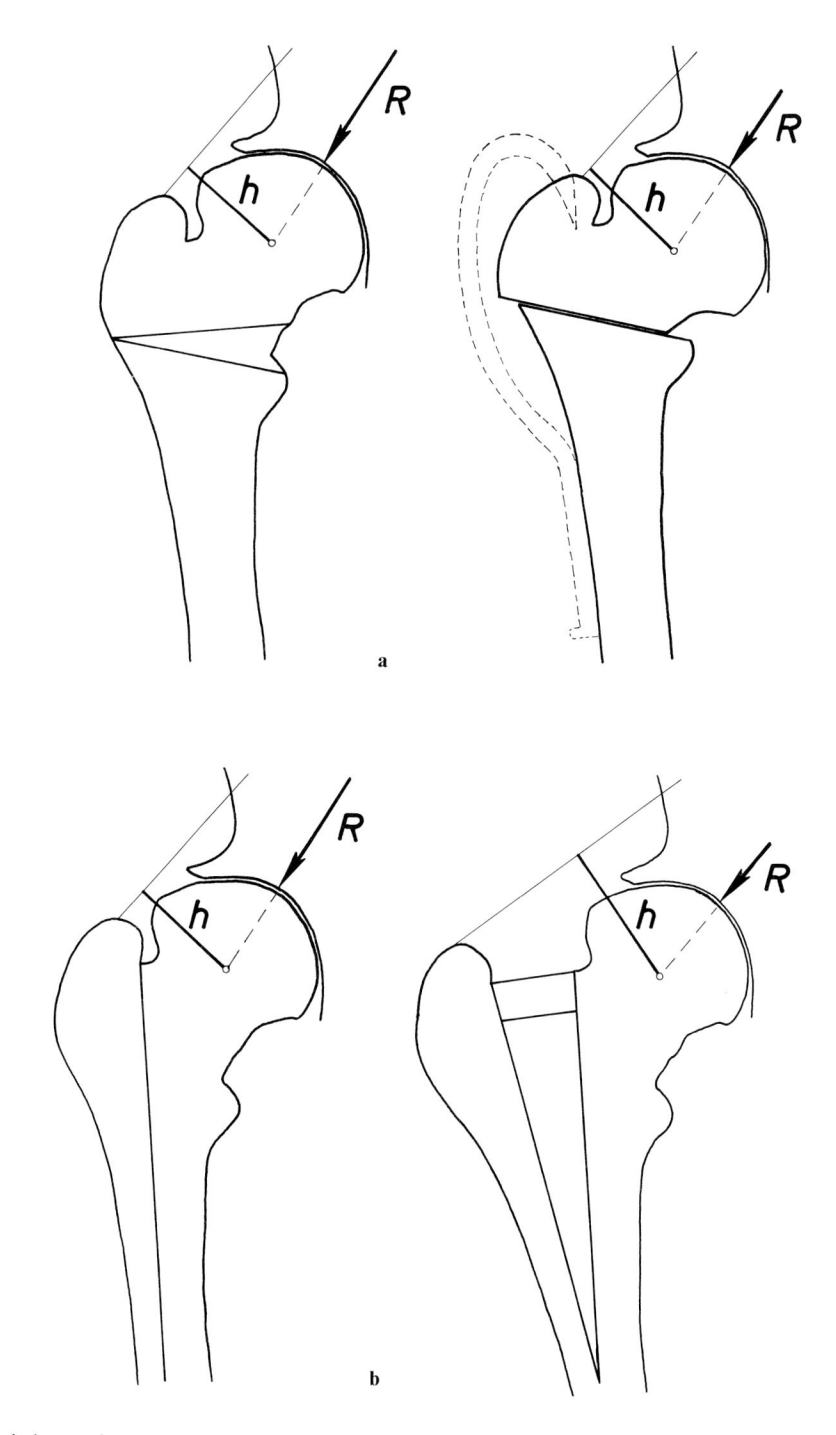

Fig. 153. Comparison of the change in the balance of forces resulting from **a** a varus osteotomy and **b** a 2-cm lateral displacement of the greater trochanter. h, lever arm of M, the force exerted by the abductor muscles; R, resultant of M and the force K exerted by the part of the body supported by the hip

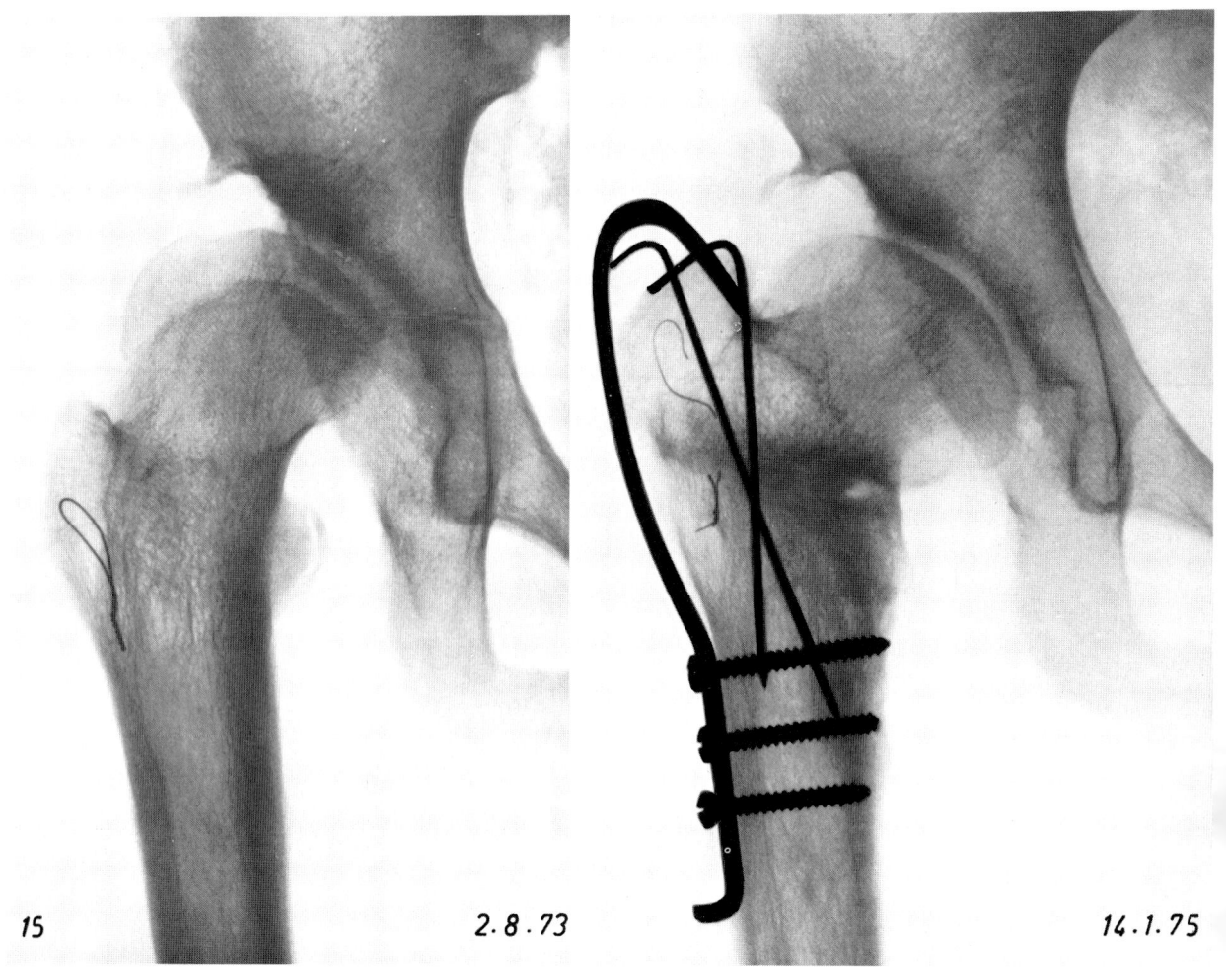

Fig. 154. a A 15-year-old male patient who had undergone a shelf operation elsewhere. **b** One year after a varus intertrochanteric osteotomy. **c** Lateral displacement of the greater trochanter. **d** Four years later

G. Lateral Displacement of the Greater Trochanter Complementing a Varus Intertrochanteric Osteotomy

In subluxated hips, the femoral head may have to be relocated in its socket. An additional lateral displacement of the greater trochanter may improve the mechanical conditions even further.

A 15-year-old boy had undergone a shelf operation elsewhere (Fig. 154a). The operation was unsuccessful and the congenital subluxation of the hip persisted; a dense triangle in the roof of the socket developed as a reaction to increased articular pressure. The affected leg was 2 cm shorter than the other. A 42° varus intertrochanteric osteotomy was planned, and was carried out by removing a 21° wedge, rotating it and replacing it between the fragments (Figs. 154 and 155). One year later the opposite femur was shortened by resection of a diaphysial fragment of 2 cm. At the same session the implant was removed from the first side and the greater trochanter was displaced laterally, using the fragment of the opposite femur as a graft (Fig. 154c). At the latest follow-up, 5 years after the beginning of the treatment, the clinical result remained excellent. The patient was a manual labourer with full working capacity. The dense triangle in the roof of the acetabulum had nearly disappeared (Fig. 154d).

It is interesting to analyse graphically the mechanical effect of the varus osteotomy (Fig. 156a, b) and that of the subsequent lateral displacement of the greater trochanter (Fig. 156b, c). One effectively complemented the other.

21.3.75

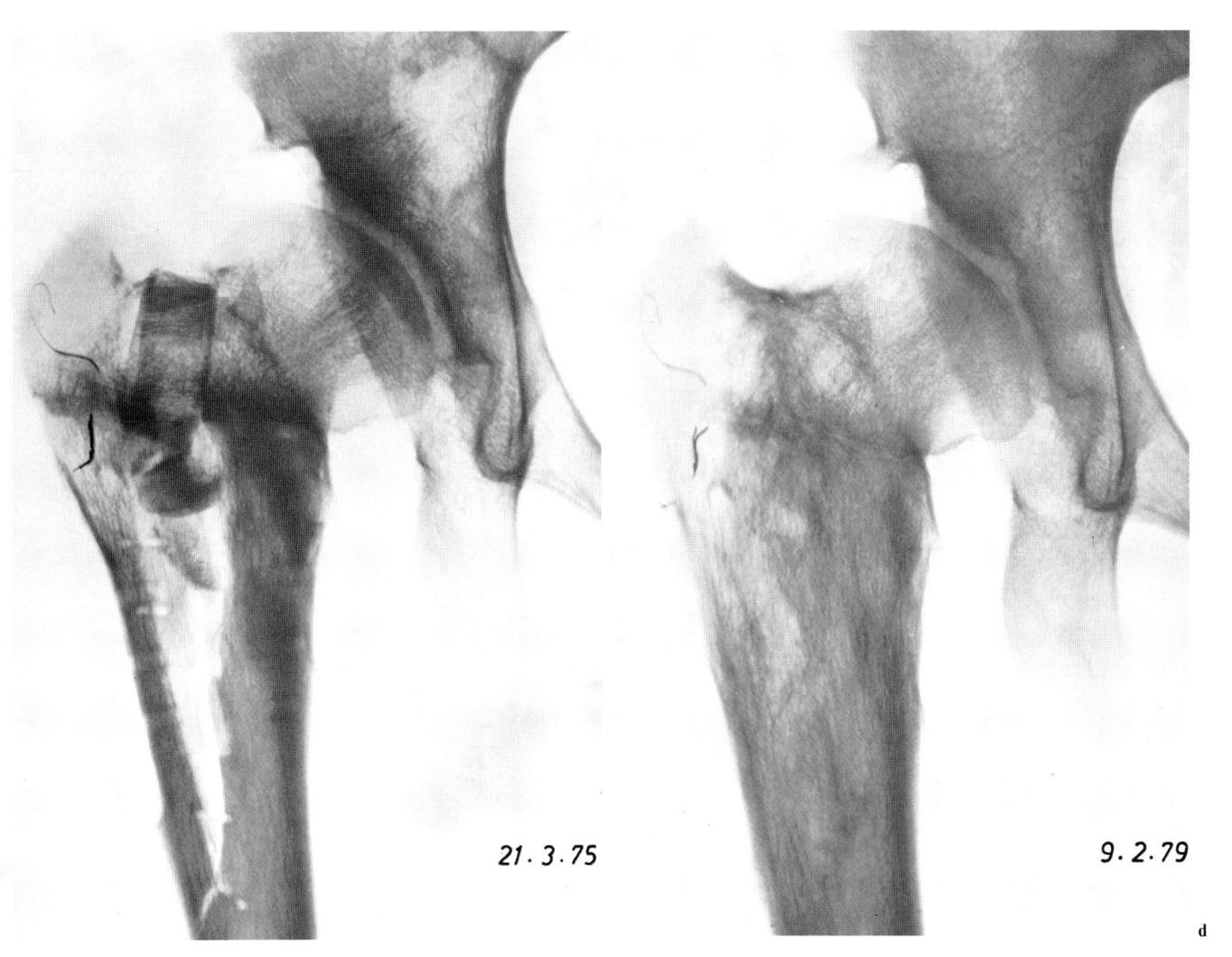

9.2.79

d

Fig. 154c, d

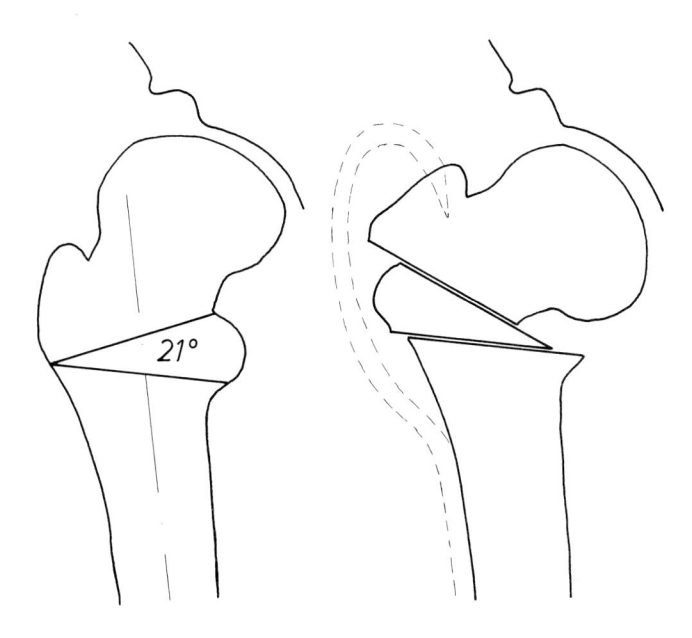

Fig. 155. Varus osteotomy: same hip as in Fig. 154

21°

145

Fig. 156 a

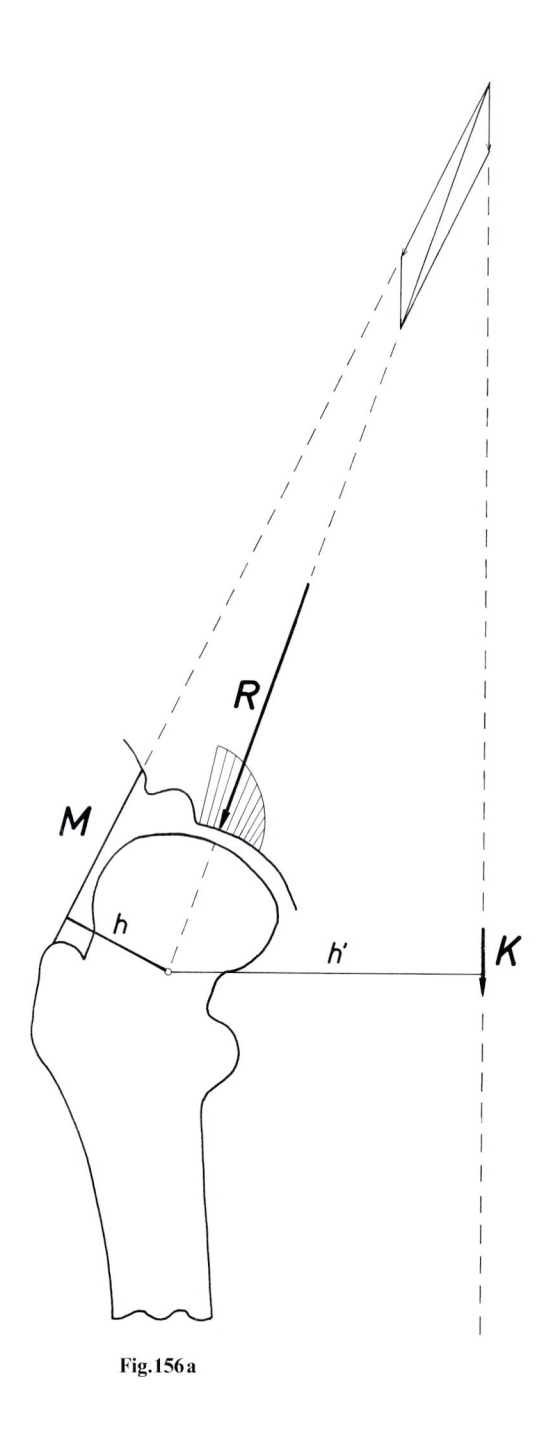

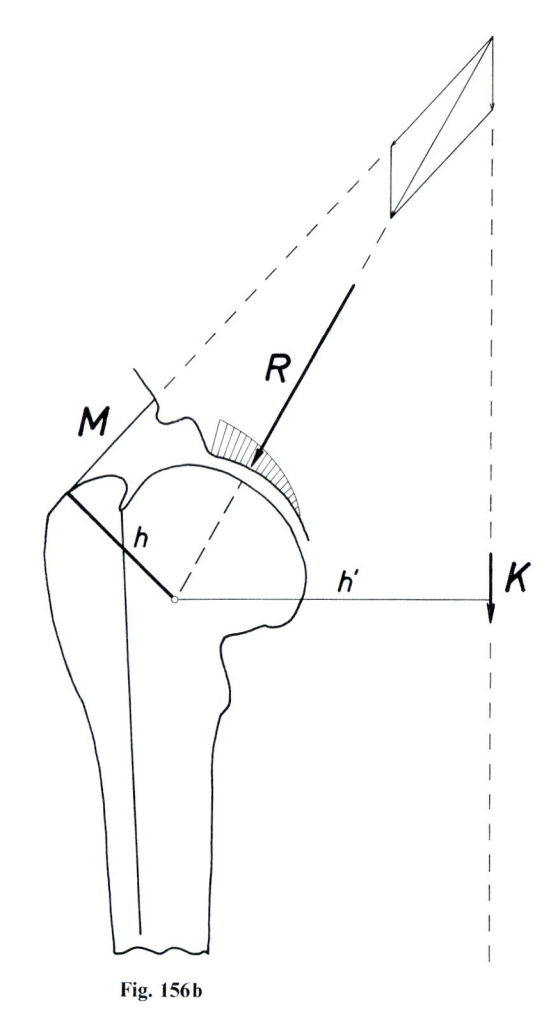

Fig. 156 b

Fig. 156c

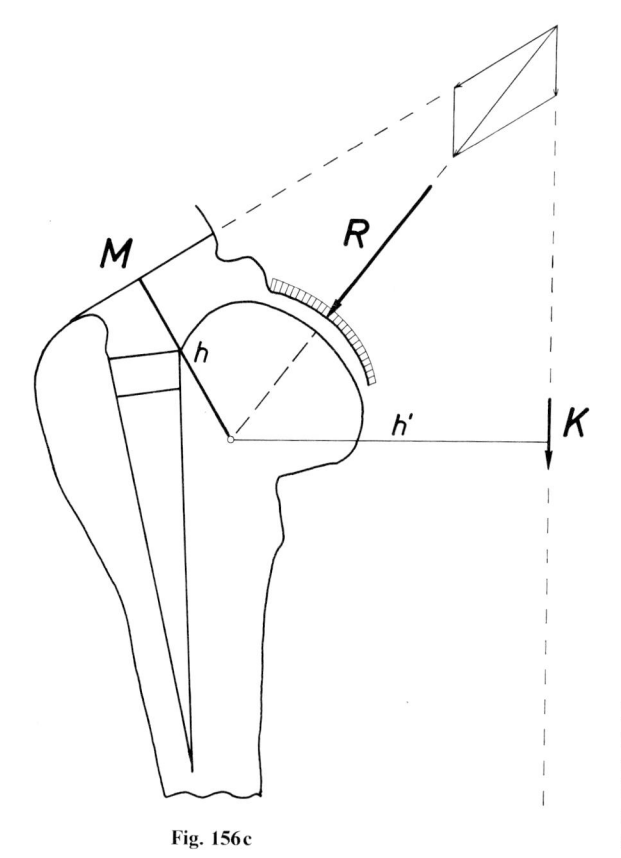

Fig. 156. Mechanical effect of the varus intertrochanteric osteotomy (**a, b**) and of the lateral displacement of the greater trochanter (**b, c**): same hip as in Figs. 154 and 155. K, force exerted by that part of the body supported by the hip; h', lever arm of K; M, force exerted by the abductor muscles; h, lever arm of M; R, resultant of K and M

Fig. 157. a A 55-year-old male patient before a Pauwels II. **b** Two years afterwards. **c** Five years after an additional lateral displacement of the greater trochanter

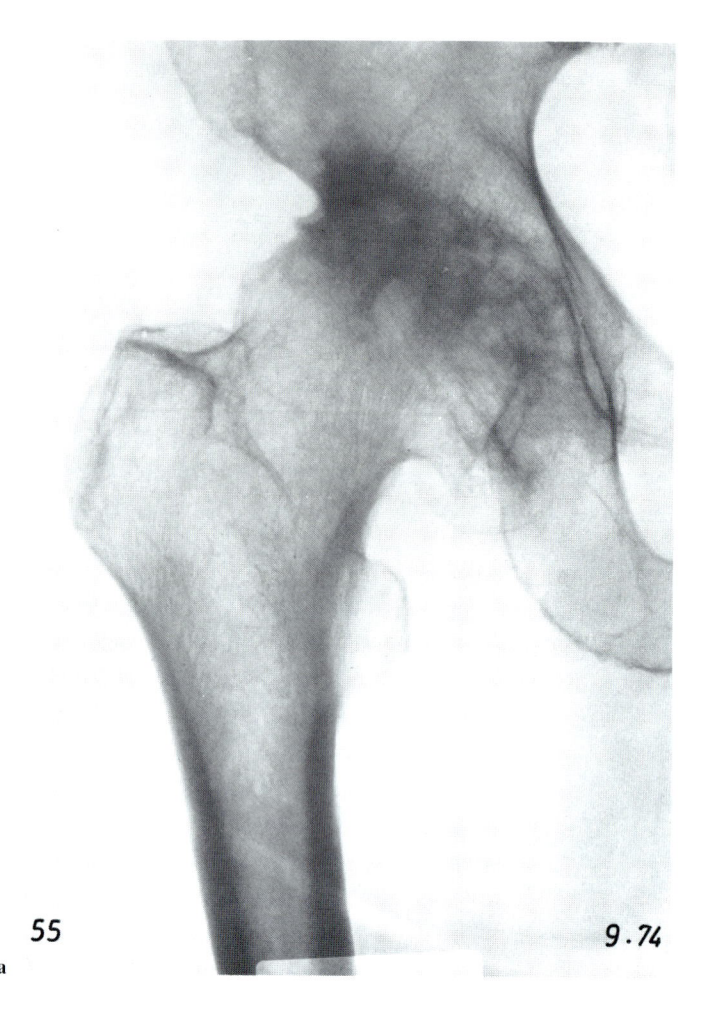

H. Lateral Displacement of the Greater Trochanter Complementing a Valgus Intertrochanteric Osteotomy

The valgus intertrochanteric osteotomy is aimed mainly at enlarging the weight-bearing surface of the joint. It may or may not shorten the lever arm of the force exerted by the abductor muscles (p. 102). In any case, displacing the greater trochanter laterally can enhance the favourable effect of the valgus osteotomy by further decreasing joint pressure.

A 55-year-old male patient with severe osteoarthritis (Fig. 157a) underwent a valgus intertrochanteric osteotomy. Two years later, the articular surfaces were congruent and the triangular subchondral sclerosis had regressed, but the joint space remained very narrow (Fig. 157b). The greater trochanter was then displaced laterally. This resulted in further regression of the pathological subchondral sclerosis and in a dramatic widening of the joint space. At the 5-year follow-up, the result remained good (Fig. 157c).

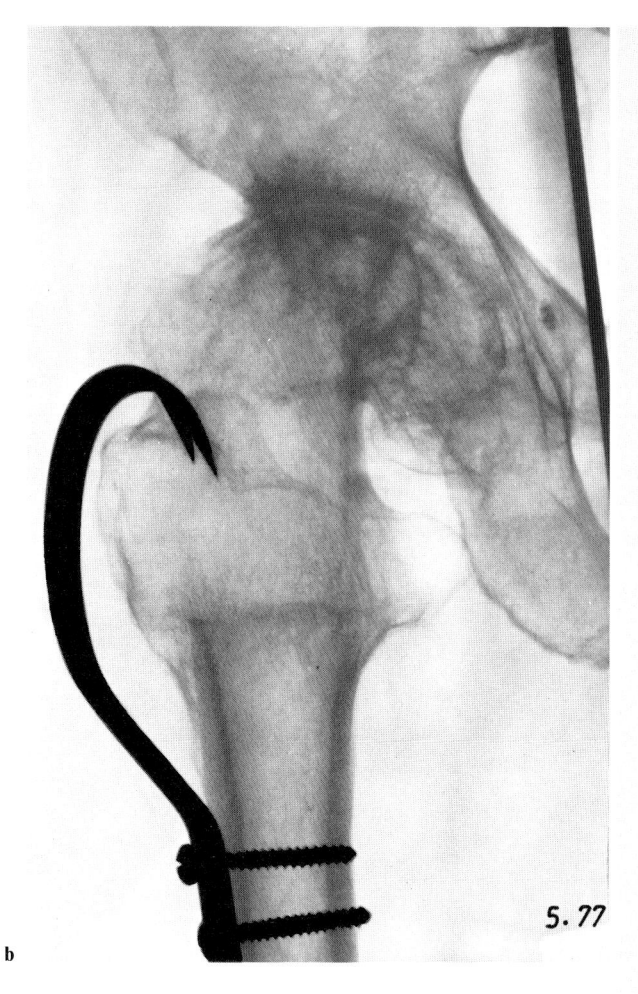

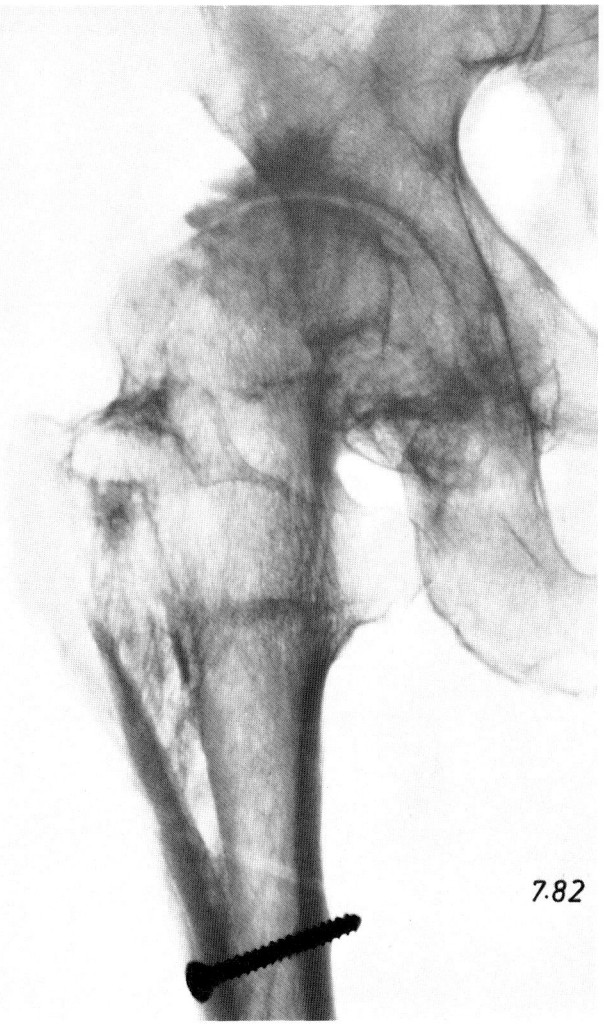

I. Conclusion

Lateral displacement of the greater trochanter combined with tenotomy of the adductor and iliopsoas muscles constitutes an alternative to varus intertrochanteric osteotomy when the greater trochanter is high or when the femoral neck is short. The articular surfaces must be congruent. Both procedures pursue the same goal and apply the same mechanical principles in two different ways. Their results are comparable as long as the indications are correct.

VI. Shortening of the Opposite Leg

A. Rationale

When the socket and femoral head are flattened, the weight-bearing area of the joint can often be increased significantly by a valgus osteotomy (p. 102). As far as the weight-bearing area of the hip is concerned, turning the socket about the femoral head, clockwise in Fig. 158a, as occurs when the opposite leg is shortened, must be equivalent to turning the femoral head in the socket, counterclockwise in Fig. 158b, as a valgus osteotomy does.

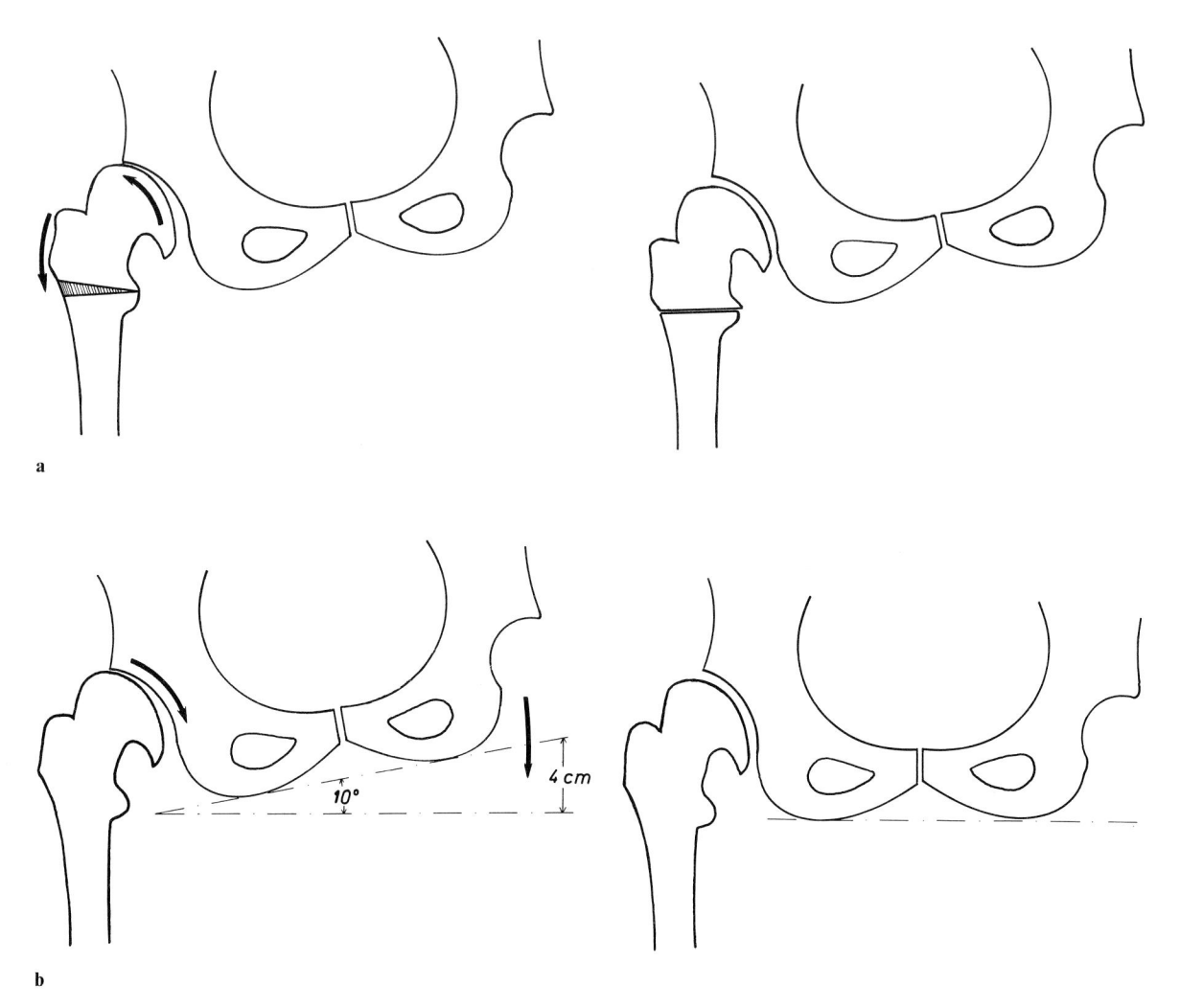

Fig. 158. Increasing the articular weight-bearing surface either **a** by turning the femoral head inside the socket or **b** by turning the socket about the femoral head

A 57-year-old female patient complaining of pain in both hips presented with bilateral dysplasia and the right femoral head articulating in a false joint more proximal than the normal socket. The pelvis was tilted to the right, resulting in an apparent discrepancy of leg length of 4 cm. The patient had developed severe bilateral osteoarthritis (Fig. 159a). A left valgus osteotomy of 55° was planned and carried out, combined with a 4-cm shortening of the left leg (Fig. 160). The shortening of the left leg compelled the pelvis to turn about the right femoral head as if a valgus osteotomy of 10° had been carried out on the right side (Fig. 161). Both hips dramatically improved. Eleven years later the result remained good, not only on the side (Table 21) which had been operated on, but also on the other side (Table 22), which did not undergo any surgery (Fig. 159b). The biological effect of the osteotomy on the left side cannot be adduced as an explanation of the good result in the right hip. Only a change in the mechanical conditions, an increase in the area of the weight-bearing surface, can have led to healing.

Table 21. Range of movement of the left hip in Fig. 159

	Before surgery	At the 11-year follow-up	Gain
Flexion	70°	85°	15°
Extension	0°	0°	
Adduction	15°	20°	40°
Abduction	5°	40°	
Int. rotation	5°	5°	5°
Ext. rotation	10°	15°	

Table 22. Range of movement of the right hip in Fig. 159

	Before surgery	At the 11-year follow-up	Gain
Flexion	90°	80°	−15°
Extension	5°	0°	
Adduction	10°	20°	55°
Abduction	0°	45°	
Int. rotation	5°	5°	60°
Ext. rotation	0°	60°	

B. Pre-operative Planning

Whole-leg X-rays in the standing position are required to enable measurement of the obliquity of the pelvis and the apparent discrepancy in leg length. When the pelvis rotates about one femoral head, it also turns about the opposite femoral head. If on one side this rotation produces the effect of a valgus osteotomy, on the other it acts as a varus osteotomy. The degree of rotation must be taken into account in determining the wedge to be resected. In the case described above (Figs. 158–161), the rotation of the pelvis about the right femoral head corresponded to a 10° valgus osteotomy on the right side and to a 10° varus osteotomy on the left side. Thus 10° were added to the valgus wedge found necessary to enlarge the weight-bearing surface on the left side. Instead of a wedge of 45°, a wedge of 55° was resected.

C. Surgical Procedure

When a significant shortening is combined with a valgus osteotomy, no tenotomy of the adductor and iliopsoas muscles is required, since the shortening releases nearly all the muscles. A trapezoid is resected instead of a wedge. If the trapezoidal fragment resected comprises the lesser trochanter, it is preferable to make the distal cut oblique rather than the proximal, in order to provide a medial support for the proximal fragment and sufficient contact surface between the fragments (p. 115).

Night traction is not used after this procedure. Otherwise the postoperative care is the same as after a valgus or a varus osteotomy.

57

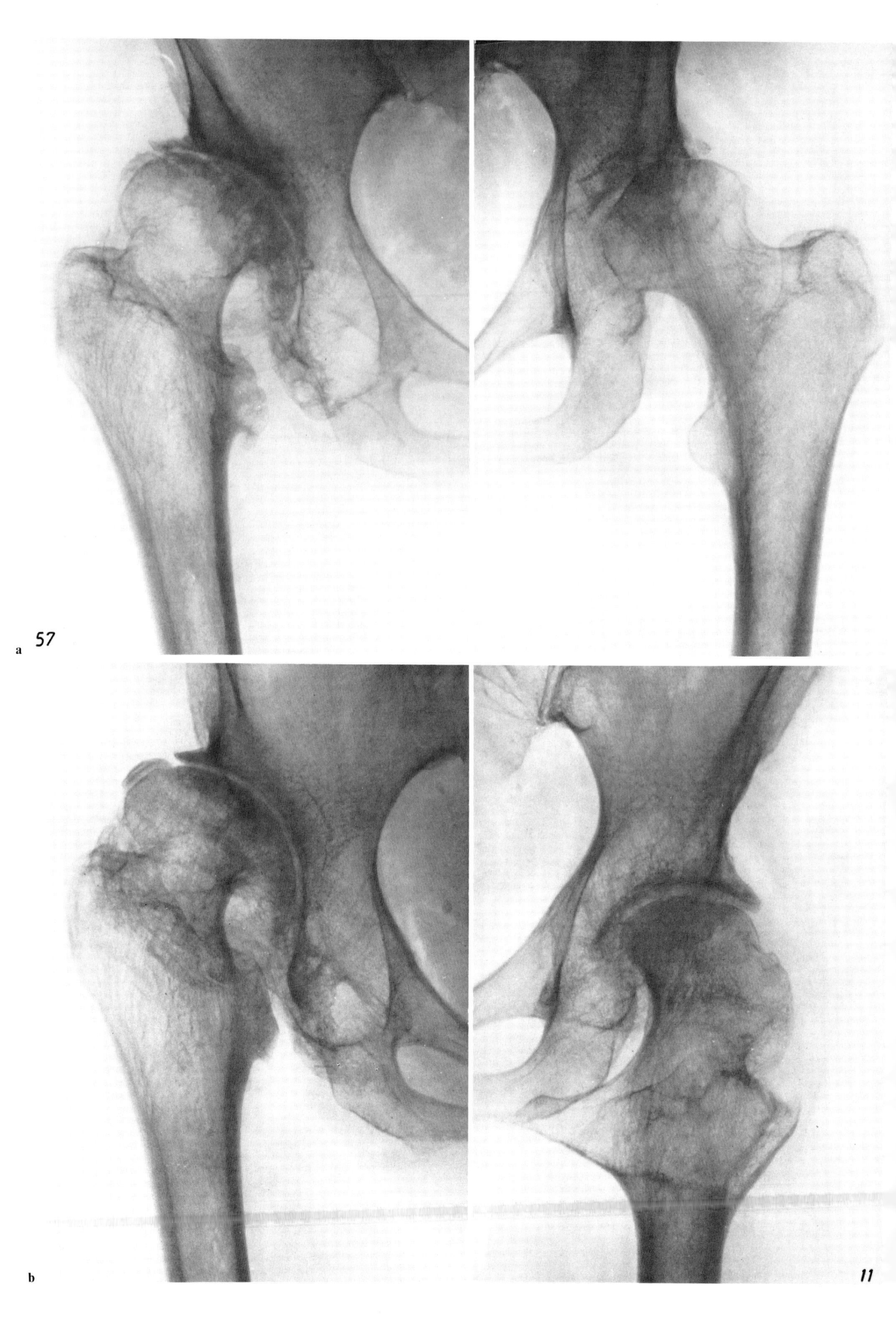

11

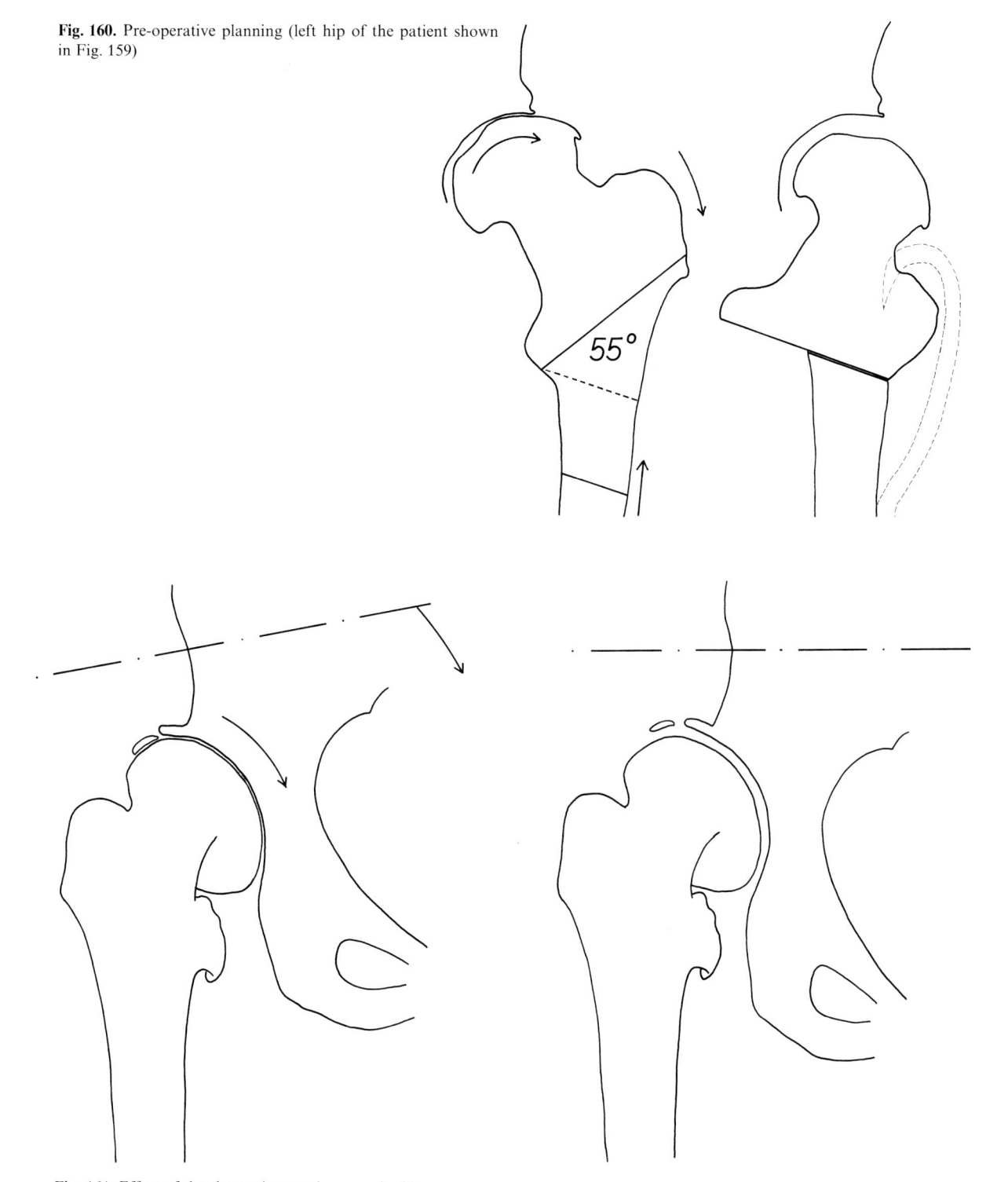

Fig. 160. Pre-operative planning (left hip of the patient shown in Fig. 159)

Fig. 161. Effect of the shortening on the opposite hip

◀ **Fig. 159. a** A 57-year-old female patient with bilateral osteoarthritis before a valgus intertrochanteric osteotomy combined with a 4-cm shortening of the longer leg. **b** Eleven years afterwards

48 a

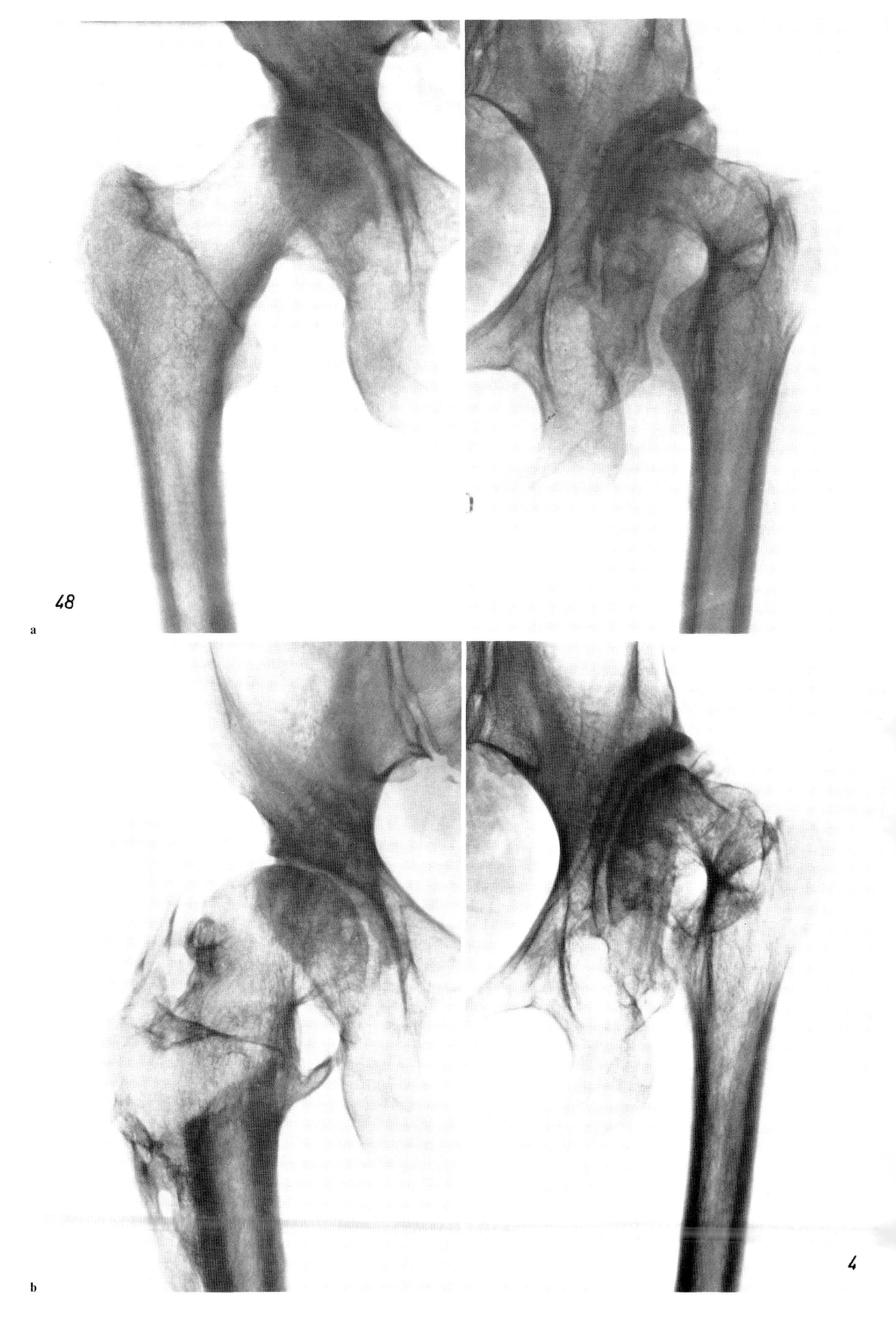

48 b

D. Results

This approach is unusual and is suitable for use only in a few patients. A 48-year-old female patient complained of pain in both hips, which were dysplastic and severely affected by osteoarthritis (Fig. 162a). The pelvis was oblique to the left, with the right leg appearing longer than the left. A 37° valgus osteotomy was carried out on the right hip, together with a 4-cm shortening (Fig. 163). At the 4-year follow-up, not only was the right hip dramatically improved but so also was the left, which had not been operated on (Fig. 162b). The left hip had also become pain-free and had regained a full range of movement.

A 40-year-old female patient had two dysplastic hips (Fig. 164a) with pain, a restricted range of movement and a severe limp. The pelvis was oblique to the left with an apparent difference in length of 4 cm between the two legs. A 30° valgus osteotomy combined with a 4-cm shortening was carried out on the right side. The diagrams show the effect that this shortening had on the pelvis. On the right side the latter turned about the femoral head, as occurs after a varus osteotomy (Fig. 165). This was taken into account in calculating the wedge to be resected. The pelvis pivoted about the left femoral head, as would have occurred after a valgus osteotomy of 10° (Fig. 166). At the 6-year follow-up both hips were improved, with reappearance of a wide joint space on the left side (Fig. 164b). The patient was relieved of pain and had a satisfactory range of movement in both hips (Tables 23 and 24). She was hardly limping and worked on a farm.

In each of the three cases presented here, the leg length discrepancy was 4 cm; this was purely coincidental. The surgical shortening must be adapted to the actual difference in length.

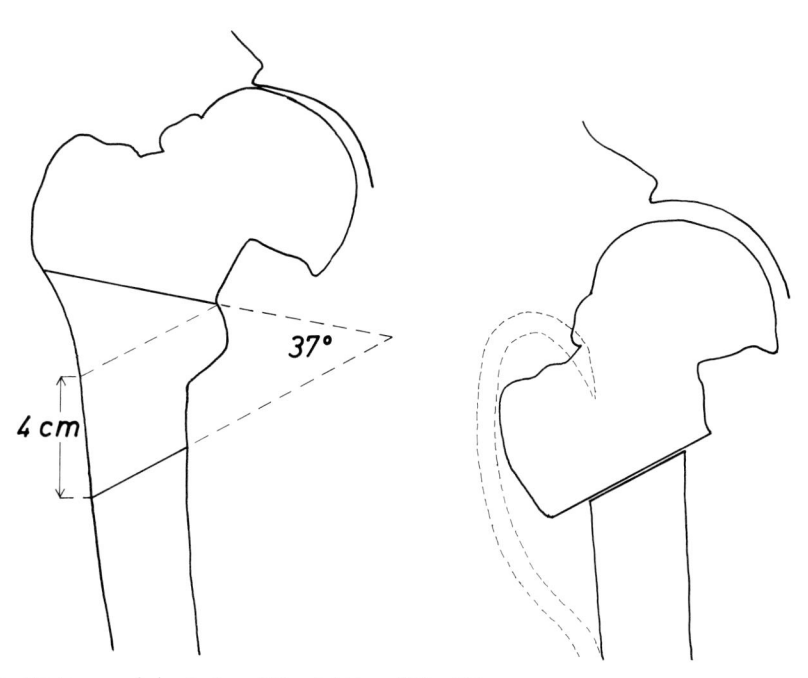

Fig. 163. Pre-operative planning of valgus osteotomy and shortening of the right leg of Fig. 162

◀ **Fig. 162. a** A 48-year-old female patient before a valgus intertrochanteric osteotomy and a 4-cm shortening of the longer leg. **b** Four years afterwards

40

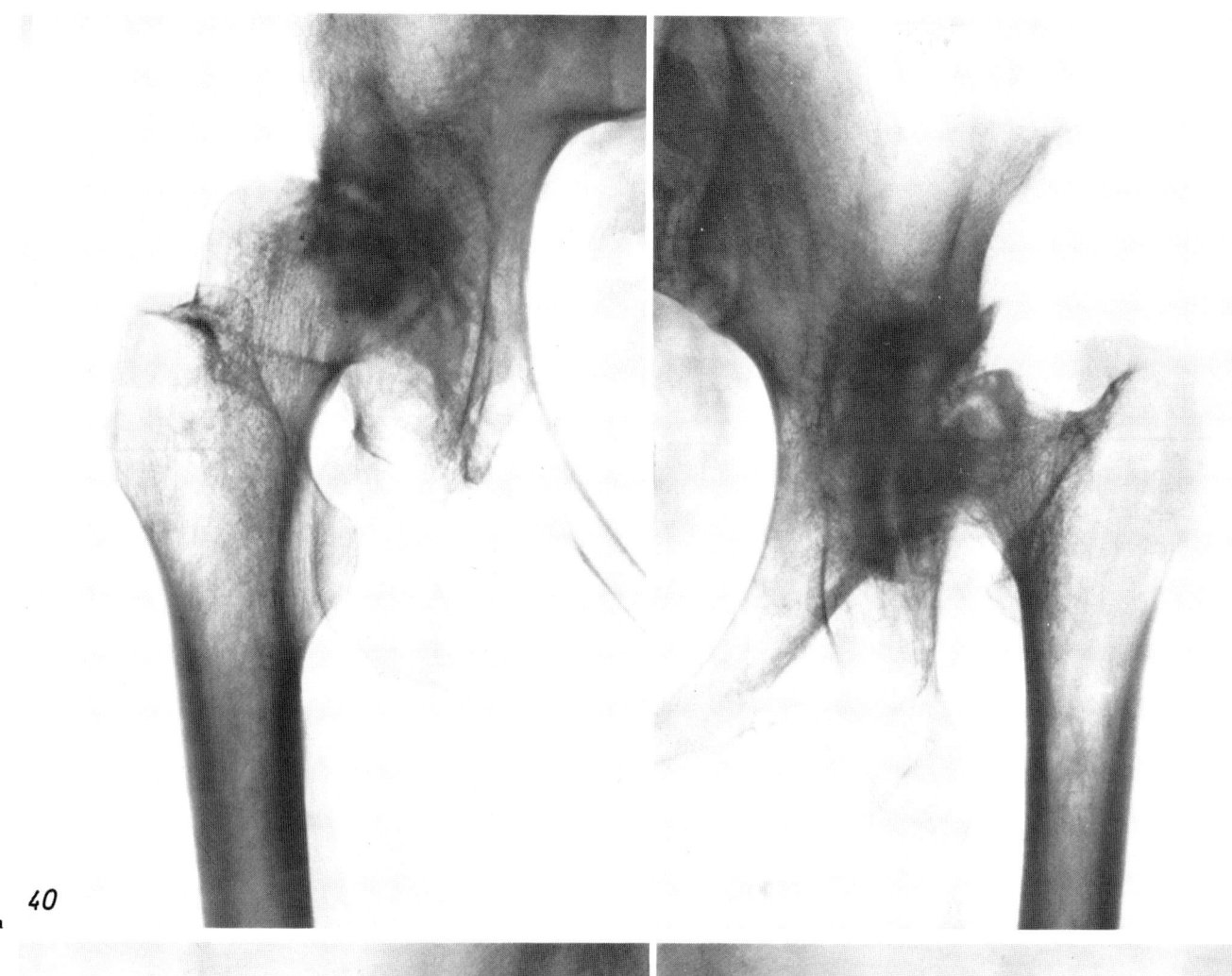

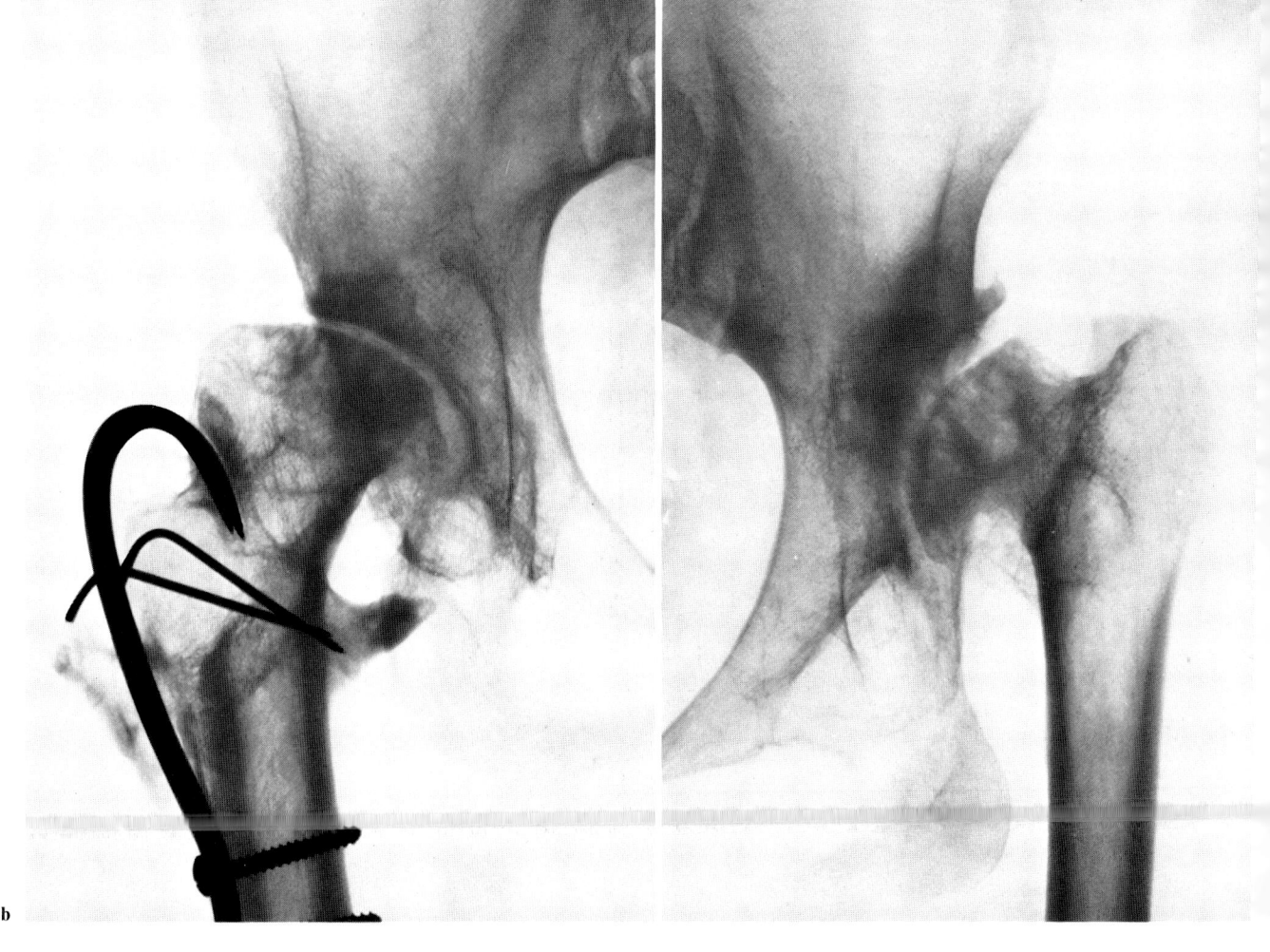

Fig. 165. Shortening a leg turns the pelvis about the ipsilateral femoral head, as does a varus osteotomy. See Fig. 164

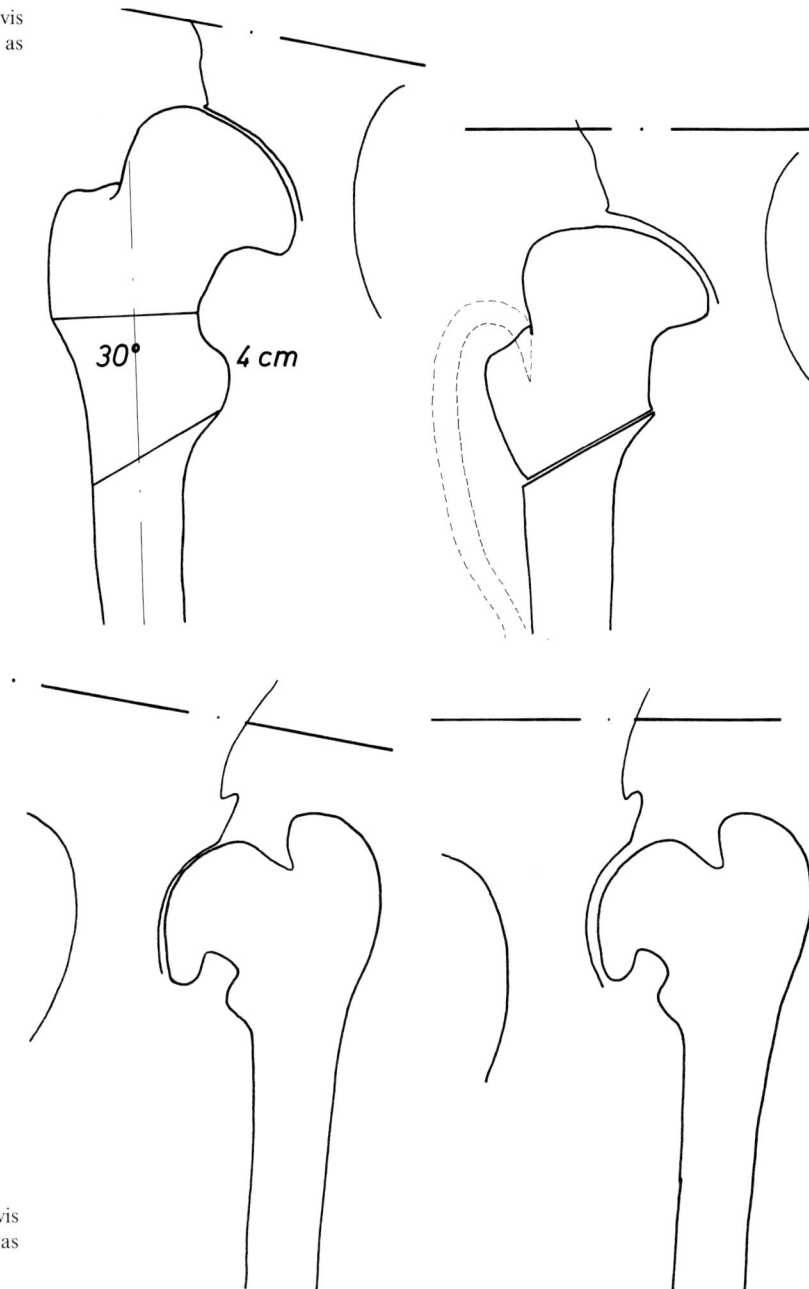

Fig. 166. Shortening a leg turns the pelvis about the contralateral femoral head, as does a valgus osteotomy. See Fig. 164

Table 23. Range of movement of the right hip in Fig. 164

	Before surgery	At the $6^1/_2$-year follow-up	Gain
Flexion	70°	80°	20°
Extension	−10°	0°	
Adduction	30°	45°	60°
Abduction	−20°	25°	
Int. rotation	− 5°	35°	70°
Ext. rotation	15°	45°	

Table 24. Range of movement of the left hip in Fig. 164

	Before surgery	At the $6^1/_2$-year follow-up	Gain
Flexion	90°	85°	5°
Extension	−10°	0°	
Adduction	25°	45°	40°
Abduction	25°	45°	
Int. rotation	5°	45°	70°
Ext. rotation	5°	35°	

◀ **Fig. 164. a** A 40-year-old female patient before a valgus intertrochanteric osteotomy and a 4-cm shortening of the longer leg. **b** Six years afterwards

157

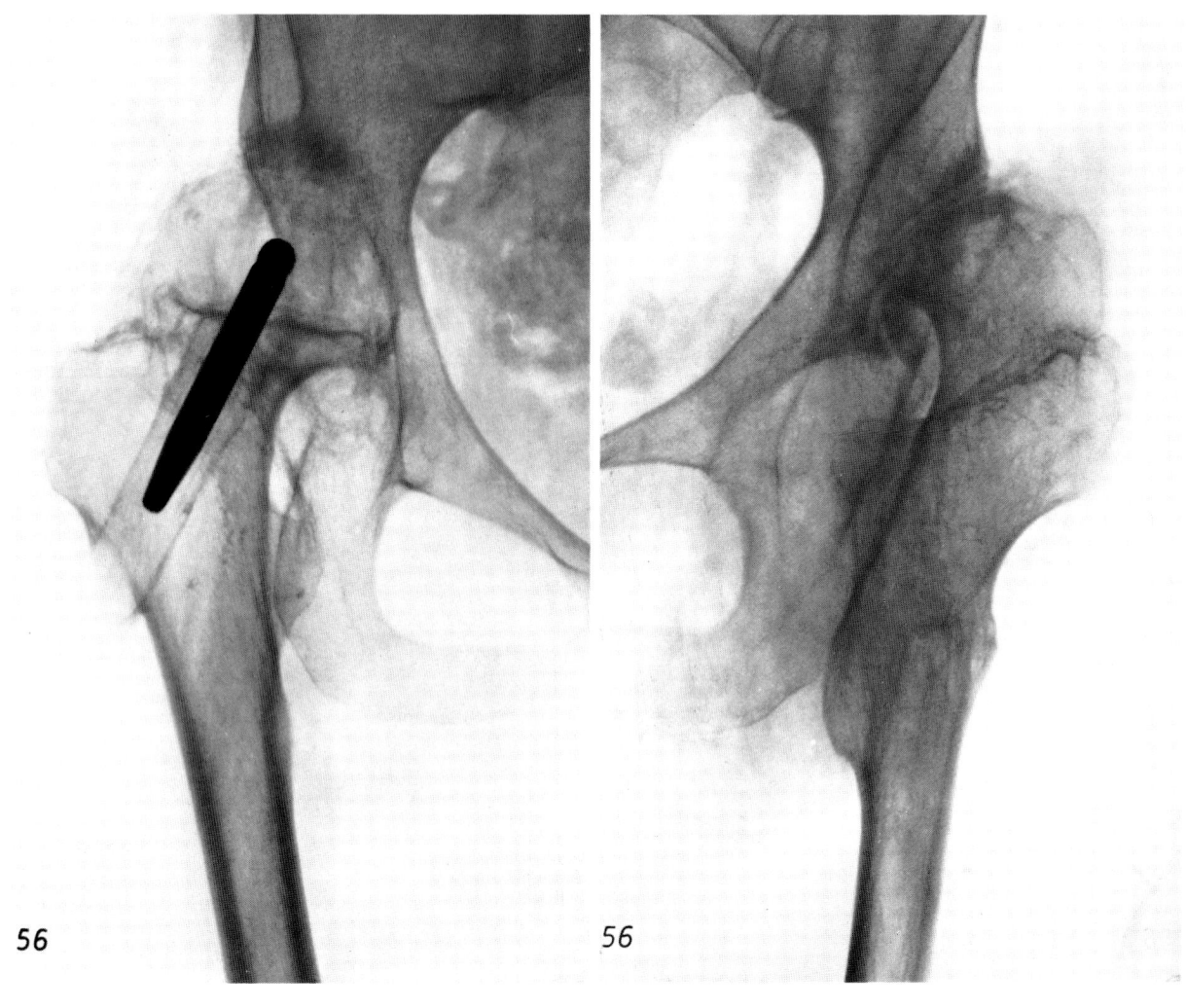

Fig. 167. a A 56-year-old female patient before a Milch osteotomy and thus a shortening of the upper end of the right femur. **b** 14 years afterwards

A 56-year-old female patient presented with two dysplastic hips. She had undergone a kind of SCHANZ osteotomy on her left side at the age of 18 and her right hip had been replaced by an acrylic prosthesis when she was 40 (Fig. 167a). The range of movement of both hips was severely restricted and she had a severe limp. A dense triangle could be observed in the socket on top of the prosthesis. On the left side a dense triangle demonstrated the increase in and concentration of the articular compressive stresses at the edge of the socket. The joint space had completely disappeared.

The prosthesis was removed and a MILCH osteotomy was carried out on the right side (see p. 201). Such an osteotomy can shorten the limb by about 5 cm. This rotated the pelvis about the opposite femoral head, which articulated with the ilium in a high false joint (Fig. 168). Osteoarthritis was severe in this joint (Fig. 167a). At the 14-year follow-up, the hips remained pain-free. The range of movement of both had considerably improved and the limp was less pronounced. On the left side the triangular subchondral sclerosis was replaced by a sclerosis of uniform width throughout and a satisfactory joint space had developed (Fig. 167b).

Here again, shortening of the right leg had turned the pelvis about the left femoral head, thus increasing the weight-bearing area of the joint as in a valgus osteotomy (Fig. 168).

The balance of the forces about the left hip was changed significantly. Tilting the pelvis to the right

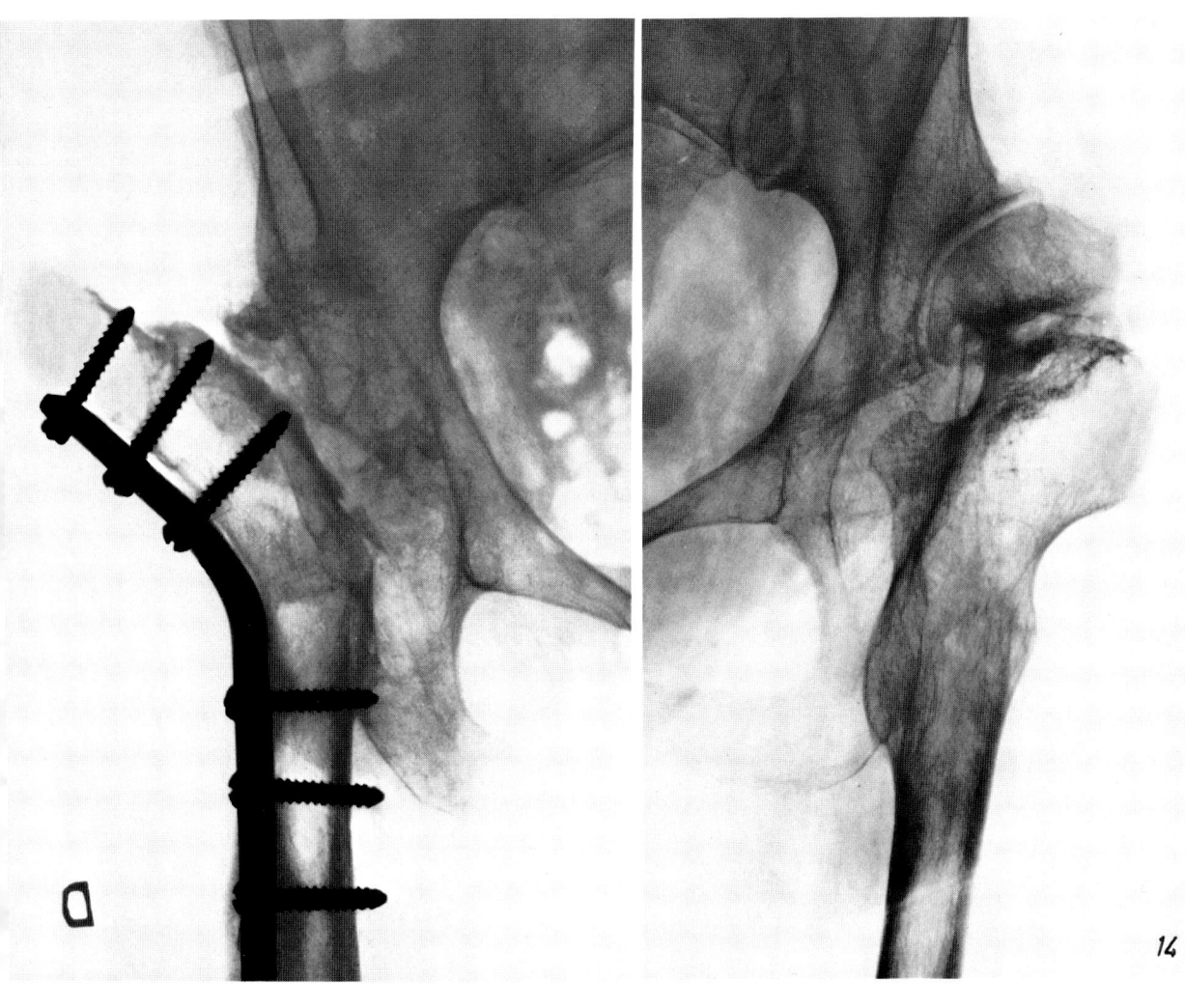

Fig. 167b

modified the direction of the abductor muscles of the left hip and brought the intersection of forces M and K downwards. This resulted in an opening of the angle $\widehat{KM}$ formed by the two forces and in a displacement of their resultant force R medially into the socket. Opening the angle $\widehat{KM}$ decreased force R. Consequently, the force R transmitted across the hip joint was reduced and distributed over a larger weight-bearing surface. This entailed a considerable decrease and a better distribution of the compressive stresses in the joint. The result was a significant regeneration of the left hip.

E. Conclusion

Shortening the opposite leg may enlarge the weight-bearing area of the hip joint in some severe cases when the pelvis is oblique and there is an apparent discrepancy in leg length. The number of cases under review is not sufficent to provide material for a statistical analysis, but the few cases in which the procedure has been carried out emphasize the validity of the mechanical approach to osteoarthritis. Hips heal when their weight-bearing area has been sufficiently increased, even without direct surgical intervention. It is, therefore the mechanical effect of the different procedures that appears to be of decisive significance.

160

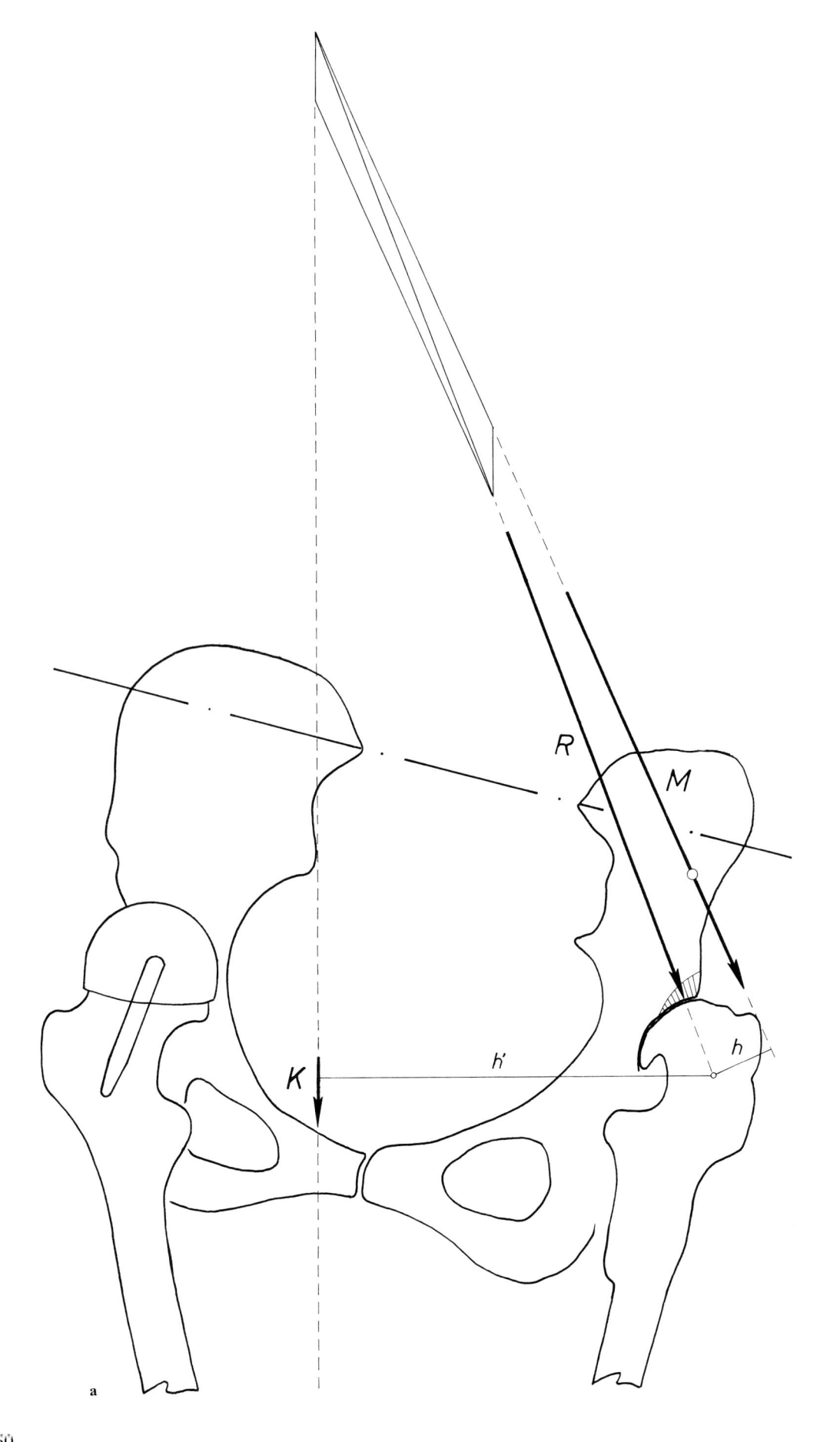

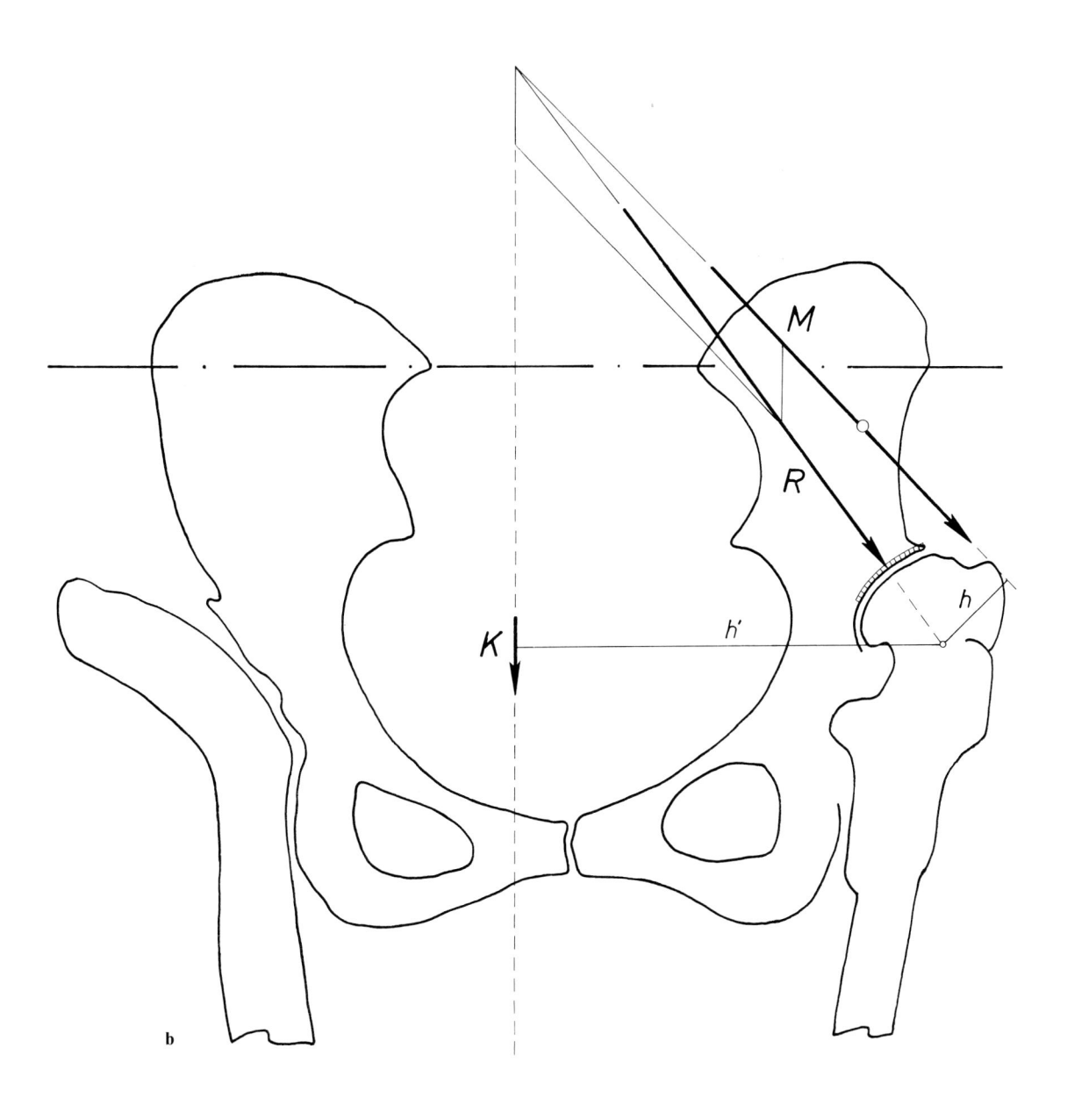

Fig. 168a, b. Shortening the leg rotates the pelvis about the left femoral head. This results in a change in the balance of forces. K force exerted by the partial mass of the body; h' lever arm of K; M force exerted by the abductor muscles; h lever arm of M; R resultant of forces K and M. **a** Before the shortening; **b** after the shortening (See Fig. 167)

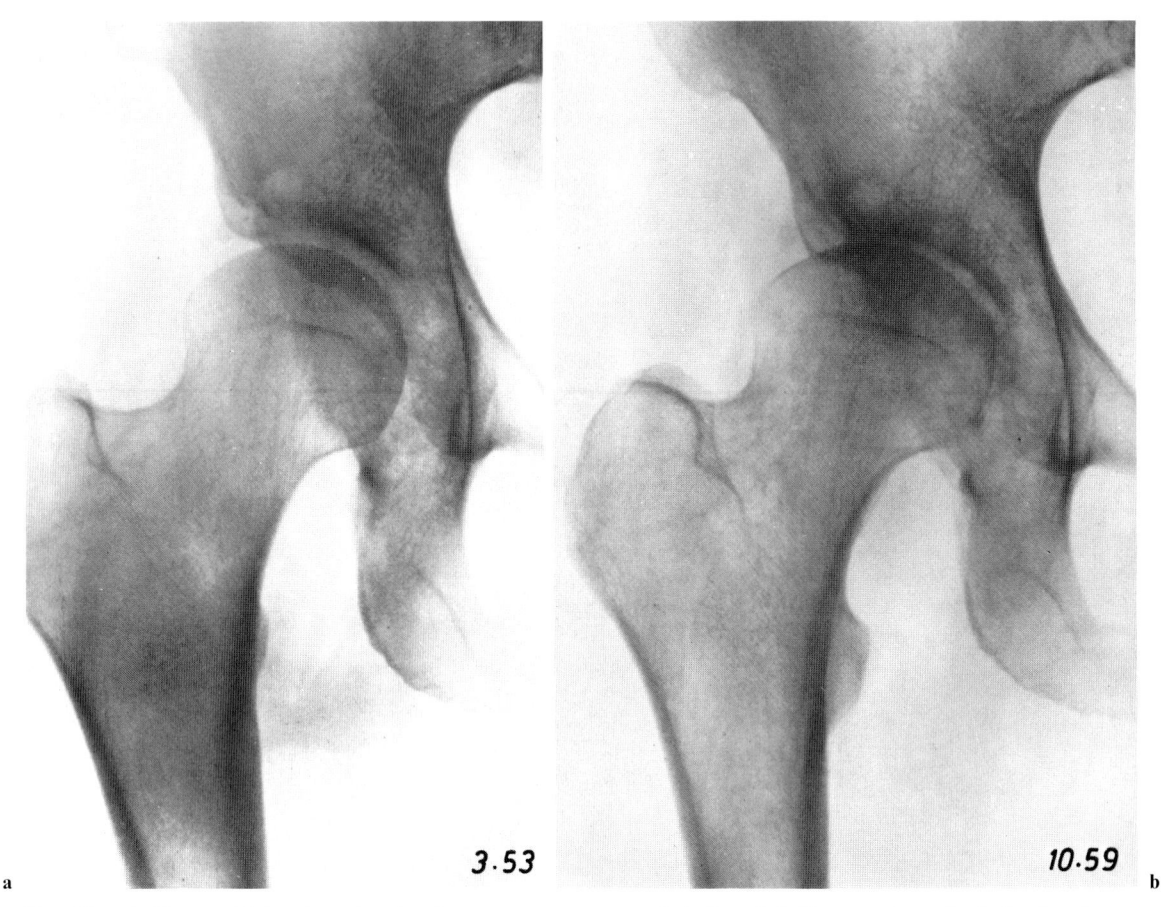

Fig. 169. a A 35-year-old female patient in whom a varus osteotomy is indicated. **b** Six years later, the indication for a varus osteotomy is no longer clear. **c** Another 10 years later a varus osteotomy would result in incongruence of the joint surfaces. **d** Two and **e** 3 years later, a valgus osteotomy is indicated. **f** One year after a valgus osteotomy. **g** Two years, **h** 5 years, **i** 7 years and **j** 9 years after the osteotomy

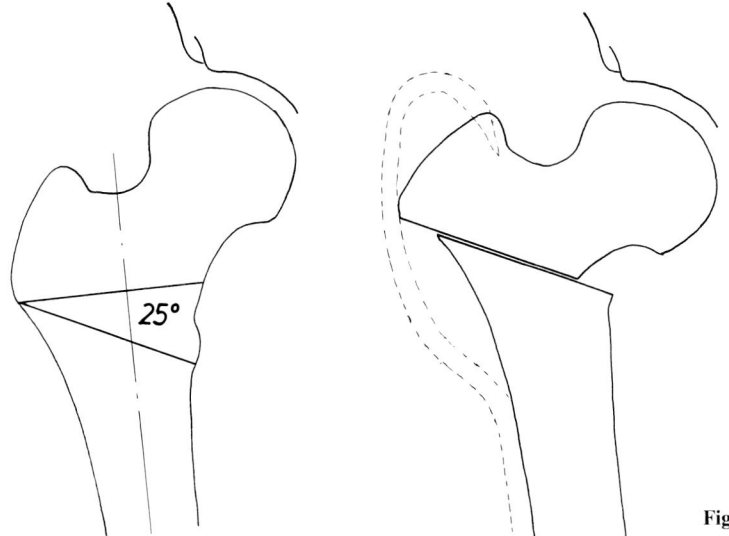

Fig. 170. For the hip shown in Fig. 169a, a varus osteotomy is clearly indicated

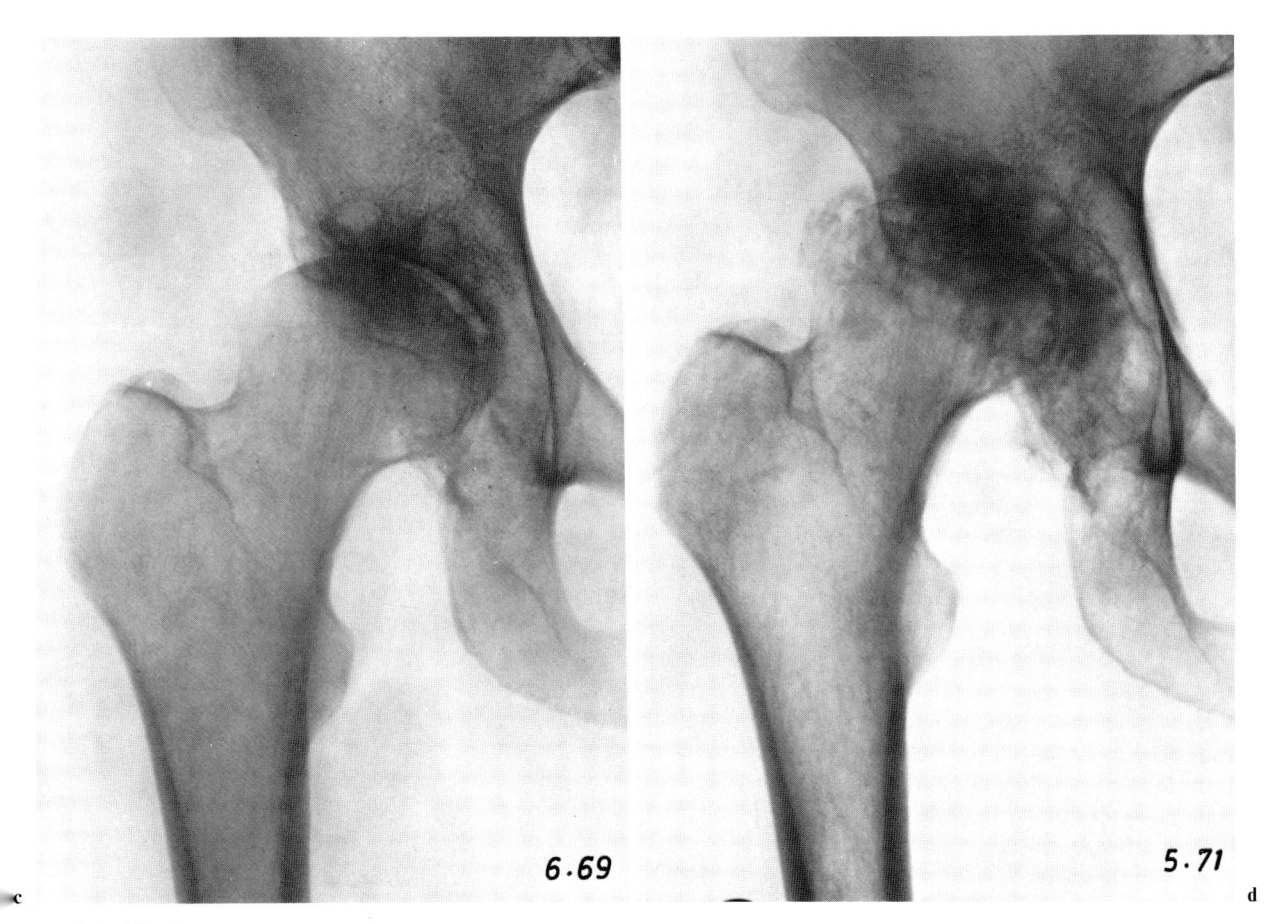

Fig. 169c, d

VII. Changing Indication

Although a varus osteotomy may often be clearly indicated in the first stages of the condition, a valgus osteotomy may come to be indicated in the course of the evolution of the disease.

A 35-year-old female patient complained of pain in her left hip, which was dysplastic. A dense triangle with a cyst showed that articular pressure was increased at the edge of the socket. The acetabulum and the femoral head were round-shaped and congruent. A varus intertrochanteric osteotomy would have constituted the treatment of choice (Figs. 169a and 170). Six years later the head and the socket were becoming flattened. It was now dubious whether varus osteotomy was indicated (Fig. 169b). Another 10 years later, a varus osteotomy would probably have resulted in incongruence of the joint surfaces (Fig. 169c). Two and three years afterwards, a valgus osteotomy was clearly indicated (Figs. 169d, e and 171). A Pauwels II was carried out, taking advantage of the huge osteophyte which had developed over the medial aspect of the femoral head. The patient was followed up for close to 10 years after the operation: during this period the abnormal subchondral sclerosis in the roof of the socket regressed and a wide joint space reappeared (Fig. 169f–i). The clinical result remained excellent (Table 25).

Table 25. Range of movement of the hip (see Fig. 169)

	Before surgery	At the 9-year follow-up	Gain
Flexion	80°	100°	20°
Extension	5°	5°	
Adduction	10°	5°	25°
Abduction	10°	40°	
Int. rotation	10°	10°	20°
Ext. rotation	5°	25°	

e

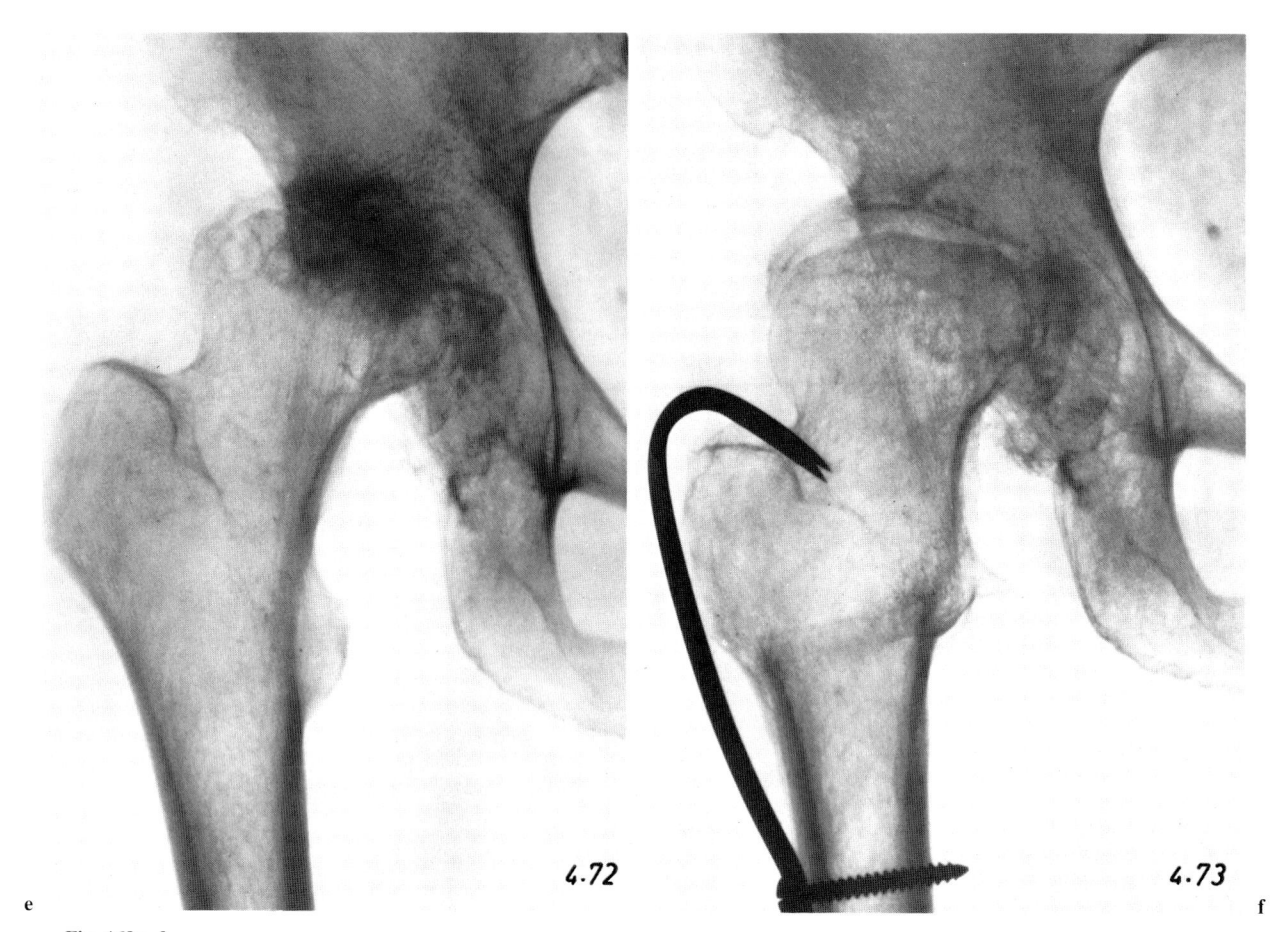

Fig. 169e, f

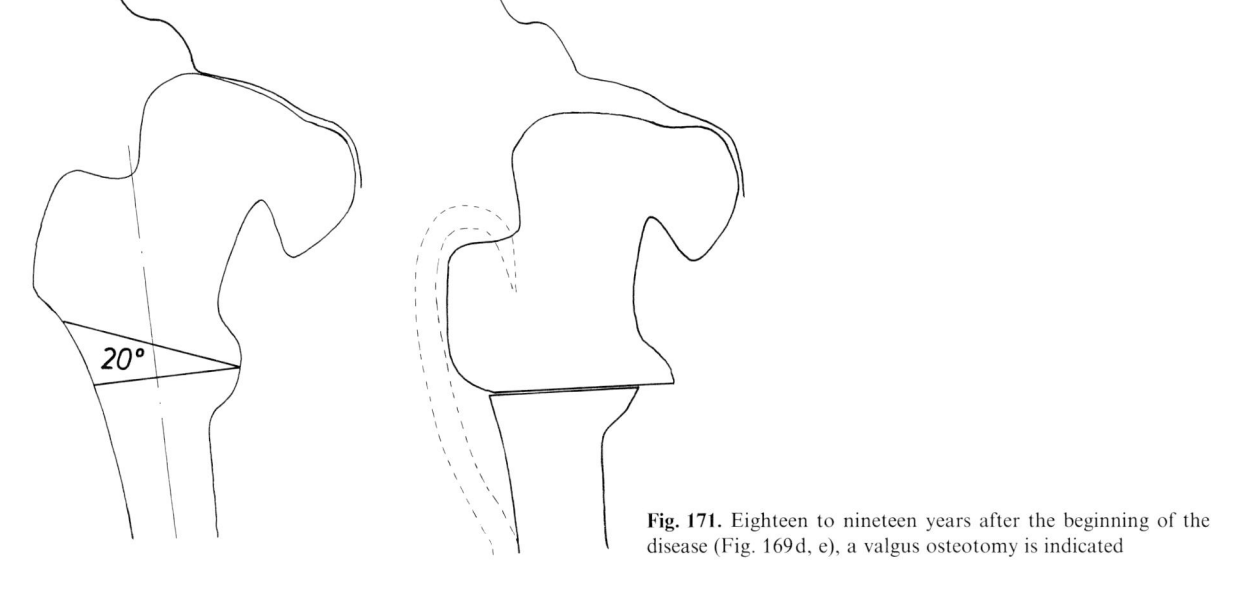

Fig. 171. Eighteen to nineteen years after the beginning of the disease (Fig. 169d, e), a valgus osteotomy is indicated

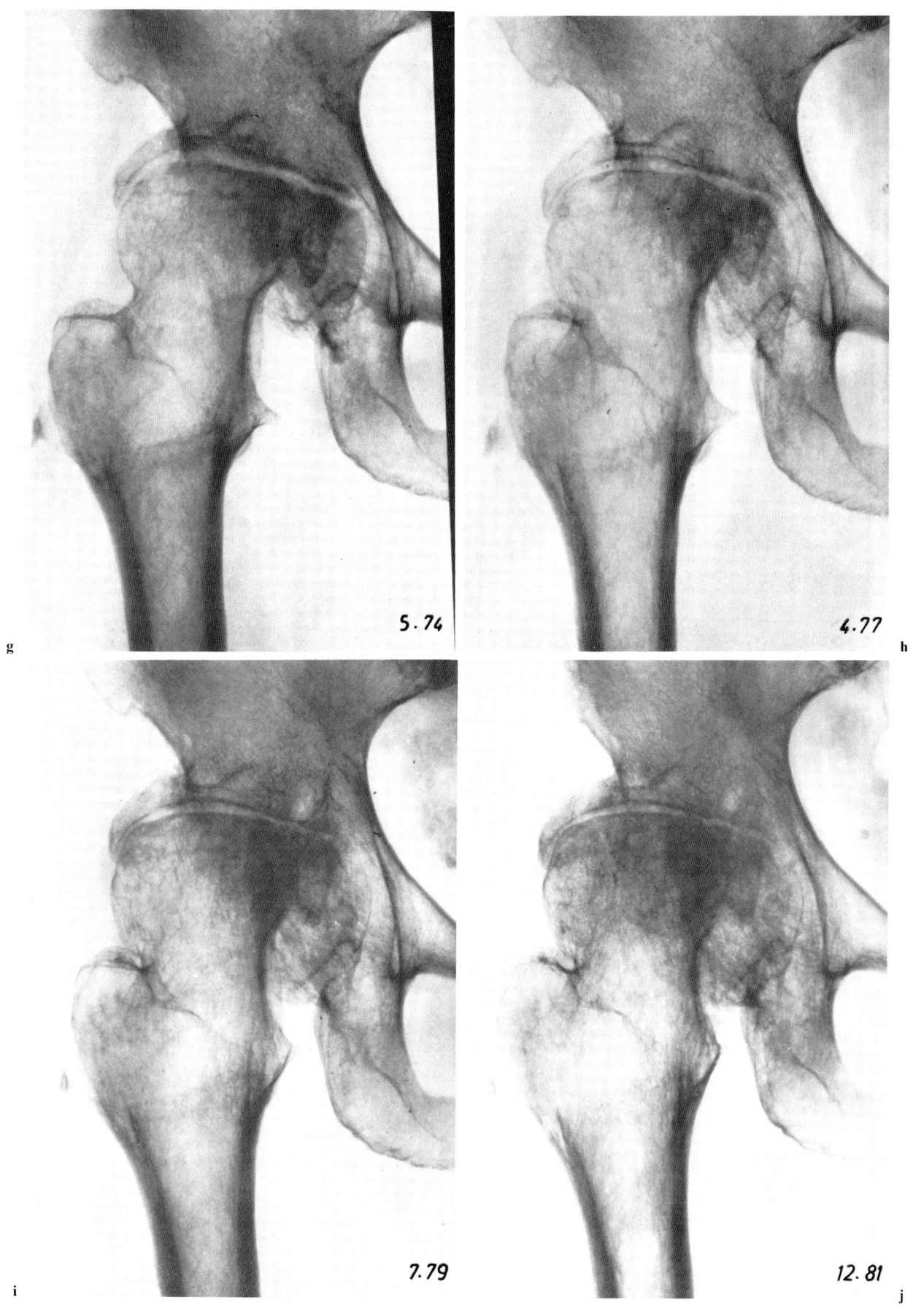

Fig. 169 g–j

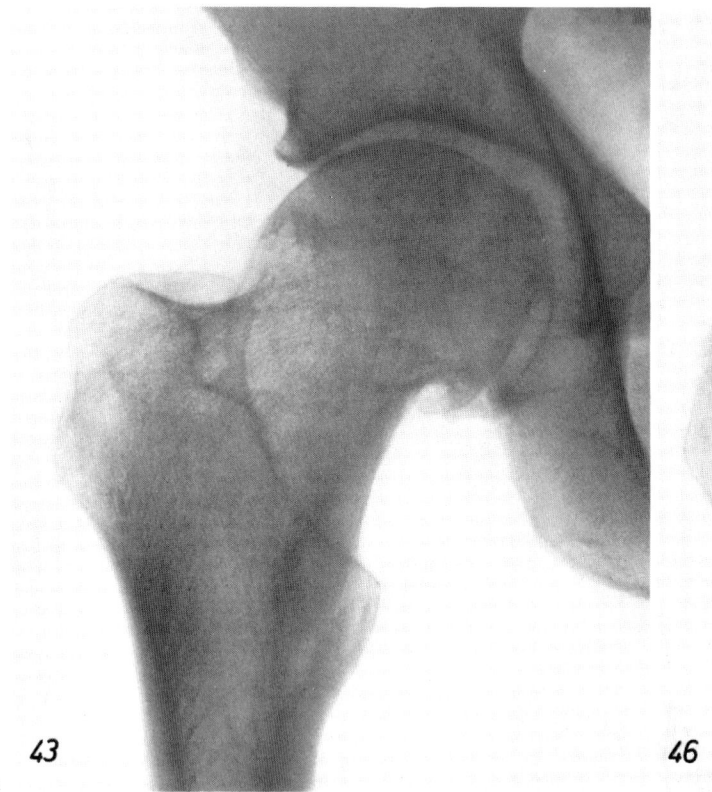

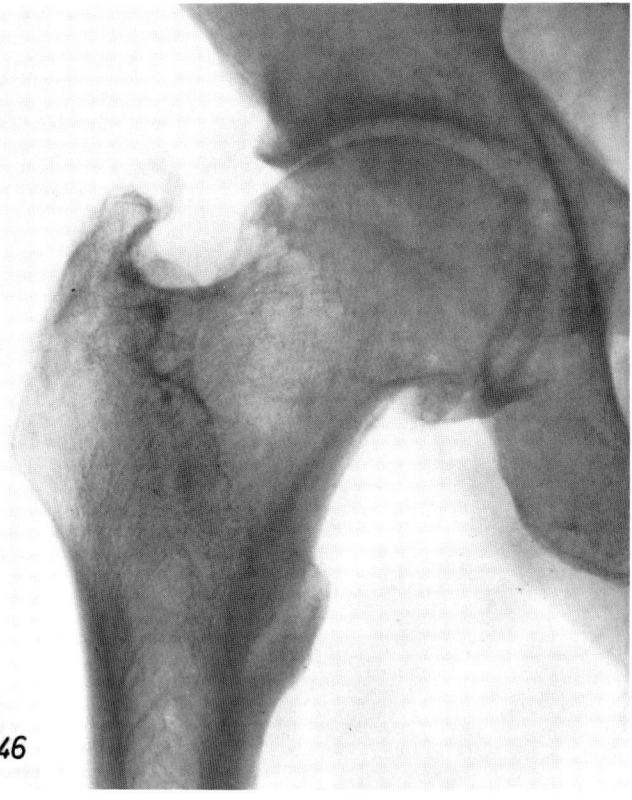

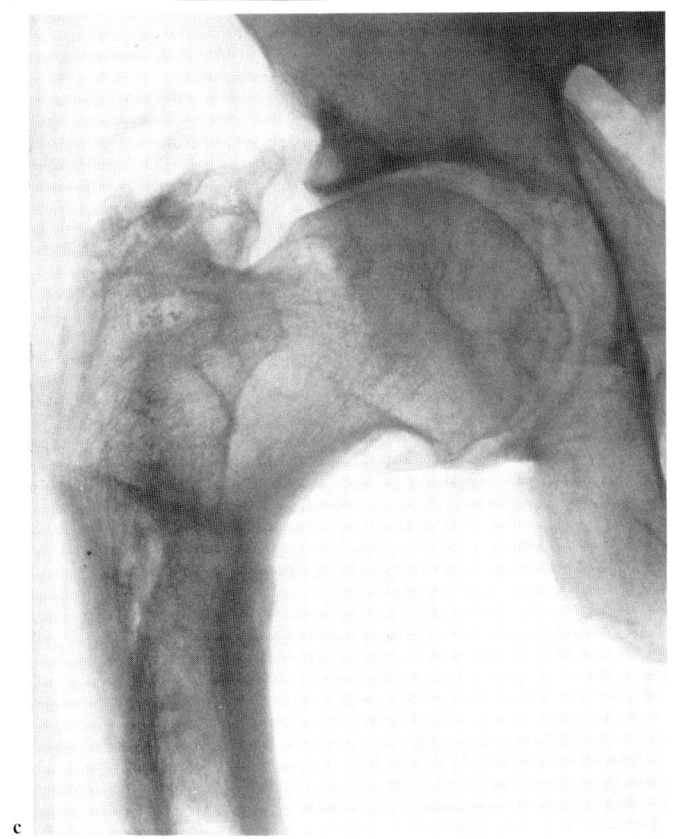

Fig. 172. a A 43-year-old male patient. In this hip joint congruence could not be achieved. **b** A hanging-hip procedure was carried out, and then **c** a varus osteotomy to no avail

VIII. No Indication for Any of the Operations Previously Described

When the articular surfaces are incongruent and congruence cannot be achieved either in full abduction or in full adduction (or in flexion) of the hip, none of the aforementioned procedures should be considered, since none of them is capable of enlarging the weight-bearing surface of the joint. This is particularly true when the femoral head has been enlarged by a medial osteophyte whilst the edge of the socket remains curved downward. Then the femoral head only pivots about the edge of the acetabulum, as on a fulcrum (Fig. 59).

The hip of a 43-year-old male patient presented these features (Fig. 172a). A hanging-hip operation was carried out elsewhere, to no avail (Fig. 172b). Two years later, a varus osteotomy was carried out and brought no improvement (Fig. 172c). In this hip there was no possibility of ensuring congruence of the articular surfaces. In such cases the edge of the acetabulum may collapse after some months or years. Then and only then can a valgus osteotomy be considered.

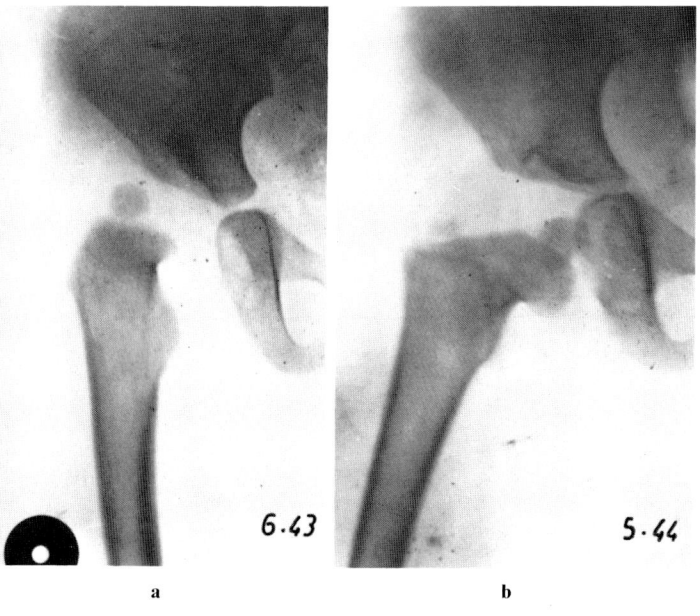

Fig. 173. a Congenital dislocation of the hip. **b** After open reduction. When the patient was 15 years old (**c**), a shelf operation was carried out (**d**). **e** At 26 years, the lateral aspect of the socket was bulging distally. **f, g** X-rays taken during operation. **h** After removal of a subchondral wedge, **i** the roof of the socket collapsed. **j** A valgus osteotomy was carried out with **k** a good result at the 12-year follow-up

In one particular instance the collapse of the edge of the acetabulum was helped to occur. The patient had undergone an open reduction of a congenitally dislocated hip (Fig. 173a, b) in her 1st year of life. At the age of 15 (Fig. 173c) a shelf operation was carried out which resulted in a lowering of the lateral margin of the acetabulum (Fig. 173d). When we saw her, she was 26 years old and was experiencing pain in the hip. The edge of the socket extended distally and the femoral head pivoted on it as on a fulcrum (Fig. 173e). We removed a wedge from above the lateral aspect of the acetabulum (Fig. 173f–h). The patient was asked to walk with her full weight on the limb. The roof of the socket collapsed (Fig. 173i). About a year after the removal of the subchondral wedge, a valgus intertrochanteric osteotomy was carried out, combined with a tenotomy (Fig. 173j). Twelve years later the result remains excellent (Fig. 173k).

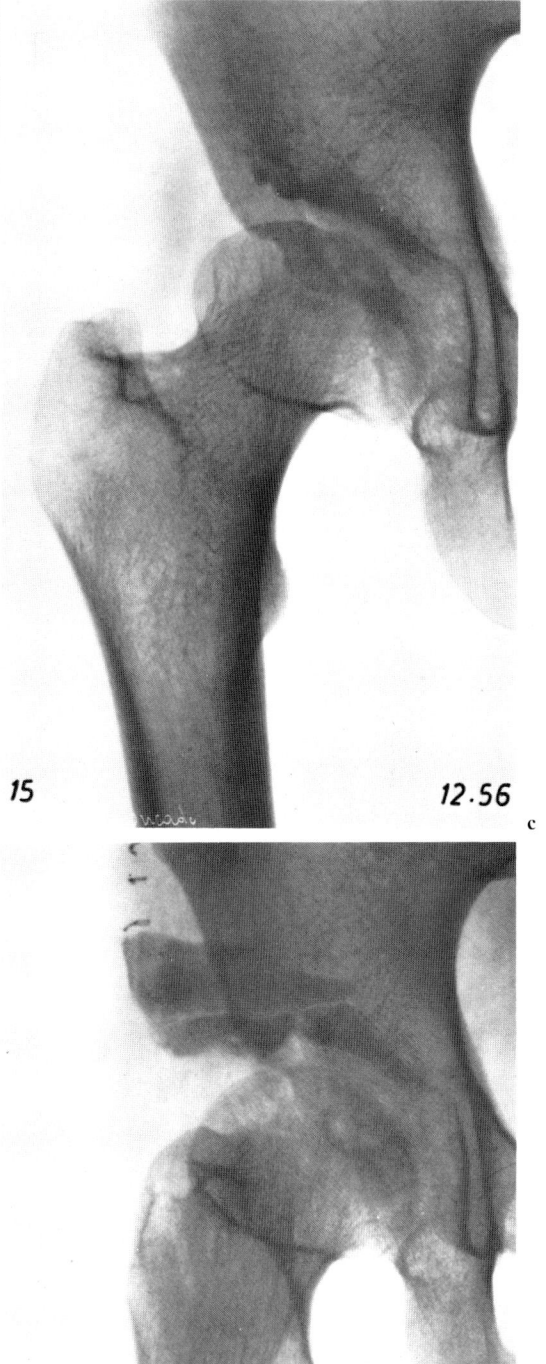

5.68

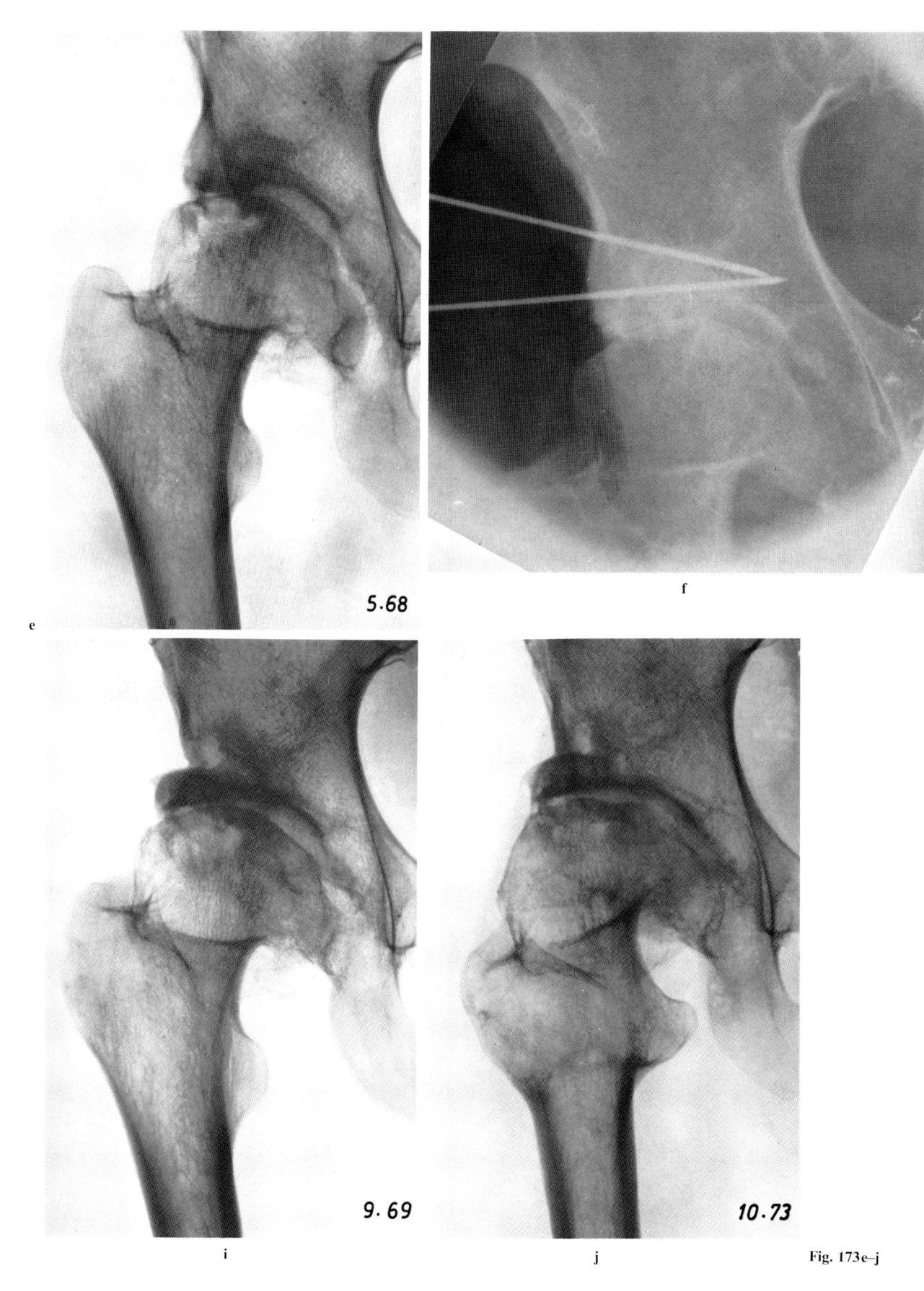

f

9.69

10.73

Fig. 173e–j

g

7.68

h

11.81

k

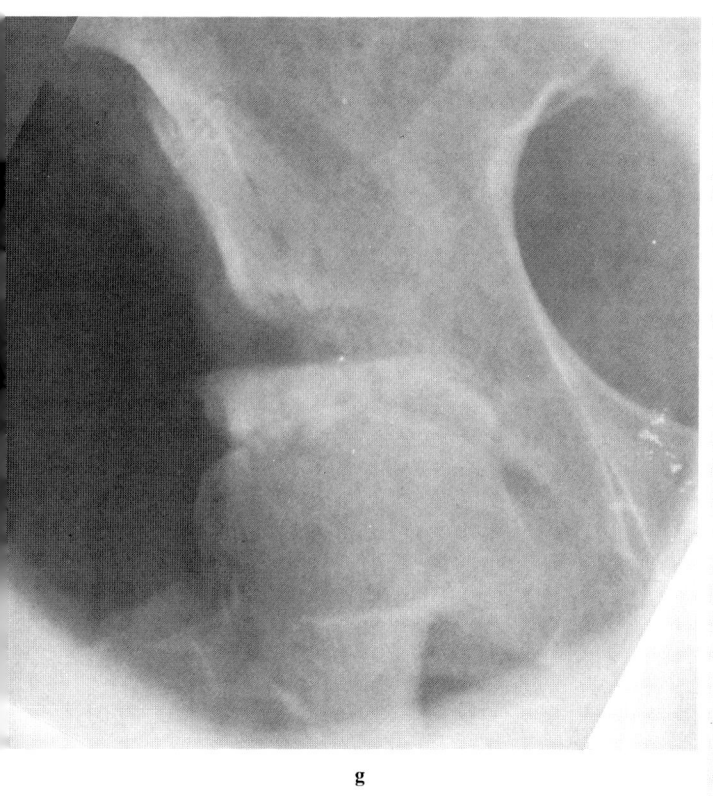

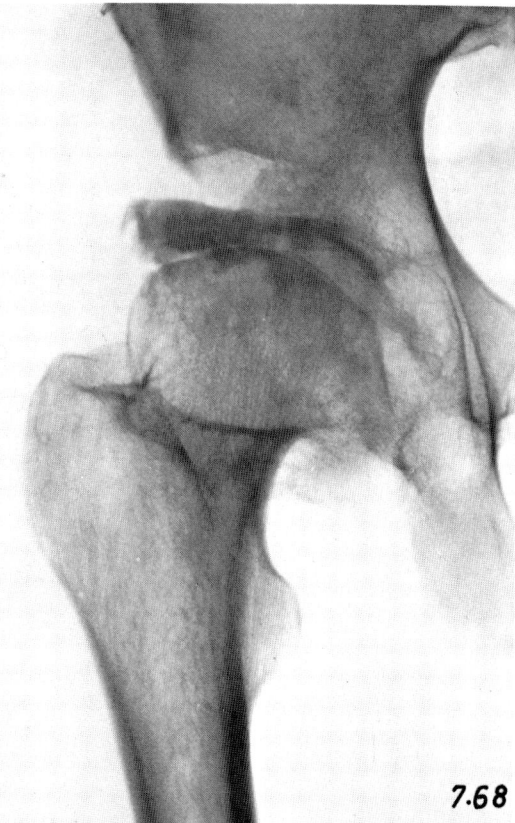

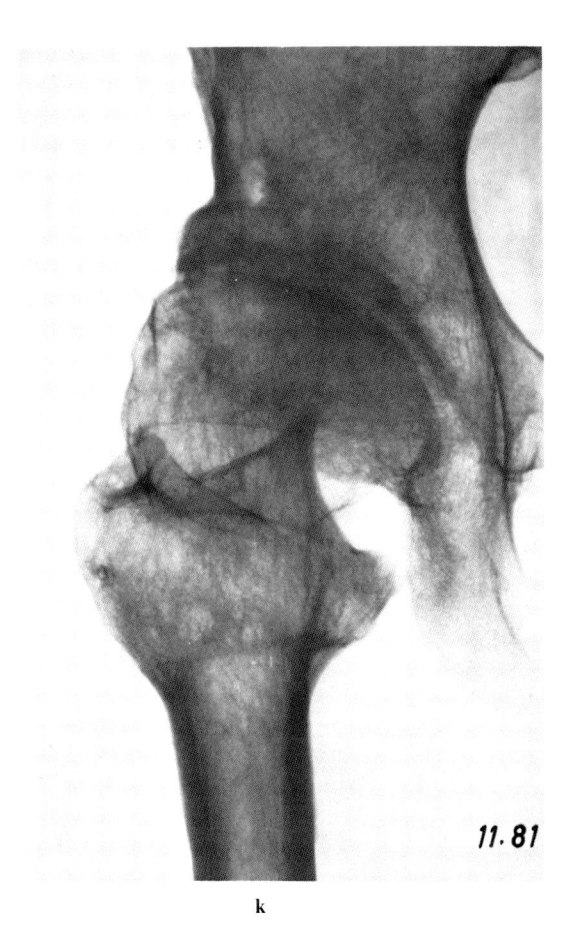

Fig. 173g–k

IX. Reoperations

When a surgical procedure carried out for osteoarthritis of the hip does not decrease joint pressure, it usually results in failure. An appropriate reoperation will often prompt healing if it decreases the joint pressure sufficiently.

A. After a Hanging-Hip Operation

A 59-year-old female patient had undergone a hanging-hip procedure 21 months previously (Fig. 174a). The femoral head was pushed outside the socket by a medial osteophyte. A triangular subchondral sclerosis at the edge of the acetabulum showed that the weight-bearing surface of the joint was reduced. A hanging-hip procedure was not indicated.

An appropriate valgus osteotomy was carried out in order to enlarge the weight-bearing surface of the joint by taking advantage of the medial cephalic osteophyte. Simultaneously, a new tenotomy of the abductor, adductor and iliopsoas muscles decreased the load transmitted across the hip. Fourteen years later the result remained good: no pain, a good range of movement (Table 26), no limp and an unlimited walking capacity. In the X-ray, the dense triangle had been replaced by a subchondral sclerosis of uniform width throughout and a wide joint space had developed (Fig. 174b).

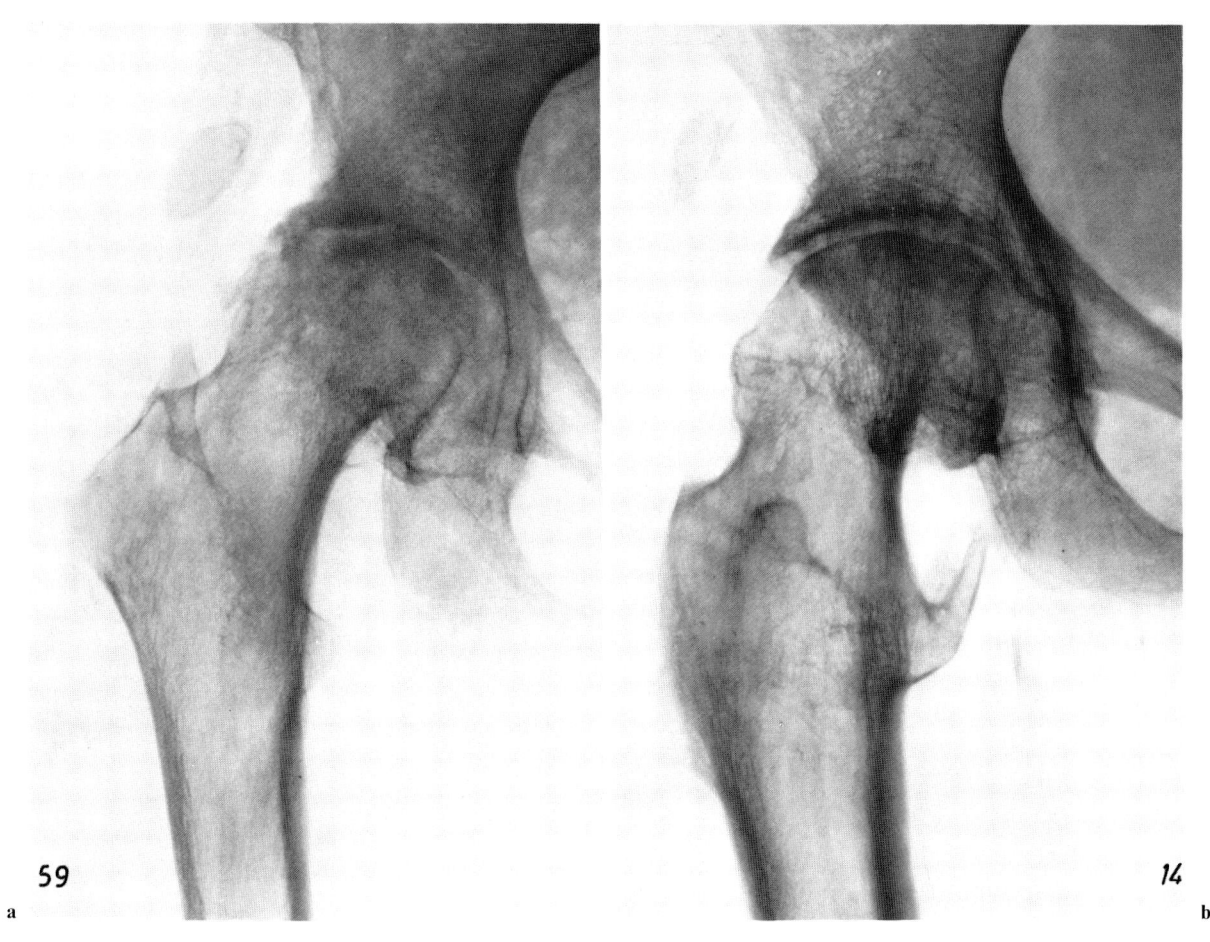

Fig. 174. a A 59-year-old female patient who had undergone a hanging-hip procedure 21 months previously. **b** Fourteen years after reoperation (valgus osteotomy)

Table 26. Range of movement of the hip (Fig. 174)

	Before surgery	At the 14-year follow-up	Gain
Flexion	60°	95°	50°
Extension	−10°	5°	
Adduction	20°	45°	60°
Abduction	−15°	20°	
Int. rotation	−5°	0°	40°
Ext. rotation	10°	45°	

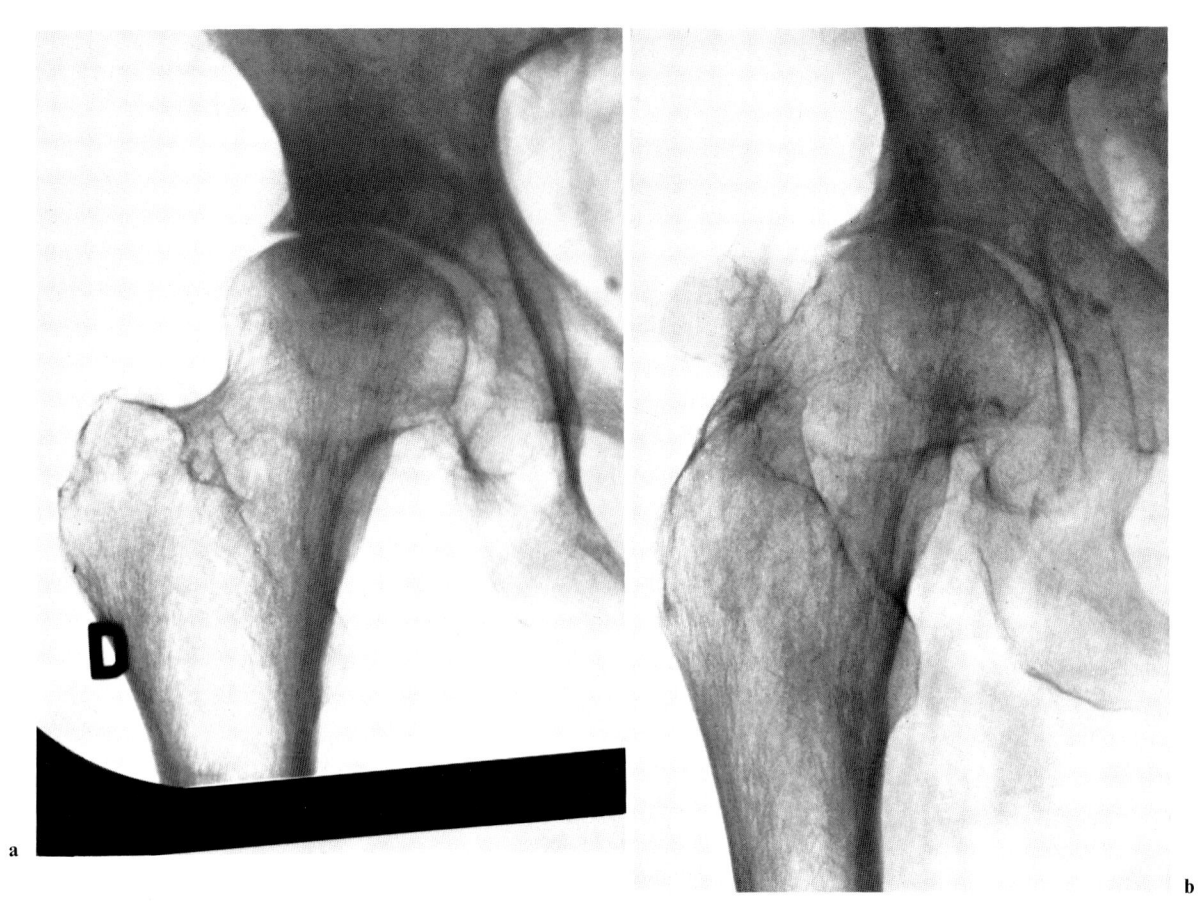

Fig. 175. a A 63-year-old female patient before a hanging-hip procedure. **b** Four years afterwards. **c** Four years after a valgus osteotomy

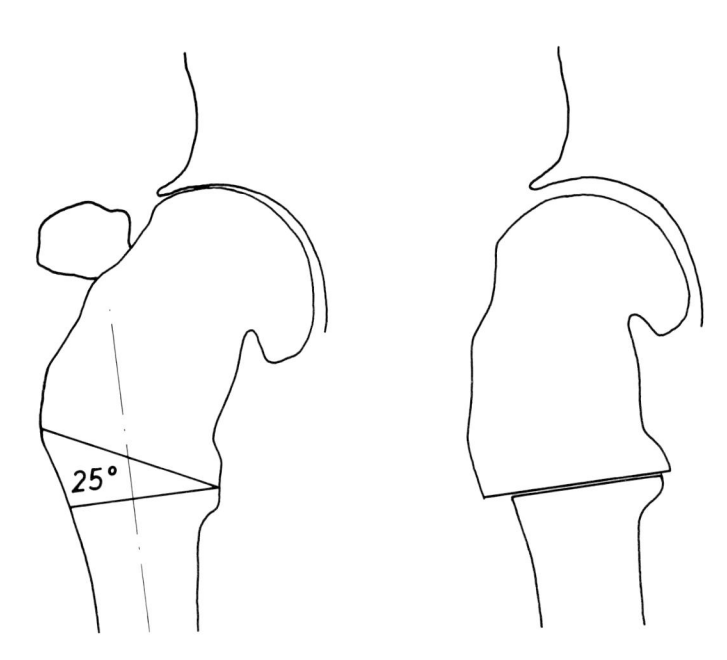

Fig. 176. Pre-operative planning: same hip as in Fig. 175

c

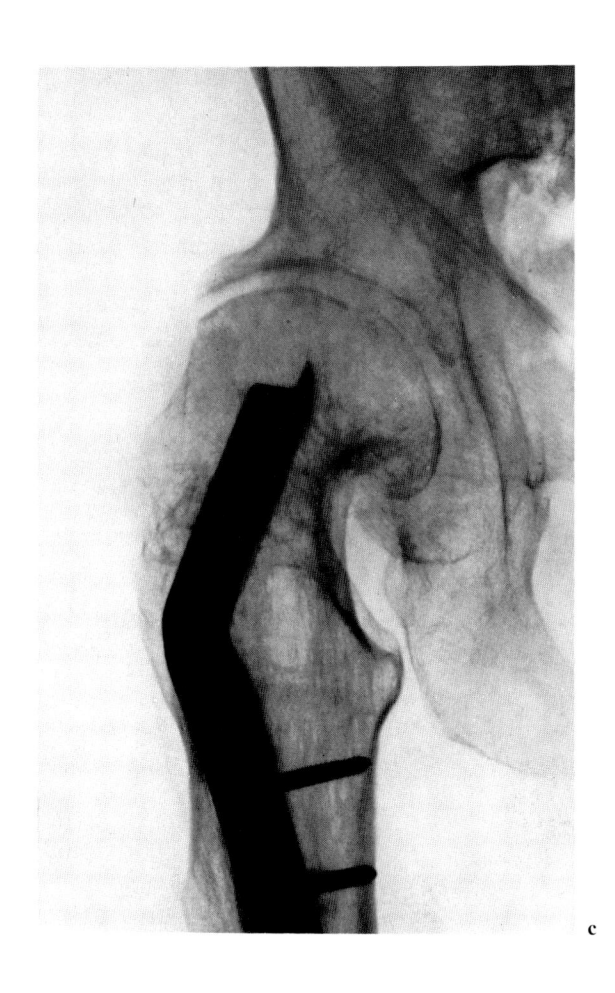

Table 27. Range of movement of the hip (Fig. 175)

	Before surgery	At the 4-year follow-up	Gain
Flexion	45°	80°	50°
Extension	0°	15°	
Adduction	25°	30°	30°
Abduction	20°	45°	
Int. rotation	−10°	30°	20°
Ext. rotation	50°	30°	

A 63-year-old female patient (Fig. 175a) had been subjected to a hanging-hip procedure 4 years previously (Fig. 175b), although the dense triangle at the edge of the socket was a contra-indication for such an operation. Pain soon recurred and the range of movement was limited (Table 27); the patient limped. The medial osteophyte which was present before, had further developed over the femoral head. A 20° valgus intertrochanteric osteotomy combined with multiple tenotomy was carried out (Fig. 176). Four years later, the clinical result was excellent: no pain, a good range of movement (Table 27), no limp and unlimited walking capacity. The X-ray showed that a wide joint space had developed between congruent articular surfaces, and a thin subchondral sclerosis of uniform width throughout could be observed in the roof of the socket (Fig. 175c). Joint pressure was now evenly distributed over a large weight-bearing surface.

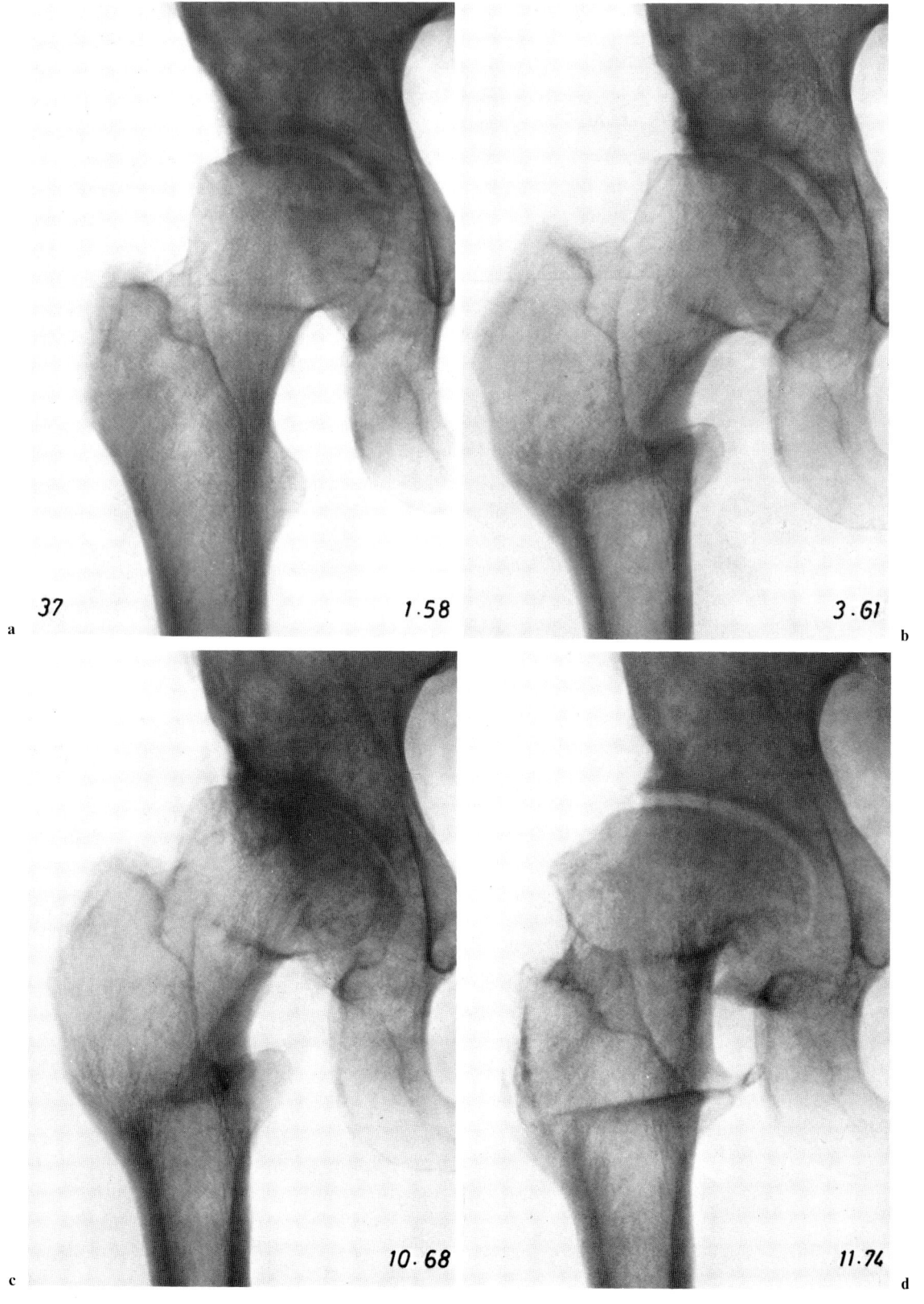

Fig. 177. A 37-year-old female patient **a** before and **b** after a varus osteotomy. **c** Ten years later the condition had worsened, a valgus osteotomy was carried out. **d** Six years later

B. After a Varus Osteotomy

Many varus osteotomies have been carried out in error in order to restore a normal anatomical shape, mainly in cases of coxa valga subluxans, despite incongruence of the articular surfaces in full abduction of the leg.

A 37-year-old female patient with coxa valga subluxans (Fig. 177a) underwent a varus osteotomy of 16° (Fig. 178a, b). After the operation the joint surfaces remained incongruent (Figs. 177b and 178b). Incongruence means reduction of the weight-bearing surface and increase in the articular compressive stresses. The increase in and uneven distribution of the articular compressive stresses is expressed in the X-ray by the dense triangle at the edge of the acetabulum. We saw the patient 10 years later (Fig. 177c). The condition had become worse. In order to reduce the joint pressure, a valgus osteotomy was planned (Fig. 178c and d) and carried out. In the years following the revision, the signs of osteoarthritis regressed and a wide joint space developed. At the 6-year follow-up the result was good (Fig. 177d).

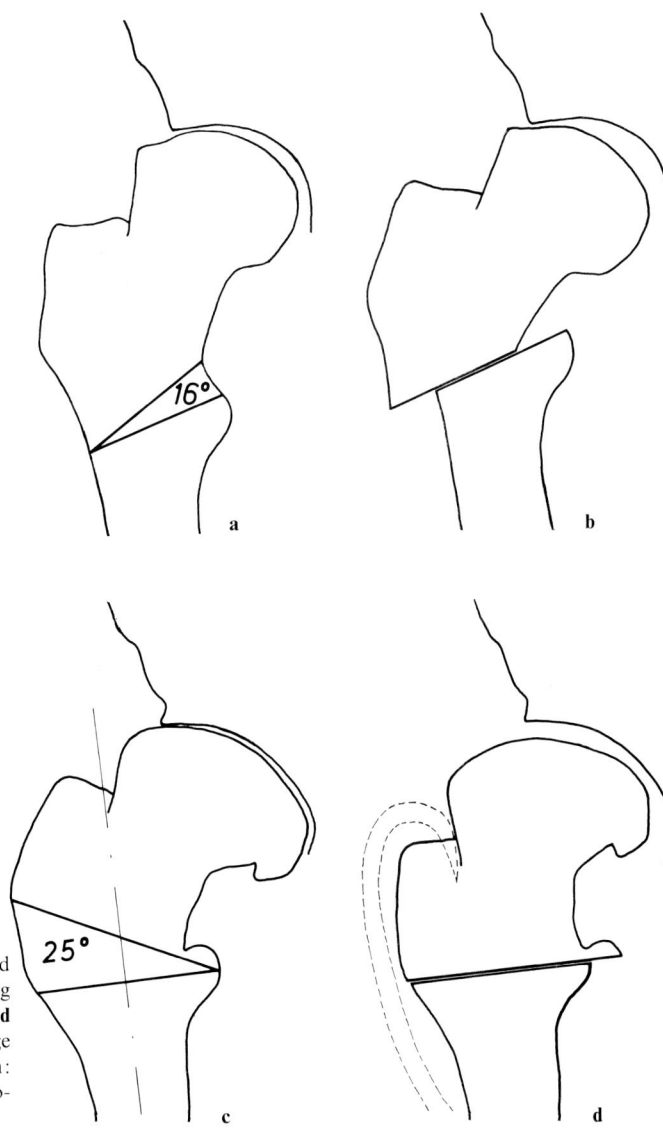

Fig. 178. a–b In the case shown in Fig. 177, it would not have been possible to enlarge the weight-bearing surface of the joint through a varus osteotomy. **c, d** A valgus osteotomy did ensure congruence and enlarge the articular weight-bearing surface. **a–b** First operation: varus osteotomy. **b–c** Second operation: valgus osteotomy

A 61-year-old female patient (Fig. 179a) had been subjected to a varus osteotomy 8 months before we saw her. After surgery the joint surface looked less congruent than before (Fig. 179b). The pain had increased and a dense triangle had developed at the edge of the acetabulum. A 40° valgus osteotomy combined with a tenotomy was carried out in order to enlarge the articular weight-bearing surface and to decrease the load supported by the joint (Fig. 180). At the 11-year follow-up, the result remained good (Table 28). The subchondral sclerosis of uniform width throughout showed that the articular stresses were evenly distributed over a large weight-bearing surface. The width of the joint space was remarkable (Fig. 179c).

Table 28. Range of movement of the hip (Fig. 179)

	Before surgery	At the $11^1/_2$-year follow-up	Gain
Flexion	70°	95°	40°
Extension	−10°	5°	
Adduction	45°	45°	25°
Abduction	−15°	10°	
Int. rotation	−20°	0°	45°
Ext. rotation	45°	70°	

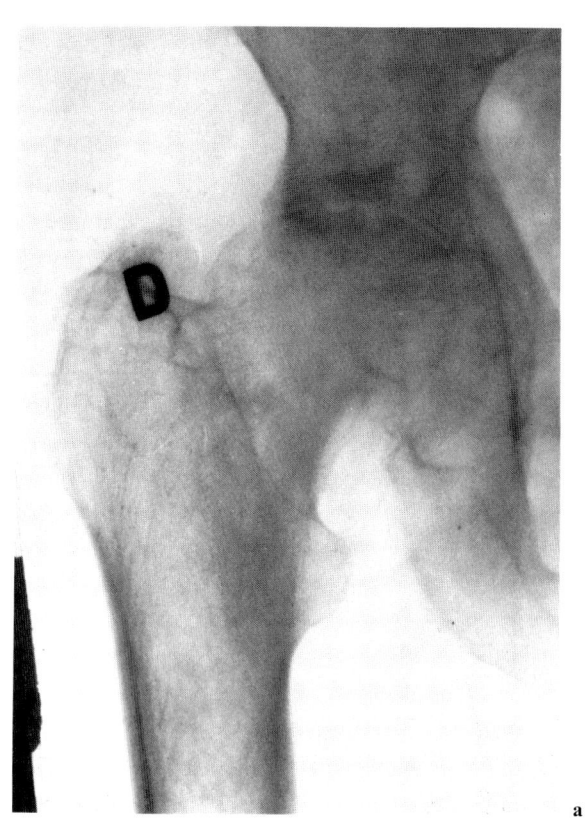

Fig. 179. A 61-year-old female patient **a** before and **b** after a varus osteotomy which did not relieve her pain. **c** Eleven years after reoperation (valgus osteotomy) which ensured congruence

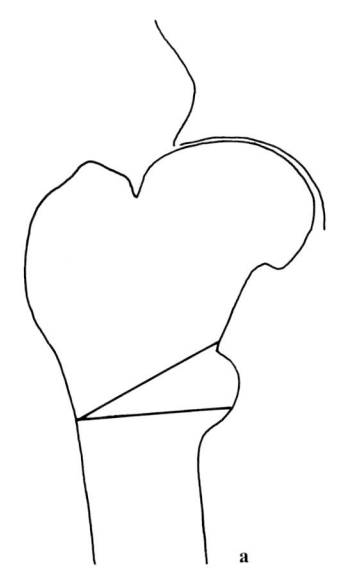

Fig. 180a–c. In the case shown in Fig. 179, a varus osteotomy was not indicated (**a, b**). A valgus osteotomy had to be carried out (**c**)

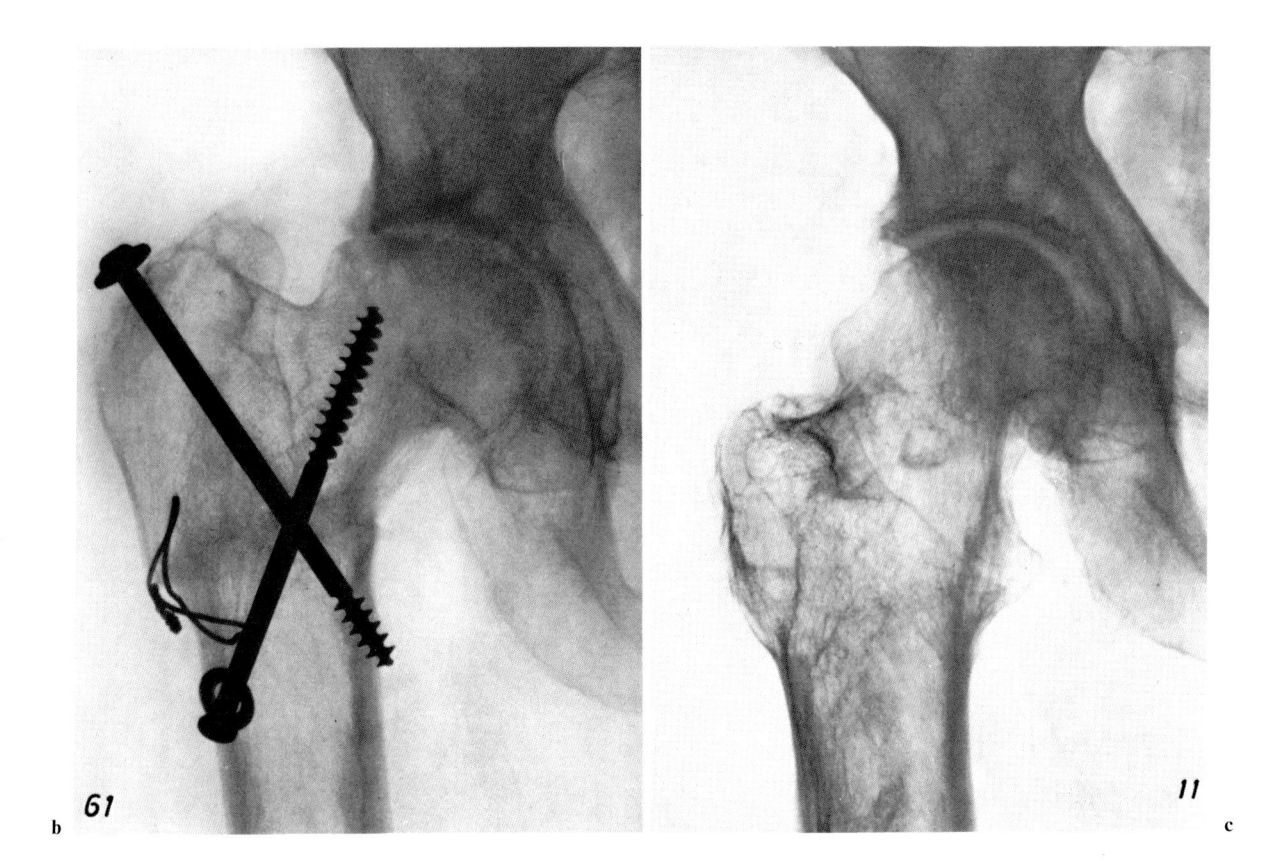

Fig. 179 b, c.

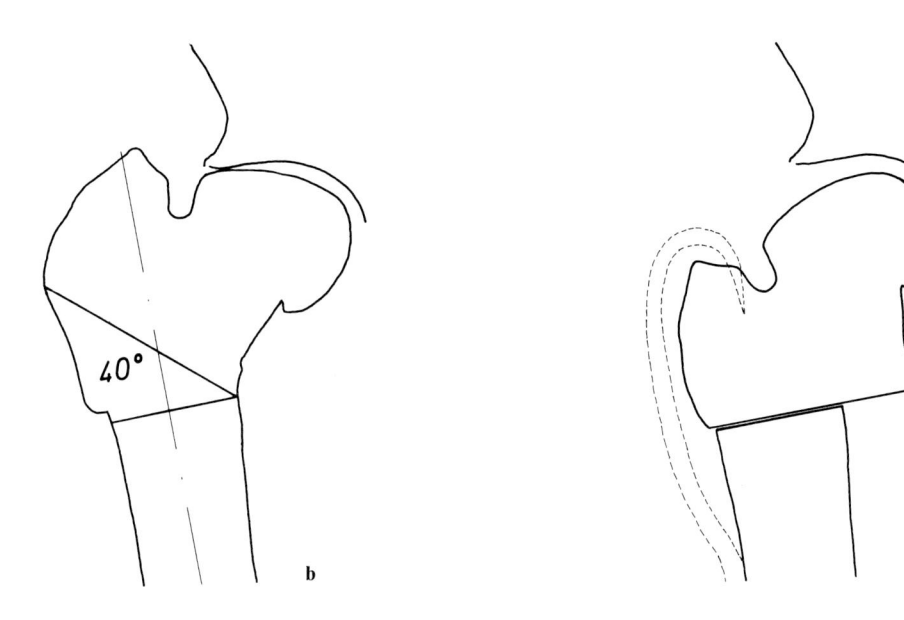

Fig. 180 b, c.

177

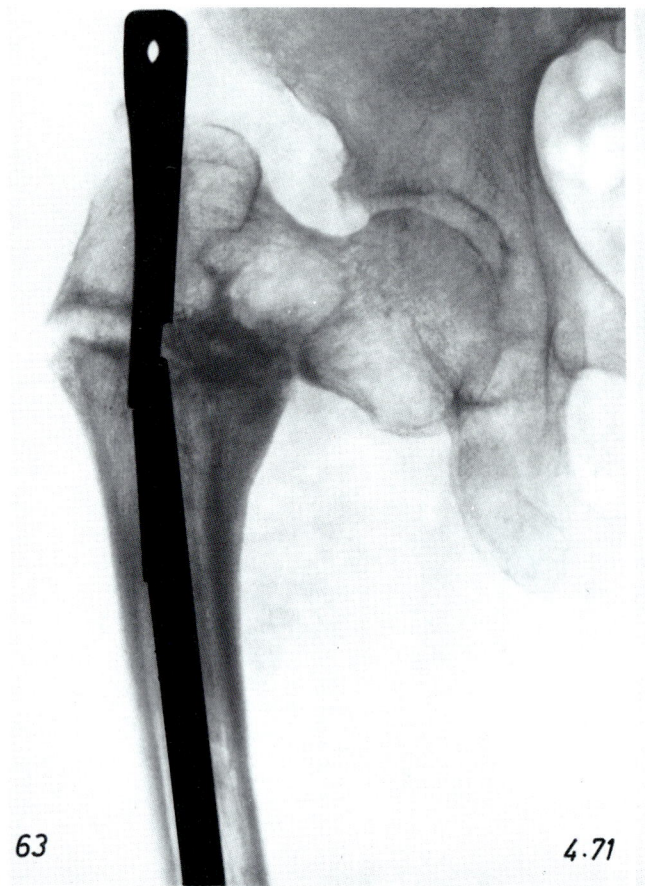

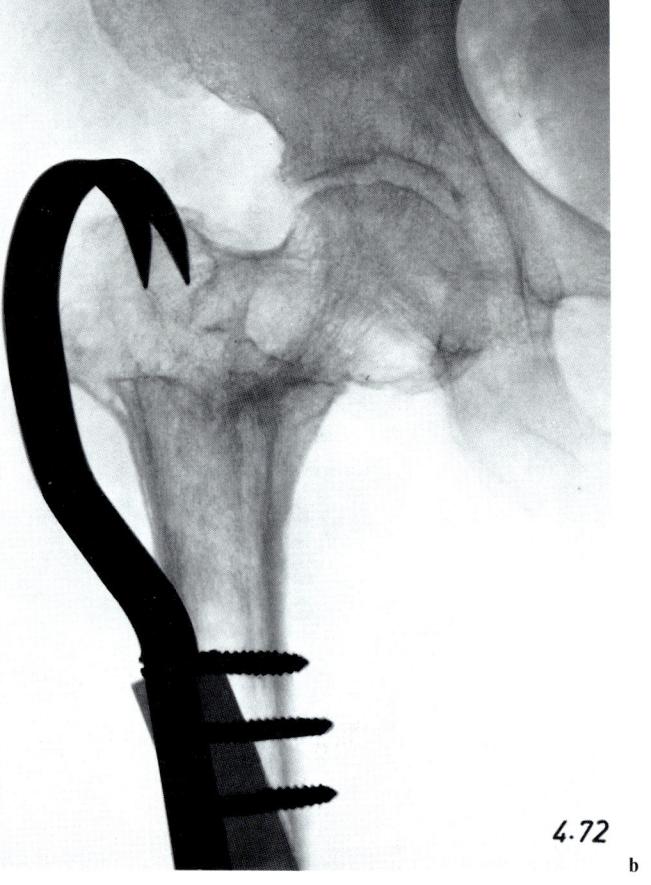

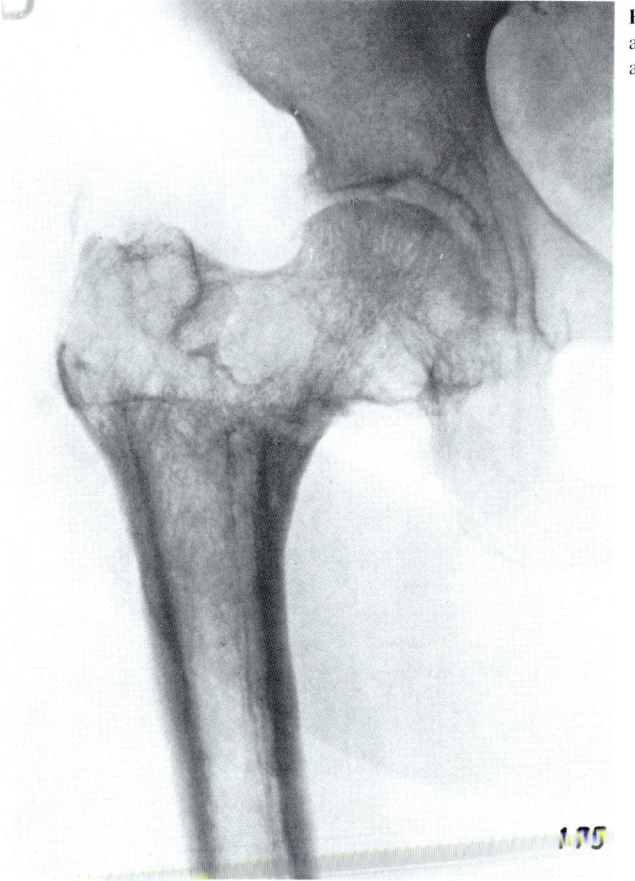

Fig. 181. a A 63-year-old female patient who had undergone a varus osteotomy 9 years previously. **b** Two years and **c** 4 years after a valgus osteotomy

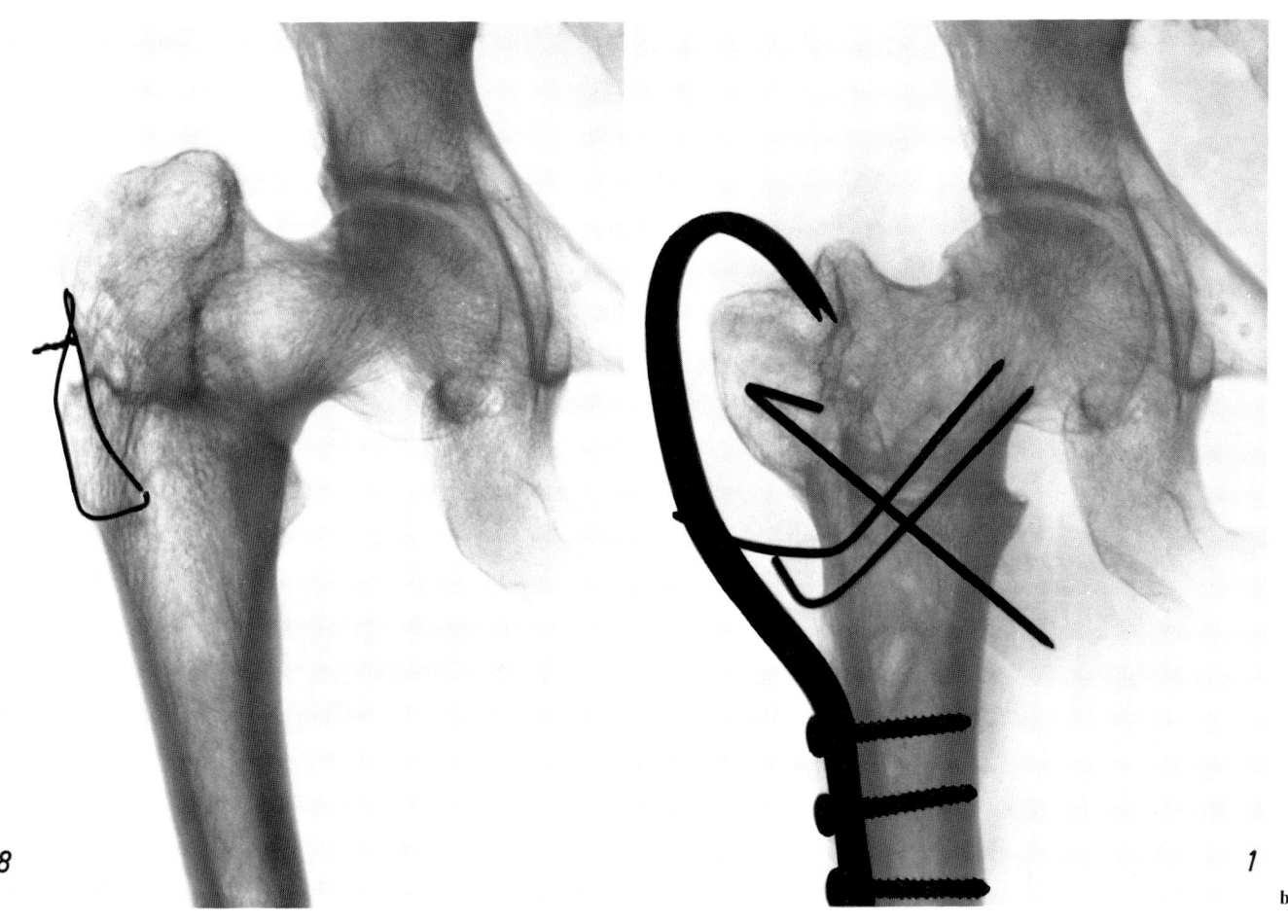

Fig. 182. a A 48-year-old female patient who had undergone a varus osteotomy 20 years previously. **b** One year after a valgus osteotomy

Some operation techniques seem not to ensure reliably the desired degree of varum. Reoperation may occasionally be necessary in order to decrease an exaggerated varum.

A 63-year-old female patient had undergone a varus osteotomy elsewhere 9 years previously. She continued to complain of pain and to limp: she had actually developed non-union with an exaggerated varus deformity (Fig. 181a). A valgus osteotomy was carried out. At the 2-year (Fig. 181b) and at the 4-year follow-ups (Fig. 181c), the result was excellent.

A 48-year old female patient had undergone a varus osteotomy 20 years previously. She did well for some years, despite some limping, and then began to complain of pain in the hip again. A dense triangle at the edge of the socket indicated that this edge acted as a fulcrum on which the femoral head pivoted (Fig. 182a). A 37° valgus osteotomy was carried out with an excellent result (Fig. 182b).

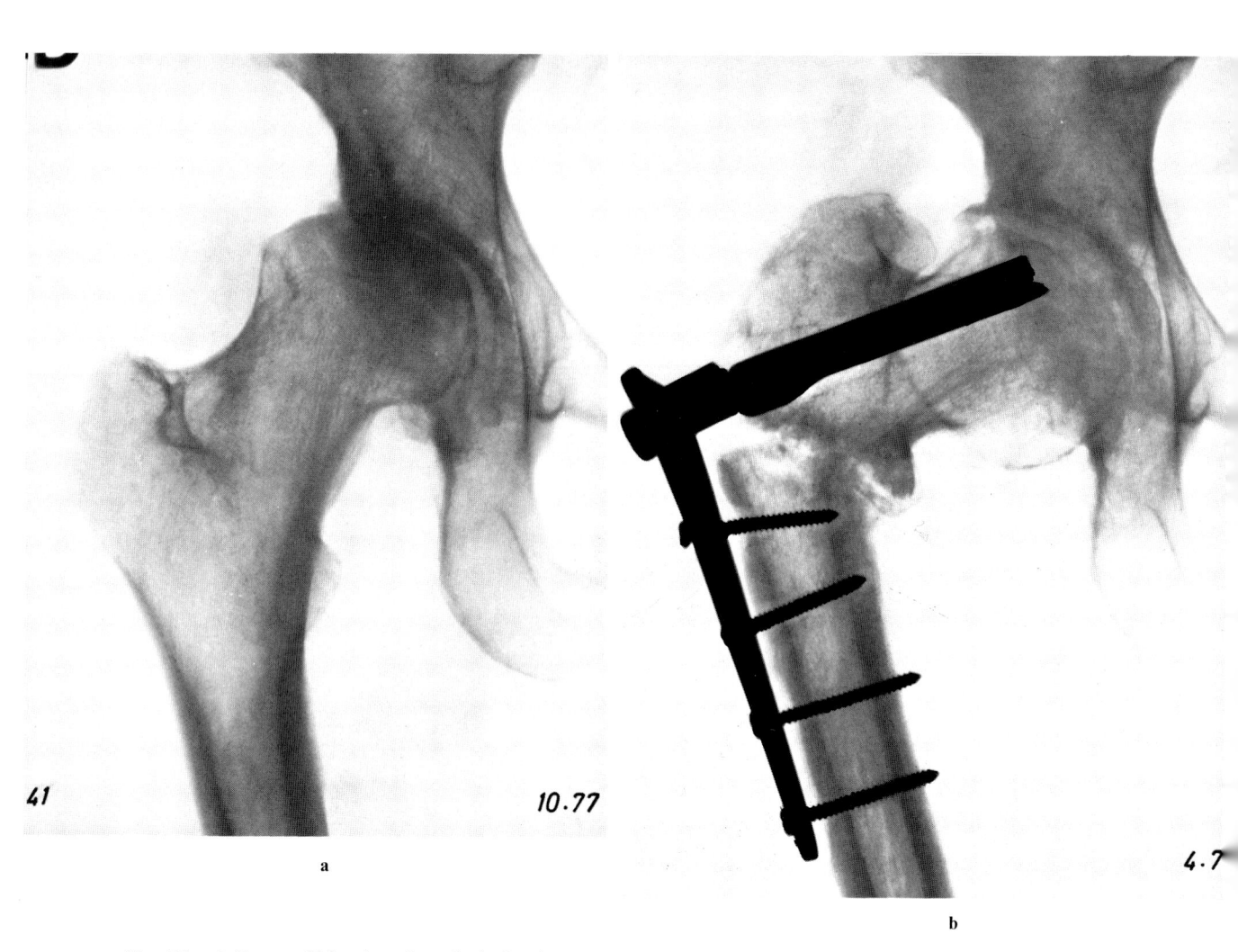

Fig. 183. a A 41-year-old female patient who had undergone a varus osteotomy 18 months previously. **b** There was a pseudarthrosis. **c** She underwent a valgus osteotomy. **d** Two-year follow-up

A 41-year-old female patient (Fig. 183a) underwent a varus osteotomy for severe osteoarthritis of the hip. When we saw her 18 months later, she had developed an exaggerated varus deformity and a non-union (Fig. 183b). The metal was removed, a 20° wedge comprising the non-union was resected and the fragments were fixed under compression (Fig. 183c). At the 2-year follow-up, the result was excellent (Fig. 183d).

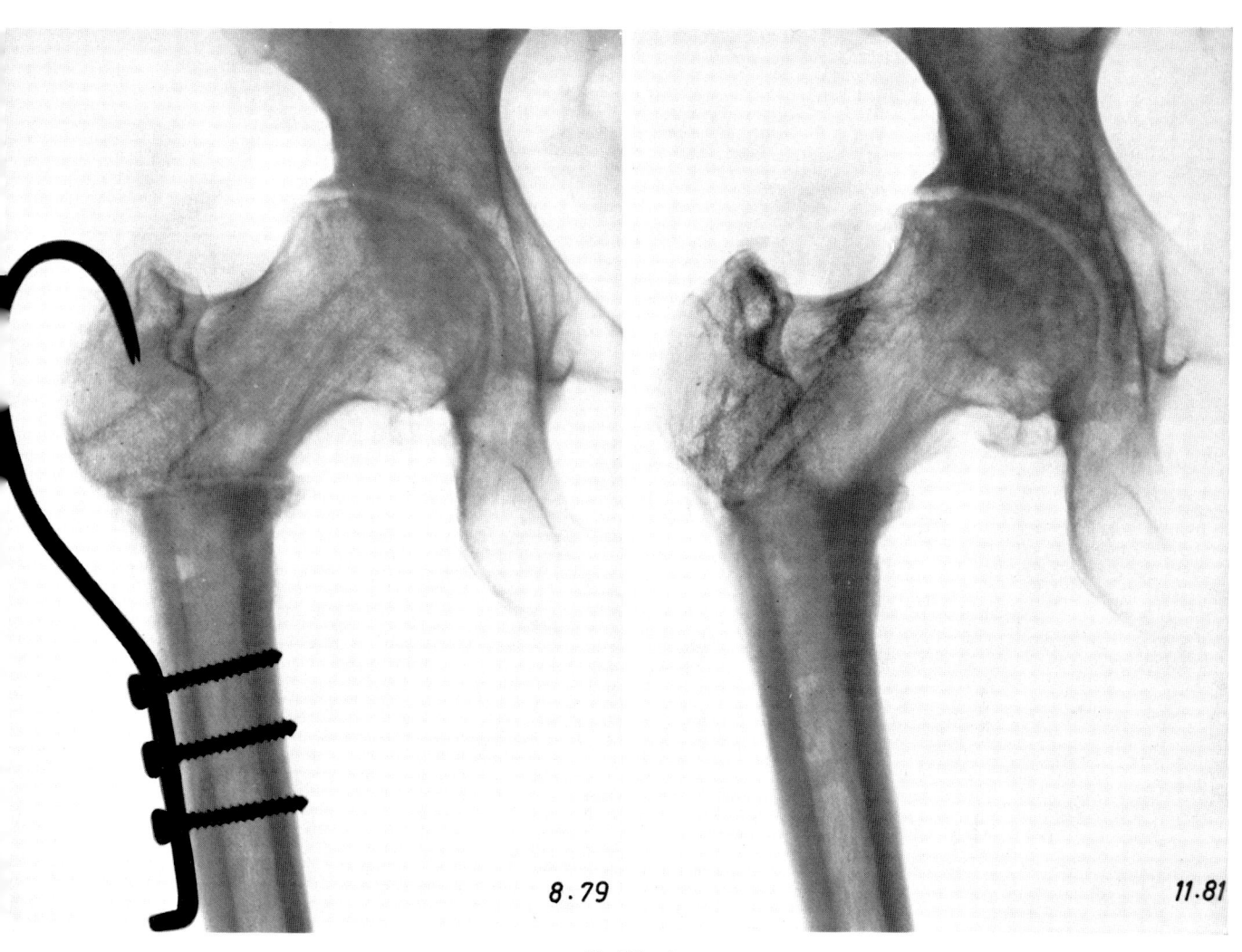

Fig. 183 c, d

C. After a Valgus Osteotomy

In some patients the degree of valgum achieved by surgery may be insufficient to enlarge the weight-bearing surface of the joint. A 54-year-old female patient (Fig. 184a) underwent a 25° valgus osteotomy (Fig. 185). Two years later (Fig. 184b) there was no improvement. Incongruence of the articular surfaces and a dense triangle at the edge of the socket showed that the weight-bearing surface remained too small. A new 32° valgus osteotomy was carried out (Fig. 186). At the 6-year follow-up (Fig. 184c) the articular surfaces appeared congruent, with a wide joint space, and the dense triangle had been replaced by a subchondral sclerosis of even width throughout. The articular compressive stresses were now uniformly distributed over a large weight-bearing surface. It must be noted that the articular surface of the head in contact with the acetabulum consisted of the medial osteophyte alone.

Fig. 184. a A 54-year-old female patient before a valgus osteotomy. **b** Two years later the weight-bearing surface remained too small. **c** Six years after a second valgus osteotomy

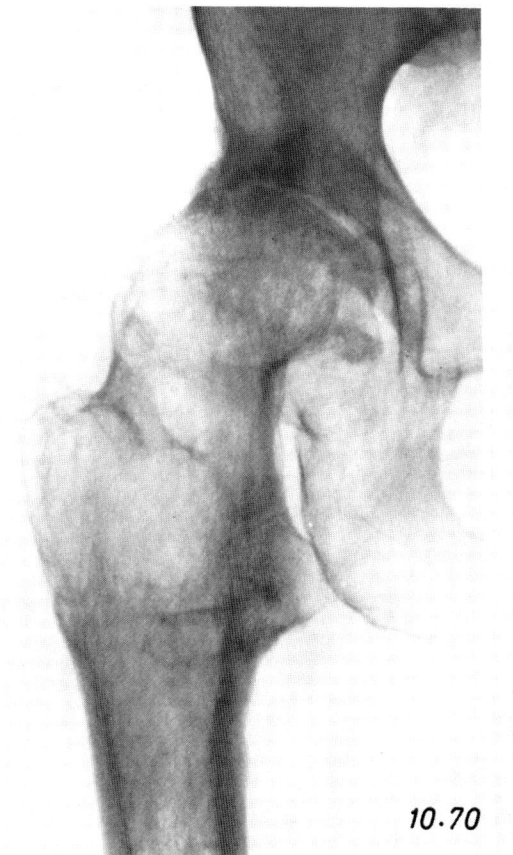

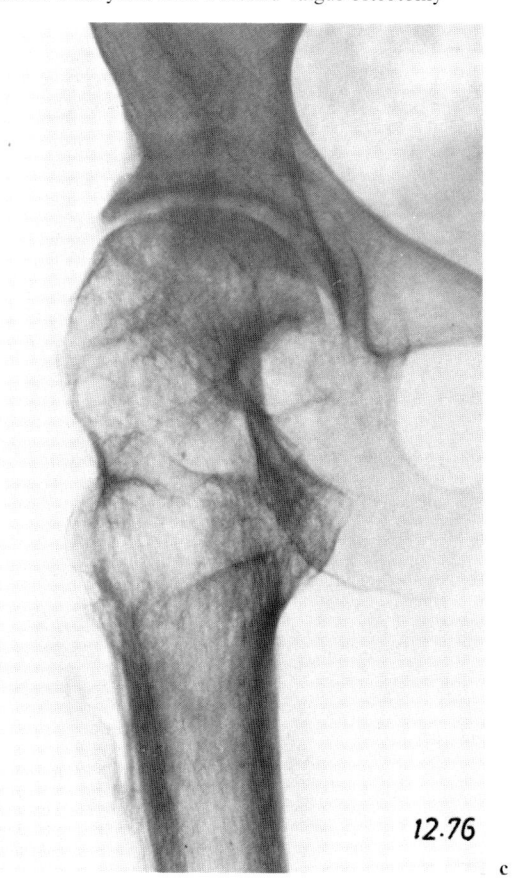

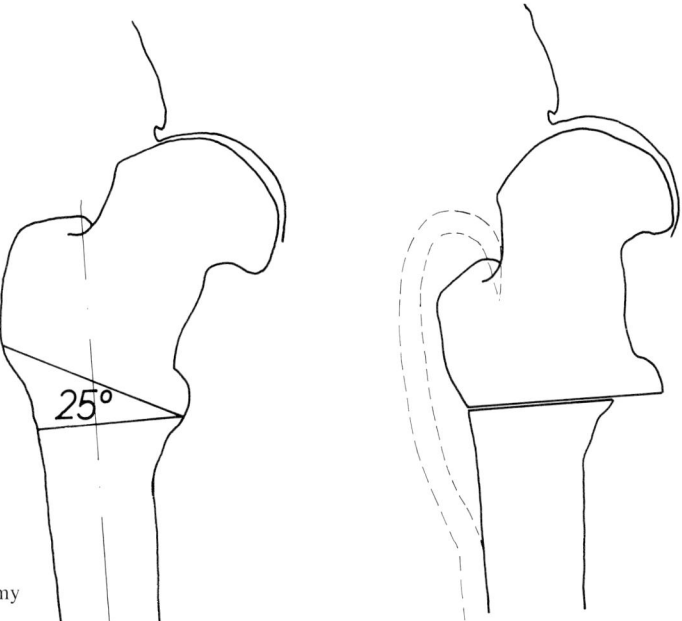

Fig. 185. Pre-operative planning of the first osteotomy on the hip shown in Fig. 184

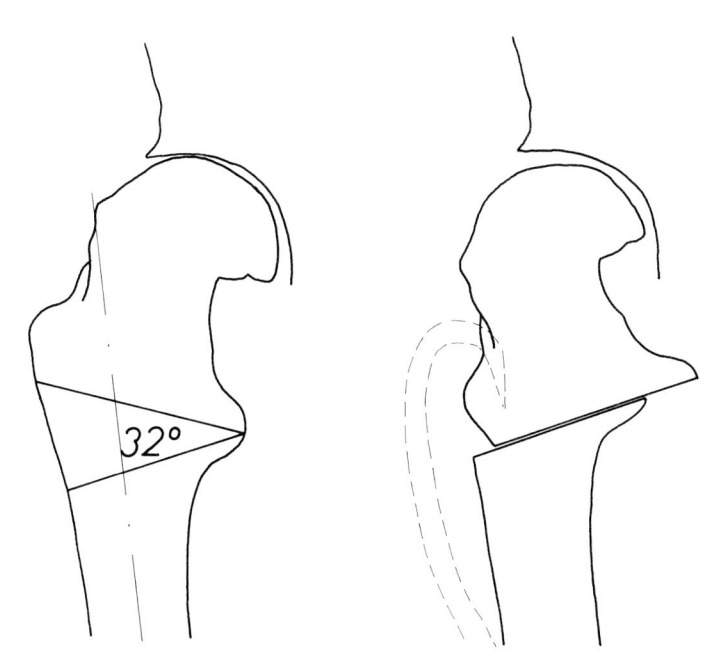

Fig. 186. Pre-operative planning of the second osteotomy on the hip shown in Fig. 184

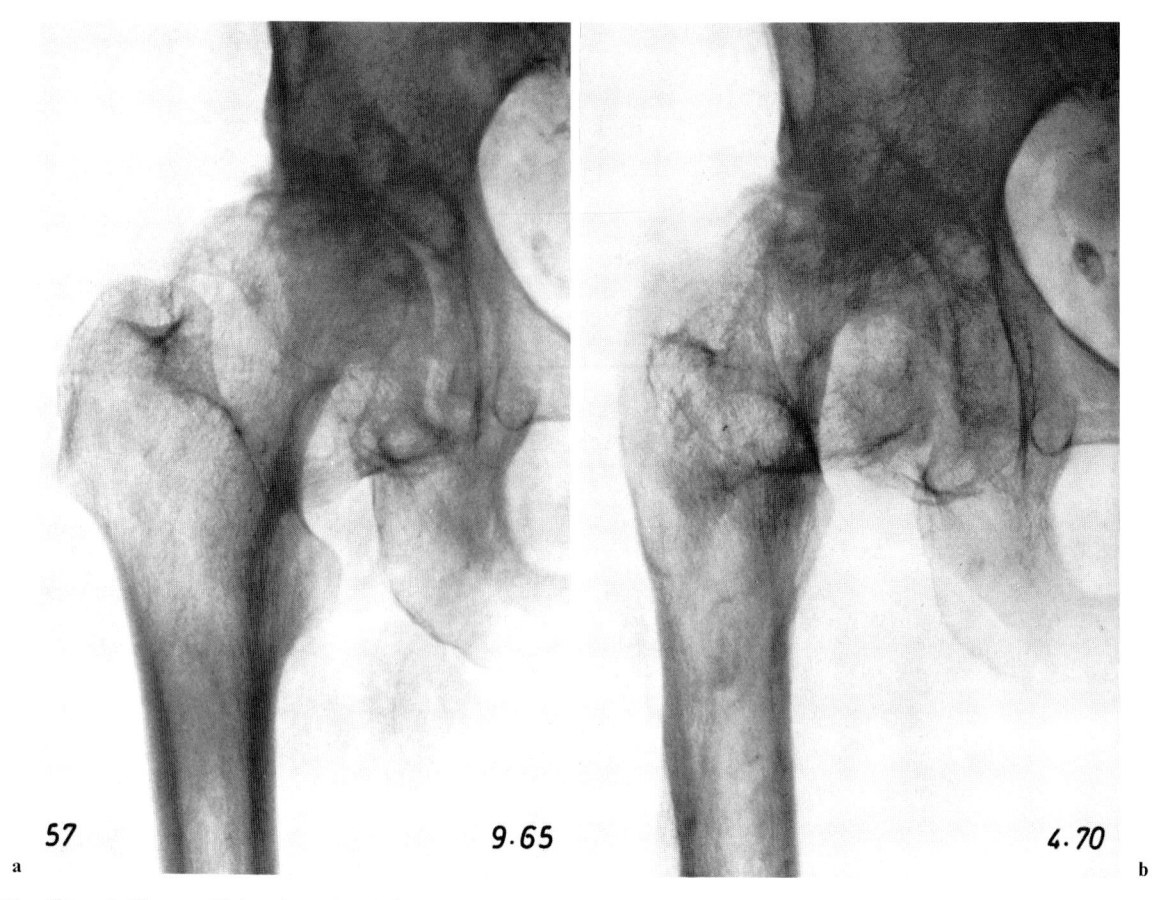

Fig. 187. a A 57-year-old female patient before a valgus osteotomy. **b** At 4 years the hip had deteriorated again. **c** Three years and **d** five years after a second valgus osteotomy

A 57-year-old female patient (Fig. 187a) underwent a 13° valgus osteotomy for severe osteoarthritis of the hip. At the 1-year follow-up the result was good. At the 4-year follow-up the hip had deteriorated again (Fig. 187b). A new valgus osteotomy was carried out with removal of a 30° wedge. Three and five years later the result was excellent (Fig. 187c, d).

5.73

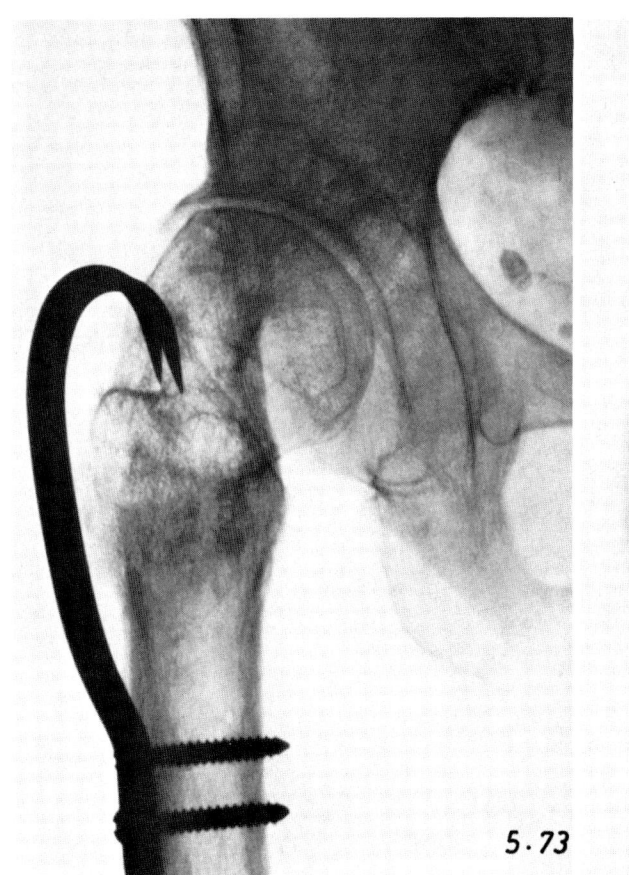

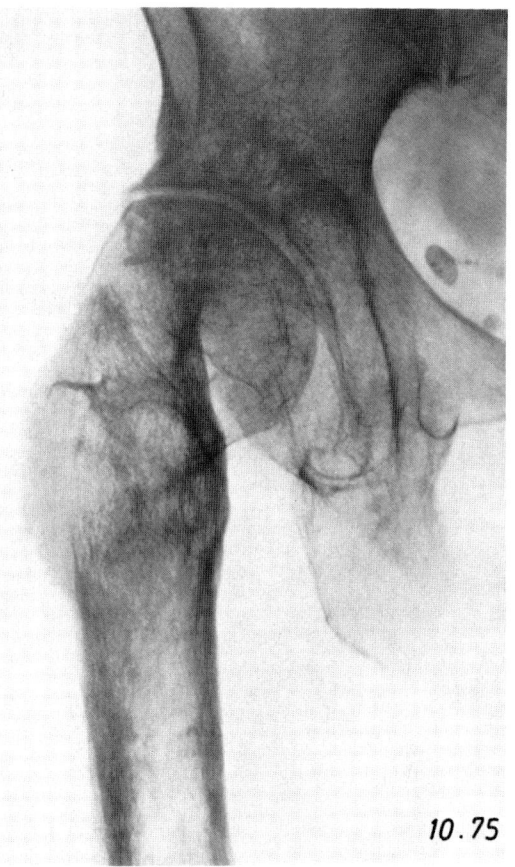

10.75

D. Conclusion

When a surgical procedure has not sufficiently enlarged a reduced articular weight-bearing surface, failure is the rule. If a revision is carried out which sufficiently enlarges the weight-bearing surface of the joint, the result is usually excellent. Dividing the tendons or even the bone is not in itself sufficient to bring about long-term improvement of the condition. The good results obtained after a significant increase in the weight-bearing surface of the joint by an appropriate operation emphasize the importance of the mechanical effect of the procedures thus proposed.

X. Age of the Patients and Duration of the Postoperative Results

Table 29. Range of movement of the hip (Fig. 188)

	Before surgery	At the 9-year follow-up	Gain
Flexion	60°	70°	15°
Extension	−5°	0°	
Adduction	15°	25°	35°
Abduction	−5°	20°	
Int. rotation	5°	5°	15°
Ext. rotation	5°	20°	

The tissues seem to retain their capacity to heal until the end of life as long as they are subjected to appropriate mechanical conditions. They also react to unfavourable circumstances and to foreign bodies, even in old people. A good example of this is described on page 93; there are others.

A 78-year-old female patient developed severe osteoarthritis which had been unsuccessfully treated with steroids (Fig. 188a). An appropriate valgus osteotomy was carried out. At the 9-year follow-up, the clinical result was excellent: no pain, good range of movement (Table 29), no limp. In the X-rays the signs of osteoarthritis had regressed and a wide joint space was present (Fig. 188b).

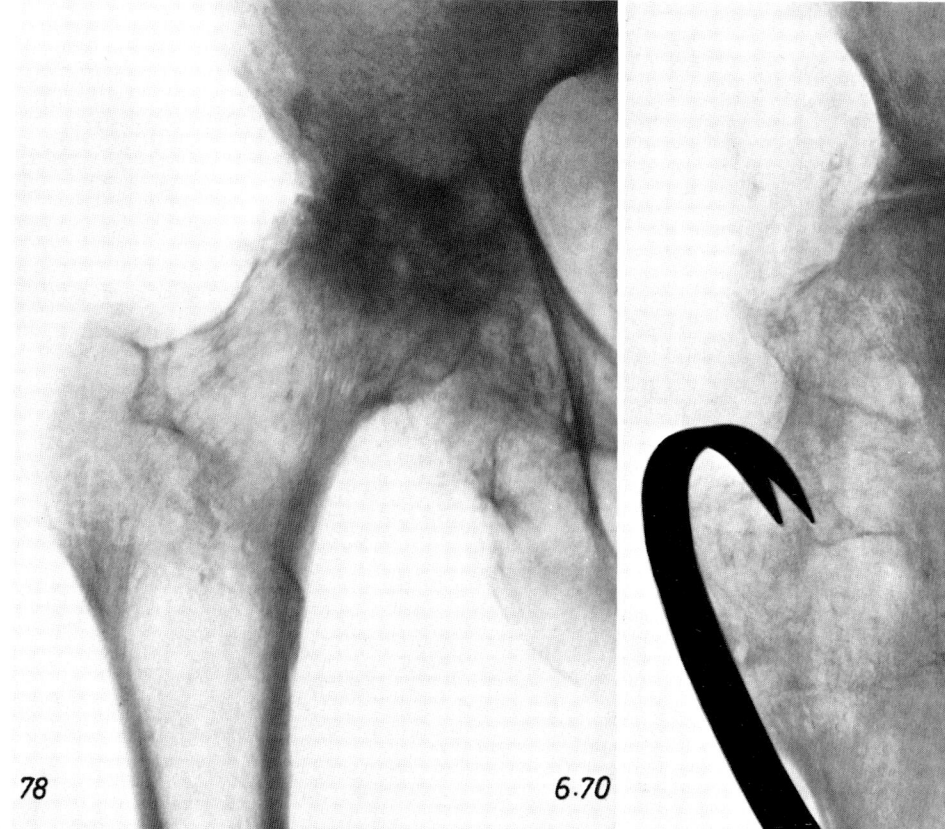

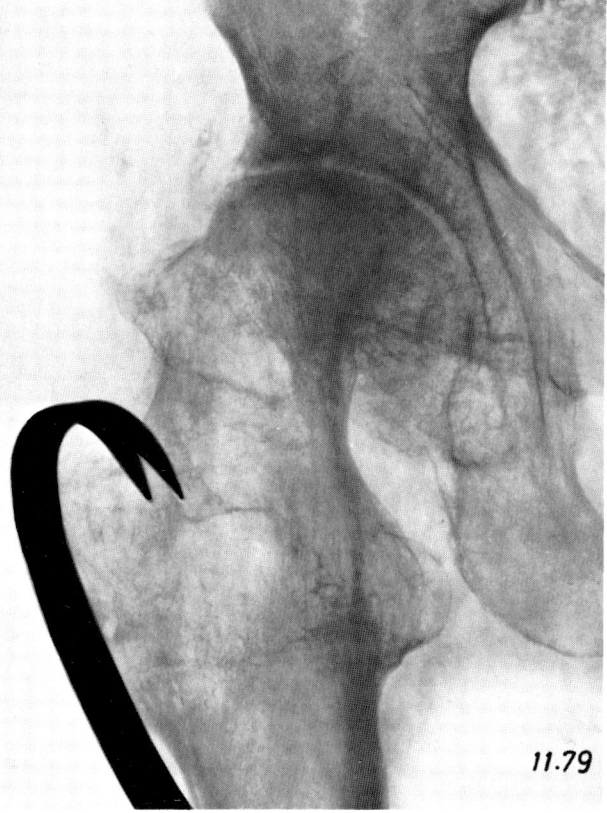

Fig. 188. a A 78-year-old female patient before a valgus osteotomy. b Nine years afterwards

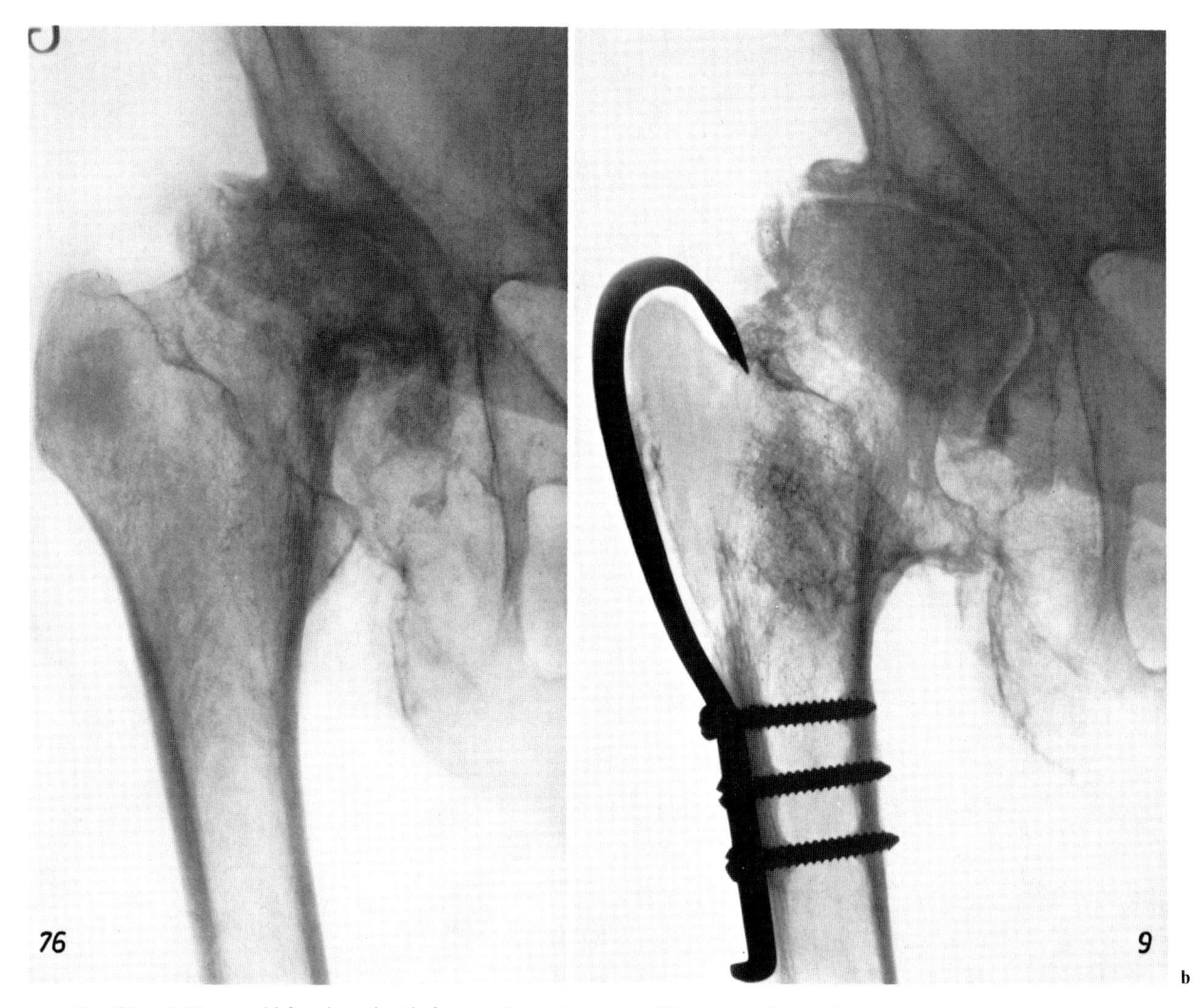

Fig. 189. a A 76-year-old female patient before a valgus osteotomy. **b** Nine years afterwards

A 76-year-old female patient presented with osteoarthritis and extensive remodelling of the femoral head and socket (Fig. 189a). The hip was painful, with a limited range of movement (Table 30). She underwent a valgus osteotomy combined with a tenotomy. At the 9-year follow-up, the clinical result was good: no pain, better range of movement than before surgery (Table 30) and only a slight limp. In the X-rays, the subchondral sclerosis had become uniform throughout and a wide joint space had reappeared (Fig. 189b).

Table 30. Range of movement of the hip (Fig. 189)

	Before surgery	At the 9-year follow-up	Gain
Flexion	25°	50°	
Extension	−5°	−5°	25°
Adduction	20°	25°	
Abduction	−5°	10°	20°
Int. rotation	−5°	10°	
Ext. rotation	10°	15°	20°

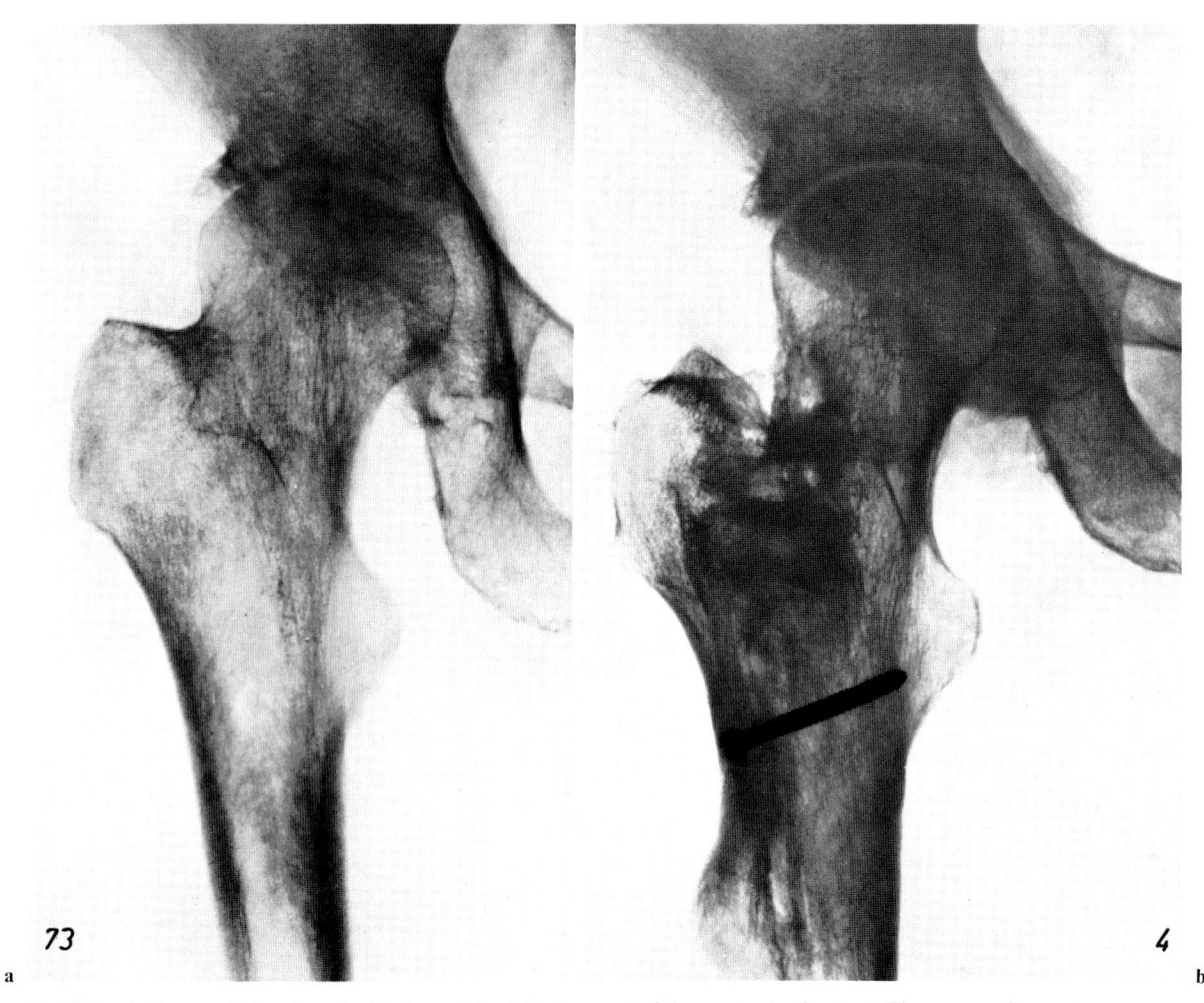

Fig. 190. a A 73-year-old female patient before a lateral displacement of the greater trochanter. **b** Three years afterwards

A 73-year-old female patient with severe osteoarthritis (Fig. 190a) underwent a lateral displacement of the greater trochanter combined with a tenotomy. At the 4-year follow-up, her hip had considerably improved (Fig. 190b). The clinical improvement was also appreciable (Table 31). Other examples of recovery in elderly patients have been described above (pp. 71–74 and 92, 94).

In old age total hip arthroplasty is often advocated because recovery is quick and improvement immediate and dramatic. However, the operative procedure is usually less benign than a tenotomy or an osteotomy. The blood loss is greater. After the joint-preserving operations, the patients get up on the 2nd day and are encouraged to walk more and more. It is true that crutches are recommended for a longer period of time than after a total replacement. But many of these elderly patients have used crutches or walking sticks before their operations anyway, and many keep them even after a total hip arthroplasty, at least for some months.

Table 31. Range of movement of the hip (Fig. 190)

	Before surgery	At the 4-year follow-up	Gain
Flexion	90°	95°	20°
Extension	−25°	−10°	
Adduction	20°	15°	20°
Abduction	0°	25°	
Int. rotation	−5°	0°	20°
Ext. rotation	15°	30°	

The theoretical inconvenience of the crutches seems to be counterbalanced by the benignity of the joint-preserving operations, the lower complication rate and the fact that living tissues are conserved. Therefore, even in elderly patients these hip-preserving operations are to be recommended in preference to total replacement, as long as the pre-operative X-rays and planning enable one unequivocally to predict a biological recovery of the joint.

XI. Long-term Results

A. Lasting Positive Results

PAUWELS (1973) published follow-up observations extending over more than 20 years. Most of the excellent results obtained in the course of the 1st postoperative year subsequently improved and remained excellent. My own experience confirms his observations. A 47-year-old female patient underwent a valgus osteotomy combined with a tenotomy (Fig. 191a). At the 17-year follow-up, the result remained excellent (Fig. 191b and Table 32). The weight-bearing surface of the femoral head was constituted by the medial osteophyte only. Other examples are mentioned on pages 98, 99 and 126, 130.

Table 32. Range of movement of the hip (Fig. 191)

	Before surgery	At the 17-year follow-up	Gain
Flexion	20°	80°	60°
Extension	0°	0°	
Adduction	10°	30°	45°
Abduction	− 5°	20°	
Int. rotation	−20°	0°	35°
Ext. rotation	30°	45°	

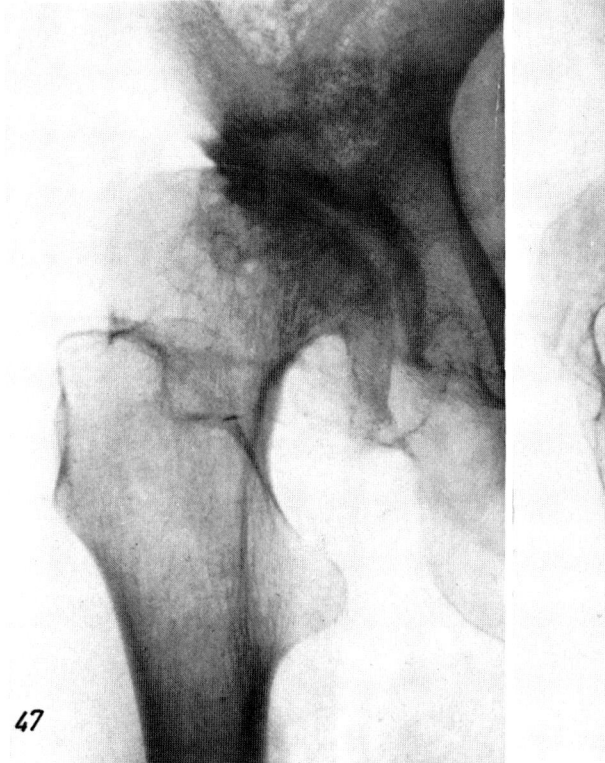

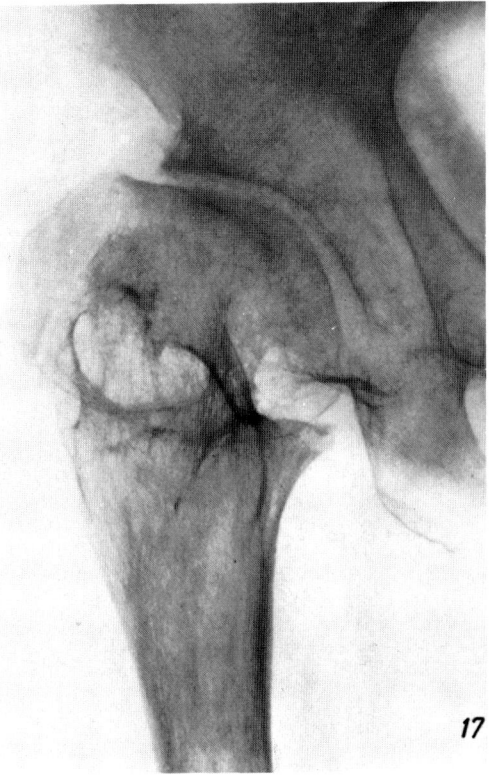

Fig. 191. a A 47-year-old female patient before a Pauwels II. **b** Seventeen years afterwards

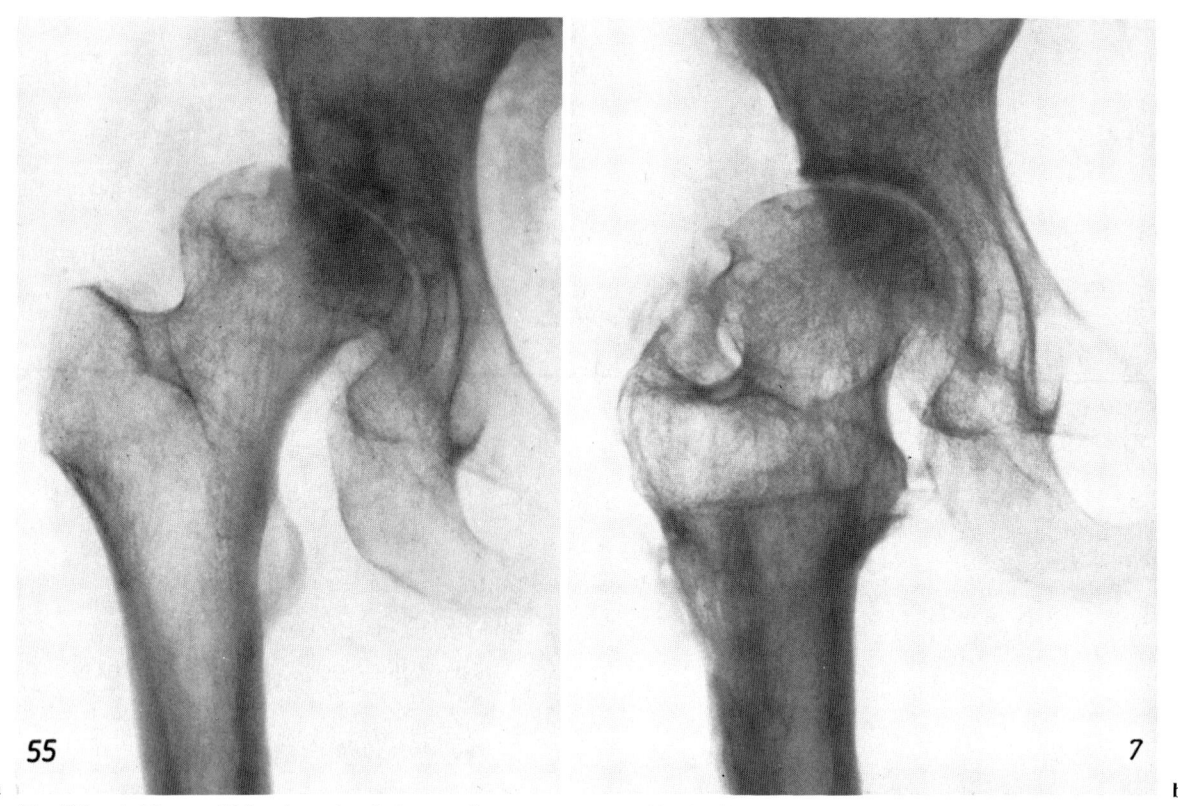

Fig. 192. a A 55-year-old female patient before a valgus osteotomy combined with a tenotomy. **b** Seven years afterwards

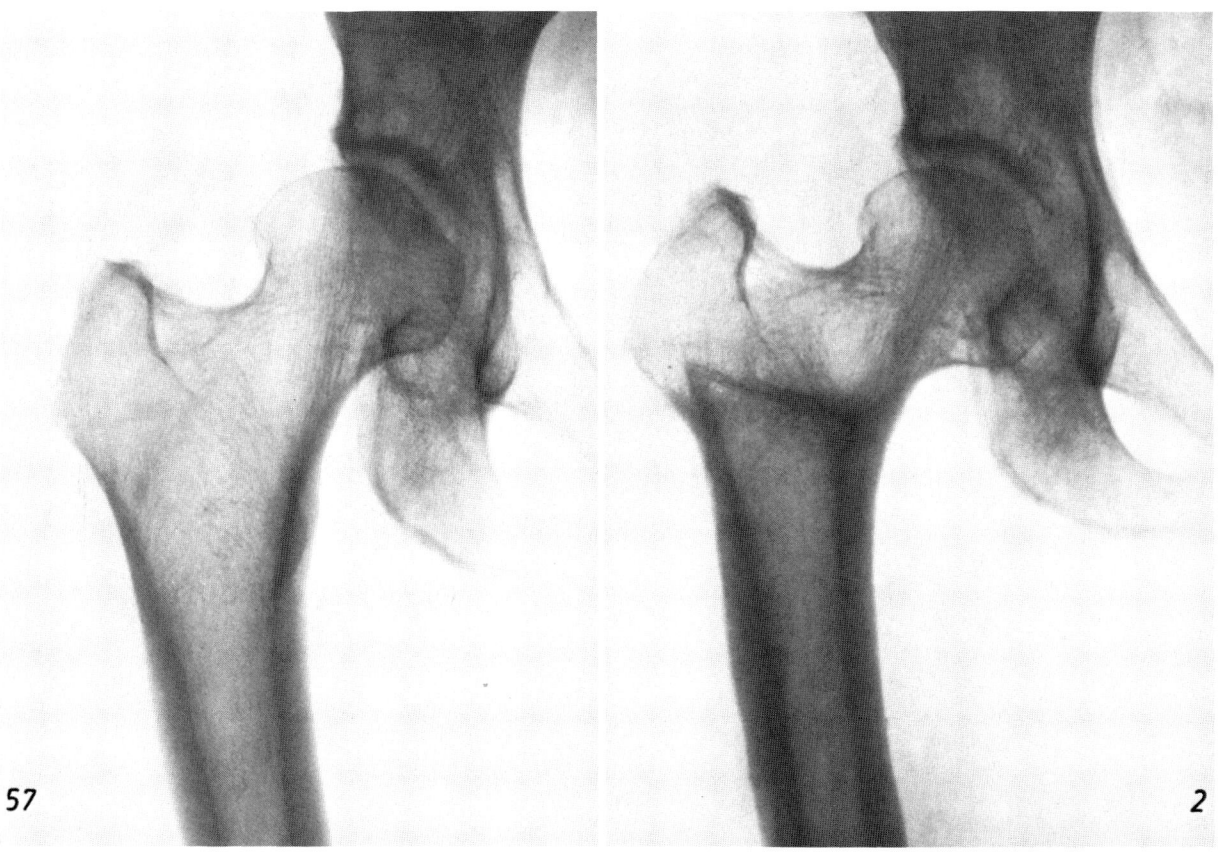

Fig. 193a, b. Same patient as in Fig. 192: opposite hip. **a** operation at age 57; **b** 2 years later

Fig. 192c. At the 11-year follow-up, deterioration was observed

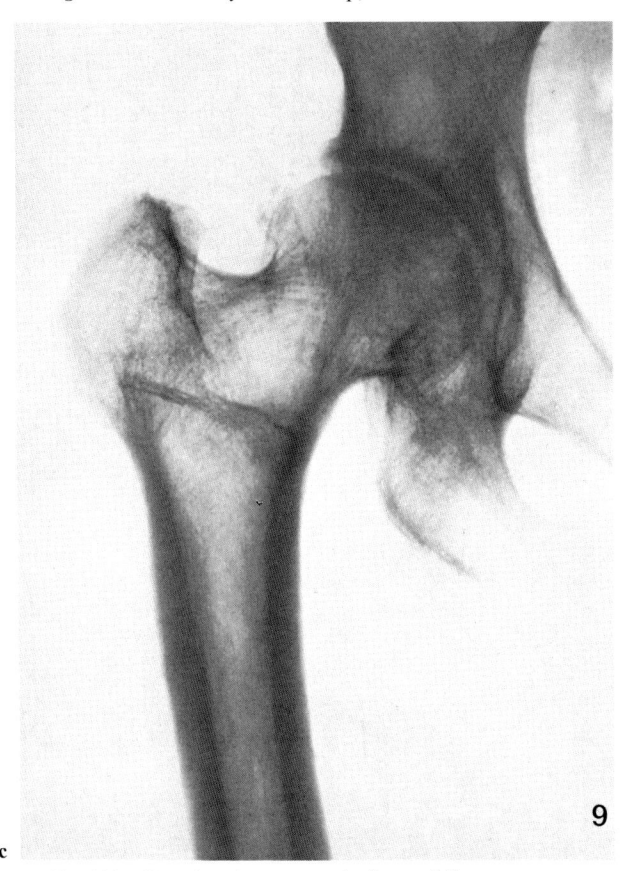

Fig. 193c. Deterioration seen at the 9-year follow-up

B. Secondary Deterioration

Some hips improve dramatically after an appropriate joint-preserving operation but degenerate again after some years. This may occur on both sides simultaneously, despite a different follow-up period for each side. Deterioration seems to coincide with a general lowering of the tissue resistance.

A 55-year-old female patient with severe osteoarthritis (Fig. 192a) underwent a valgus osteotomy of the right femur combined with a tenotomy. At the 7-year follow-up, the clinical result was good (Table 33). In the X-rays a subchondral sclerosis of uniform width throughout had replaced the pre-operative dense triangle at the edge of the acetabulum and a wide joint space had developed (Fig. 192b). Four years later, at the 11-year follow-up, the joint space had disappeared and a new dense triangle had developed at the edge of the socket (Fig. 192c). The clinical picture had also worsened: pain with weather changes, some restriction of movement (Table 34) and a limp.

Table 33. Range of movement of the hip (Fig. 192)

	Before surgery	At the 7-year follow-up	Gain
Flexion	95°	90°	−5°
Extension	0°	0°	
Adduction	20°	45°	60°
Abduction	10°	45°	
Int. rotation	0°	25°	60°
Ext. rotation	10°	45°	

Table 34. Range of movement of the hip (Fig. 192)

	Before surgery	At the 11-year follow-up	Gain
Flexion	95°	85°	10°
Extension	0°	0°	
Adduction	20°	15°	10°
Abduction	10°	25°	
Int. rotation	0°	25°	40°
Ext. rotation	10°	25°	

At the age of 57 the same patient underwent a varus osteotomy for osteoarthritis of the opposite hip (Fig. 193a). Two years later the left hip looked very satisfactory (Fig. 193b) and the clinical result was excellent, but by the 9-year follow-up the joint space had become narrower (Fig. 193c) and the hip ached when the weather changed. Both hips seemed to deteriorate simultaneously, although they had been operated on at an interval of 2 years.

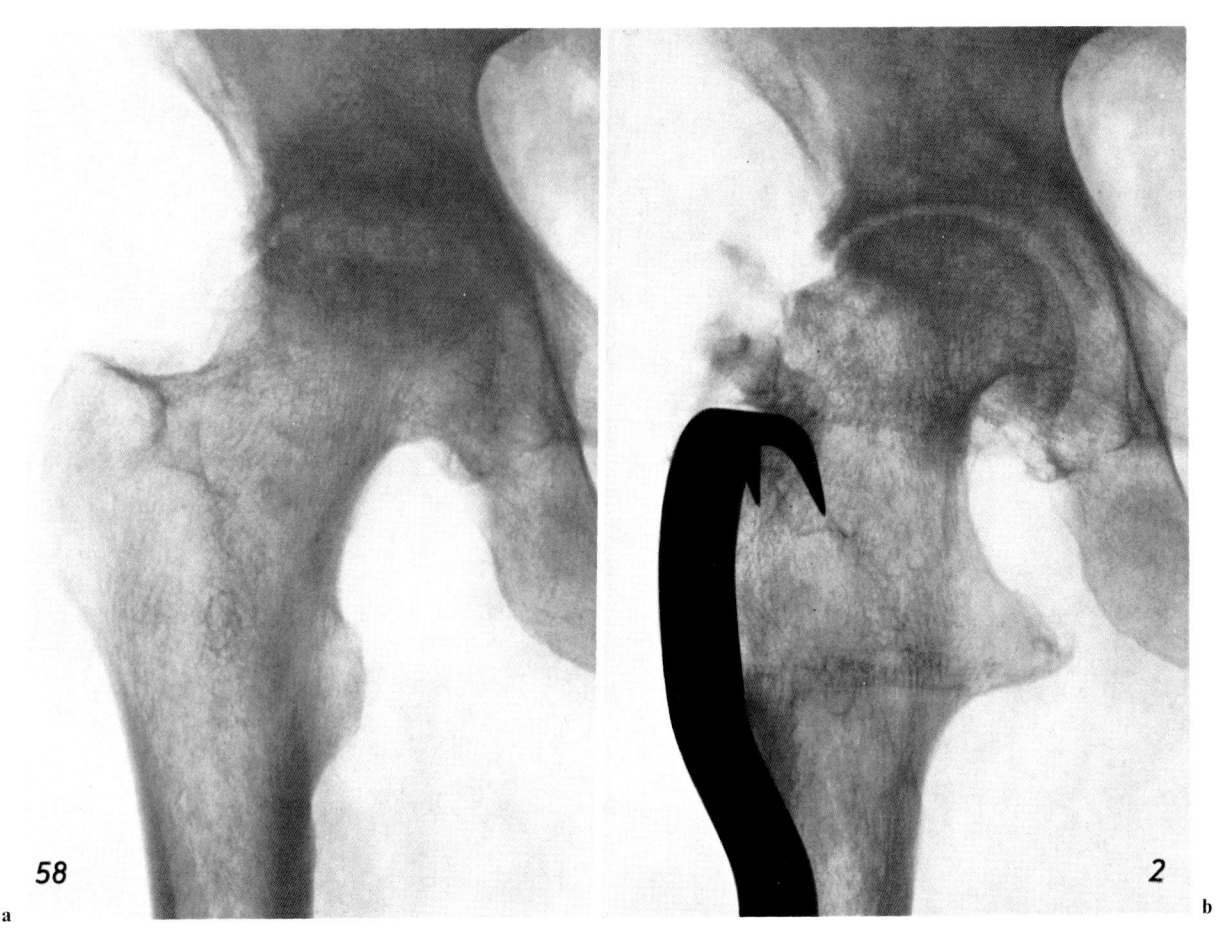

Fig. 194. a A 58-year-old male patient with necrosis of the femoral head following a traumatic dislocation of the hip. **b** Two years after a valgus intertrochanteric osteotomy combined with a tenotomy. **c** Seven years after the operation. **d** Deterioration seen at the 10-year follow-up. **e** At the 11-year follow-up total hip replacement was decided upon. Eleven years had been gained

A 58-year-old male patient presented with very severe osteoarthritis of the hip (Fig. 194a) secondary to an ischaemic necrosis of the femoral head, the consequence of a traumatic dislocation of the hip. He underwent a valgus osteotomy combined with a tenotomy, and was subsequently able to resume his work as a games teacher. At the 2-year follow-up, the signs of osteoarthritis had dramatically regressed (Fig. 194b). At 7 years, the joint space was a little narrower but the subchondral sclerosis remained uniform throughout (Fig. 194c). At 10 years, the joint space was further narrowed and a dense triangle had appeared at the edge of the socket (Fig. 194d); the patient again complained of pain. A total hip arthroplasty was carried out 11 years after the osteotomy (Fig. 194e). The patient was then 69 years old, and had been pain-free with good hip function for about 10 years.

Fig. 194c–e.

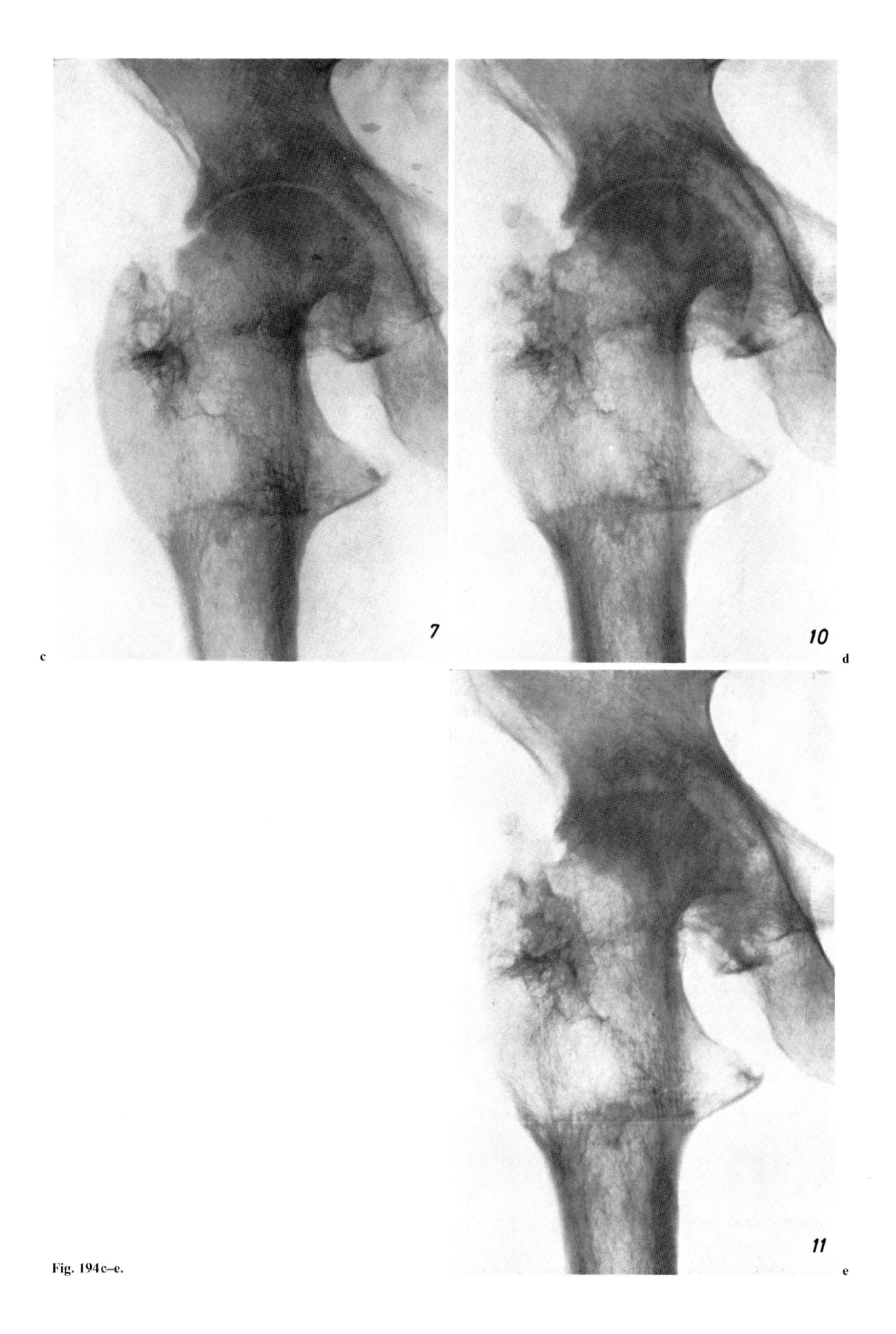

| a | b |

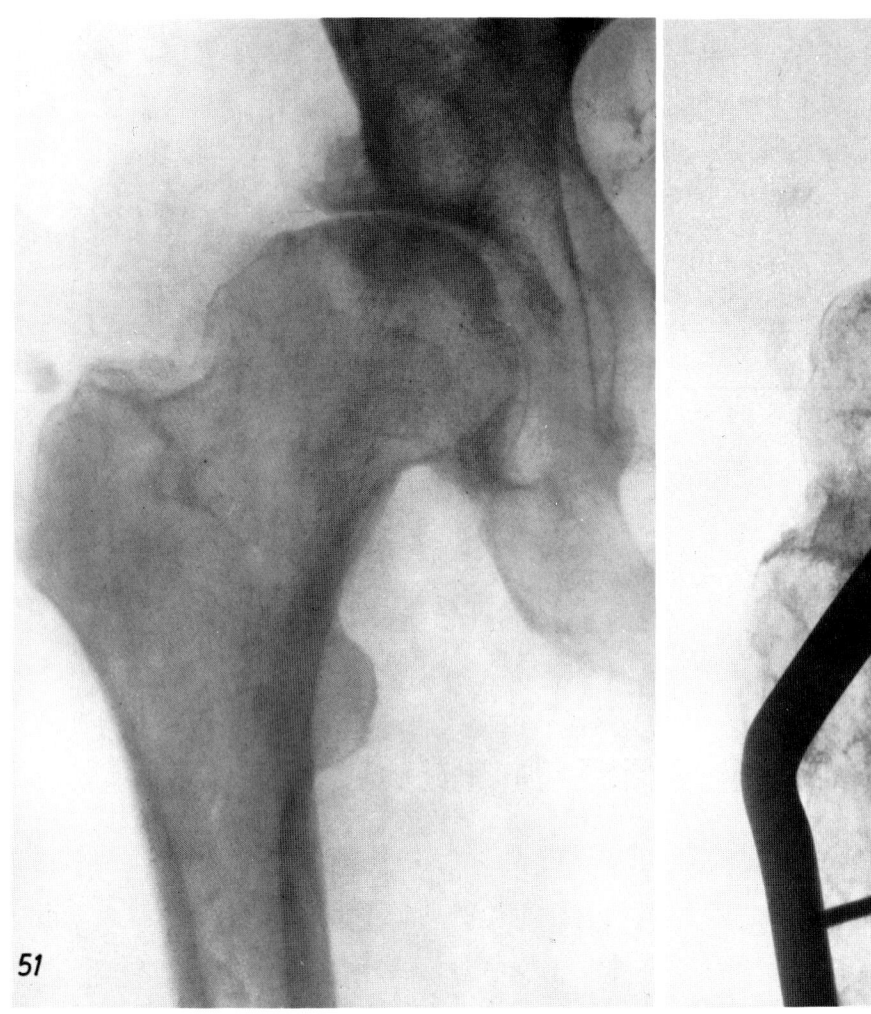

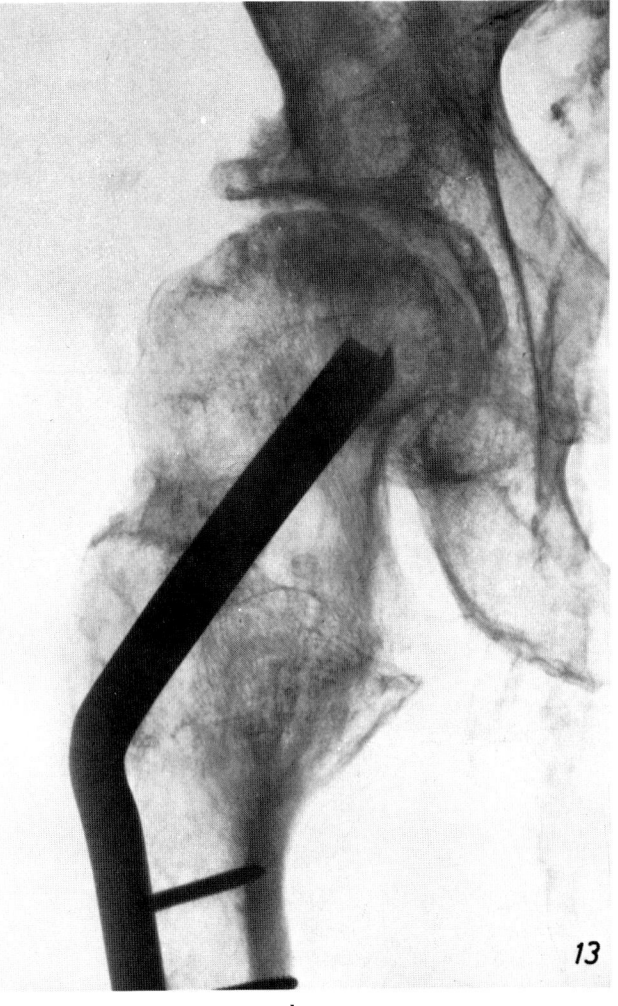

In some patients the cause of the deterioration can only be suspected. For example, a 51-year-old male patient underwent a valgus osteotomy combined with a tenotomy for severe osteoarthritis of the right hip (Fig. 195a). At the 13-year follow-up, the clinical result remained excellent and the X-rays showed far-reaching regeneration of the joint (Fig. 195b). At the 15-year follow-up, the hip had deteriorated (Fig. 195c). At the age of 57, the same patient underwent a valgus osteotomy on the opposite side (Fig. 196a). At the 7-year follow-up, the result looked satisfactory (Fig. 196b). Two years later the left hip had deteriorated, although it remained almost pain-free (Fig. 196c). The patient had developed endarteritis with obstruction of the iliac arteries, and these had to be by-passed by artificial grafts before a total hip arthroplasty could be carried out on the painful right hip. The vascular condition may have provoked the deterioration. In some other patients a cerebral thrombosis precedes the deterioration.

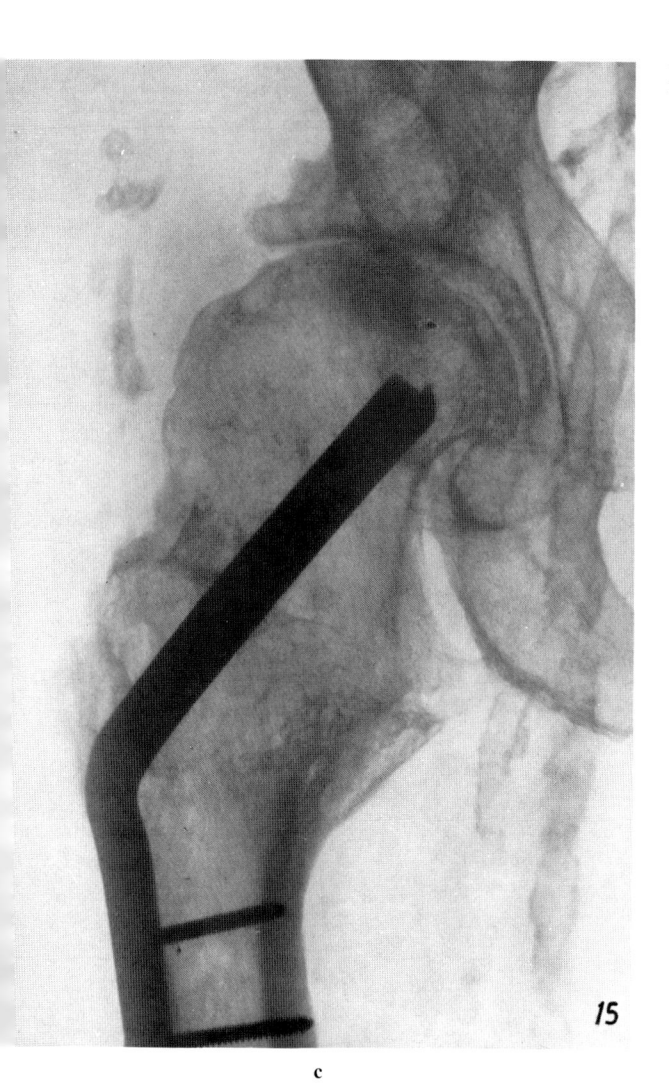

Fig. 195. a A 51-year-old male patient before a Pauwels II. **b** Thirteen years afterwards. **c** Deterioration observed after 15 years

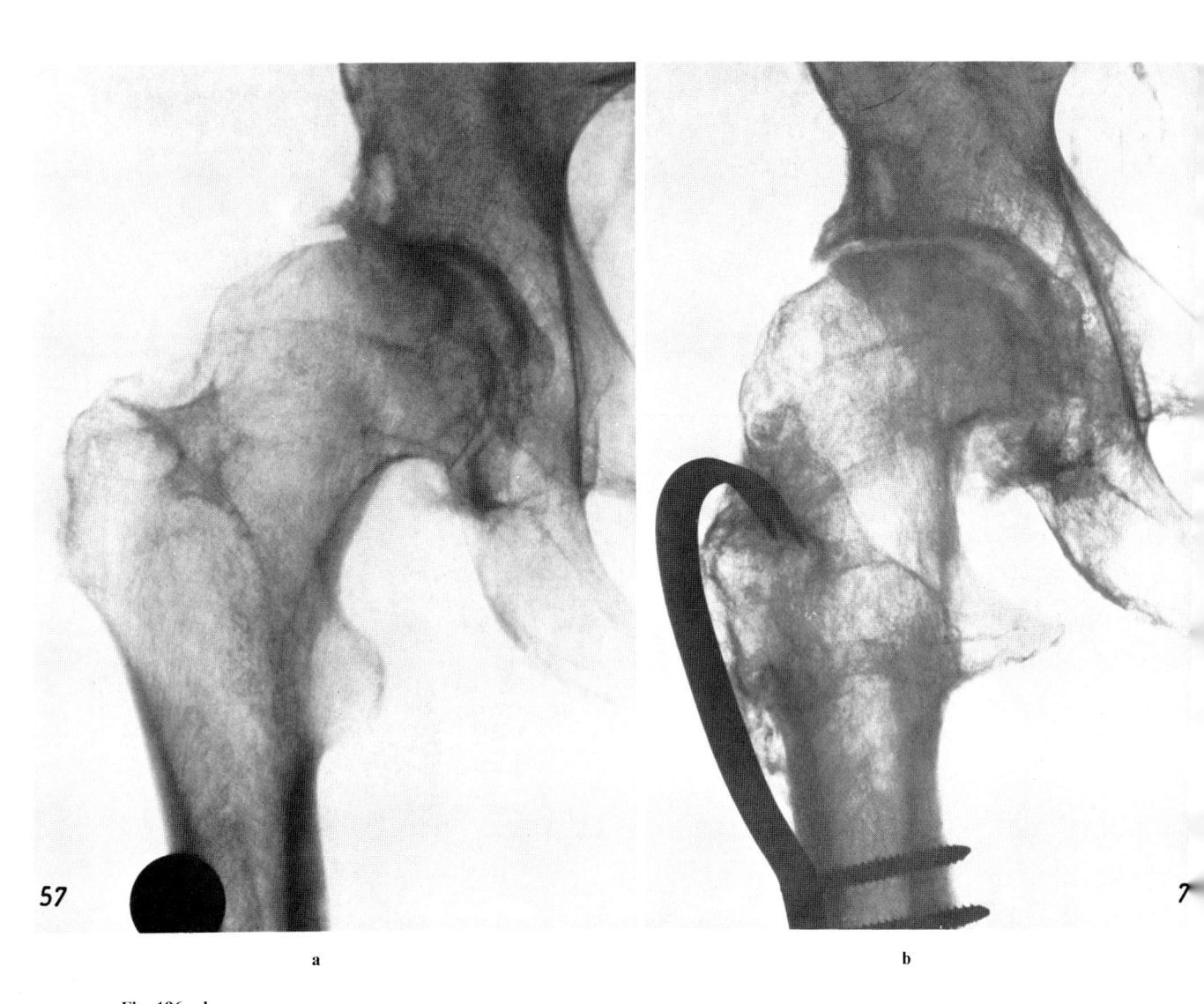

Fig. 196a, b

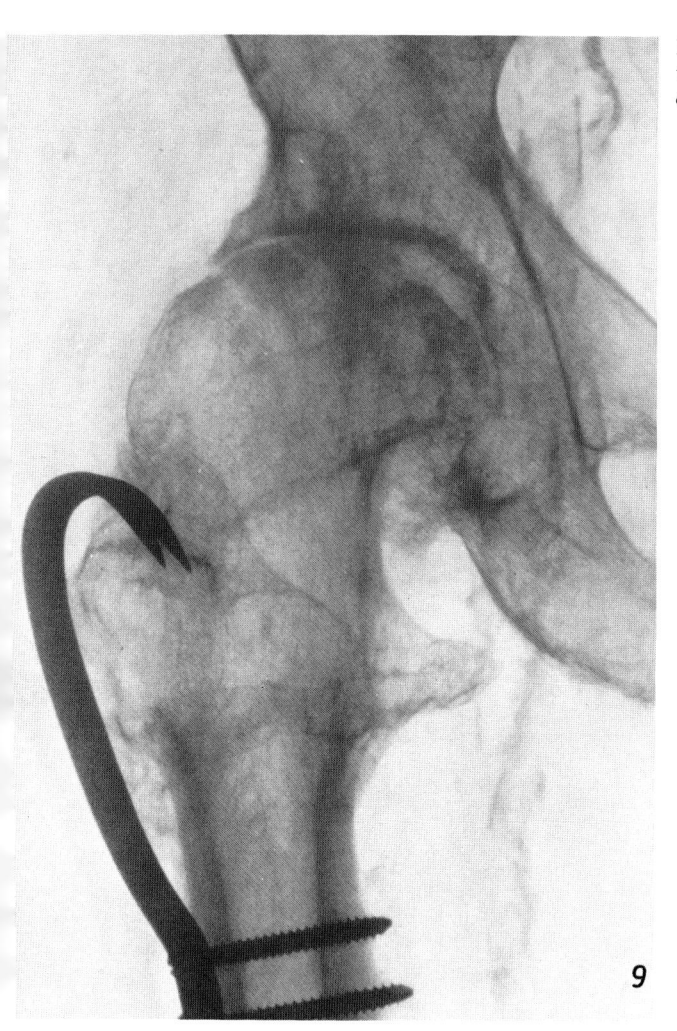

Fig. 196a–c. Same patient as in Fig. 195: opposite hip. **a** operation at age 57; **b** good result seen at the 7-year follow-up; **c** deterioration seen at the 9-year follow-up

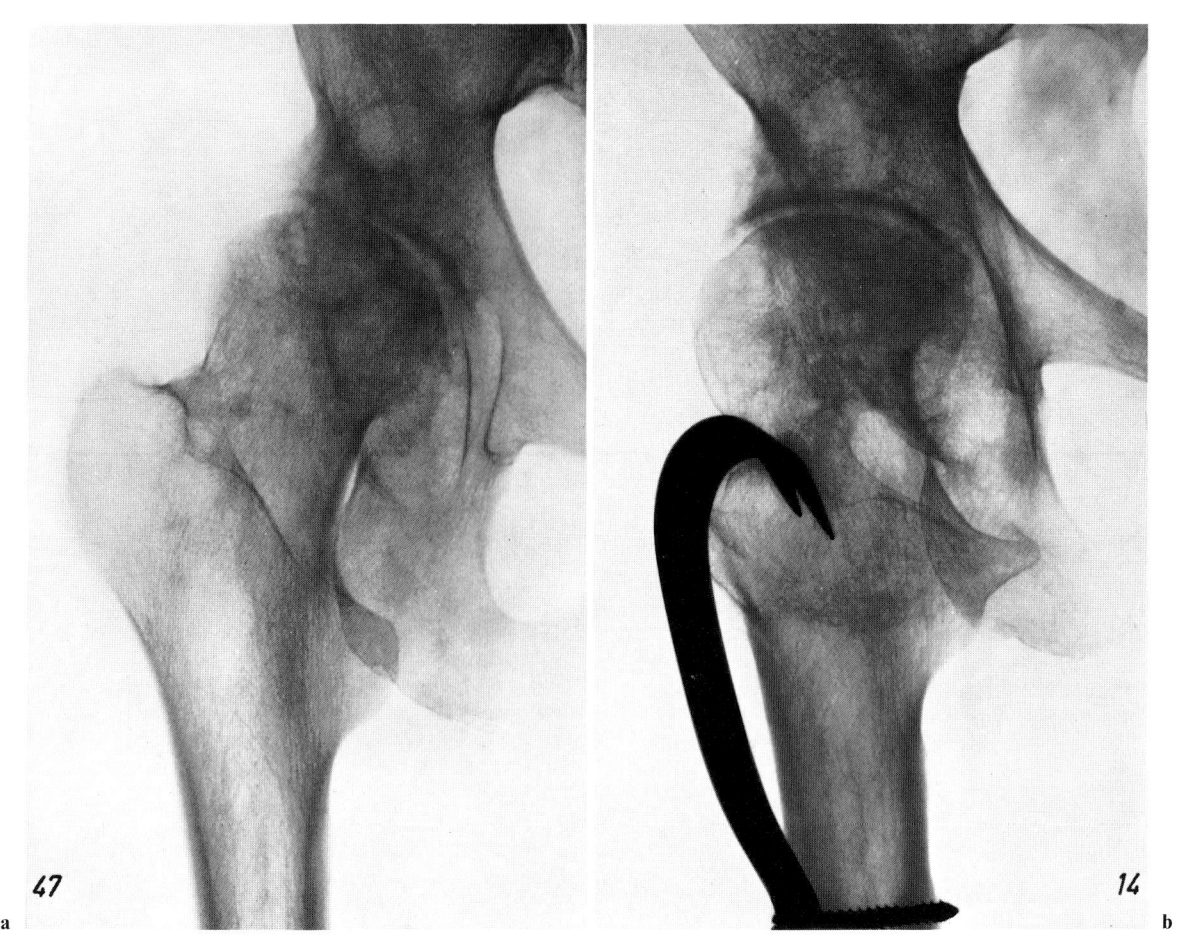

Fig. 197. a A 47-year-old female patient before a Pauwels II. b Fourteen years afterwards

Secondary deterioration may be attributed to a critical lowering of the tissue resistance, and in certain patients a cause for this can be found. In some other patients, overstressing of the joint can be blamed. But sometimes there is no obvious explanation. However, after a secondary deterioration, a total hip replacement can be carried out without any difficulty, and the patient has gained some years before undergoing this drastic treatment. In other patients, further joint-preserving operations may be considered.

A 47-year-old female patient developed osteoarthritis in both hips, which were dysplastic. On the right side (Fig. 197a), a 28° valgus osteotomy was carried out. Despite reversal of the neck-shaft angle, the result was excellent after 14 years (Fig. 197b). The left hip (Fig. 198a) underwent a 20° valgus osteotomy (Fig. 199) 3 years after the right. The result was fair for some years (Fig. 198b) and then deteriorated (Fig. 198c). Seven years after the first osteotomy on this left side, a second valgus osteotomy (25°) was carried out (Fig. 200). At the 5-year follow-up, the result was excellent (Fig. 198d).

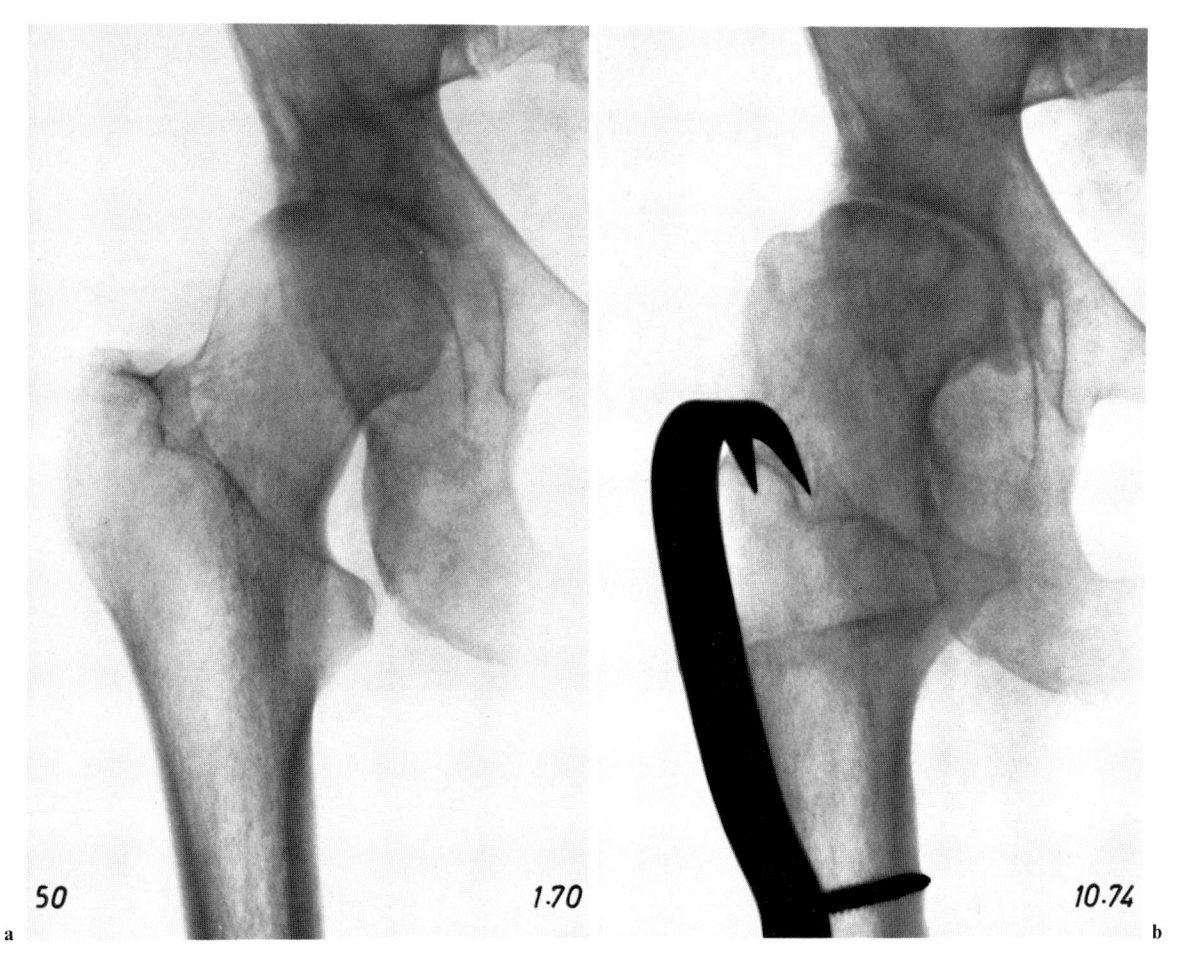

Fig. 198a–d. Same patient as in Fig. 197: opposite hip. **a** valgus osteotomy at 50 years of age; **b** after 4 years; **c** after 7 years; **d** 5-year follow-up after a second valgus osteotomy (**c, d** see page 200)

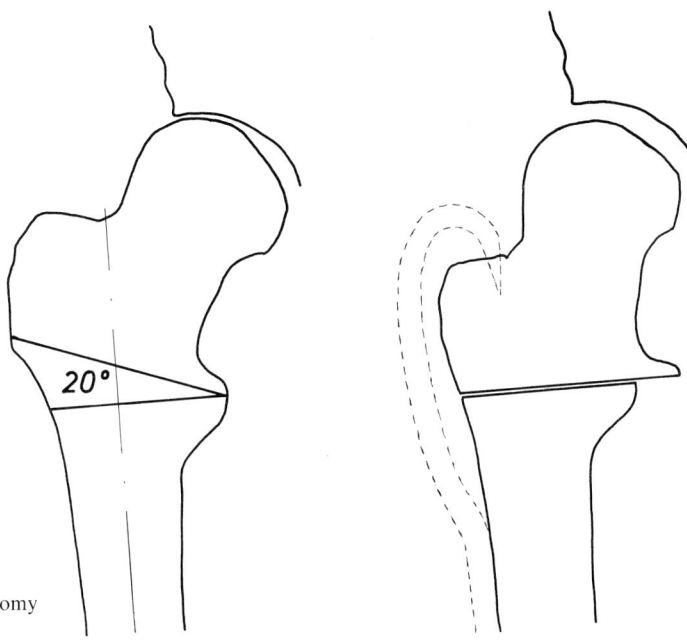

Fig. 199. Pre-operative planning of the first osteotomy carried out on the hip shown in Fig. 198

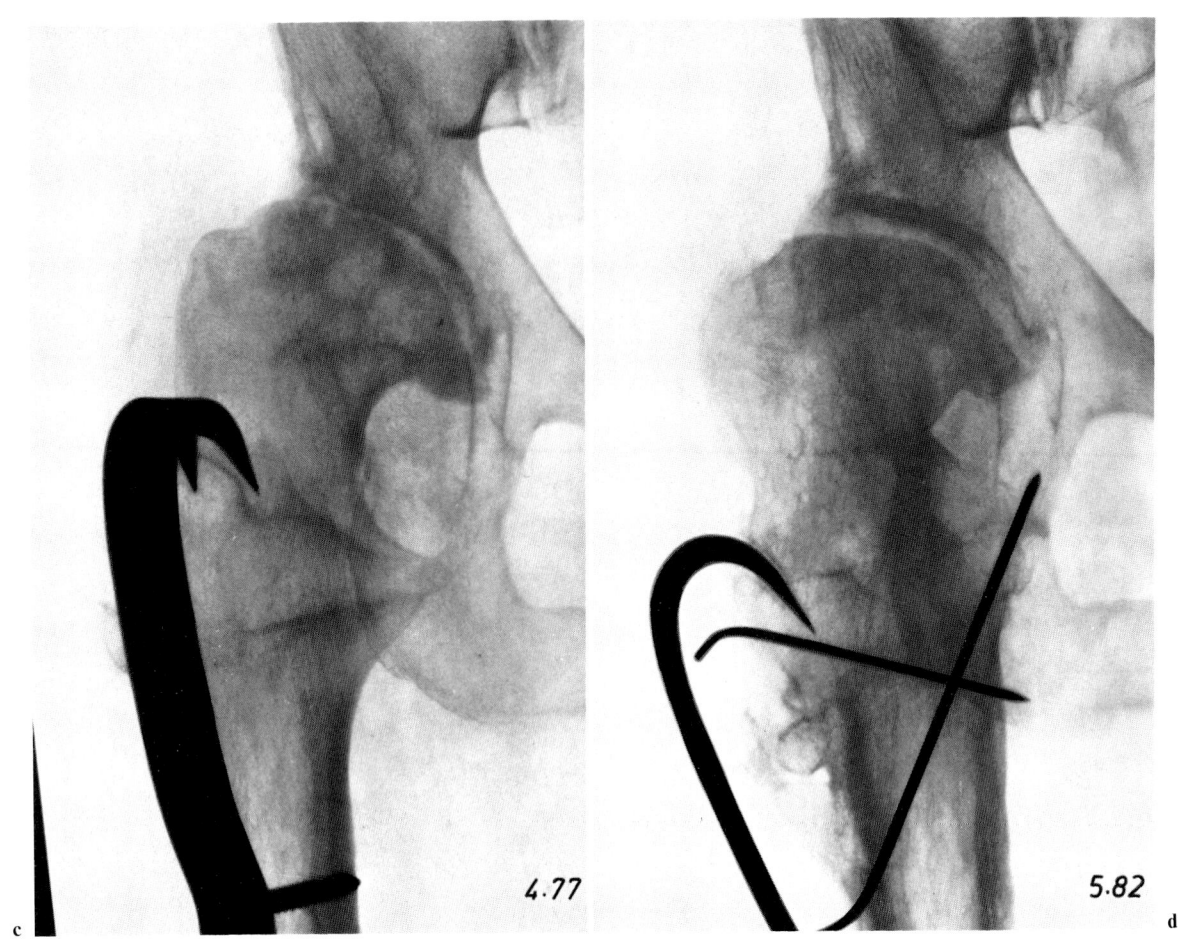

Fig. 198c, d

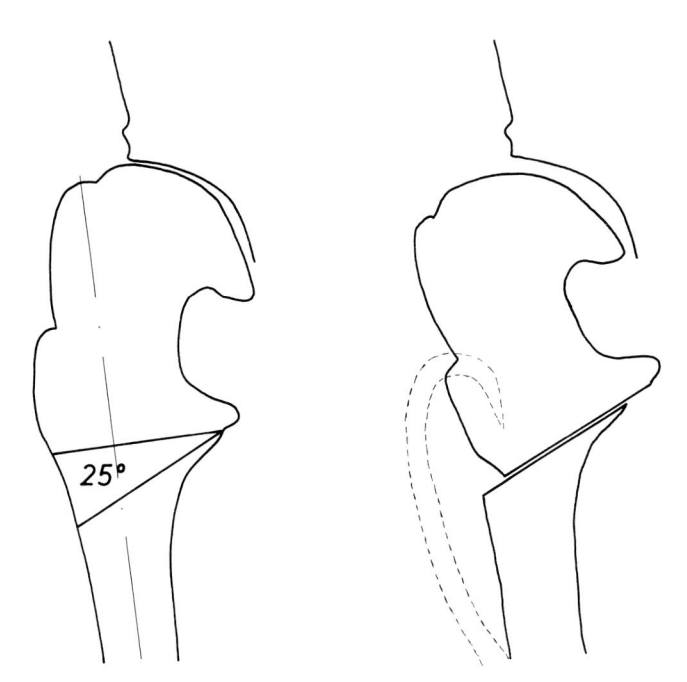

Fig. 200. Pre-operative planning of the second osteotomy carried out on the hip shown in Fig. 198

200

XII. Osteotomies Distal to the Lesser Trochanter (Lorenz, Schanz, Milch)

A. Rationale

A transverse beam (Fig. 201a) supports a weight which is counterbalanced by a tension band. The tension band is attached to the column and to the extremity of the transverse beam opposite to the weight; it is subjected to tension Z. Equilibrium can also be ensured by a strut between the column and the extremity of the transverse beam on which the weight lies (Fig. 201b). This strut is subjected to compression D.

The pelvis, supporting part of the body weight, acts as does the transverse beam. The weight, exerted eccentrically, tends to tilt it in adduction on the thigh (Fig. 202a). The abductor muscles hold the pelvis horizontal. They act as a tension band, thanks to the neck-shaft angle. The angle between the neck and the shaft provides the tension band with a lever arm. One can imagine reverse angle of the upper femur bringing the femoral shaft into contact with the pelvis. The femur, being angulated at the level of the ischial tuberosity, would then tend to act as a strut supporting the pelvis (Fig. 202b). It would be subjected to compression in its supporting area.

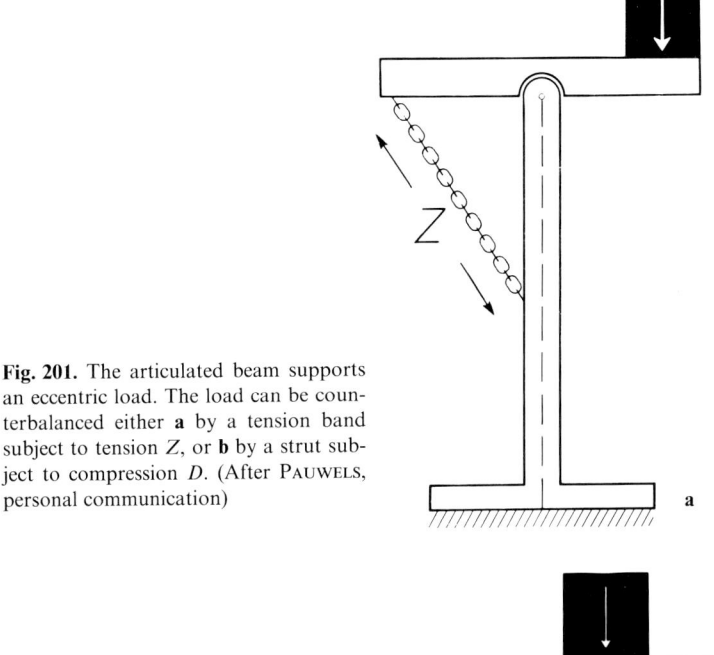

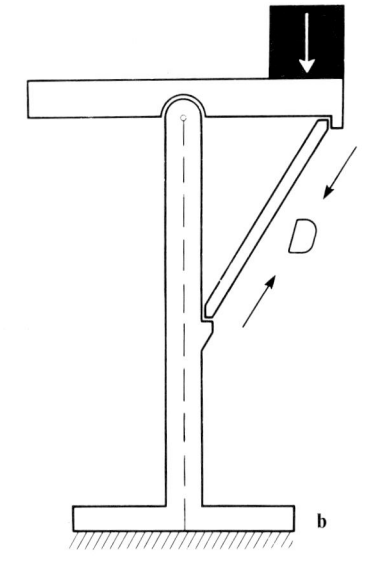

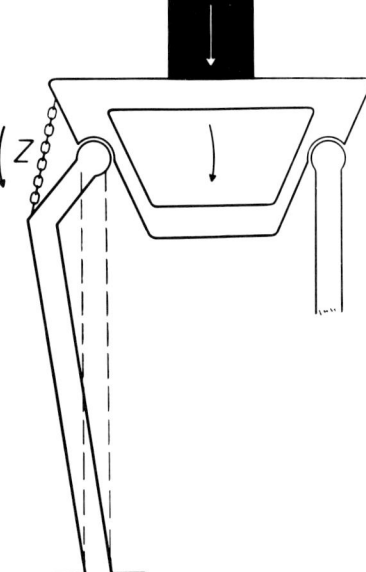

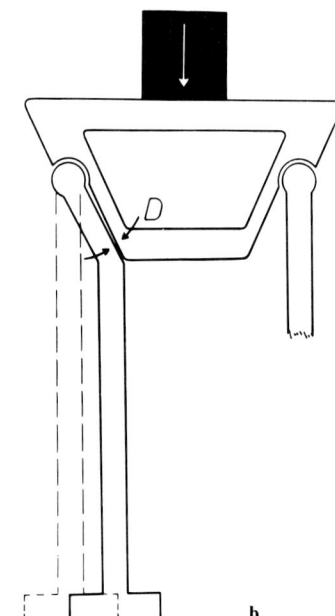

Fig. 201. The articulated beam supports an eccentric load. The load can be counterbalanced either **a** by a tension band subject to tension Z, or **b** by a strut subject to compression D. (After Pauwels, personal communication)

Fig. 202. a A muscular tension band ensures equilibrium. **b** The pelvis abuts on the femoral shaft. Z, tension; D, compression. (After Pauwels, personal communication)

In the dislocated hip, the pelvis tilts in adduction on the thigh under the partial body weight K (body weight minus the supporting leg), which acts with the long lever arm OC (Fig. 203a). The TRENDELENBURG sign is positive. Equilibrium is (poorly) ensured by the capsule and the abductor muscles M stretched over the femoral head. The force M acts with the very short lever arm OB. The femoral head supports the resultant R of the two forces K and M.

LORENZ proposed a "bifurcation" of the femur (Fig. 203b). After an oblique intertrochanteric osteotomy, the lesser trochanter is pushed into the acetabulum. After union, the fragments form an angle open laterally. The centre of rotation of the hip is now at the lesser trochanter. The lever arm OC of the partial body weight K is thus shortened, and that, OB, of the force M exerted by the abductor muscles is lengthened. The abductor muscles can ensure equilibrium with a much smaller force. Consequently, the resultant force R transmitted from the pelvis to the femur is diminished (Fig. 203b).

Some LORENZ osteotomies have given excellent long-term results. PAUWELS carried out a LORENZ osteotomy in a 26-year-old female patient with a congenital high dislocation of the hip (Fig. 204). When we saw her 42 years later, she was well, without pain and with a satisfactory range of movement. Actually, she came to us for an operation on the opposite hip.

However, the weight-bearing surface provided by the lesser trochanter is small. Therefore, the articular pressure in the joint formed by the lesser trochanter and the socket can be high despite the reduction of the load R.

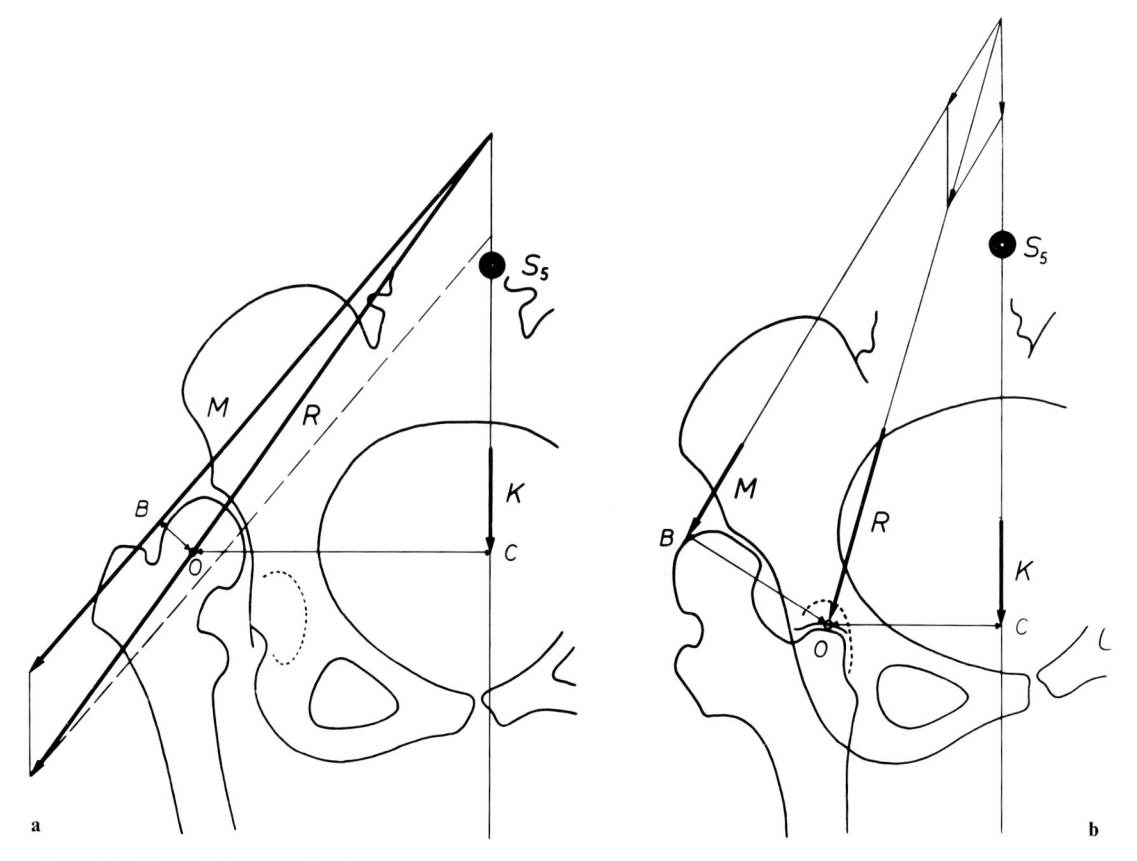

Fig. 203. a The hip is dislocated. The force K exerted by the part of the body supported by the hip acts with the long lever arm OC, the capsule and the abductor muscles M with the short lever arm OB. **b** The "bifurcation" of Lorenz shortens OC and lengthens OB. This considerably decreases the resultant R. However, the weight-bearing surface provided by the lesser trochanter is small. S_5, centre of gravity of that part of the body acting on the hip during the single-support period of gait. (After PAUWELS, personal communication)

Fig. 204. Lorenz osteotomy in a 26-year-old female patient: 42-year follow-up

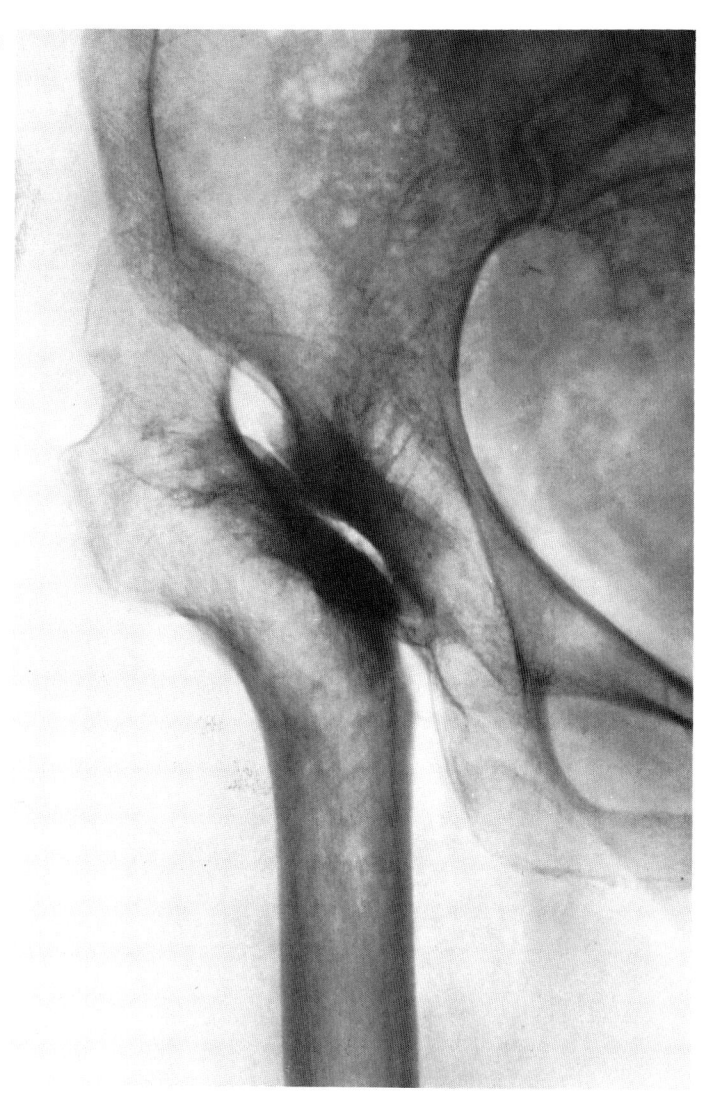

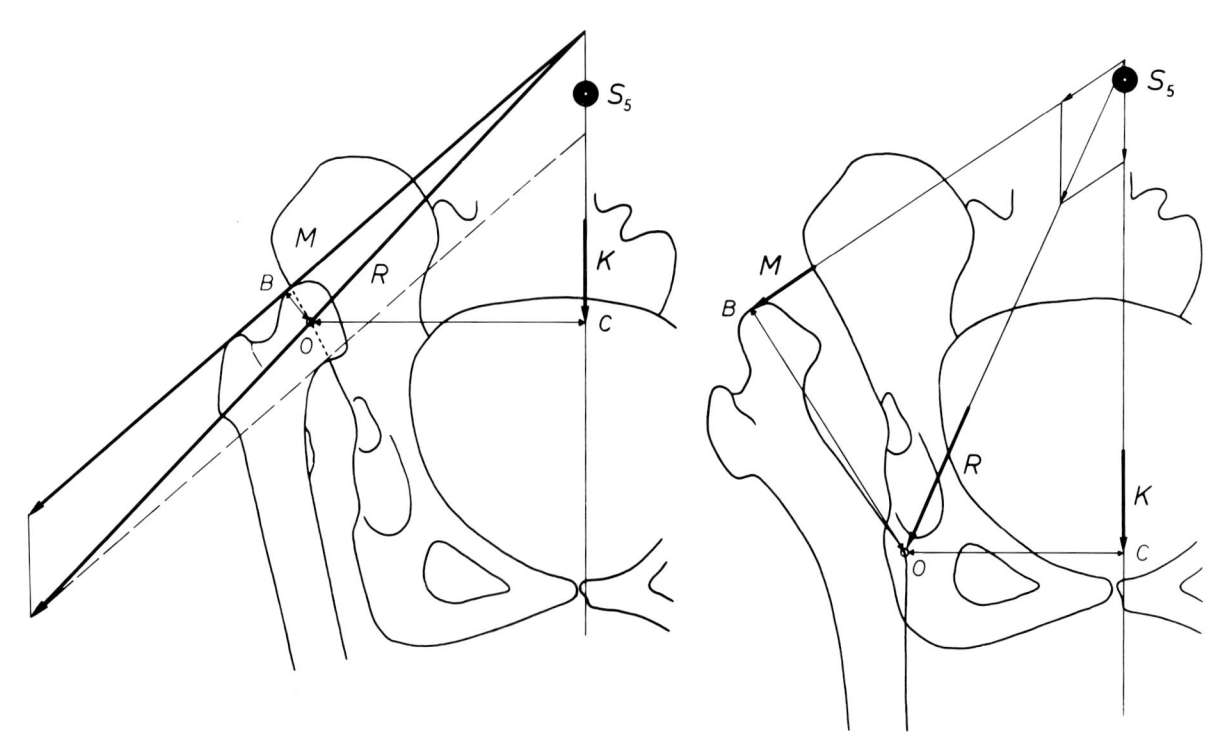

Fig. 205. The Schanz osteotomy is carried out at the level of the ischial tuberosity. The femur is angulated. This shortens the lever arm OC of the force K exerted by the part of the body supported by the femur and considerably lengthens the lever arm OB of the force M exerted by the abductor muscles. Consequently, the resultant force R transmitted from the pelvis to the femur through the soft parts is impressively decreased. S_5, centre of gravity of that part of the body acting on the hip during the single-support period of gait. (After Pauwels, personal communication)

Schanz proposed the division of the femur at the level of the ischial tuberosity and the displacement of the femoral shaft medially. The fragments form an angle open laterally. After this low osteotomy, the pelvis rests on the femoral shaft with the soft parts intervening (Fig. 205). The medial displacement of the support shortens the lever arm OC of the body weight K. Because of the angulation of the fragments, the femoral head is forced away from the ilium, thus stretching the abductor muscles M. These act now with a much longer lever arm, OB. Because of the shortening of the lever arm OC of the partial body weight K and because of the lengthening of their own lever arm OB, the abductor muscles M can counterbalance K by exerting a much smaller force. This considerably reduces the load R transmitted from the pelvis to the femur across the soft parts. The surfaces which transmit this load R are large and vary continuously.

$$M \cdot OB = K \cdot OC \quad M = \frac{K \cdot OC}{OB}$$

$$R = \sqrt{M^2 + K^2 + 2 \cos \widehat{MK}}$$

where $\widehat{MK}$ is the angle formed by the lines of action of forces K and M. K is constant. Consequently, a shortening of OC and a lengthening of OB decrease M. The vectorial sum R of K and M is thus diminished.

Milch combined a Schanz osteotomy with a resection of the femoral head and neck. The mechanical action of a Milch osteotomy is similar to that of a Schanz osteotomy.

B. Indications

Bilateral high congenital dislocation of the hip often causes no pain and limping may be very slight. When unilateral the dislocation causes a limp, and pain may also occur. The opposite hip often develops osteoarthritis, either because it is also dysplastic initially or as a consequence of the subluxation resulting from the obliquity of the pelvis. In the adult, the congenitally dislocated hip, whether it abuts against the pelvis or not, should be treated only if painful. In this case a Schanz osteotomy may be considered.

When a hip prosthesis has to be removed and a fresh total replacement does not seem possible or desirable, the same kind of osteotomy can be carried out. Since the femoral neck and head have been removed, it has to be a MILCH osteotomy. This type of osteotomy will probably have increasingly greater value in the future, in view of the huge number of total prostheses now being implanted in younger and younger patients.

C. Pre-operative Planning

An anteroposterior view of the pelvis with the dislocated femur in full adduction will give an idea of the angulation of the fragments of the femur that will be necessary. The hemipelvis and the upper half of the femur are traced on a sheet of transparent paper (Fig. 206a). The hemipelvis is traced on a second sheet of transparent paper (Fig. 206b). The second sheet is rotated over the first until the upper half of the femur on the first sheet appears parallel or nearly parallel to the wing of the ilium on the second sheet. The angle formed by the edges of the two sheets is measured (Fig. 206c). About 10° are added to this angle. The angle thus obtained is drawn on the first sheet in the femoral shaft at the level of the ischial tuberosity. The apex of this angle is medial (Fig. 206d). The drawing on the second sheet is then completed using the first sheet (Fig. 206e). The angle of the wedge to be removed usually attains at least 35°–45°. The drawing is displayed in the operating-theatre (Fig. 206f).

D. Operative Procedure

The operation is carried out under general anaesthesia with tracheal intubation. The patient lies prone; the surgeon sits at the level of the hip and the first assistant stands at the level of the patient's knees. A second assistant stands near the patient's feet, as for the varus or valgus osteotomy or lateral displacement of the greater trochanter. The image-intensifier is positioned opposite the surgeon on the other side of the patient.

The approach is posterolateral, through a 15-cm incision centred at the level of the ischial tuberosity. At this level a wedge is delineated by two KIRSCHNER wires drilled into the femur, after the second assistant has flexed the knee of the patient and rotated the leg internally by 10°–15°. The lower leg thus forms an angle of 10°–15° from the vertical. The wedge is removed from the femur with a reciprocating saw. The leg, still internally rotated, is brought into abduction in order to coapt the osteotomy surfaces. The fragments are fixed under compression with a properly moulded plate and six screws. The tissue layers are sutured separately using suction drainage.

The MILCH osteotomy is planned like a SCHANZ osteotomy. We have used this procedure when a prosthesis had to be removed and it did not seem desirable to replace it. In such a case the incision must be long enough to allow for the removal of the prosthesis. The osteotomy itself is carried out exactly like the SCHANZ osteotomy.

After removal of a prosthesis the MILCH osteotomy seems mechanically preferable to a GIRDLESTONE resection of the femoral head and neck. It seems to ensure better stability for the hip, and it has given us consistently satisfactory results. However, larger series of both procedures with adequate follow-up periods should be compared. Like the SCHANZ osteotomy, the MILCH osteotomy leads to a valgus deformity of the leg. The correction of this deformity may require a varus supra-condylar osteotomy of the femur. On the other hand, shortening after a MILCH osteotomy may be less than after a GIRDLESTONE.

E. Postoperative Care

As suggested by BERTRAND et al., the ankle and lower leg are put in a plaster splint which is fitted with a transverse axle and two small wheels. This allows the movement of flexion and extension of the hip and knee, and controls rotation while the patient lies in bed, the wheels rolling over a wooden board. The splint is removed after 6 weeks. The patient then starts walking with part of his weight on the hip but with the help of two crutches. These are discarded as soon as bony union has taken place.

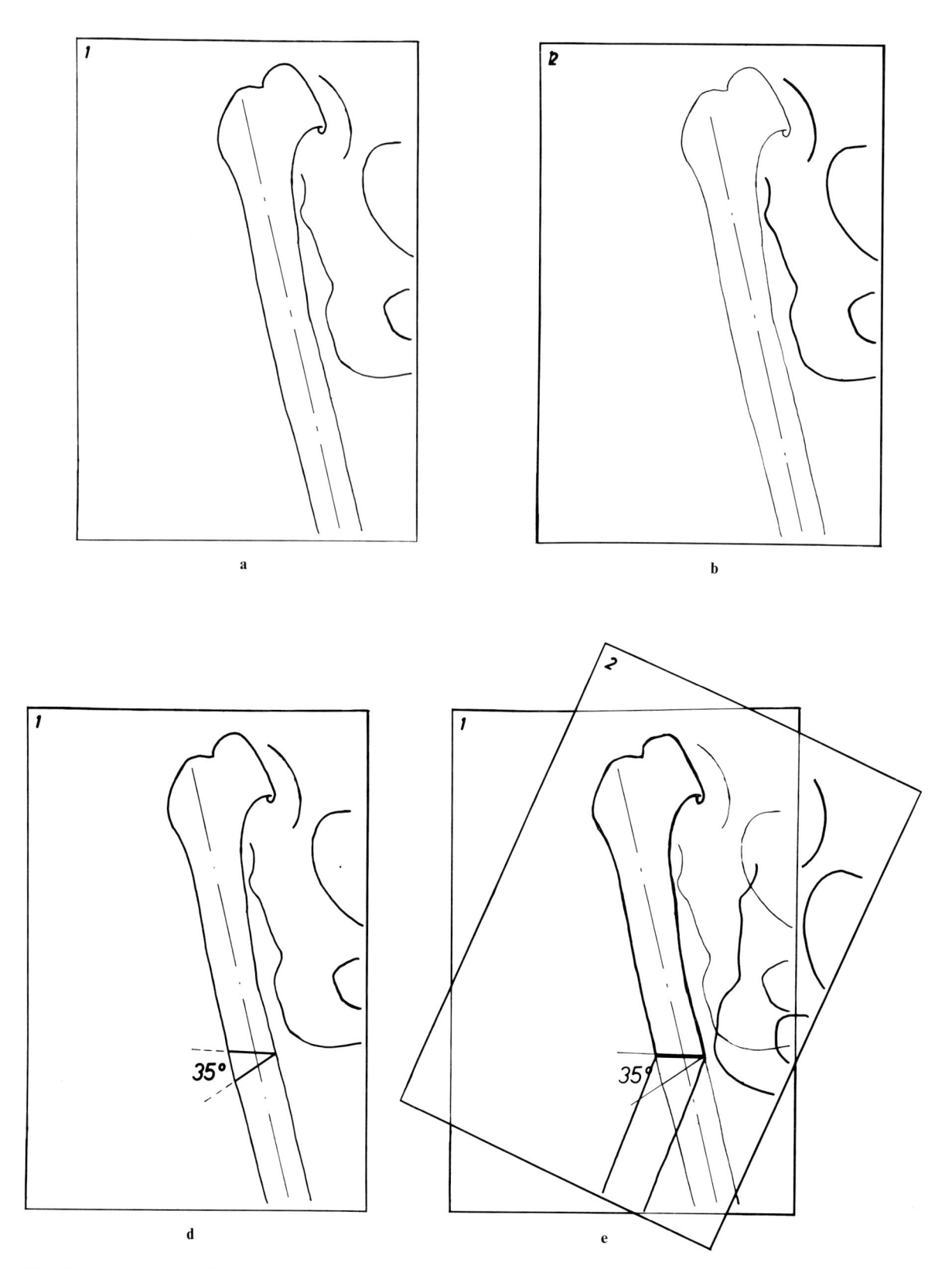

Fig. 206a–f. Planning of a Schanz osteotomy. *1, 2*, first and second half-sheets of transparent paper

35°

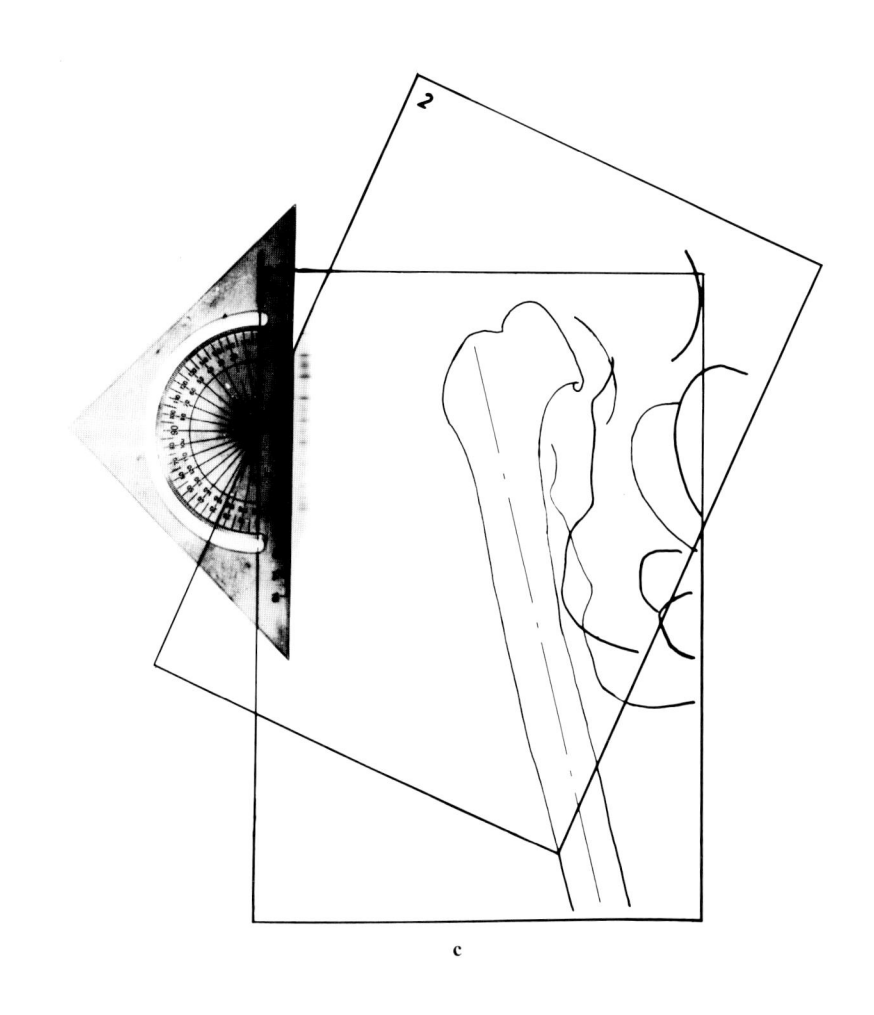

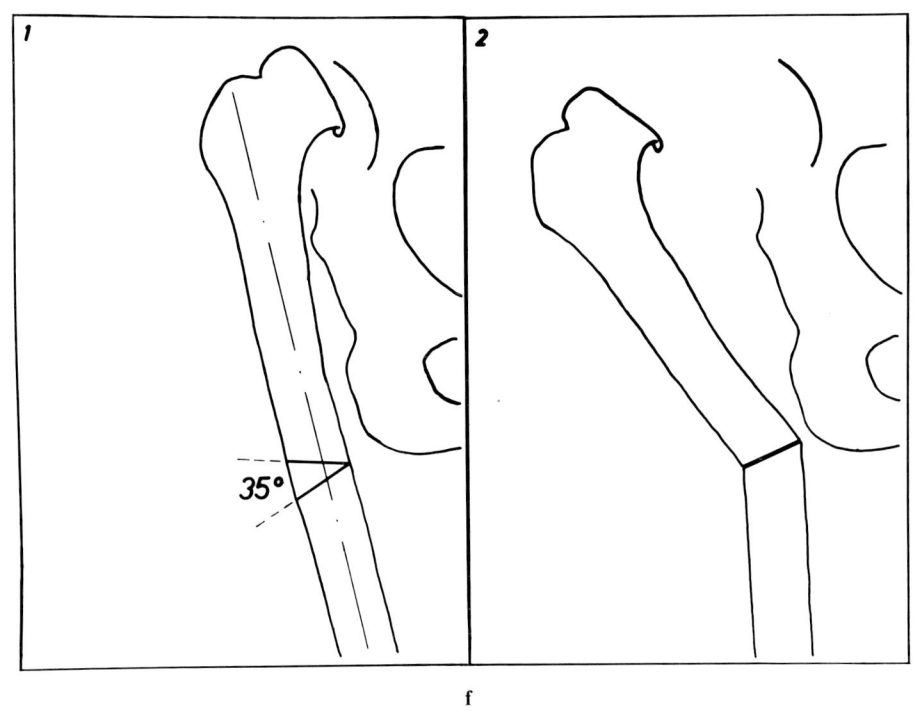

c

f

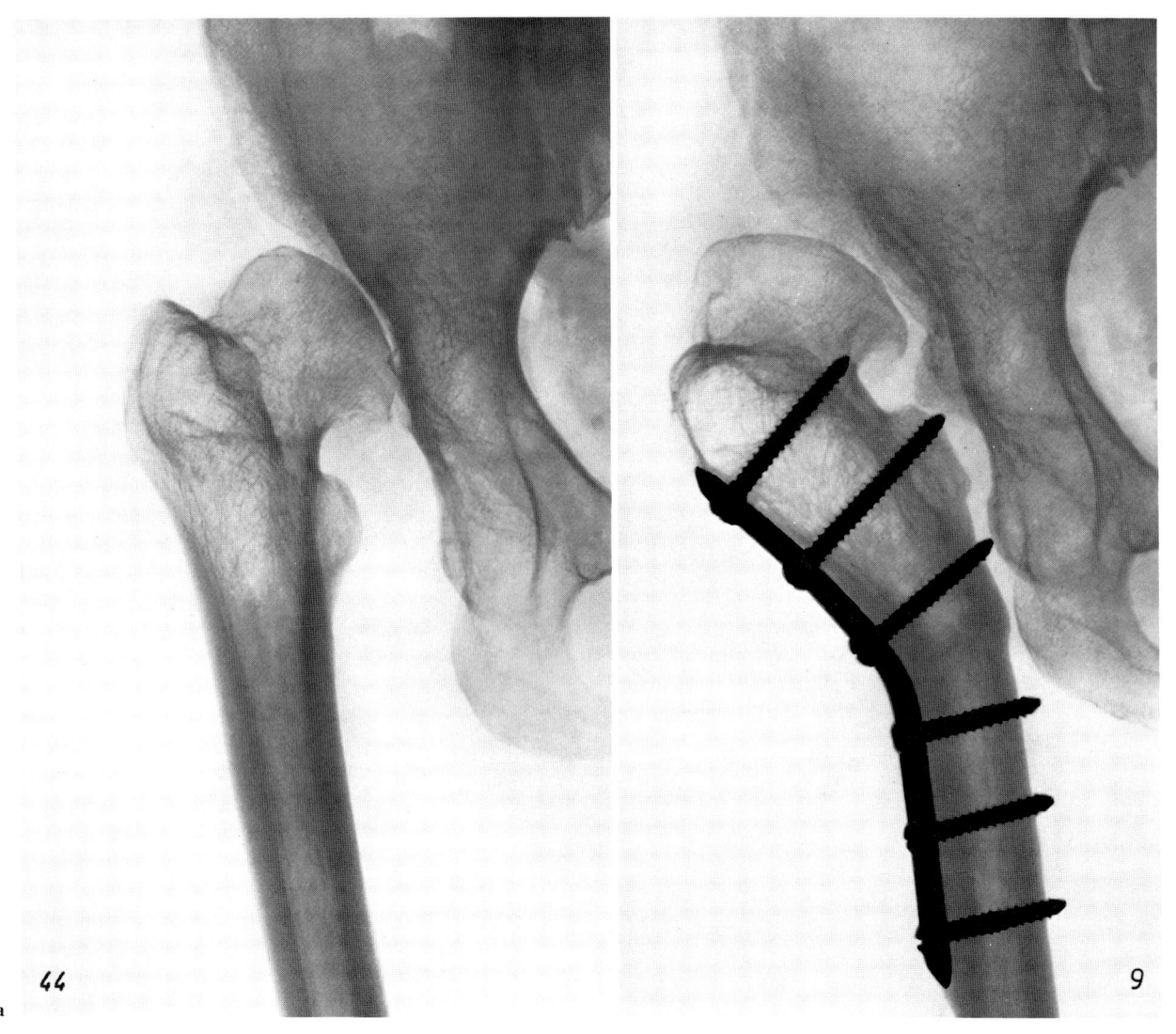

Fig. 207. a A 44-year-old female patient before a Schanz osteotomy. **b** Nine years afterwards

F. Postoperative Evolution

Remarkably enough, some patients stop limping after a few months. The results will be analysed in detail in Chap. VI. A 44-year-old female patient had developed a painful false articulation in a congenitally dislocated hip (Fig. 207a). The range of movement was satisfactory (Table 35). Nine years after a SCHANZ osteotomy her hip was still pain-free with a good range of movement (Table 35). The patient no longer limped and was fully active (Fig. 207b).

A 51-year-old female patient had had a JUDET prosthesis of the femoral head implanted 20 years previously (Fig. 208a). The hip had been painful and stiff for years. The prosthesis was removed and a MILCH osteotomy was carried out (Fig. 208b). At the 10-year follow-up, the patient was pain-free and the hip was mobile (flexion 60°; extension 0°; adduction 20°; abduction 40°; internal rotation 10°; external rotation 45°). She was not limping.

Table 35. Range of movement of the hip (Fig. 207)

	Before surgery	At the 9-year follow-up	Gain
Flexion	85°	85°	− 5°
Extension	20°	15°	
Adduction	30°	15°	0°
Abduction	45°	60°	
Int. rotation	30°	50°	− 20°
Ext. rotation	60°	20°	

Fig. 208. a A 51-year-old female patient who had been with a Judet prosthesis, before a Milch osteotomy. **b** Ten years afterwards

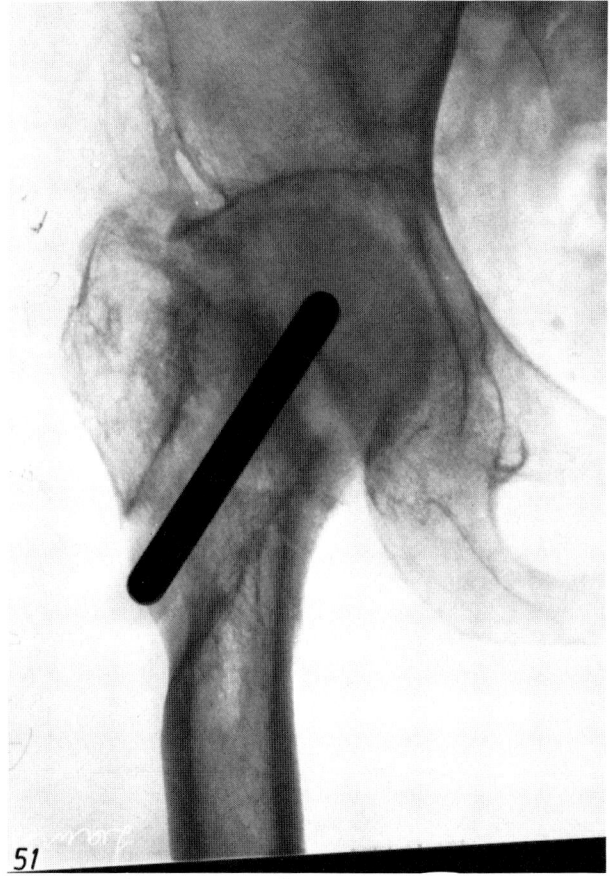

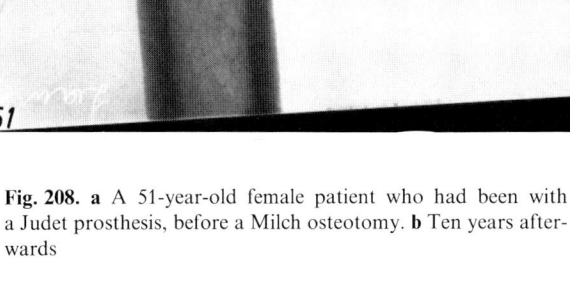

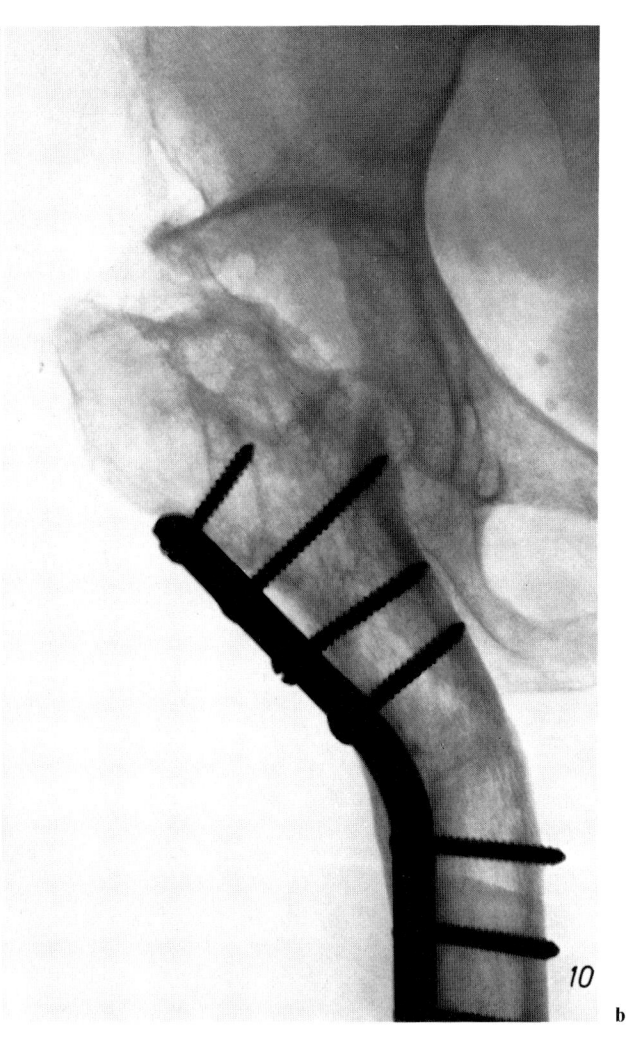

G. Additional Procedures

After surgery, movement of the hip is as a rule maintained. This movement may be greater than in a normal hip. Pain usually disappears. Some patients no longer limp, and some others limp less than before.

Medial displacement of the femoral shaft entails a valgus deformity of the knee (Fig. 49), which in turn may cause overloading of the lateral aspect of this joint. Such overloading is made apparent by the increase of the subchondral sclerosis and of the density of the cancellous structure beneath the lateral tibial plateau. A varus supracondylar osteotomy is then indicated in order to shift the load back to the centre of the knee and to distribute it evenly over the two plateaux (MAQUET 1976).

When the dislocation is unilateral, the dislocated leg is shorter than the other. To avoid disturbing the spine and the other hip, the patient should either wear a shoe high enough to render the pelvis level or undergo a shortening of the sound femur or a lengthening of the dislocated femur. Most young and female patients prefer a surgical shortening. This is carried out either by resecting part of the shaft and nailing the fragments, or by a varus intertrochanteric osteotomy in the case of coxa valga subluxans without deformation of the femoral head and socket. Osteoarthritis may indicate a valgus intertrochanteric osteotomy, which is then combined with the shortening procedure.

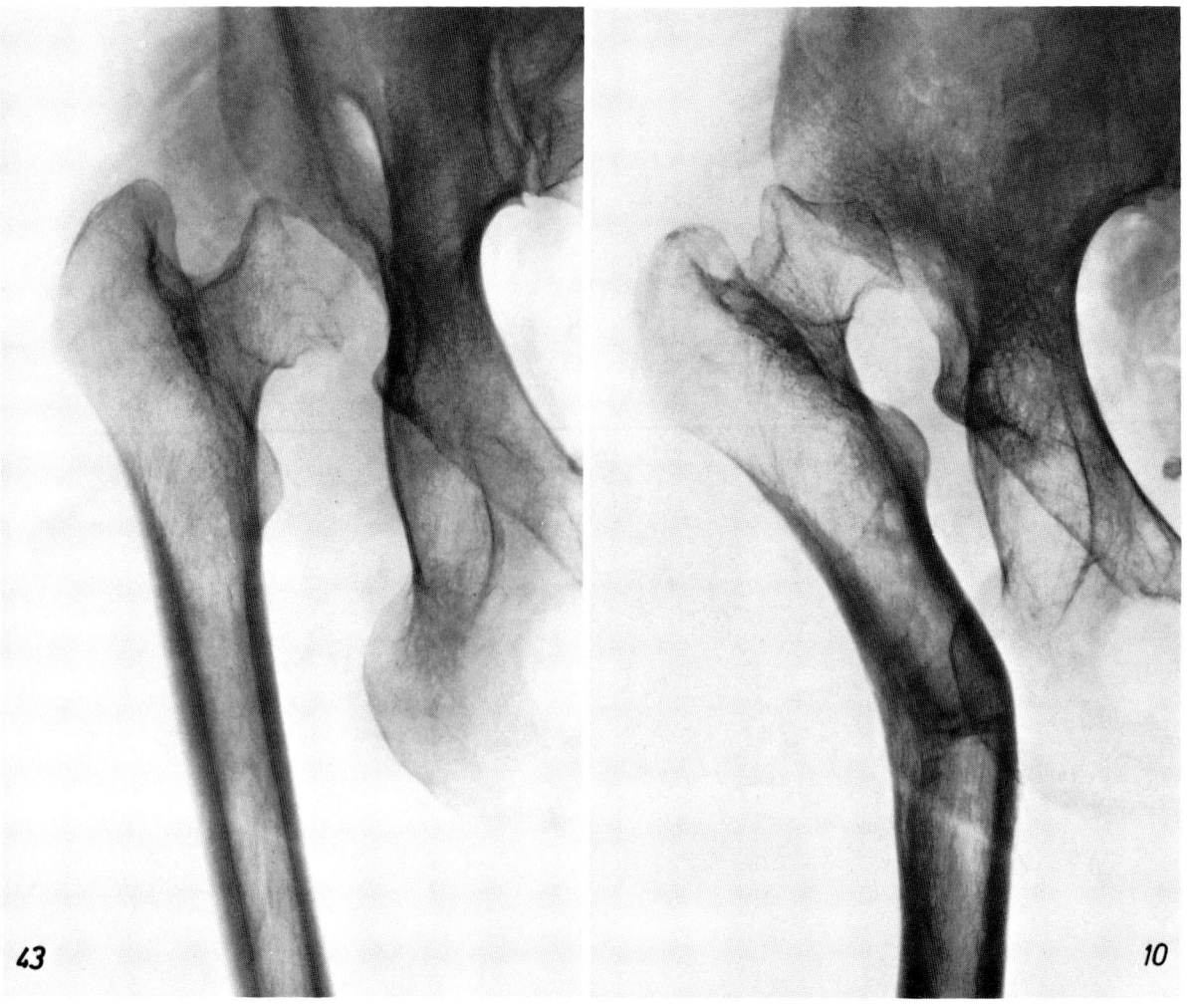

Fig. 209. a A 43-year-old female patient before a Schanz osteotomy. b Ten years afterwards

A 43-year-old female patient with a painful congenitally dislocated hip underwent a SCHANZ osteotomy (Fig. 209). One year later the opposite femur was shortened by 5 cm to make the pelvis level but by that time the knee on the osteotomy side had developed a valgus deformity. The increased subchondral sclerosis beneath the lateral tibial plateau and the fading away of the subchondral sclerosis and cancellous structure beneath the medial plateau pointed to an abnormal distribution of the compressive stresses in the knee (Fig. 210). The valgus deformity was corrected by a supracondylar osteotomy of the femur (Fig. 211; MAQUET 1976). At the latest follow-up, 8 years after the supracondylar osteotomy, the patient was free from pain and very active, with no limp. The subchondral sclerosis had regressed beneath the lateral tibial plateau and was more pronounced beneath the medial plateau (Fig. 210b).

H. Conclusion

In adults the SCHANZ osteotomy may offer an elegant and lasting solution to the problem of the congenitally dislocated hip which has become painful. It must often be complemented by a supracondylar osteotomy of the femur necessary to correct a valgus deformity of the knee. It can be followed by shortening of the opposite femur to make the pelvis horizontal and thus straighten the spine. This solution offers the advantage of using living tissues, and therefore seems preferable to total arthroplasty, at least in relatively young patients who have retained a good range of movement.

The MILCH osteotomy may represent a good salvage procedure when a hip prosthesis has to be removed and cannot be replaced.

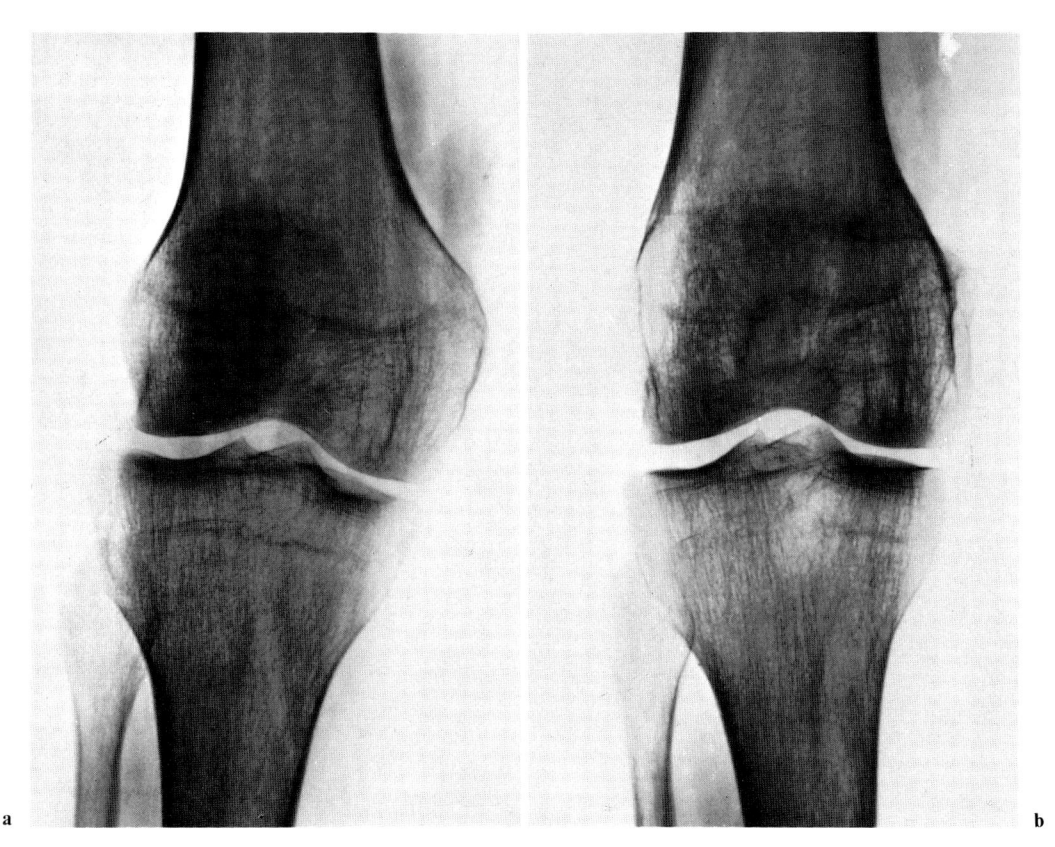

Fig. 210a, b. Same patient as in Fig. 209: the leg developed a valgus deformity after the Schanz osteotomy. **a** Increase in the subchondral sclerosis beneath the lateral tibial plateau. **b** Eight years after a femoral supracondylar osteotomy correcting the deformity, the subchondral sclerosis was more pronounced beneath the medial tibial plateau and less beneath the lateral

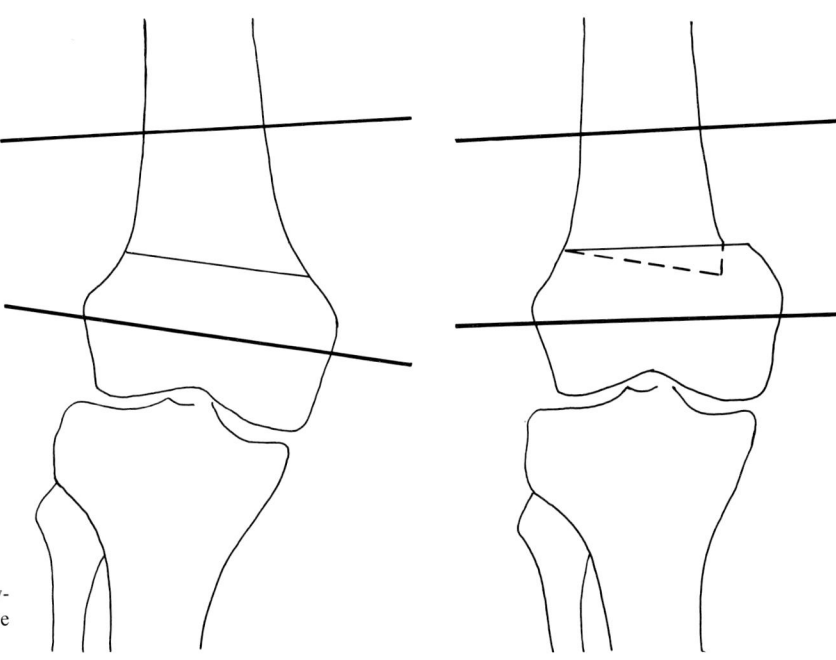

Fig. 211. Planning of the supracondylar osteotomy carried out for the knee shown in Fig. 210

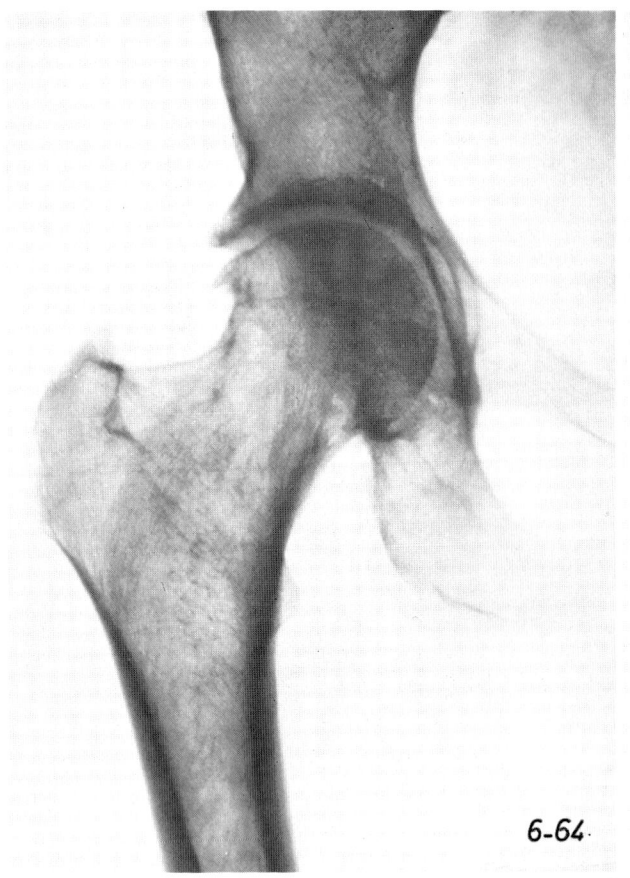

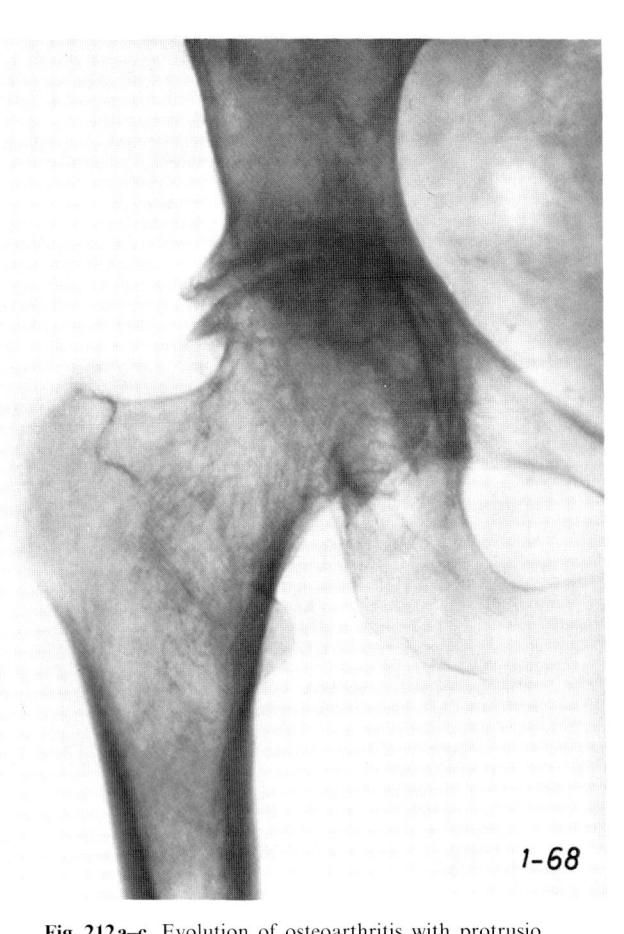

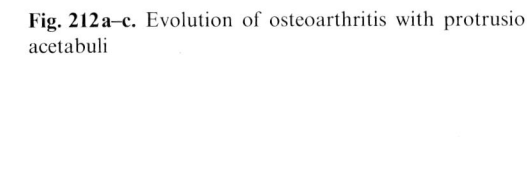

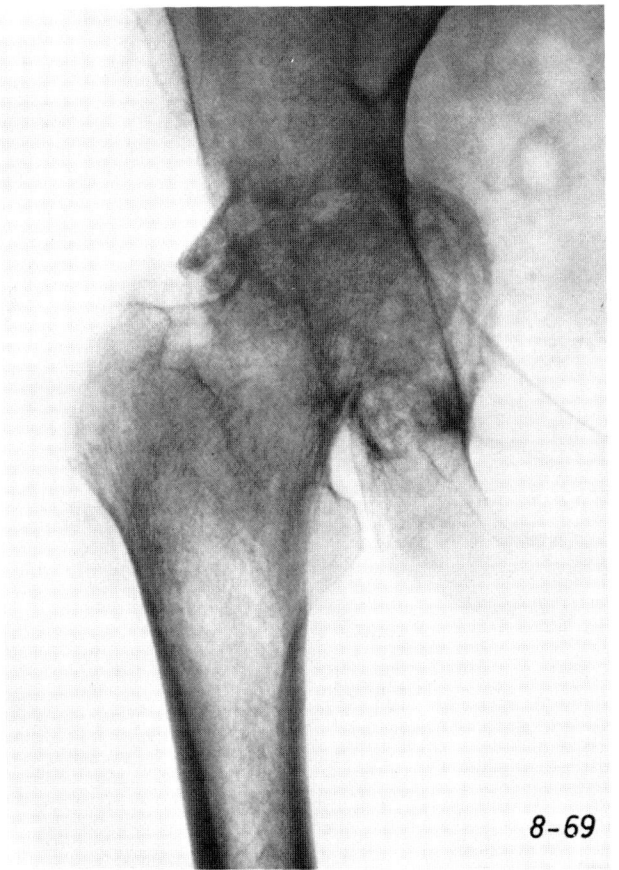

Fig. 212a–c. Evolution of osteoarthritis with protrusio acetabuli

Chapter IV. Osteoarthritis with Protrusio Acetabuli

In osteoarthritis with protrusio acetabuli, the joint space tends to be narrowed in the depths of the socket. Often the condition at first appears as a primary osteoarthritis with a cup-shaped sclerosis in the roof of the acetabulum (Fig. 212a). Later, this cup-shaped sclerosis is replaced by a dense triangle in the depths of the joint (Fig. 212b), where the articular stresses are increased and unevenly distributed. Cysts may develop in this triangular subchondral sclerosis. The femoral head seems to be pushed into the pelvis (Fig. 212c).

I. Rationale

The resultant force R or its counter-force R_1 can be resolved into a longitudinal component L and a transverse component Q (Fig. 213a). The longitudinal component of R_1 pushes the femoral head upwards; the transverse component pushes the head medially. In protrusio acetabuli, everything that occurs indicates that the tissues are unable to withstand the transverse component Q. The latter can be decreased either by reducing the resultant force R by tenotomy of the abductor, adductor and iliopsoas muscles (page 68) or by valgus intertrochanteric osteotomy (page 102). A valgus intertrochanteric osteotomy modifies the direction of R, which is brought closer to the vertical (Fig. 213b). Both these procedures decrease Q. If force R were vertical, Q would be zero. Tenotomy and valgus osteotomy thus relieve pressure in the depths of the socket.

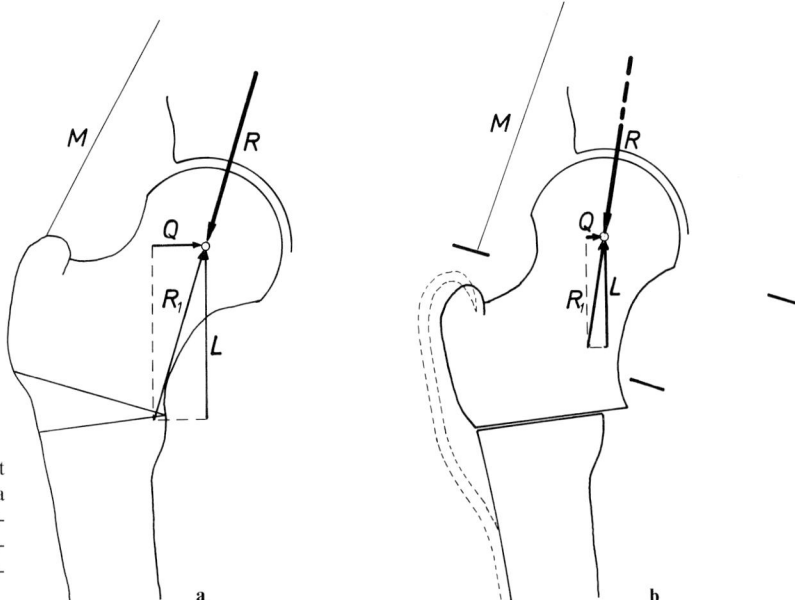

Fig. 213a, b. Resolving the resultant force R or its reaction force R_1 into a longitudinal component L and a transverse component Q. **a** protrusio acetabuli; **b** after a Pauwels II. M, force exerted by the abductor muscles

II. Indications

When there is no dense triangle in the depths of the acetabulum, a hanging-hip procedure may be sufficient.

A 57-year old female patient presented with an impressive protrusio acetabuli with significant degeneration of the joint (Fig. 214a). The hip was painful and its range of movement limited as could be expected from seeing the X-ray. A hanging hip procedure was carried out. Eighteen years later the hip remains pain-free although the range of movement has not been improved. In the X-ray a joint space separates two articular surfaces which appear smooth (Fig. 214b).

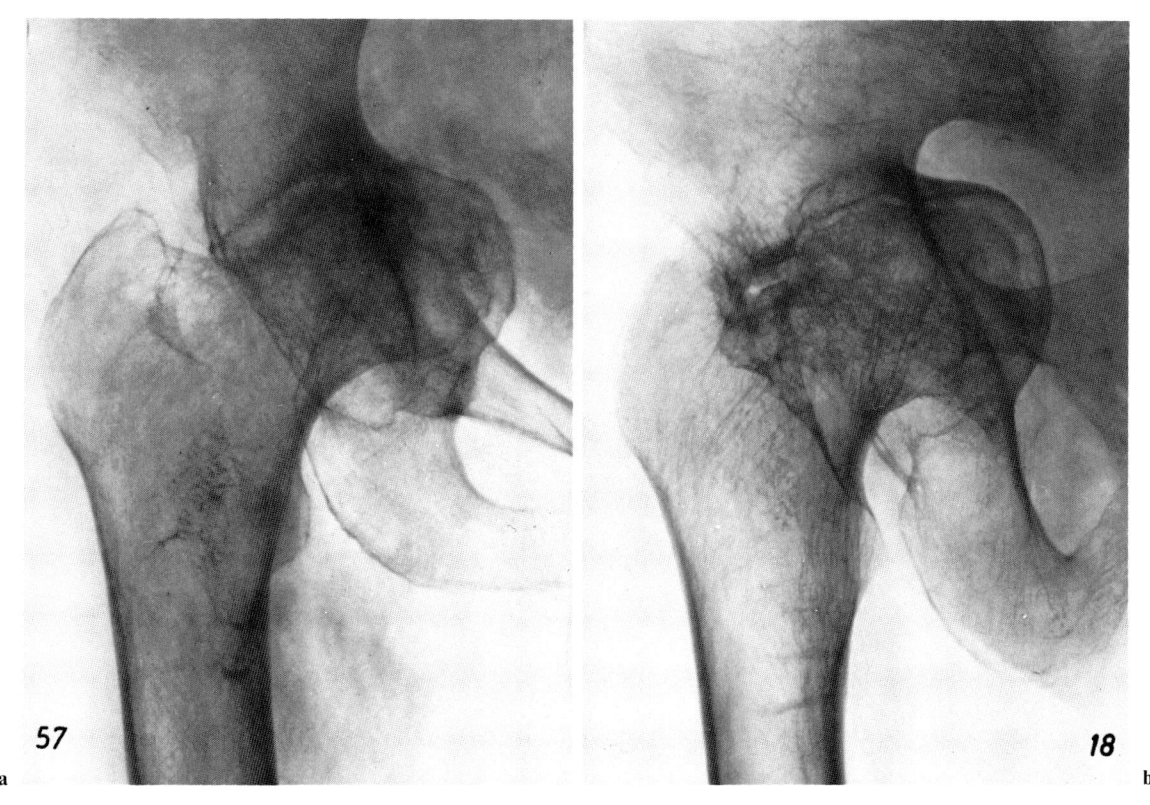

Fig. 214. a A 57-year-old female patient before a hanging-hip procedure. **b** Eighteen years afterwards

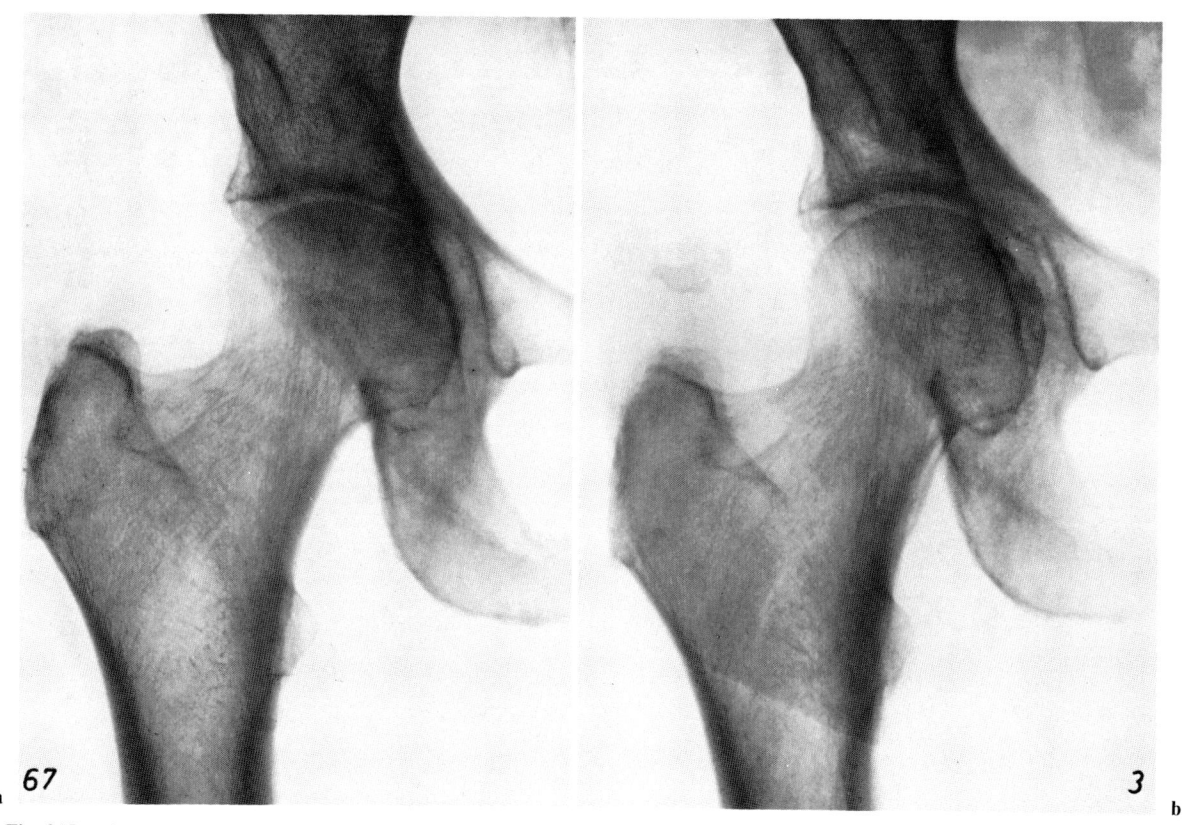

Fig. 215. a A 67-year-old female patient before a hanging-hip procedure. **b** Three years afterwards

A 67-year-old female patient presented with protrusive osteoarthritis of the hip with narrowing of the joint space and cysts in the roof of the acetabulum (Fig. 215a). Three years after a hanging-hip procedure, the hip had a full range of movement (Table 36), and the patient was free from pain and was not limping. The X-ray shows that the cysts had disappeared and a wide joint space had developed (Fig. 215b).

Table 36. Range of movement of the hip (Fig. 215)

	Before surgery	At the 3-year follow-up	Gain
Flexion	95°	130°	35°
Extension	0°	0°	
Adduction	0°	20°	40°
Abduction	25°	45°	
Int. rotation	40°	30°	10°
Ext. rotation	20°	40°	

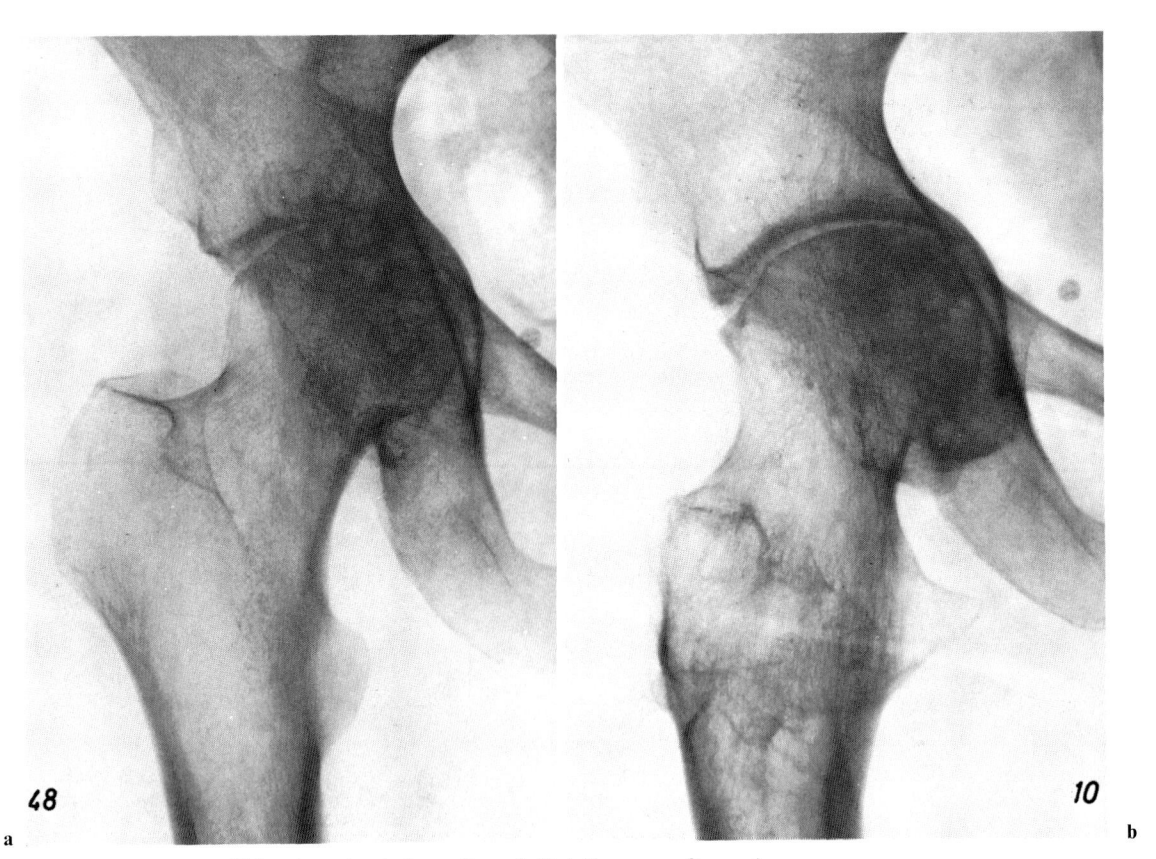

Fig. 216. a A 48-year-old female patient before a Pauwels II. **b** Ten years afterwards

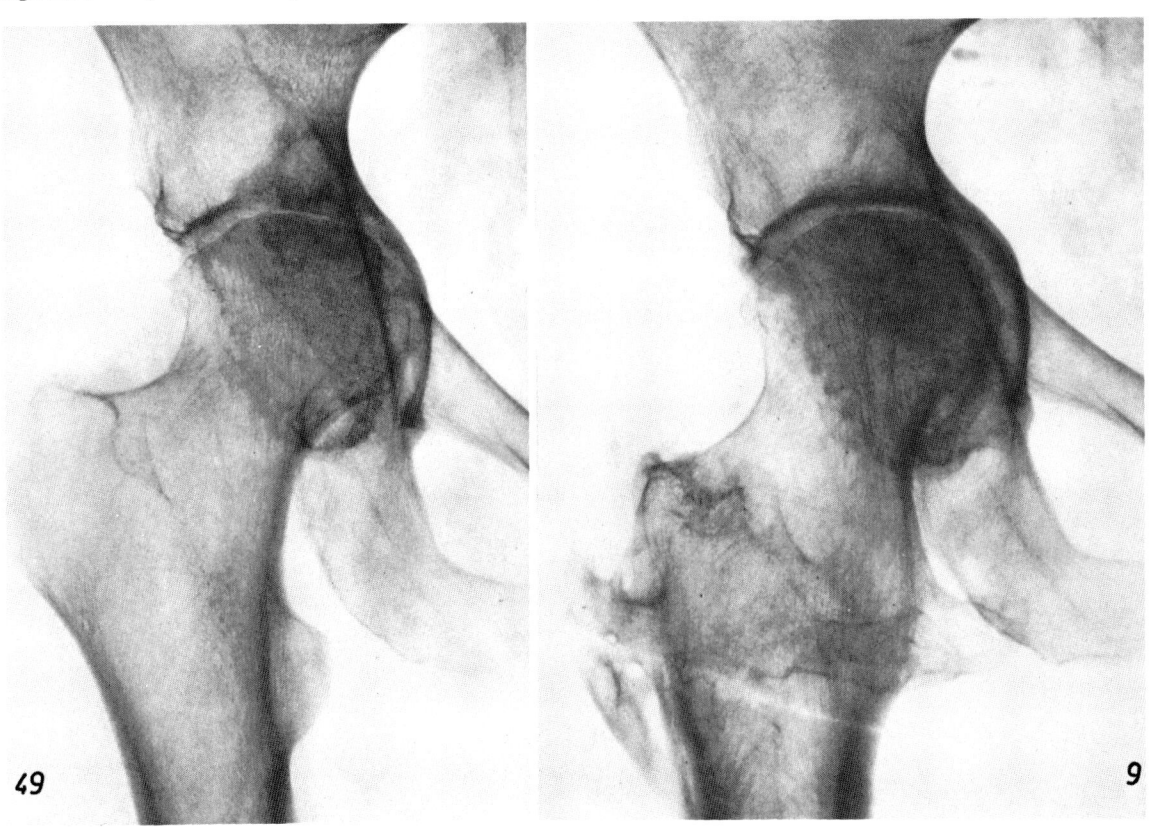

Fig. 217. a Same patient as in Fig. 216: opposite hip. Age at operation: 49 years. **b** Nine-year follow-up

When there is a dense triangle in the depths of the acetabulum, the hanging-hip operation alone is not sufficient, since it does not enlarge the weight-bearing area of the joint. It is then combined with a valgus intertrochanteric osteotomy. The procedure must be planned carefully on paper. Here the degree of valgum necessary depends on the possibility of adduction under anaesthesia, since in protrusio adduction may be restricted by bony obstacles.

A 48-year-old female patient complained of pain in both hips, which were protrusive (Figs. 216a and 217a). The two hips were successively operated on at a 1-year interval. At the 10-year follow-up for the left hip (9-year follow-up for the right hip), the results remained excellent: no pain or limping and a full range of movement. In the X-ray, the pathological subchondral sclerosis had disappeared. A thin ribbon of even width throughout underlined both sockets, and a wide joint space had reappeared (Figs. 216b and 217b).

In a 58-year-old female patient, the femoral head was bulging into the pelvis (Fig. 218a). A valgus osteotomy was carried out with a hanging-hip procedure. Ten years later, the result remained good (Fig. 218b).

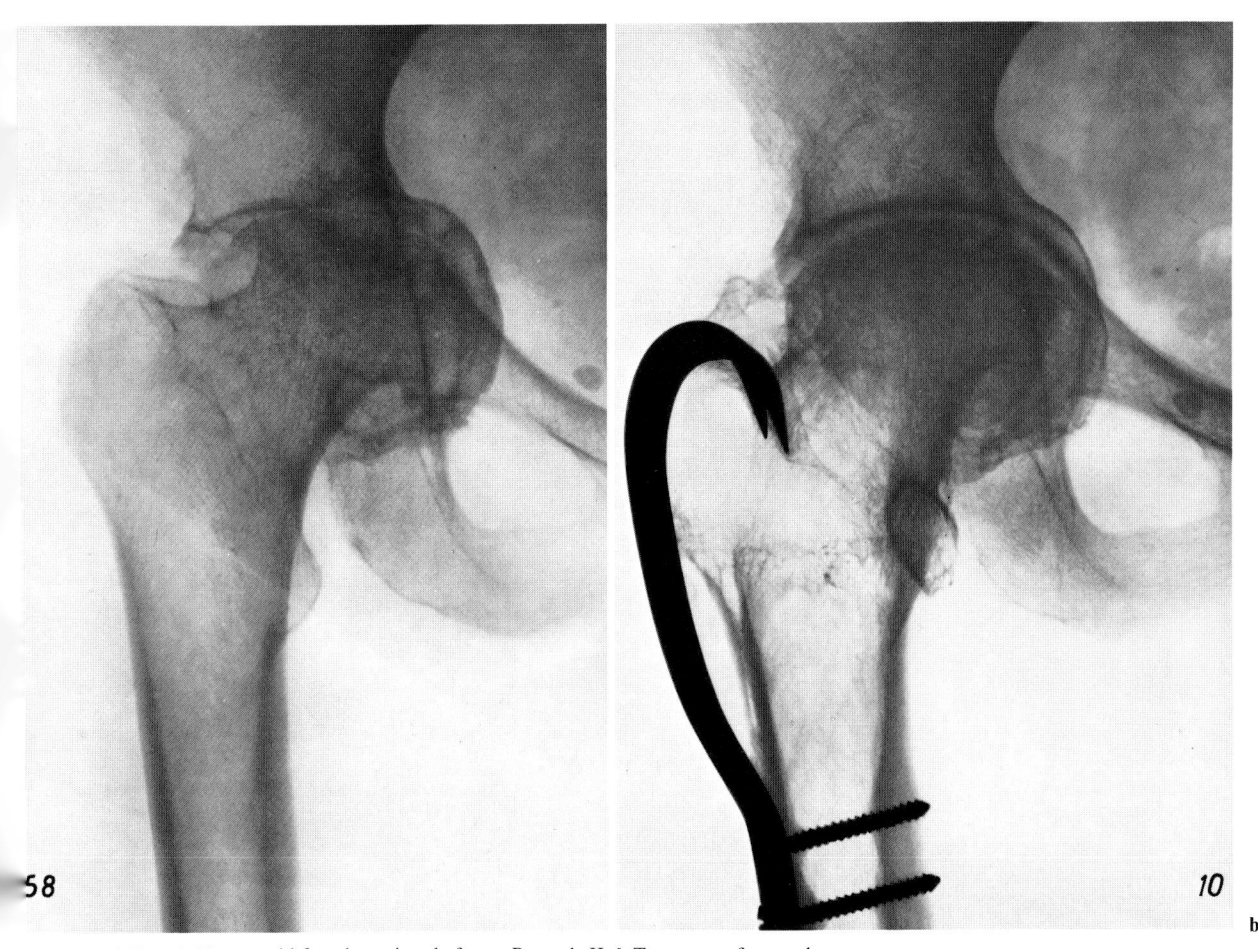

Fig. 218. a A 58-year-old female patient before a Pauwels II. **b** Ten years afterwards

III. Abduction Contracture

In exceptional instances, protrusio acetabuli seems to result from an abduction contracture. The abduction contracture rotates the pelvis about the femoral head, counter-clockwise if we consider the coronal projection of a right hip (Fig. 219a). This rotation of the pelvis has the following consequences.

1. The centre of gravity S_5 is displaced towards the hip as in limping. Therefore, the lever arm h' of force K is shortened and the resultant force R is decreased.

2. The lateral displacement of the line of action of force K and the change in direction of the abductor muscles change the direction of the line of action of the resultant force R, which becomes less inclined from the vertical.

3. Despite the change in direction of its line of action, the resultant force R no longer intersects the facies lunata at its centre of gravity but closer to its medial border. Therefore, the stresses are no longer evenly distributed over the weight-bearing surface of the joint. The stress diagram appears as a triangle with its base medially.

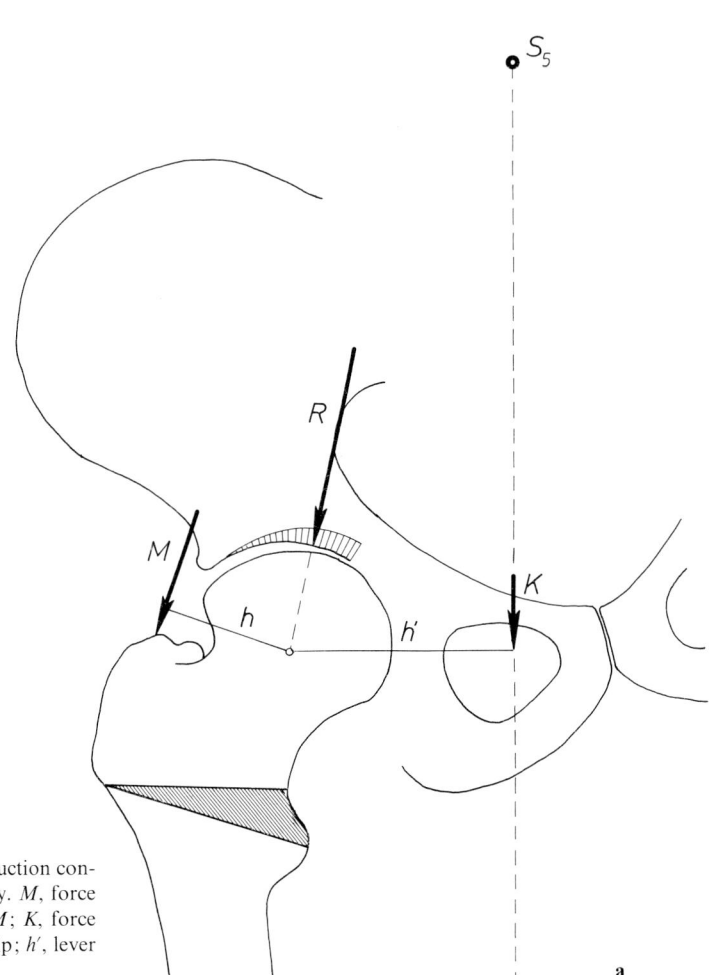

Fig. 219. a Protrusio acetabuli resulting from an abduction contracture. **b** After a varus intertrochanteric osteotomy. M, force exerted by the abductor muscles; h, lever arm of M; K, force exerted by that part of the body supported by the hip; h', lever arm of K; R, resultant of M and K

Force R, although decreased, evokes higher compressive stresses than normal in the depths of the acetabulum because it acts off-centre on the weight-bearing surface. However, the height of the triangle in the depths of the acetabulum is small in comparison to the dense triangle which often appears in subluxated dysplastic hips. This difference seems to result from the fact that force R is not increased as it is in a subluxated hip.

In such instances, a valgus osteotomy would increase the tilt of the pelvis further. A varus intertrochanteric osteotomy can be considered (Fig. 219b). The consequent return of the pelvis to the horizontal lengthens the lever arm h' of force K and somewhat increases the resultant force R, but R then acts at the centre of gravity of the weight-bearing surface of the joint. This ensures an even distribution of the articular compressive stresses and eliminates their medial peak.

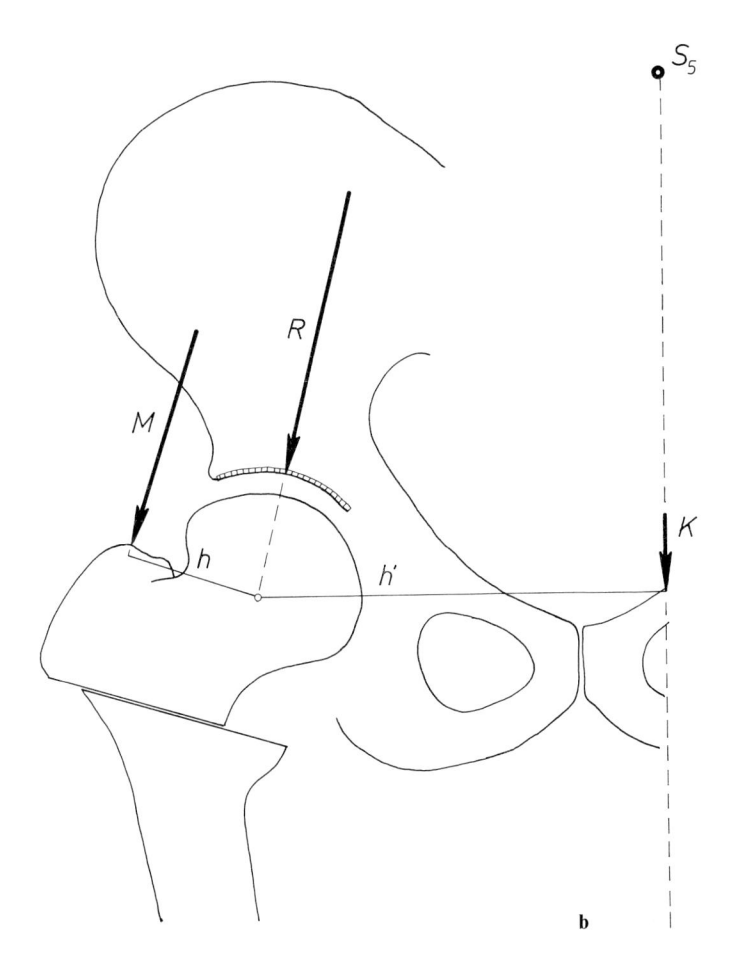

Fig. 219b

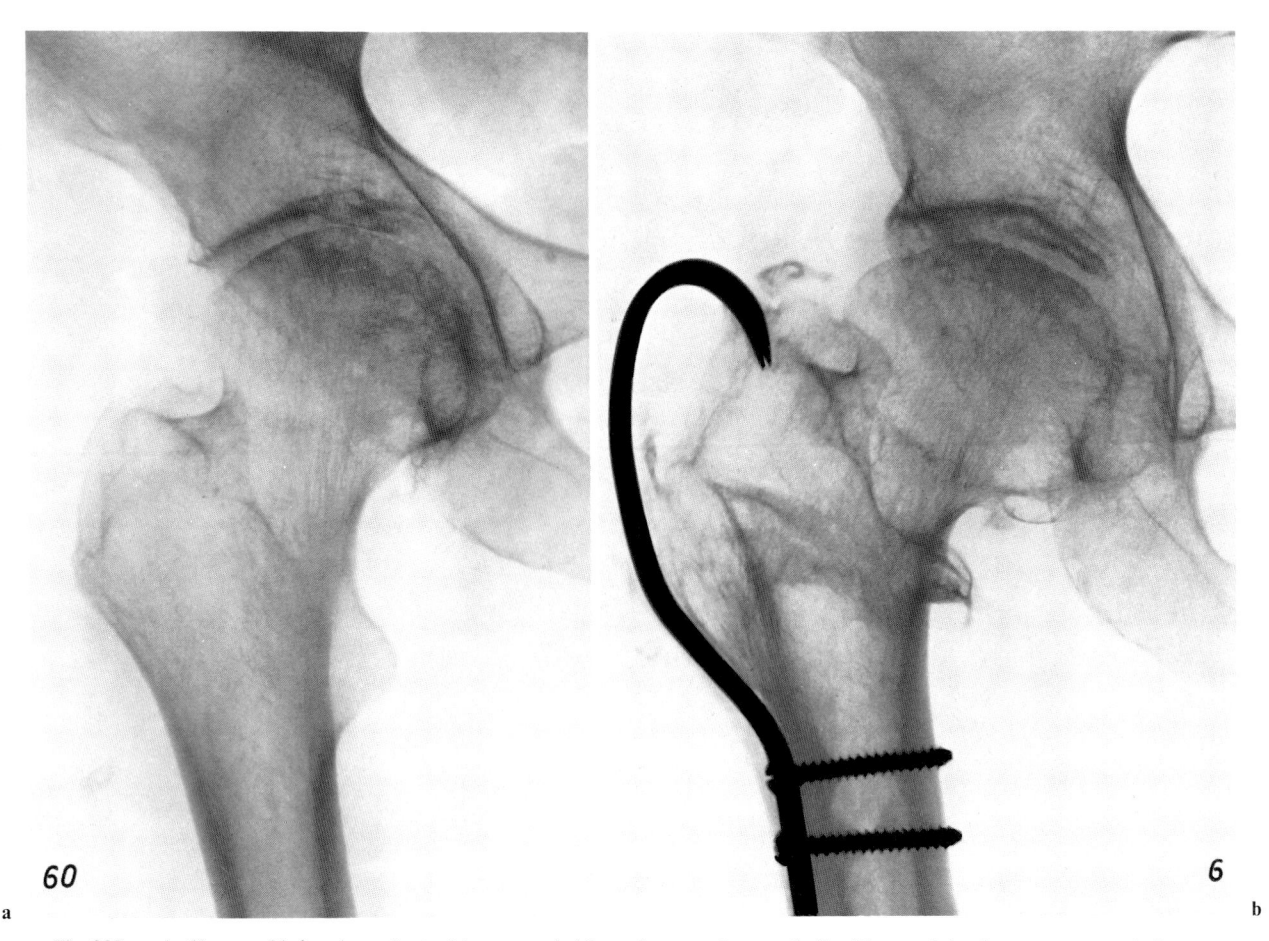

Fig. 220. a A 60-year-old female patient with osteoarthritis and protrusio acetabuli with an abduction contracture before a varus intertrochanteric osteotomy. **b** Six years afterwards

This concept is illustrated by the case of a 60-year-old female patient presenting with protrusive osteoarthritis with an abduction contracture (Fig. 220a). There was a dense triangle in the depths of the acetabulum corresponding to the stress diagram, and the joint space was narrowed. Six years after a varus intertrochanteric osteotomy, the pelvis was level. The dense triangle had been replaced by a subchondral sclerosis of uniform width throughout, and a normal joint space had reappeared (Fig. 220b).

IV. Conclusion

In osteoarthritis developing with protrusio acetabuli, a hanging-hip procedure may be sufficient if the X-rays show no sign of stress concentration. However, in many instances the condition is characterized by an increase in the stresses in the depths of the socket. A dense subchondral triangle appears with its base medial. Then, as a rule, a valgus intertrochanteric osteotomy combined with a hanging-hip procedure constitutes the treatment of choice. However, in exceptional instances the protrusio acetabuli seems to result from an abduction contracture. In such cases a varus intertrochanteric osteotomy may have to be considered.

Chapter V. Avascular Necrosis of the Femoral Head

I. Legg-Calvé-Perthes' Disease

In LEGG-CALVÉ-PERTHES' disease, the femoral head always becomes revascularized. The problem consists in preserving its shape and in avoiding its collapse. It seems sensible to contain as much as possible of the "head at risk" in a mould, the acetabulum, and to reduce the pressure exerted on this head. Both prerequisites can be fulfilled by means of a varus intertrochanteric osteotomy in many cases, as the following three examples show.

In a 6-year-old boy with LEGG-CALVÉ-PERTHES' disease which seemed to involve three-quarters of the femoral head (Fig. 221a), a 30° varus osteotomy was carried out. To this end, a 15° wedge was resected, rotated and reinserted. It is interesting to follow the evolution and the reorientation of the epiphysial cartilage (Fig. 221 b–j). At the latest follow-up, the hip looked normal and was functioning normally. The boy plays basketball for a renowned team.

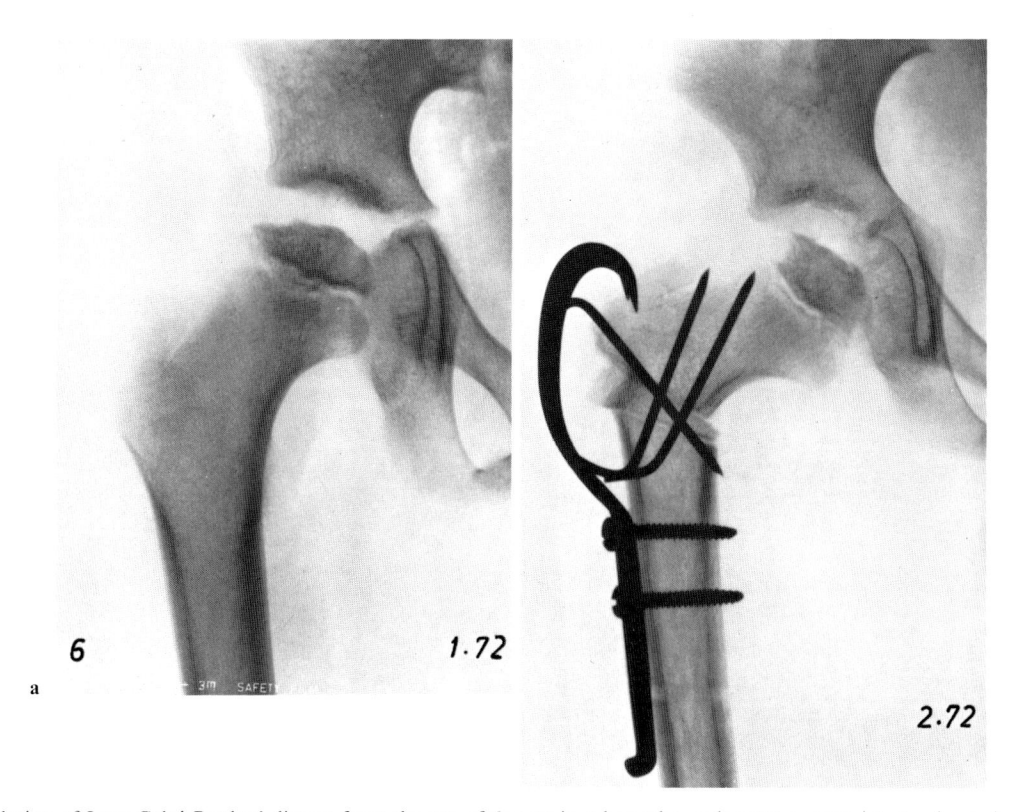

Fig. 221 a–j. Evolution of Legg-Calvé-Perthes' disease from the age of 6 years in a boy who underwent a varus intertrochanteric osteotomy. Fig. 221 e–j see pages 222–223

c   4.72

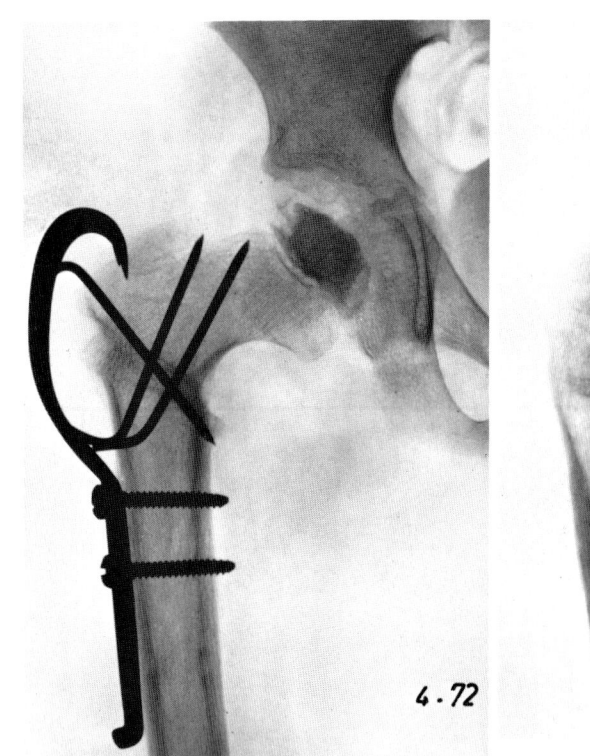

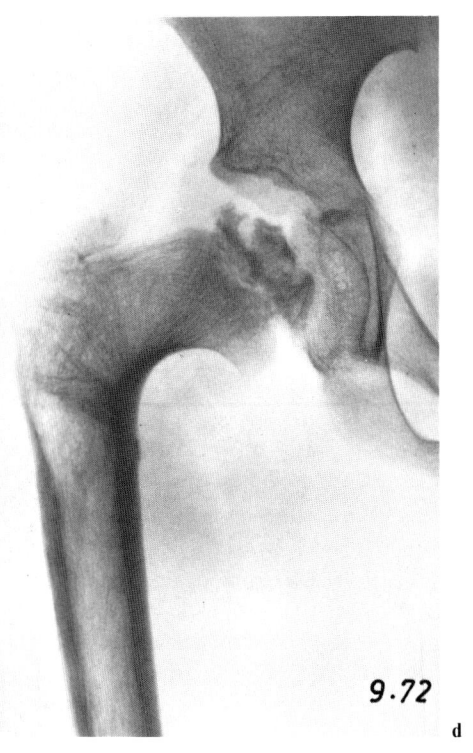

d   9.72

g   12.72

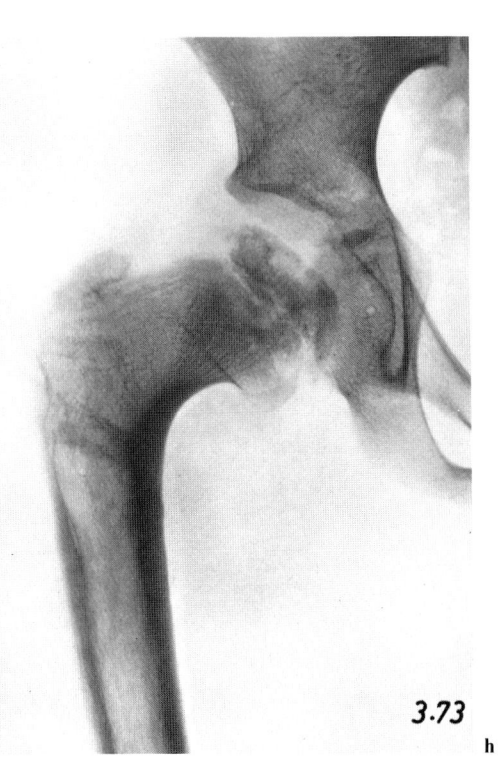

h   3.73

Fig. 221

12.73

8.74

e

f

8.76

8.78

i

j

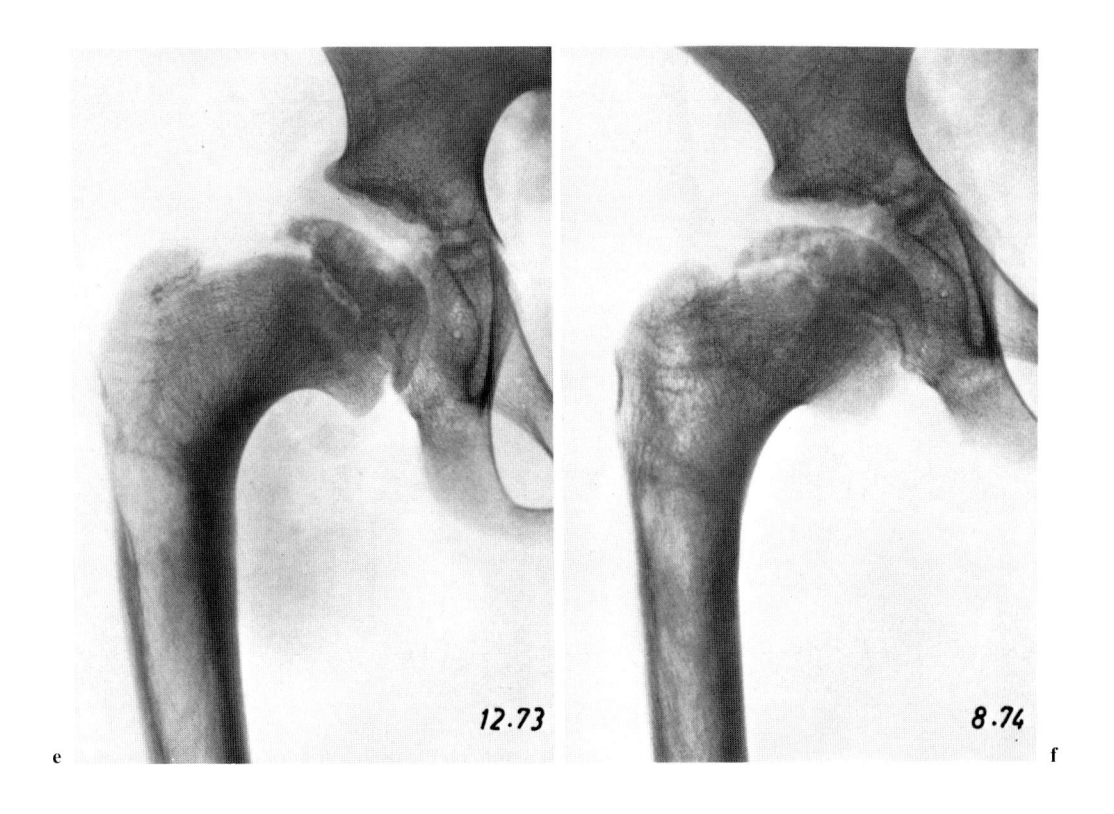

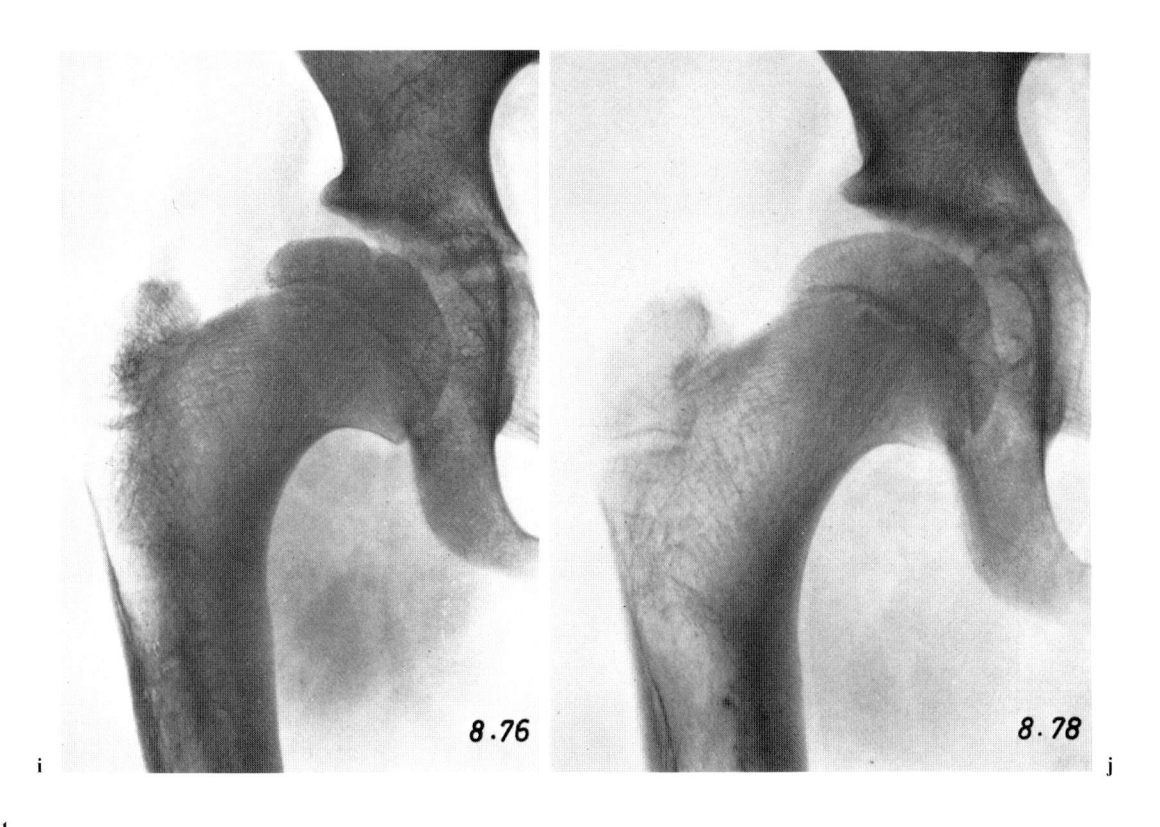

Fig. 221

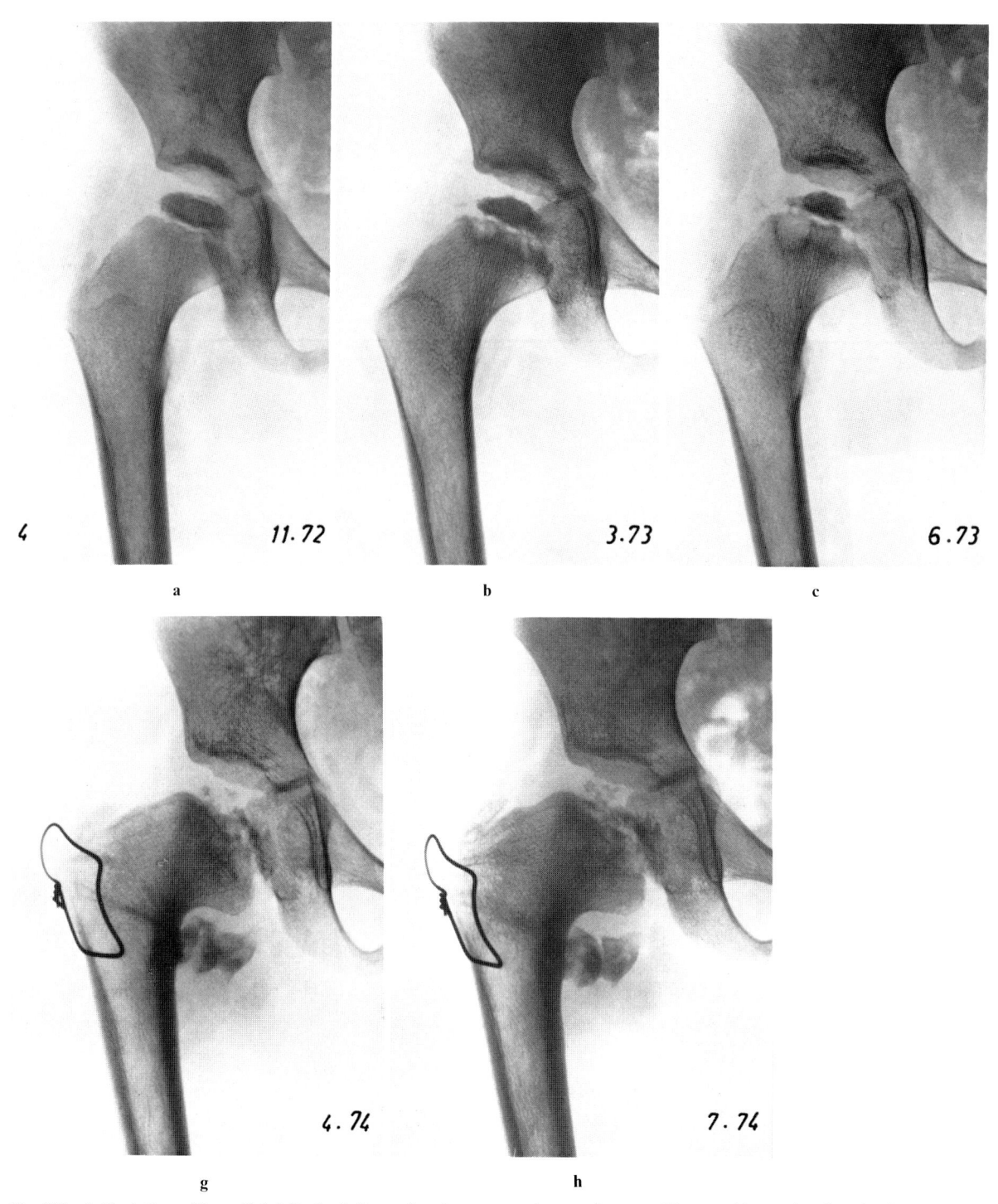

Fig. 222a–l. Evolution of Legg-Calvé-Perthes' disease in a boy operated on at the age of 5 years, 11 months after the first X-rays were taken

The same evolution was observed in a boy who was operated on at the age of 5, 11 months after the first X-rays were taken (Fig. 222). Here the whole femoral head was involved. At the 9-year follow-up, the X-ray appearance was normal and the hip was functioning normally.

9.73

d

11.73

e

1.74

f

1.75

i

9.76

j

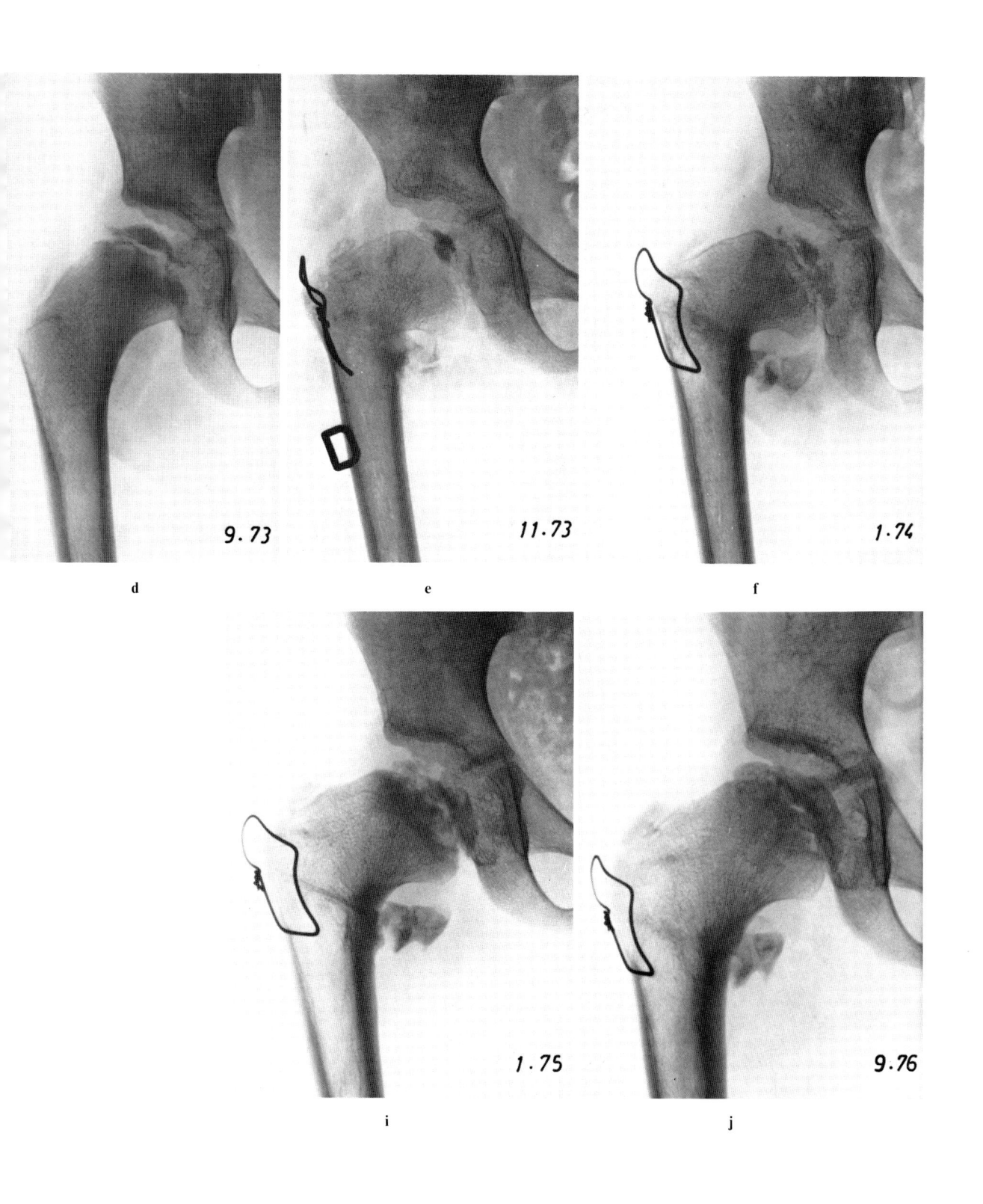

Fig. 222k, l see next page

Fig. 222   k   10.78

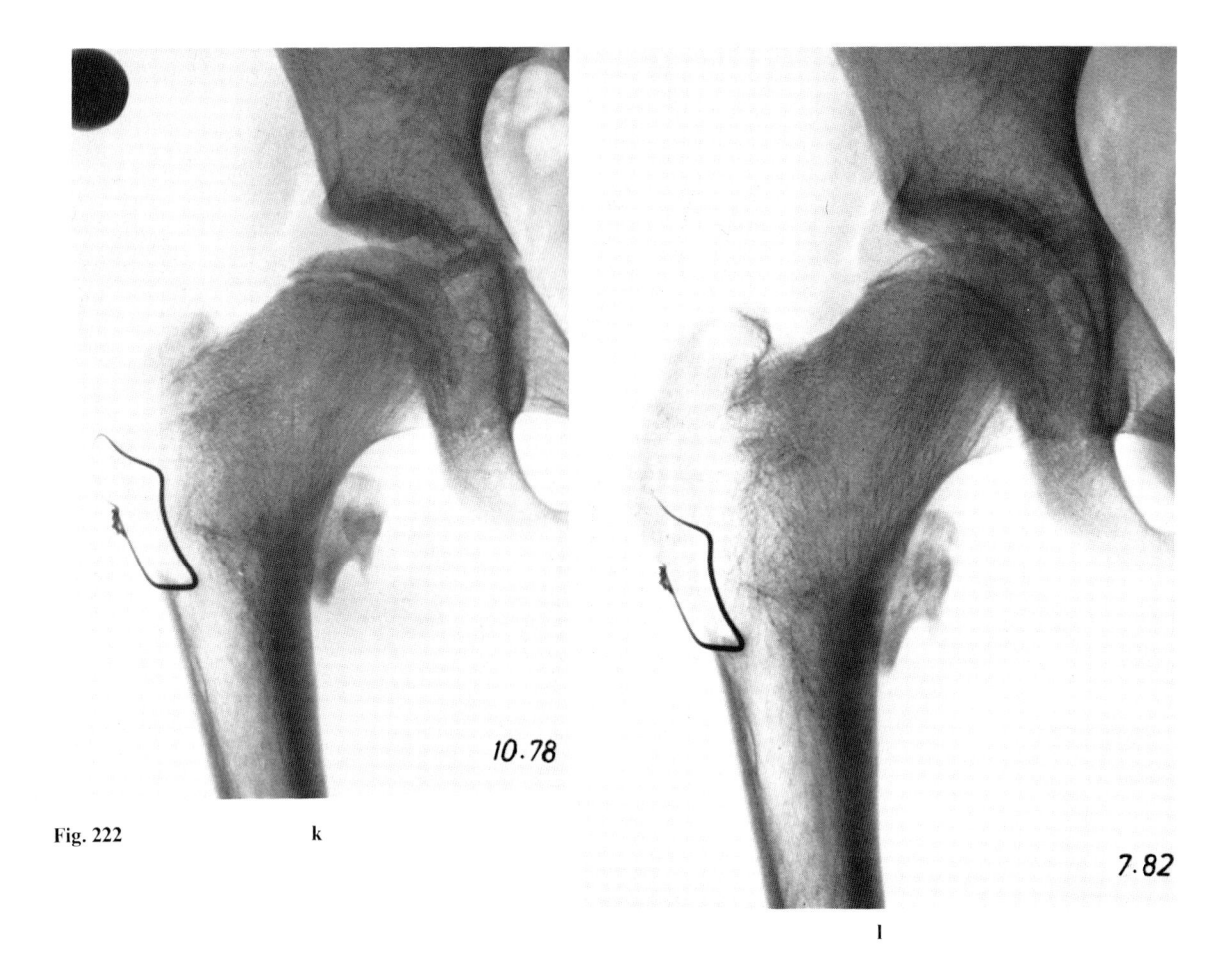

7.82

l

A 7-year-old patient was operated on 9 months after the first diagnostic X-ray (Fig. 223a). Nearly all the femoral head and the metaphysis were involved. At the latest follow-up, more than 12 years after the operation, the hip joint appeared normal and was functioning normally (Fig. 223j).

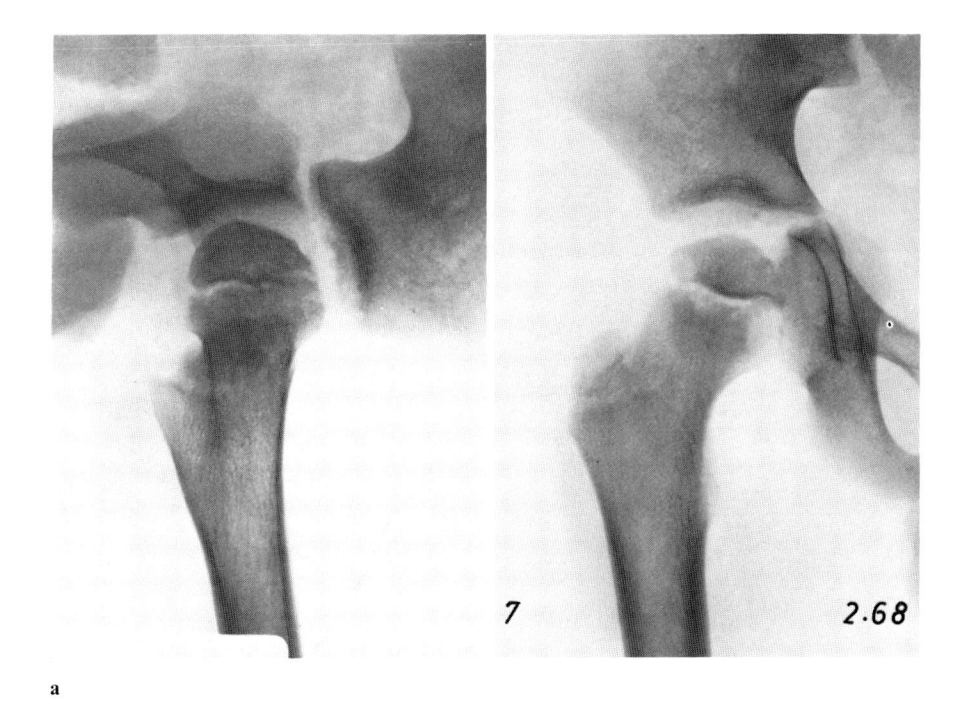

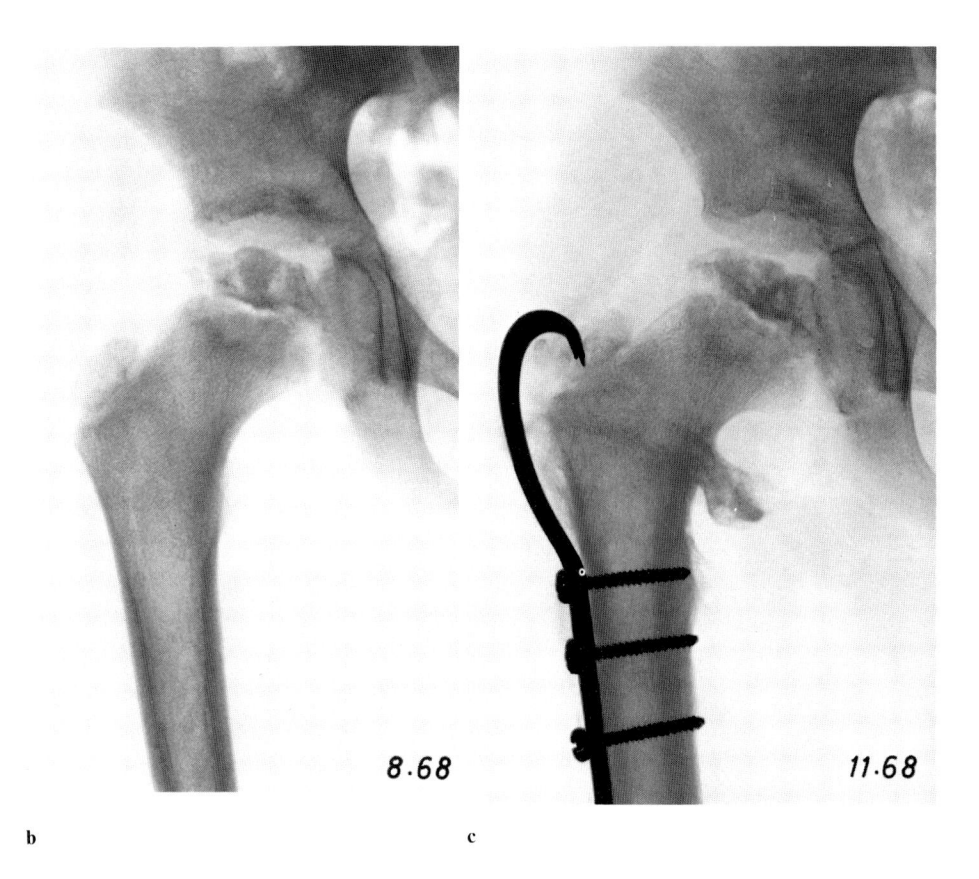

Fig. 223a–j. Evolution of Legg-Calvé-Perthes' disease from the age of 7 years in a boy who underwent a varus intertrochanteric osteotomy. Fig. 223e–j see pages 228–229

d

2.69

e

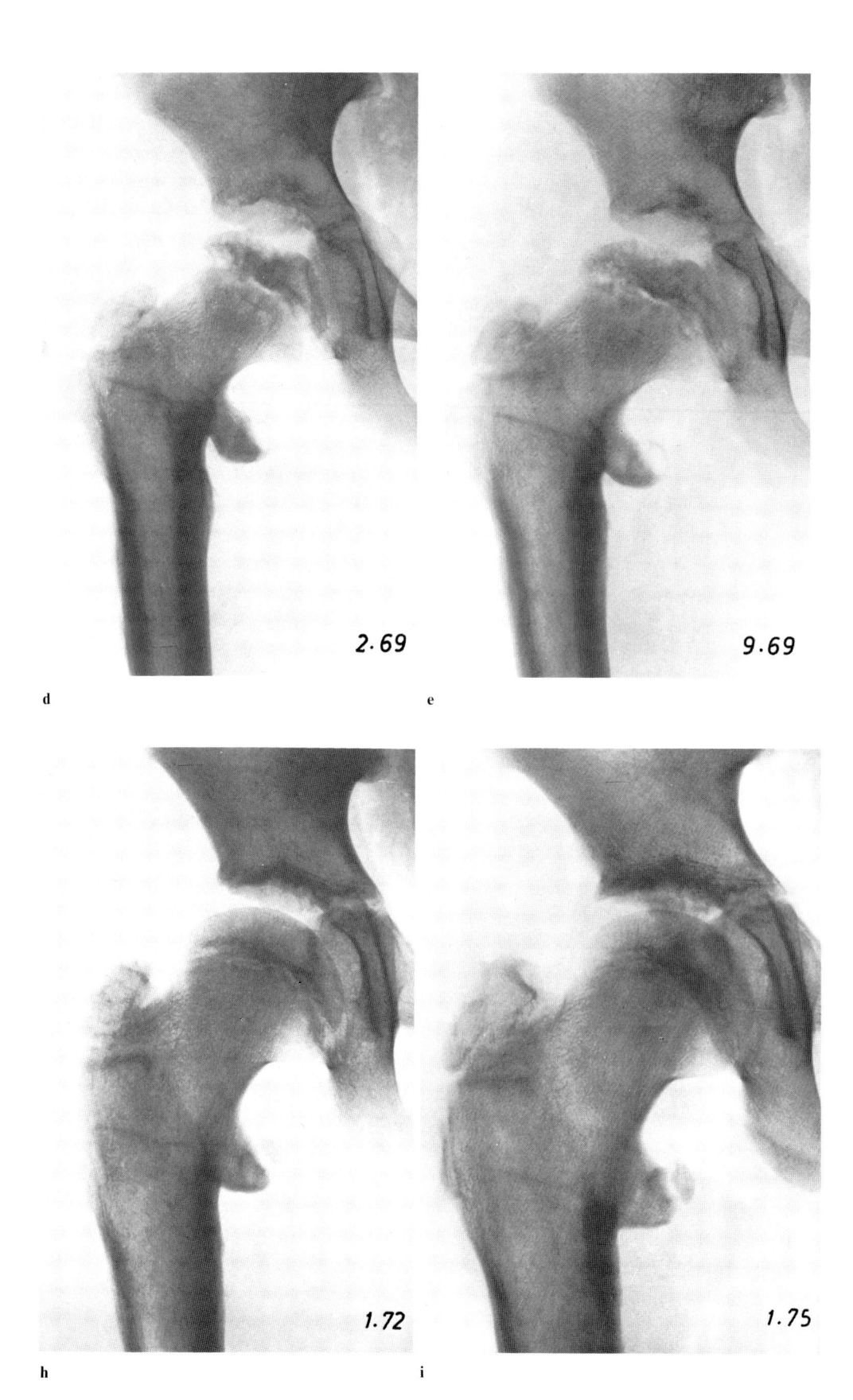

9.69

h

1.72

i

1.75

Fig. 223

4.70 1.71

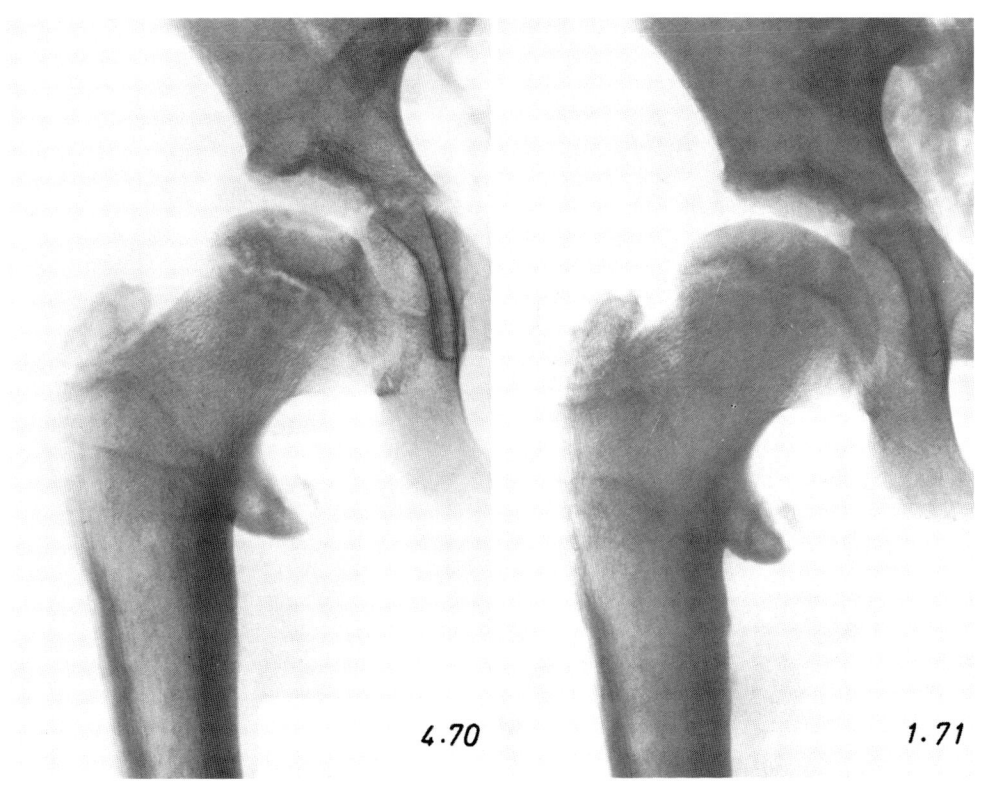

3.81

Fig. 223   f   g   j

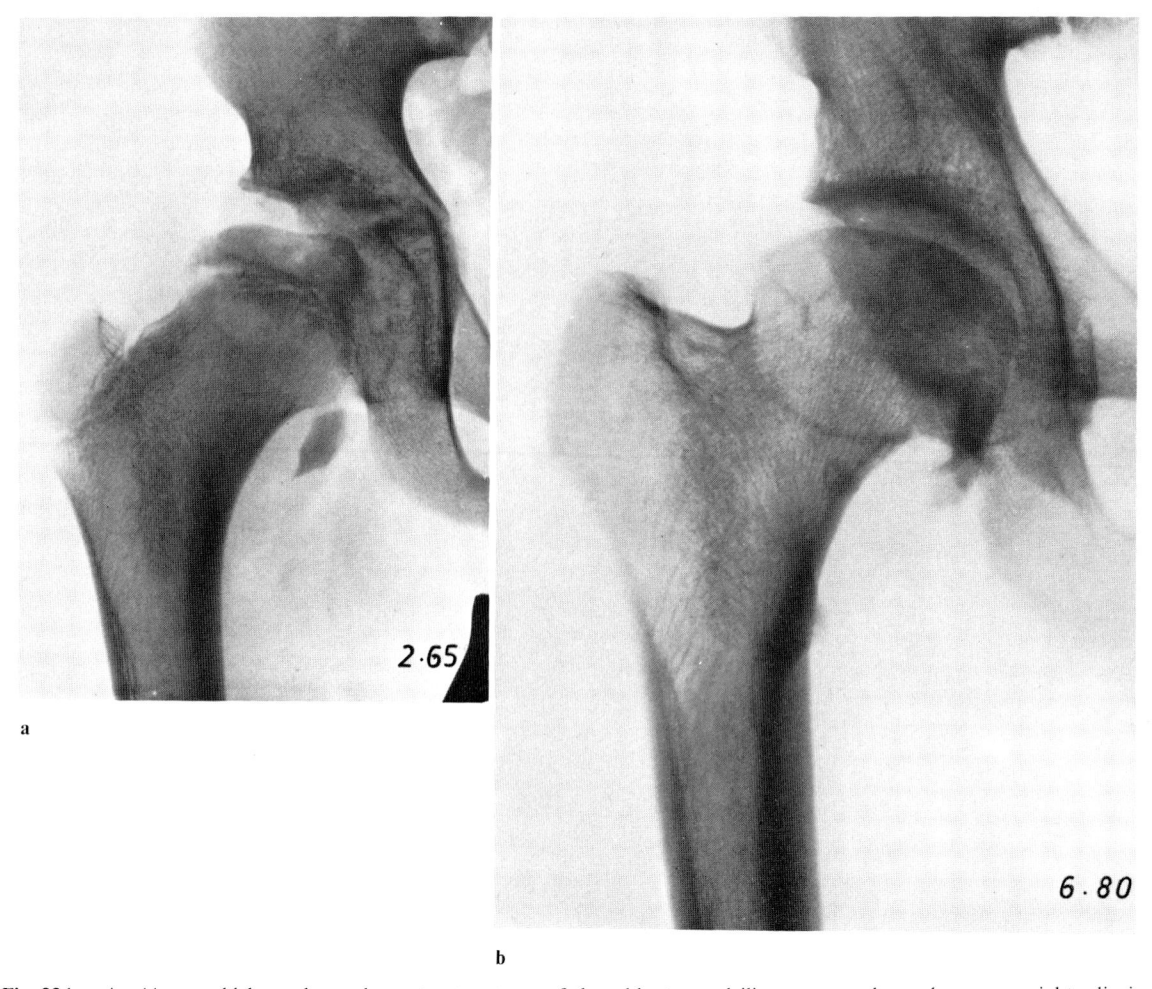

Fig. 224. a An 11-year-old boy who underwent a tenotomy of the adductor and iliopsoas muscles and wore a weight-relieving calliper. **b** Seventeen-year follow-up

The hanging-hip operation does not seem to be sufficient in this condition. It does not provide the weakened femoral head with a covering mould in which it can become revascularized without collapsing. An 11-year-old boy underwent a tenotomy of the adductor and iliopsoas muscles for LEGG-CALVÉ-PERTHES' disease involving about three-quarters of the femoral head (Fig. 224a). After the operation, he was given a weight-relieving calliper. Seventeen years later, he had developed an osteophyte on the medial side of the femoral head, which was flattened (Fig. 224b).

The articular pressure in the hip may be reduced sufficiently by an abduction walking-frame or by a weight-relieving calliper. Each case must be carefully analysed before the form of treatment is decided upon. A 5-year-old boy was first treated by traction in the recumbent position (Fig. 225a–d). We saw him at the stage of revascularization and prescribed a weight-relieving calliper, which was used for 14 months. Eventually, complete healing took place (Fig. 225e–j). At the latest follow-up, he was 20 years old and the clinical result was excellent. In the X-ray, the hip looked satisfactory despite some shortness of the femoral neck (Fig. 225k).

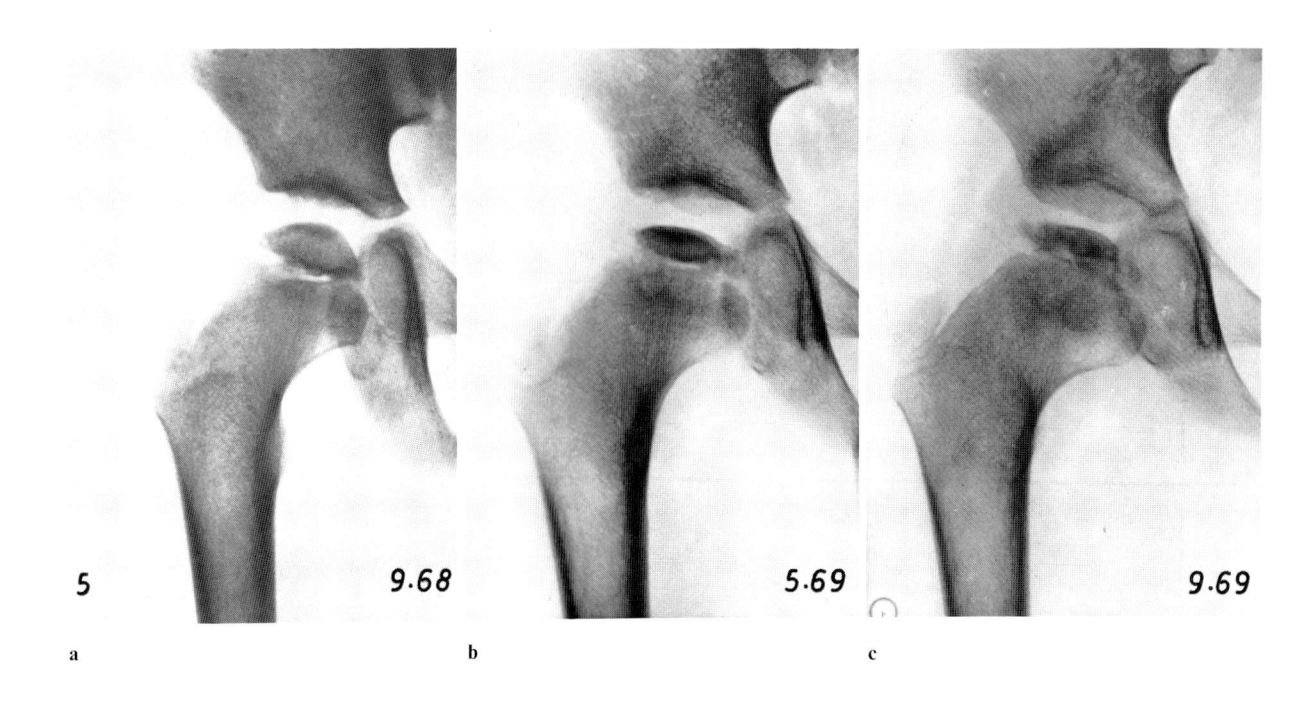

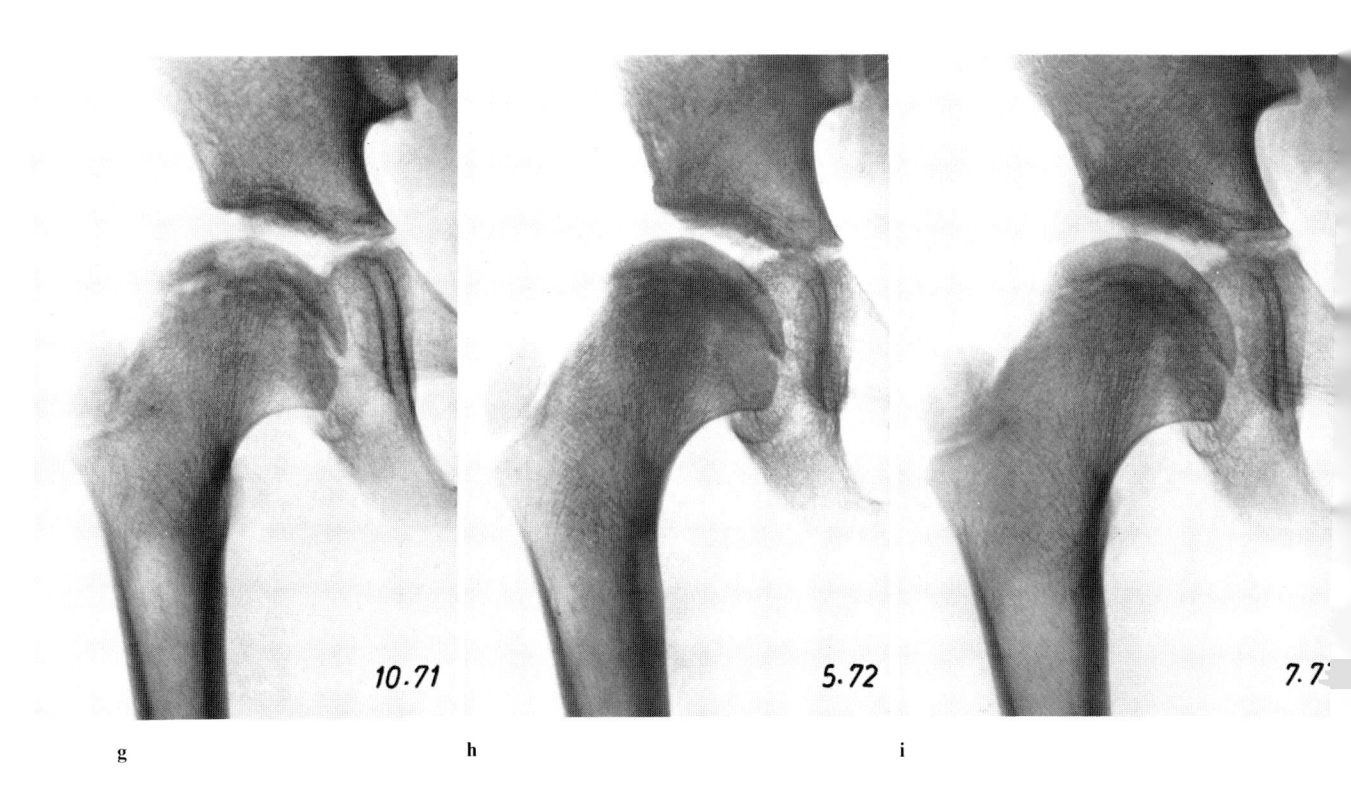

Fig. 225a–k. Evolution of Legg-Calvé-Perthes' disease from the age of 5 years in a boy treated by means of a weight-relieving calliper

d

e

1.70

7.70

f

1.71

j

8.75

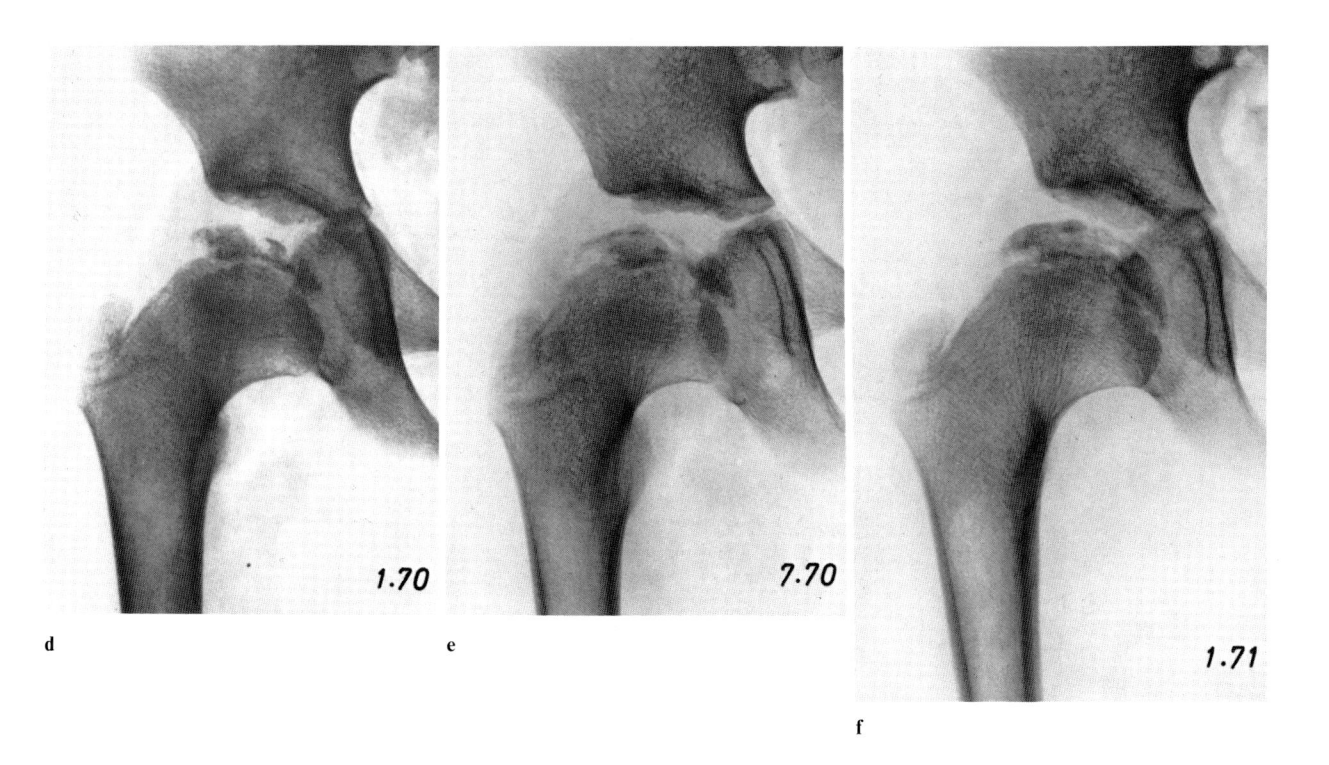

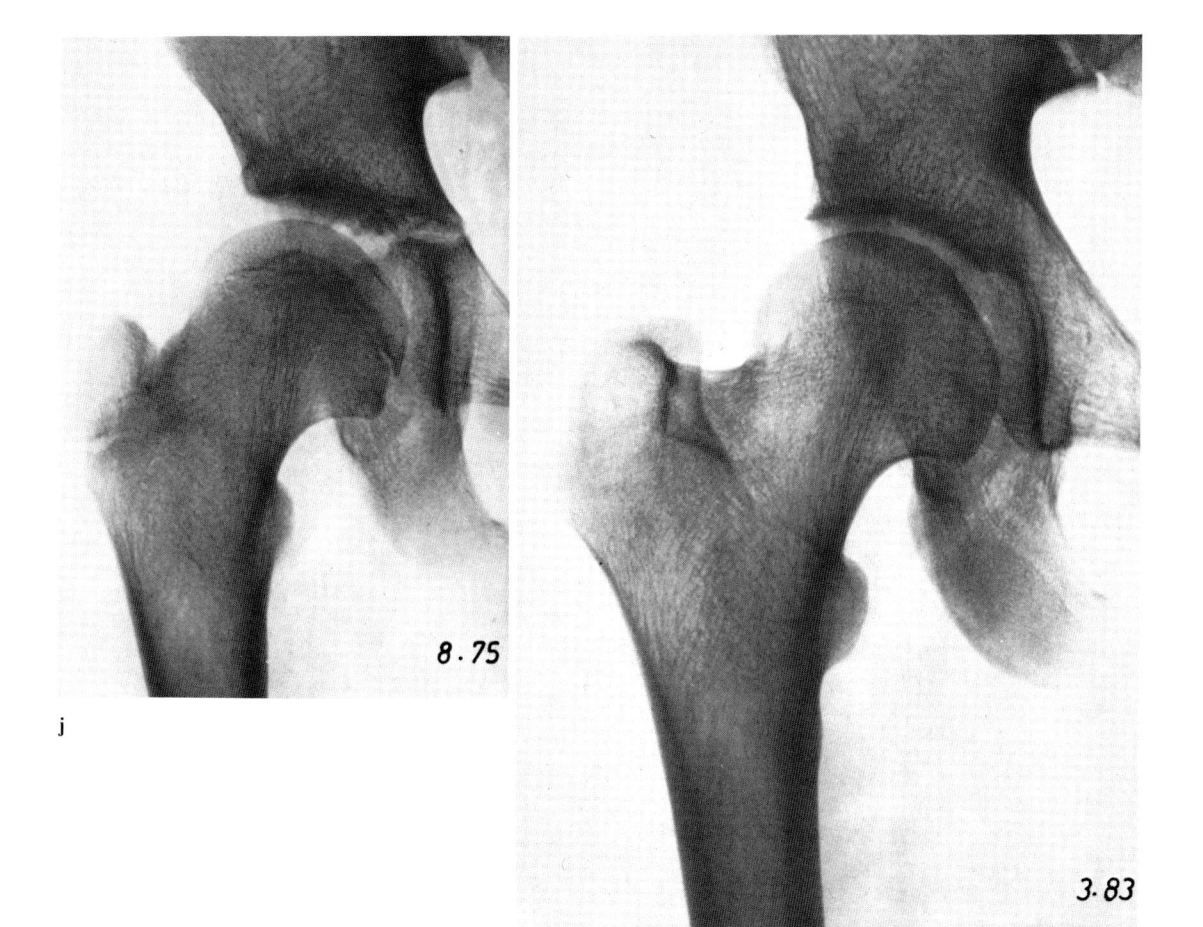

k

3.83

Fig. 225

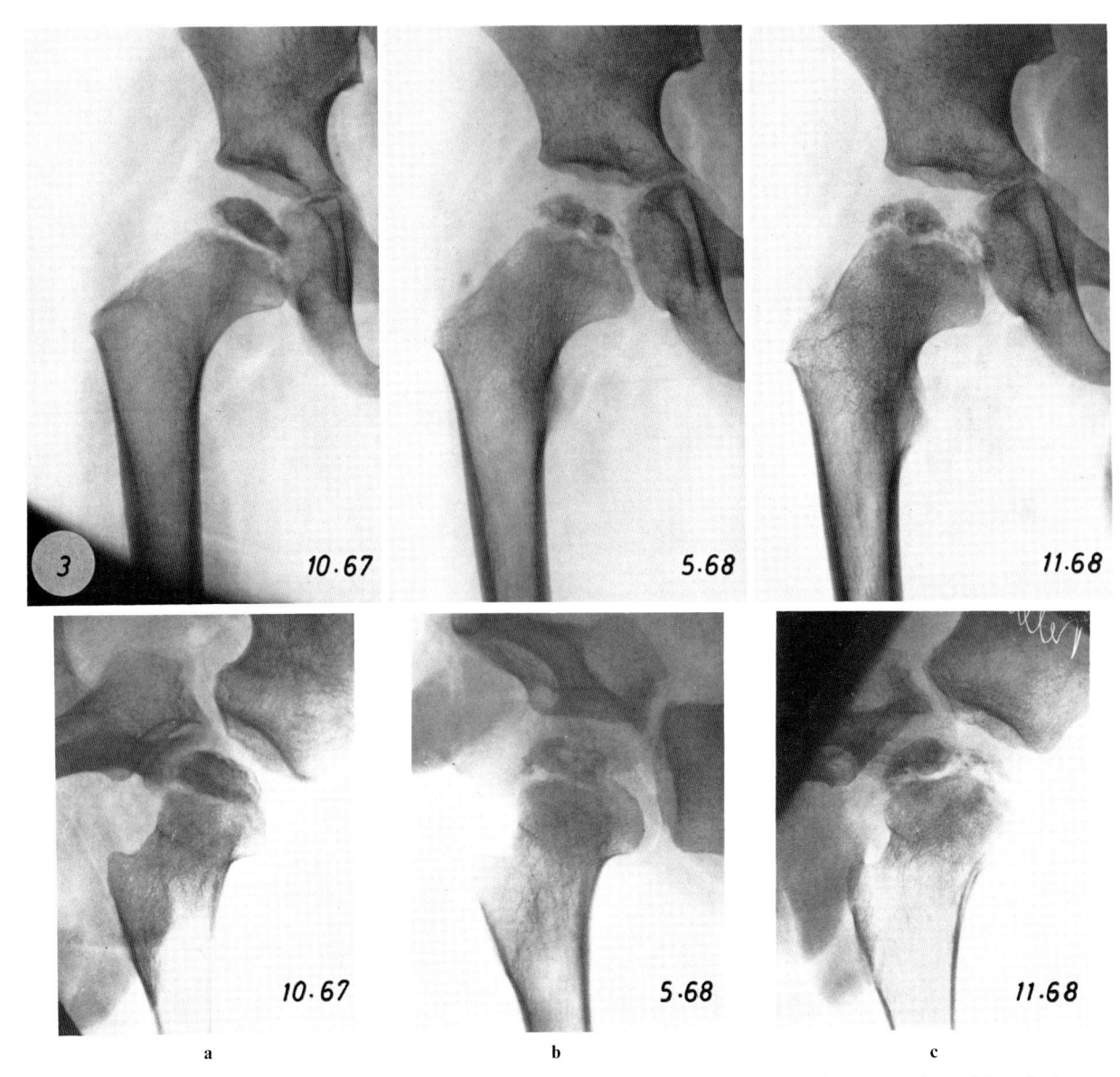

Fig. 226a–j. Evolution of Legg-Calvé-Perthes' disease from the age of 3 years in a boy treated by means of a weight-relieving calliper. Fig. 226g–j see pages 236–237

Following diagnosis of the disease, a 3-year-old boy was treated with a calliper for 32 months (Fig. 226a–i). The femoral head seemed to be contained in its acetabular mould. At the latest follow-up he was 14 years old and the hip looked normal. In such instances there is some doubt as to whether any treatment is necessary.

Both non-surgical treatment using an abduction frame or a weight-relieving calliper and varus osteotomy result in a reduction of the joint pressure. The condition progresses through its successive stages whatever the treatment, but a varus osteotomy seems to accelerate the evolution, which is thus brought to its conclusion much more quickly.

The choice of treatment depends on the age of the patient, the information derived from X-rays of the hip (hips at risk) and the attitude of the parents. A varus osteotomy is more likely to be considered in a patient older than 5 years, with involvement of more than half the femoral epiphysis and at the beginning of the period of fragmentation. It is also recommended when the condition affects both hips.

2.69	5.69	11.69
2.69	5.69	11.69
d	e	f

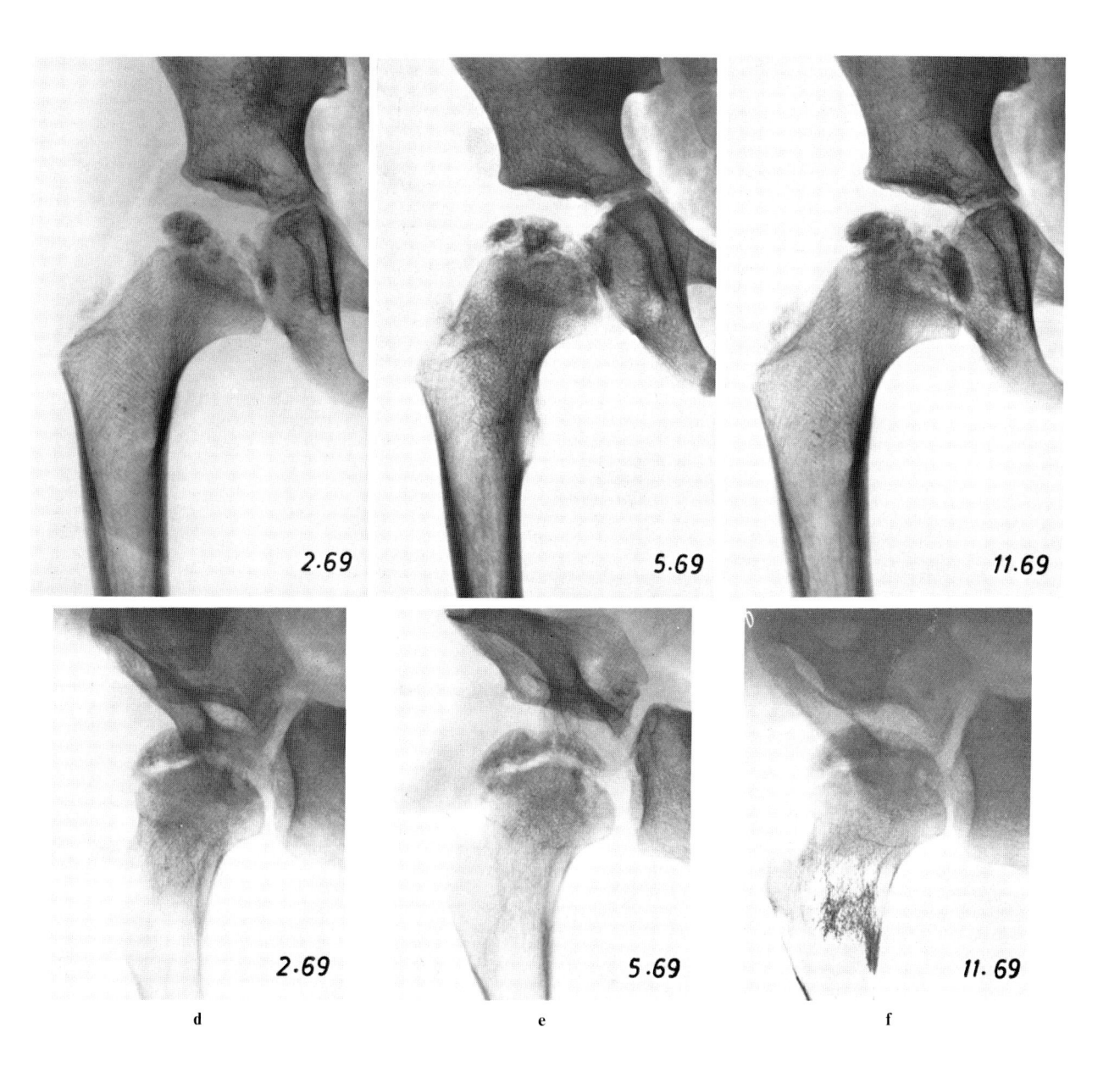

Fig. 226

235

g h Fig. 226g, h

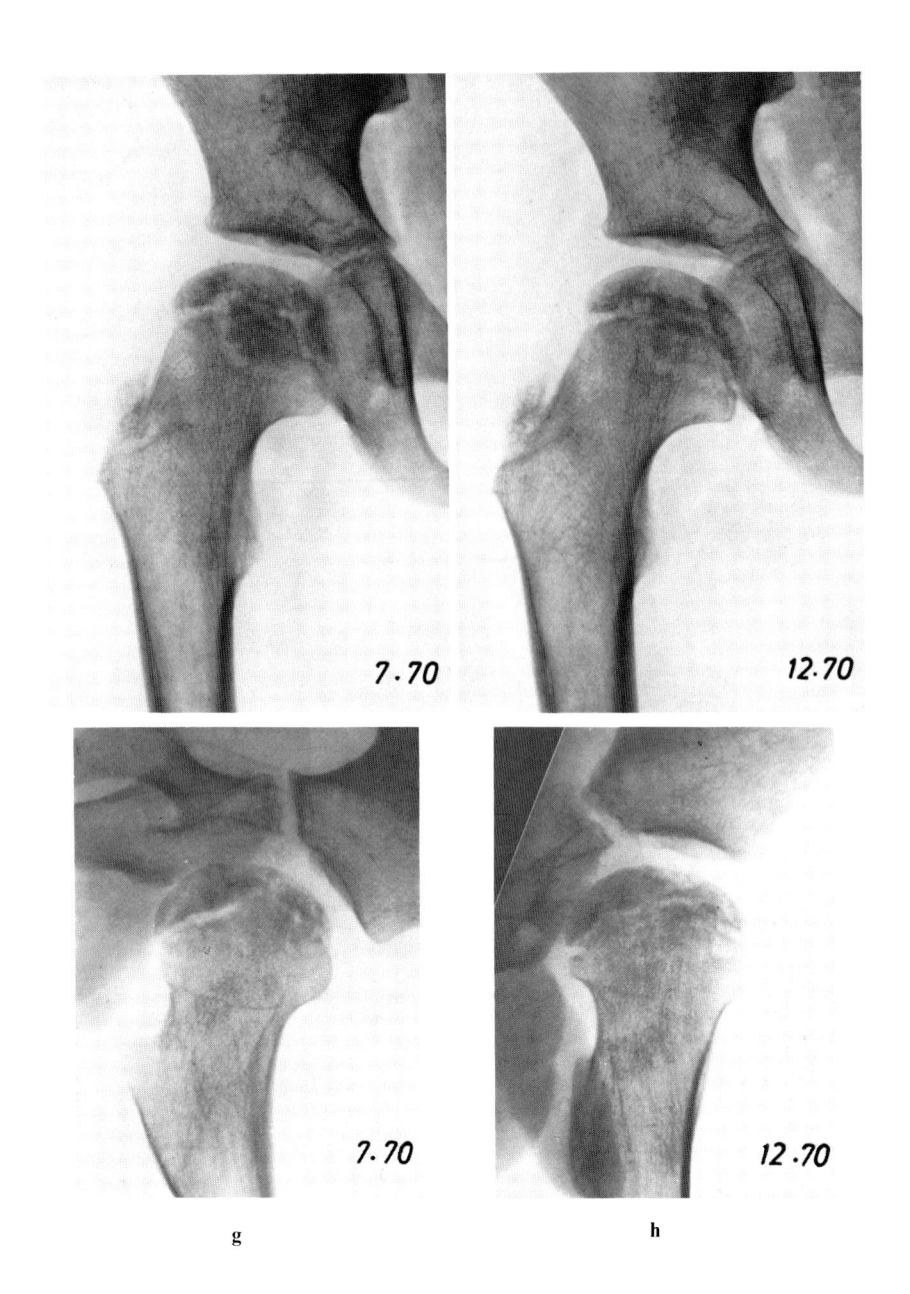

Fig. 226i, j

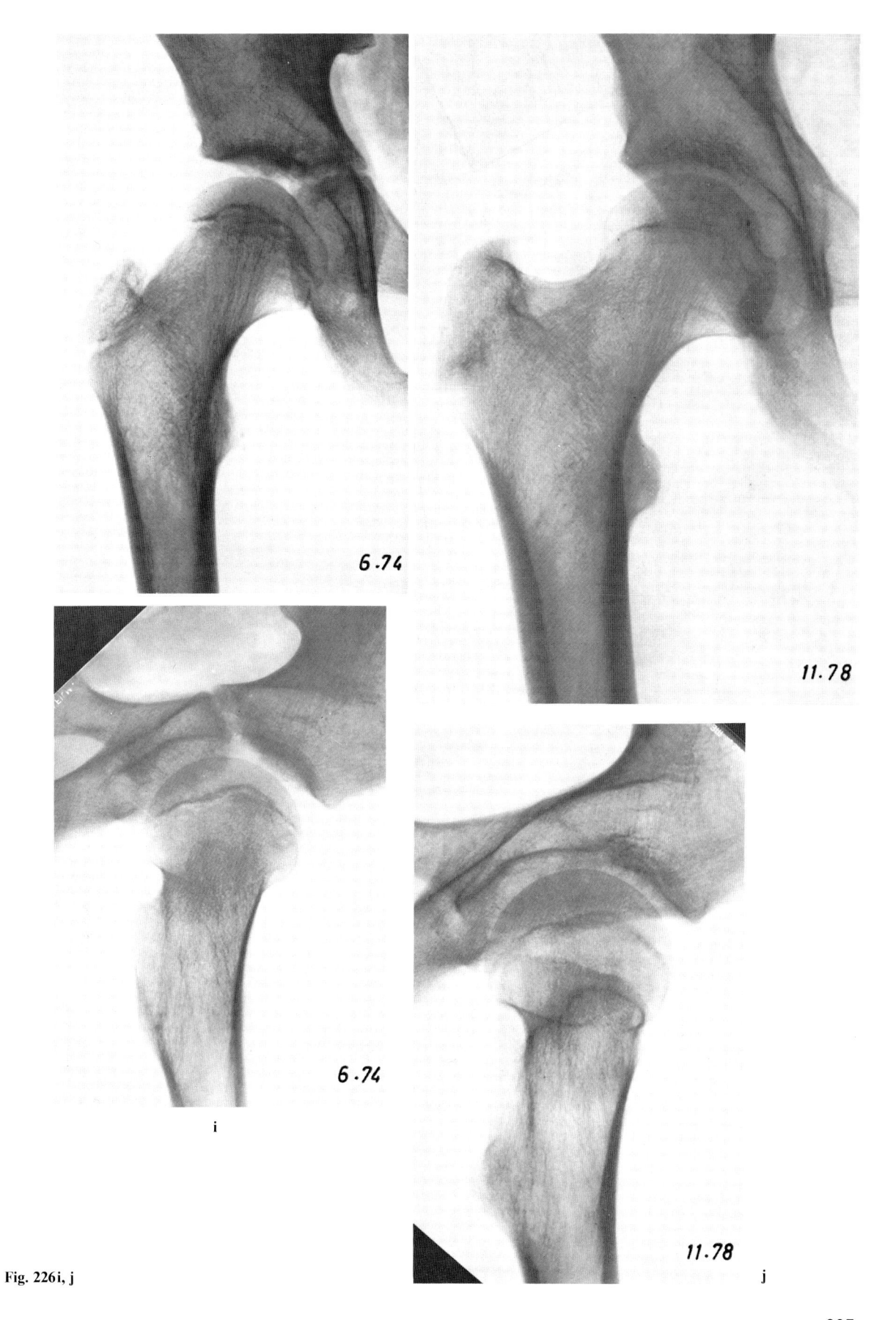

II. Avascular Necrosis of the Femoral Head in Adults

A. Rationale

Whatever its initial cause, ischaemic necrosis seems to lower the resistance of the femoral head to mechanical stress. The femoral head can no longer withstand the physiological articular pressure, and collapses. This collapse leads to incongruence of the joint surfaces and a reduction of the articular weight-bearing area. As a consequence of this diminution of the weight-bearing area, the compressive stresses are increased and unevenly distributed in the joint. Pain due to necrosis and aggravated by increased articular pressure can cause contracture of the muscles spanning the hip, and this further increases joint pressure. The joint becomes progressively deformed and degenerates, as it does in osteoarthritis.

A large osteophyte develops over the medial aspect of the femoral head, which is pushed laterally in the socket, thus decreasing the weight-bearing area of the joint. The acetabulum becomes enlarged and flattened. The evolution in a 57-year-old patient treated with corticosteroids illustrates this sequence (Fig. 227).

The resistance of the tissues depends on biological factors which we do not understand. Some of these factors, such as the blood supply, seem to

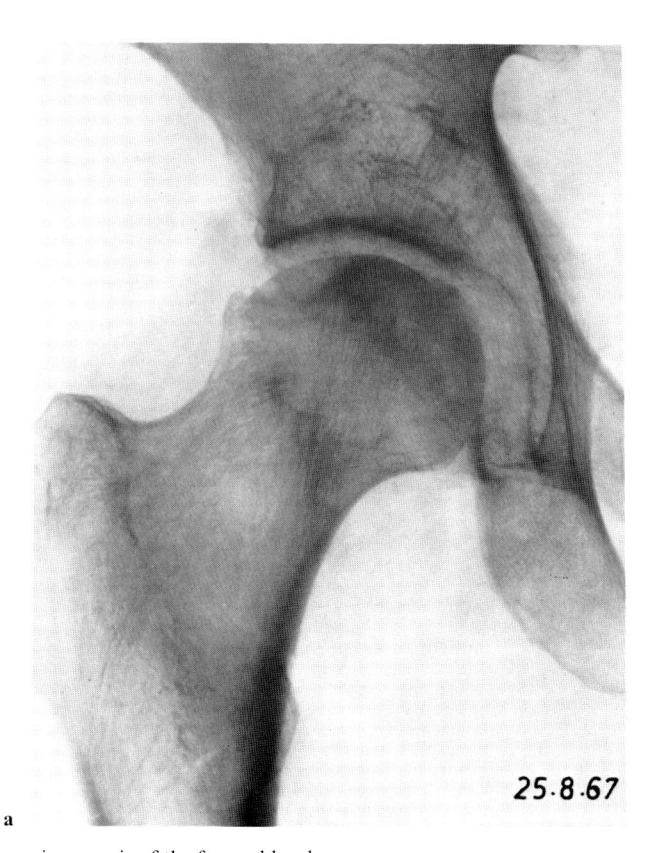

Fig. 227. a A 57-year-old male patient. **b, c** Evolution of ischaemic necrosis of the femoral head

be favourably influenced by an osteotomy through the proximal end of the femur or even by a tenotomy of periarticular muscles. However, this biological effect cannot be reliably predicted and does not last if the mechanical conditions are not improved.

The rotational osteotomy of SUGIOKA attempts to replace the necrotic part of the femoral head by an intact part in the weight-bearing area of the joint. This procedure is supposed to restore the tissue resistance in the weight-bearing area to normal. We have not as yet used this operation, however.

An alternative to improving the tissue resistance consists in reducing the compressive stresses in the joint. This can be achieved either by a multiple tenotomy, or by a varus osteotomy, or by a lateral displacement of the greater trochanter combined with a tenotomy or, more often, by a valgus osteotomy combined with a tenotomy.

It seems sensible to expect better results in post-traumatic than in idiopathic necrosis of the femoral head. In the former case, the resistance of the tissues was probably normal before the trauma and time should restore it to normal. In idiopathic necrosis, the biological cause of the necrosis may persist and thus keep the tissue resistance low even after surgery. However, we have not observed any significant difference in the postoperative evolution.

The indications and surgical procedures are similar to those which apply in cases of osteoarthritis.

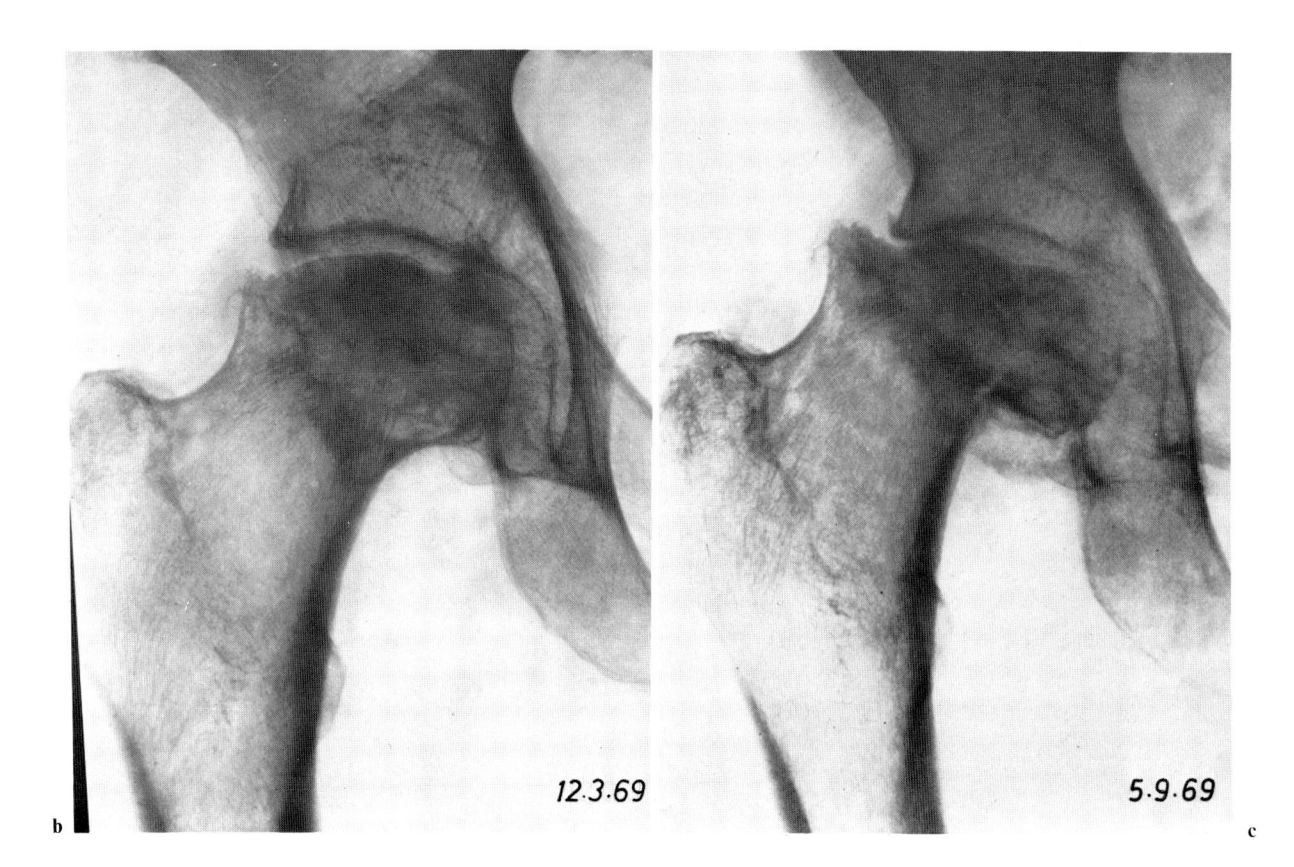

B. Hanging-Hip Procedure

When congruence of the articular surfaces is maintained in the neutral position as well as in adduction and in abduction of the leg, a hanging-hip operation may be sufficient.

A 26-year old male patient was seen 3 years after a traumatic dislocation of the hip with a fracture of the socket. Necrosis of the femoral head had developed with narrowing of the joint space and a cup-shaped sclerosis in the roof of the acetabulum (Fig. 228a). Two years after a hanging-hip procedure the hip remained pain-free with a full range of movement and the patient was not limping. A joint space had developed and the subchondral sclerosis was of uniform width throughout in the roof of the socket (Fig. 228b).

A 46-year-old female patient had had a fracture of the femoral neck 19 months before we saw her. This fracture had been poorly nailed and necrosis of the femoral head developed with chondrolysis (Fig. 229). Eight years after a hanging-hip operation, the clinical result remained excellent (Table 37). In the X-ray, a large joint space had reappeared (Fig. 229g).

Table 37. Range of movement of the hip (Fig. 229)

	Before surgery	At the 8-year follow-up	Gain
Flexion	80°	95°	15°
Extension	10°	10°	
Adduction	30°	45°	10°
Abduction	20°	15°	
Int. rotation	−5°	5°	−15°
Ext. rotation	60°	35°	

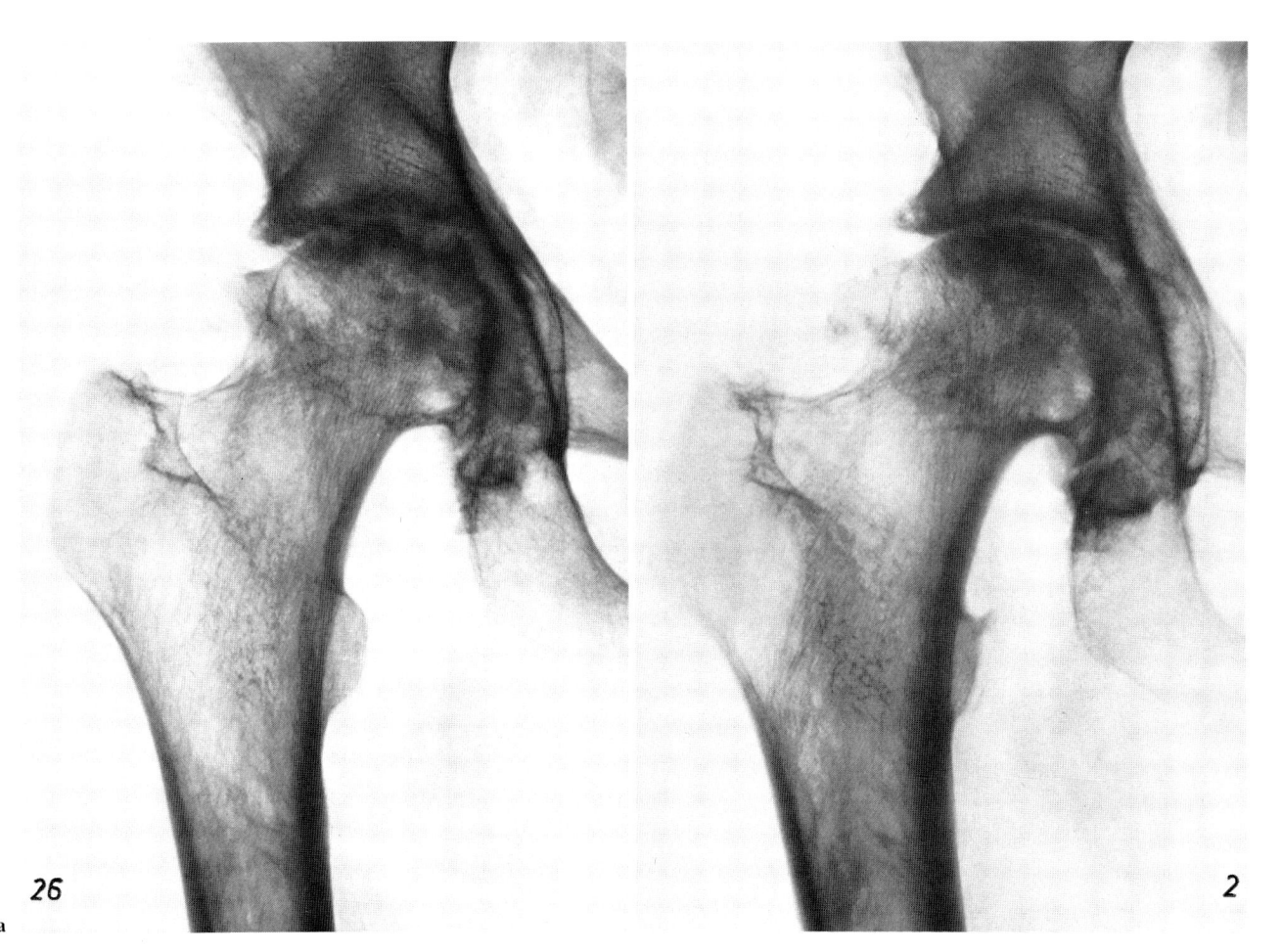

Fig. 228. a A 26-year-old male patient with post-traumatic necrosis of the femoral head before a hanging-hip operation. **b** Two years afterwards

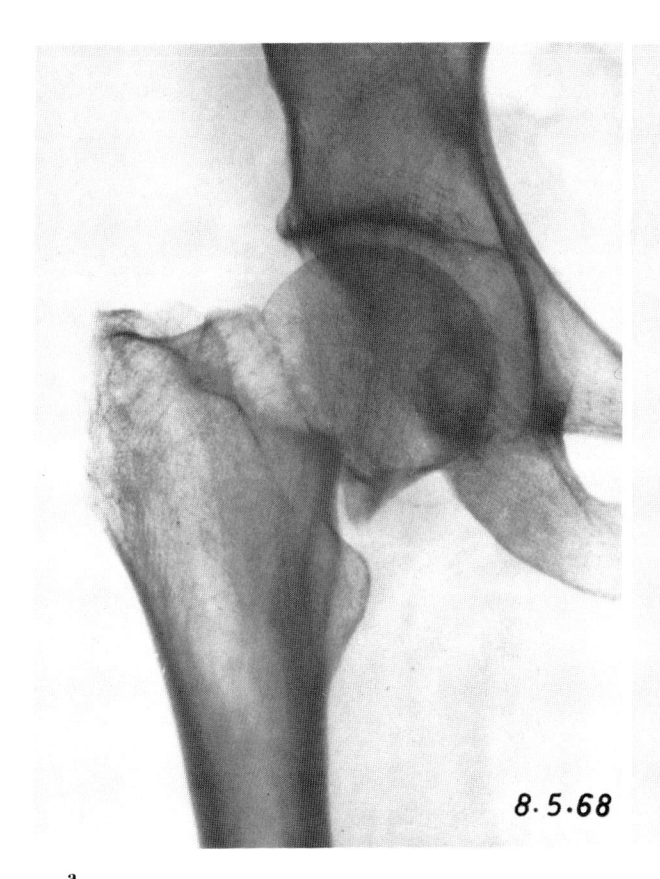

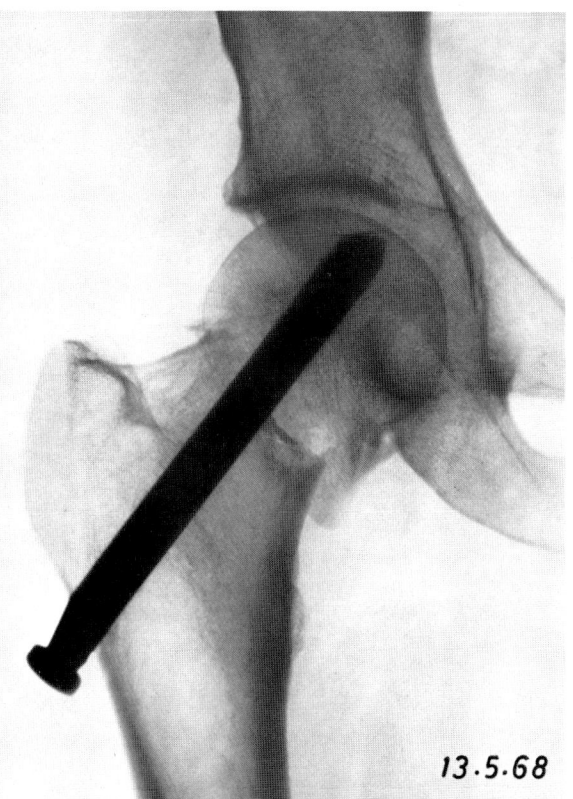

Fig. 229. a, b Poorly nailed fracture of the femoral neck. **c** Subsequent displacement. **d** Development of chondrolysis. **e–g** Evolution after a hanging-hip procedure. Fig. 229c–g see pages 242–243

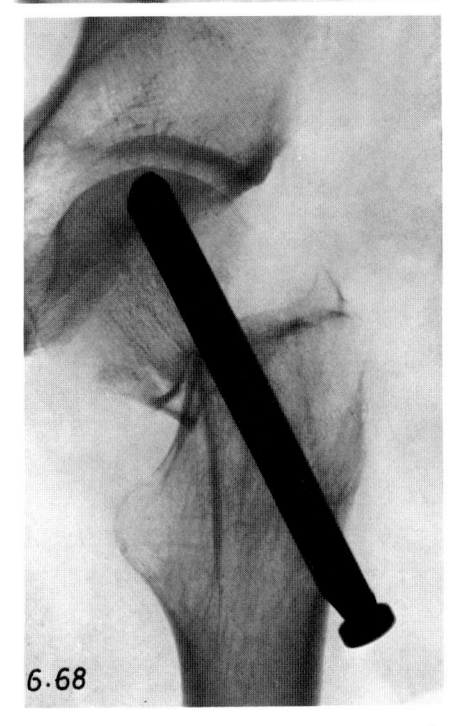

4.7.68

12.11.69

11.69

c

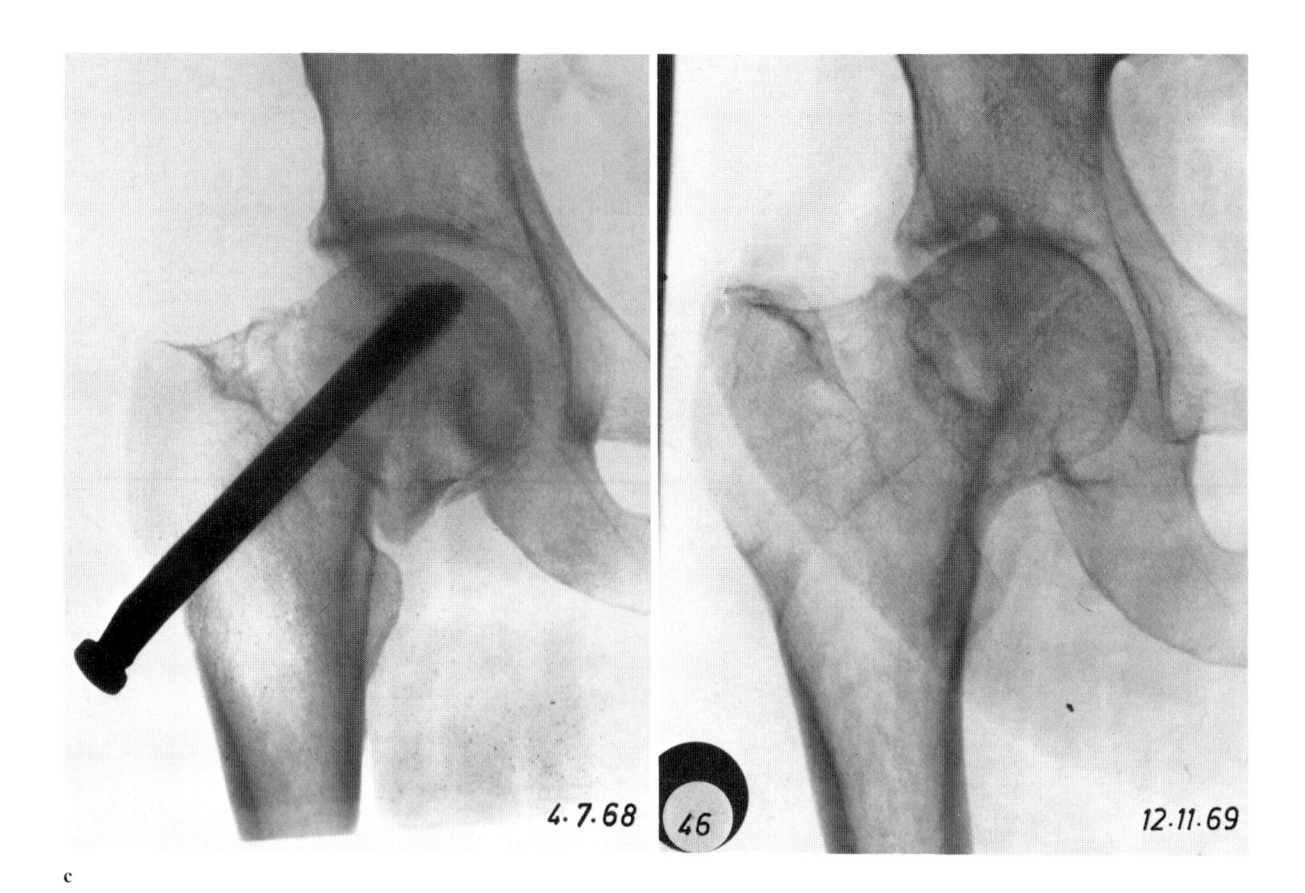

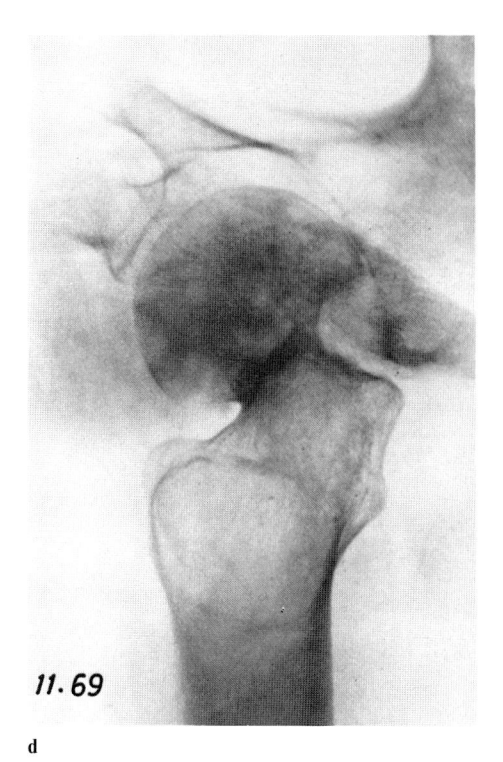

d

Fig. 229 c, d

242

3.8.71

15.5.73

e

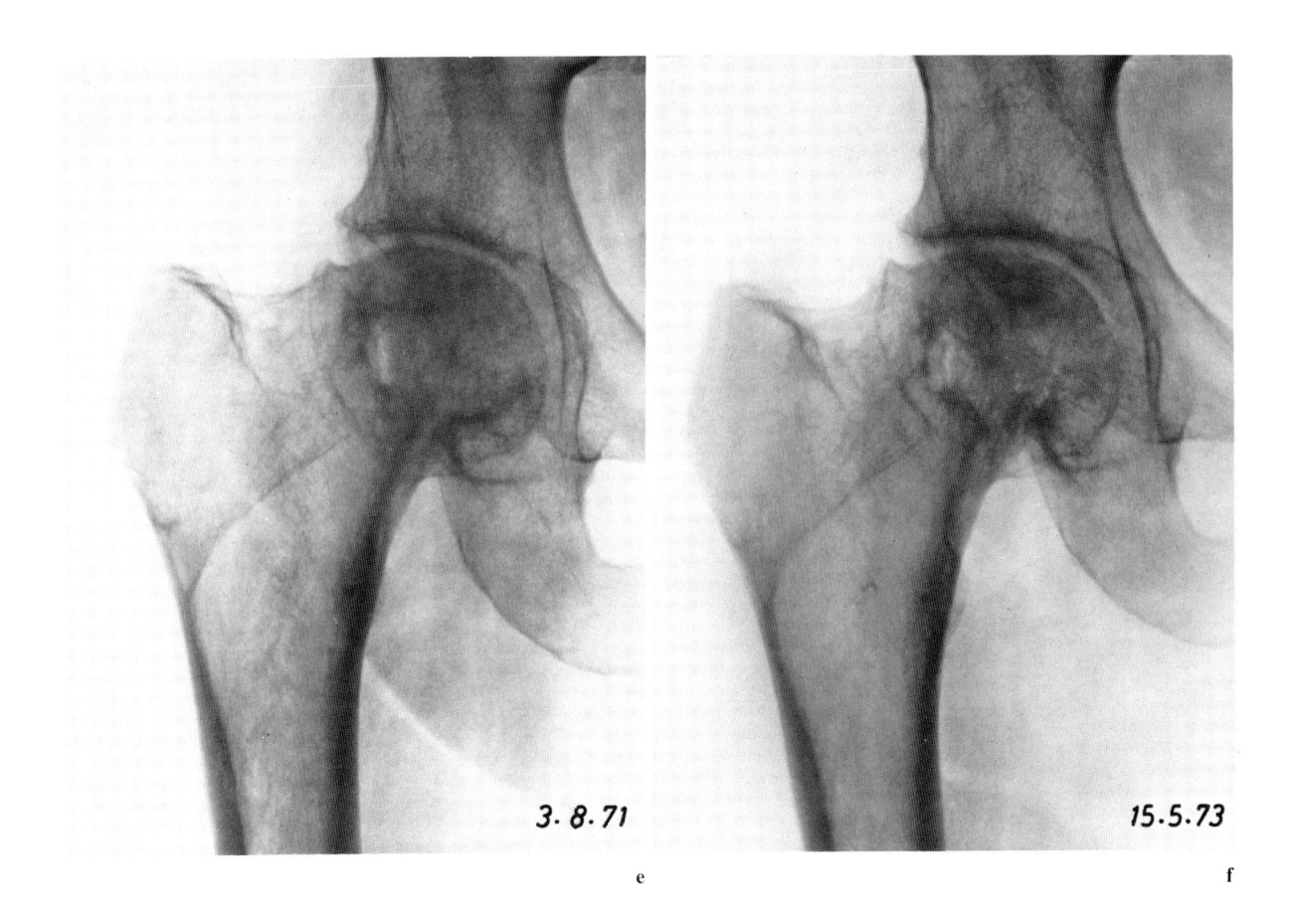

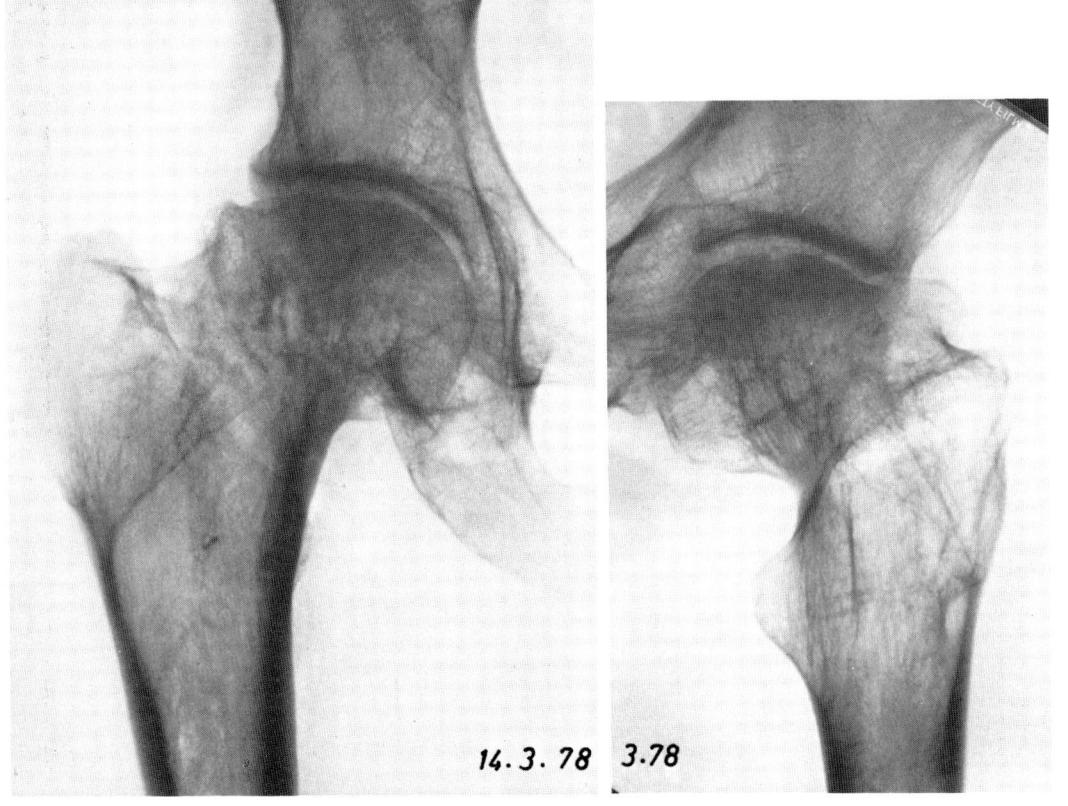

f

14.3.78

3.78

Fig. 229 e–g

g

243

C. Varus Intertrochanteric Osteotomy

When the joint surfaces are congruent, as long as the greater trochanter is not too high a varus osteotomy will probably be more effective than a hanging-hip operation in providing more of the femoral head with a covering mould in which the tissues can heal under low pressure.

D. Lateral Displacement of the Greater Trochanter

When the joint surfaces are congruent and the femoral neck is short with a relatively high greater trochanter, and if there is a sclerotic triangle at the edge of the acetabulum, a lateral displacement of the greater trochanter combined with a tenotomy of the adductor and iliopsoas muscles should be considered. Such a case has been described on page 42.

E. Valgus Intertrochanteric Osteotomy

When the weight-bearing surface of the joint is reduced as a consequence of flattening and lateral extrusion of the femoral head and of shallowing of the socket, only the X-rays in full adduction show a tendency to articular congruence. Then a well-planned valgus intertrochanteric osteotomy combined with a tenotomy of the abductor, adductor and iliopsoas muscles will be able to enlarge the weight-bearing surface of the joint and to decrease the load supported. The wedge to be resected may be very large, in some instances significantly larger than in the usual cases of osteoarthritis.

A 37-year-old patient had suffered a traumatic dislocation of his hip with fracture of the acetabulum in a car accident 2 years before we saw him. He developed severe osteonecrosis of the femoral head (Fig. 230a) with a painful hip, restricted range of movement (Table 38) and severe limping. Eight years after a 30° valgus intertrochanteric osteotomy, the result remained good. The range of movement had considerably improved (Table 38), and the patient was free from pain and was not limping. In the X-rays, the signs of necrosis had regressed and a wide joint space had developed (Fig. 230b).

The wedge to be resected may be very large indeed. A 22-year-old male patient developed necrosis of the femoral head after a traumatic dislocation of the hip. We saw him 5 years after the initial accident, when he was 17. The articular surfaces were incongruent, with narrowing of the joint space and a dense triangle at the edge of the socket (Fig. 231a). A 55° wedge was resected (Fig. 232). Despite this valgus osteotomy, the joint surfaces remained incongruent (Fig. 231b). About a year later, an additional 20° wedge was removed (Fig. 233). This ensured better congruence of the articular surfaces (Fig. 231c). Nine years later, the clinical result remained excellent: no pain, nearly full range of movement, no limp and unrestricted walking capacity. The patient was working full-time as a mechanic. In the X-rays, a thin ribbon of sclerosis of even width throughout demonstrated an ideal distribution of the articular compressive stresses over a large weight-bearing surface. A wide joint space had reappeared (Fig. 231d).

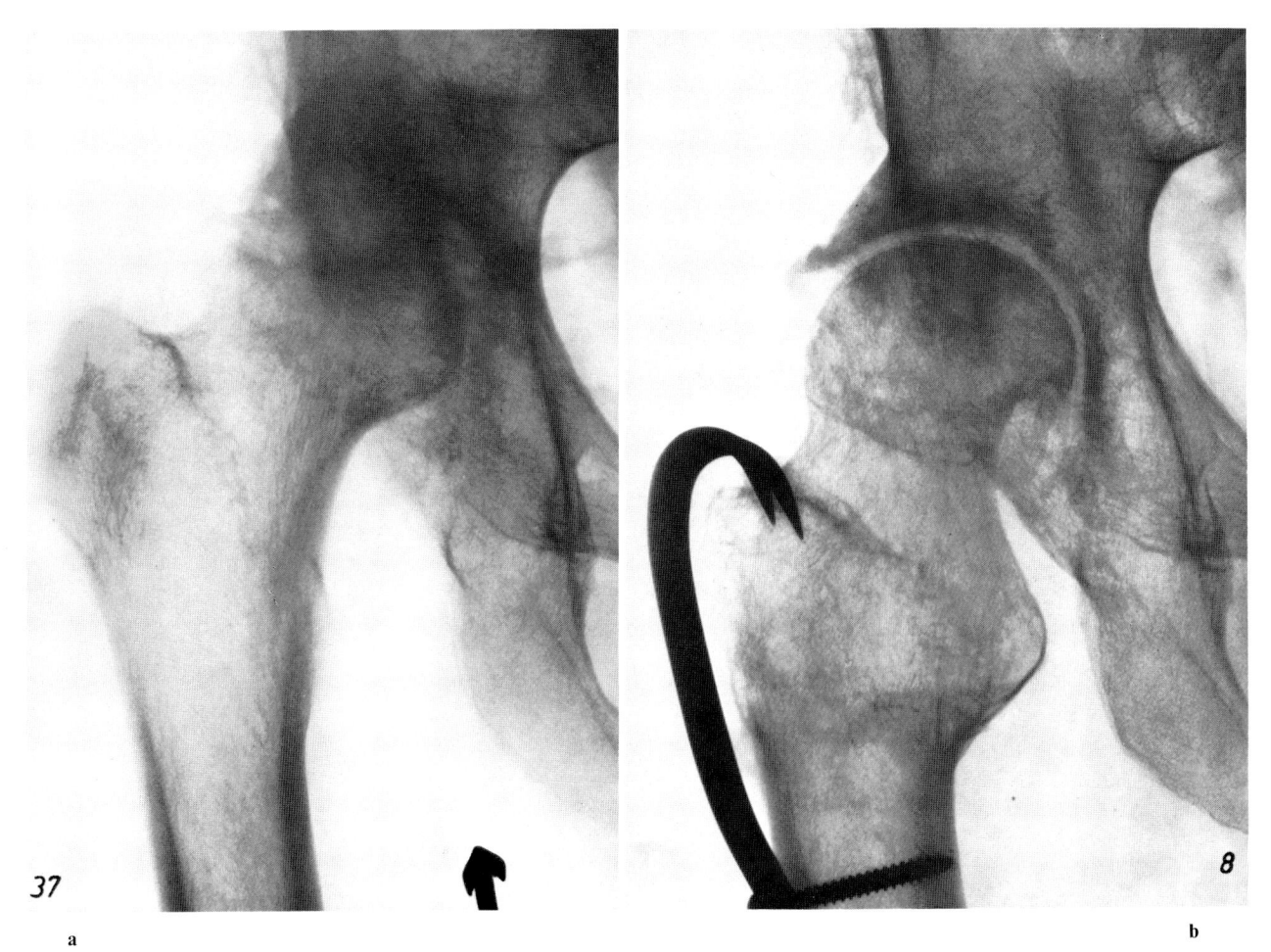

Fig. 230. a Post-traumatic ischaemic necrosis of the femoral head in a 37-year-old male patient. **b** Eight years after a valgus intertrochanteric osteotomy combined with a tenotomy

Table 38. Range of movement of the hip (Fig. 230)

	Before surgery	At the 8-year follow-up	Gain
Flexion	45°	85°	45°
Extension	0°	5°	
Adduction	20°	30°	50°
Abduction	0°	40°	
Int. rotation	0°	5°	40°
Ext. rotation	15°	50°	

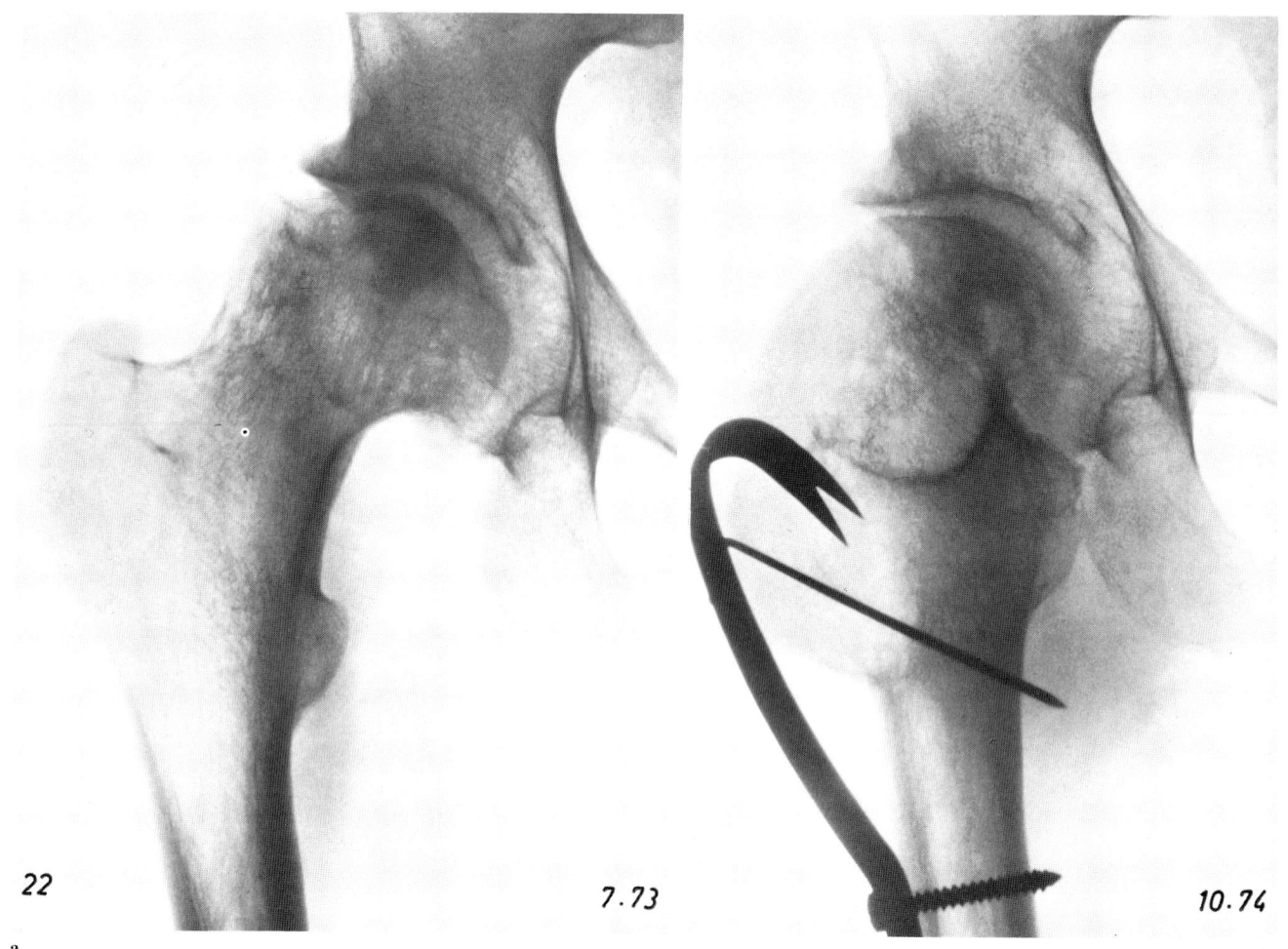

Fig. 231. a Post-traumatic necrosis of the femoral head in a 22-year-old male patient 5 years after a dislocation. **b** One year after a first valgus osteotomy. **c** A second valgus osteotomy was then carried out. **d** Nine years later

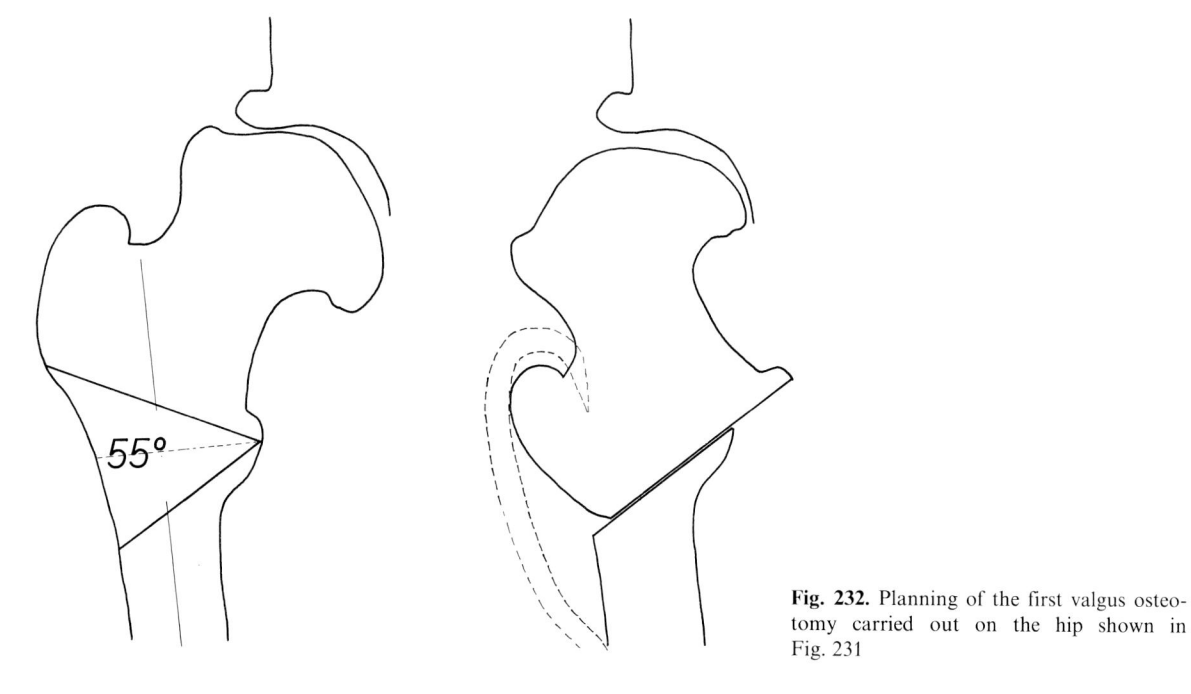

Fig. 232. Planning of the first valgus osteotomy carried out on the hip shown in Fig. 231

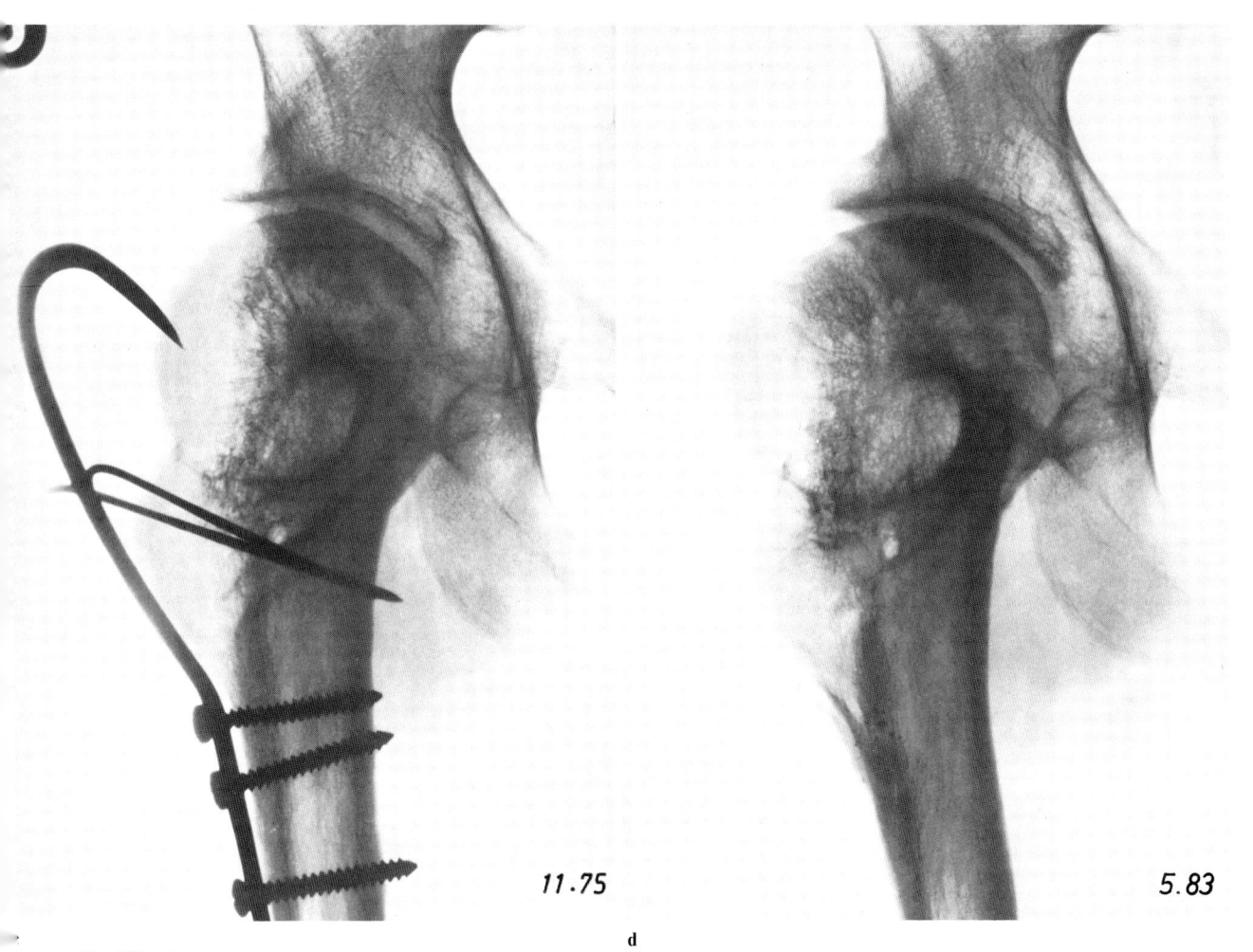

Fig. 231 c, d

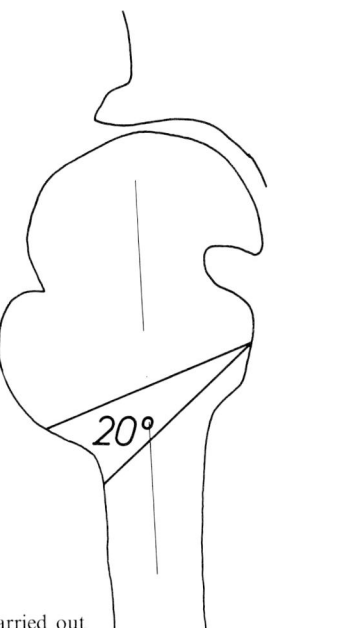

11.75

5.83

Fig. 233. Planning of the second valgus osteotomy carried out on the hip shown in Fig. 231

The same good results may be obtained in idiopathic necrosis of the femoral head. This is illustrated by the hip of a 55-year-old male patient (Fig. 234a). Six years after a valgus intertrochanteric osteotomy, the signs of necrosis had regressed and a wide joint space had developed (Fig. 234b).

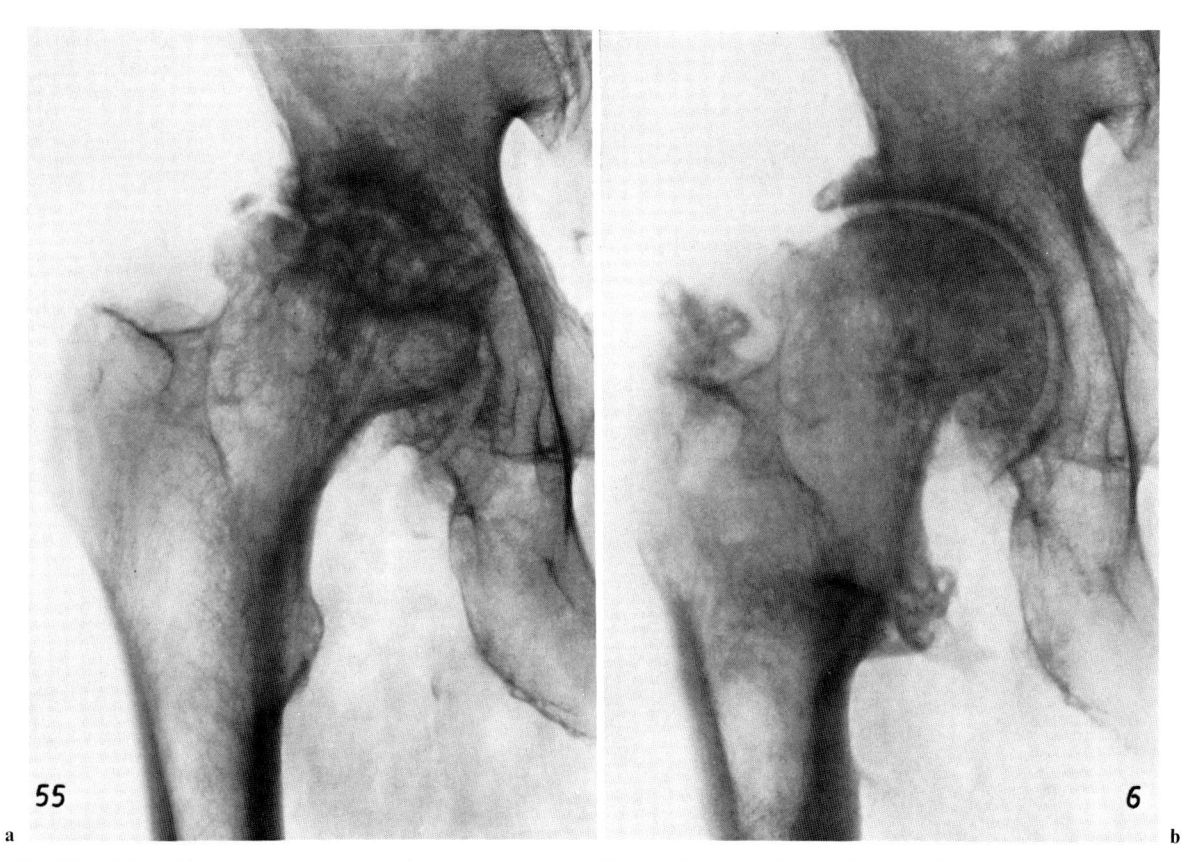

Fig. 234. a Idiopathic avascular necrosis of the femoral head in a 55-year-old male patient. **b** Six years after a Pauwels II

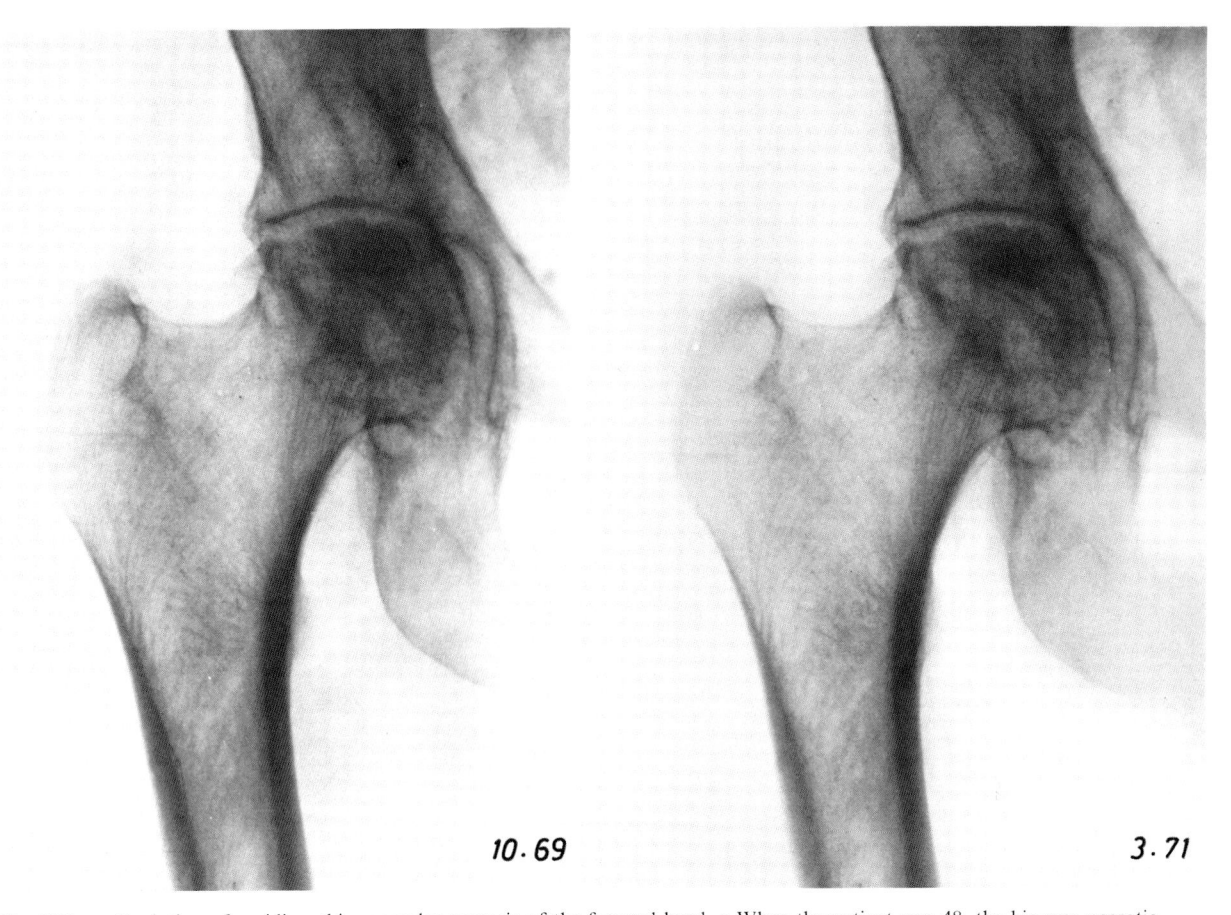

Fig. 235a–e. Evolution of an idiopathic avascular necrosis of the femoral head. **a** When the patient was 48, the hip was necrotic but remained spherical. **b** One and a half years later the head had begun to collapse. **c** By the time the patient was 52, further collapse had occurred and the joint space was narrowed. A Pauwels II operation was performed. **d** Four years later

It is interesting to follow the evolution of non-traumatic avascular necrosis in a patient who was operated on at the age of 52. When he was 48, the hip was necrotic but remained spherical (Fig. 235a). One and a half years later, the head had begun to collapse (Fig. 235b). By the time the patient was 52, further collapse had occurred and the joint space was narrowed (Fig. 235c). Four years after a valgus intertrochanteric osteotomy, the signs of necrosis were regressing and a wide joint space had reappeared (Fig. 235d). The clinical result was excellent. It was also excellent in the other hip, which had been operated on when the patient was 50 and had been followed-up for 6 years (Fig. 236).

6.72 52   10.73

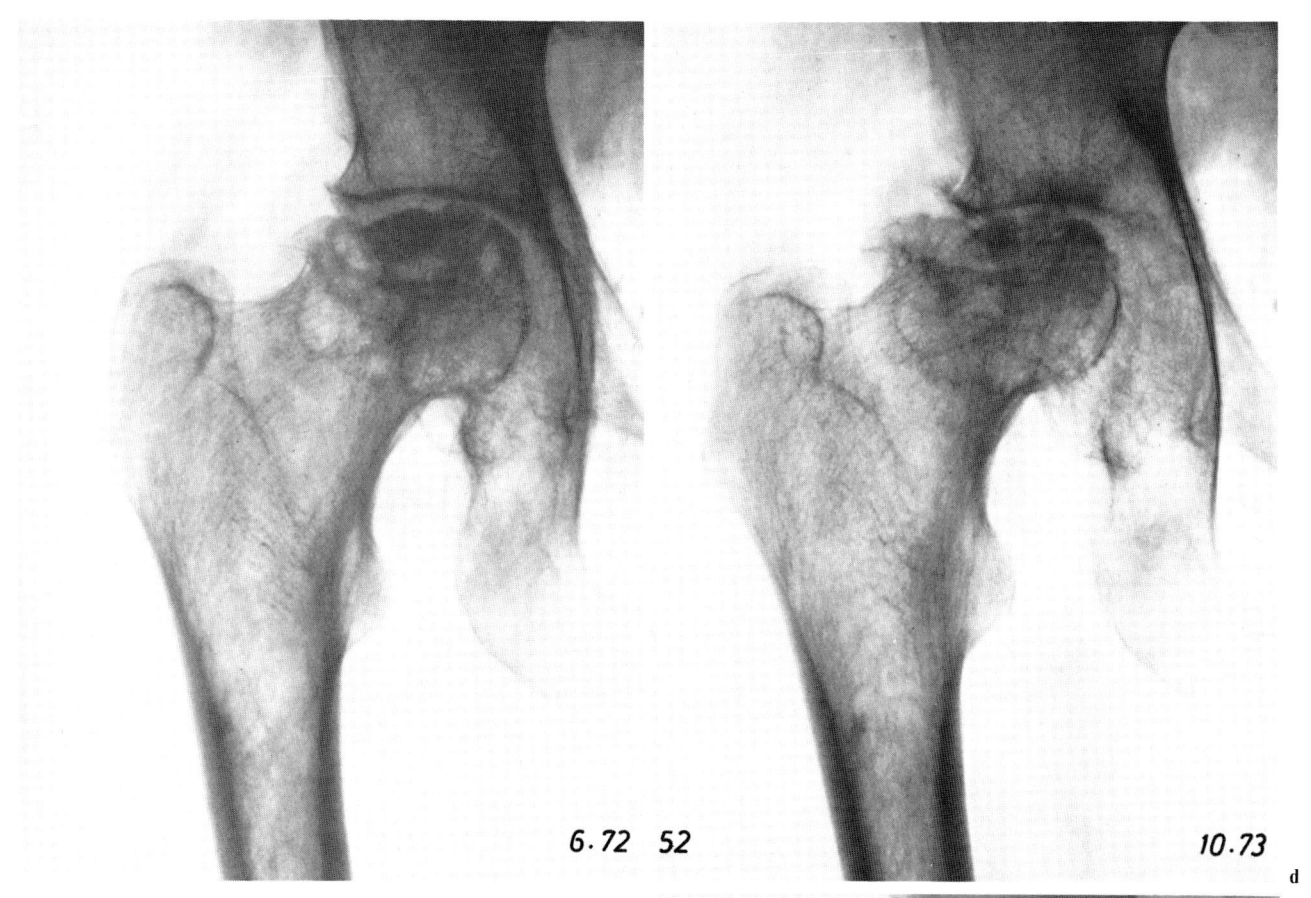

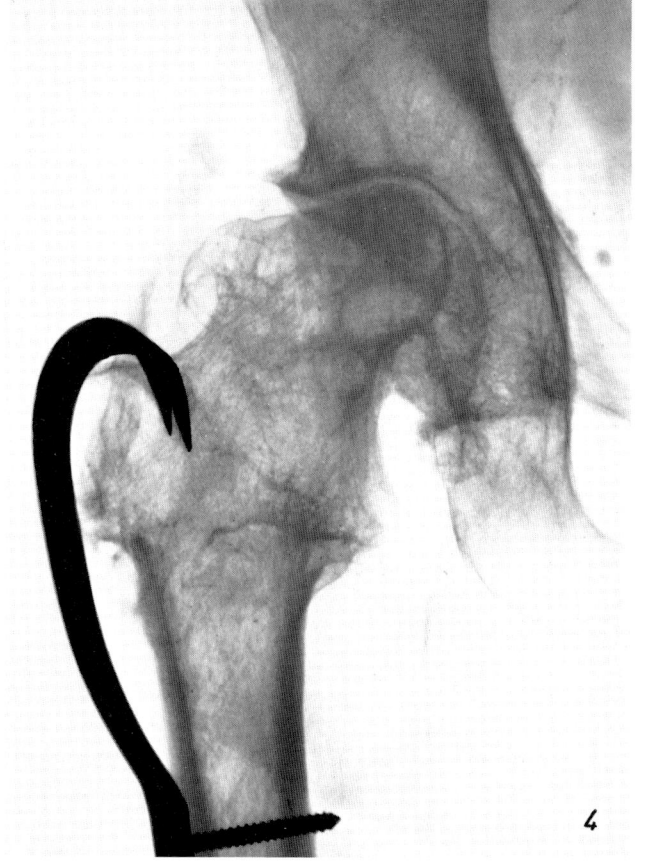

Fig. 235c–e.

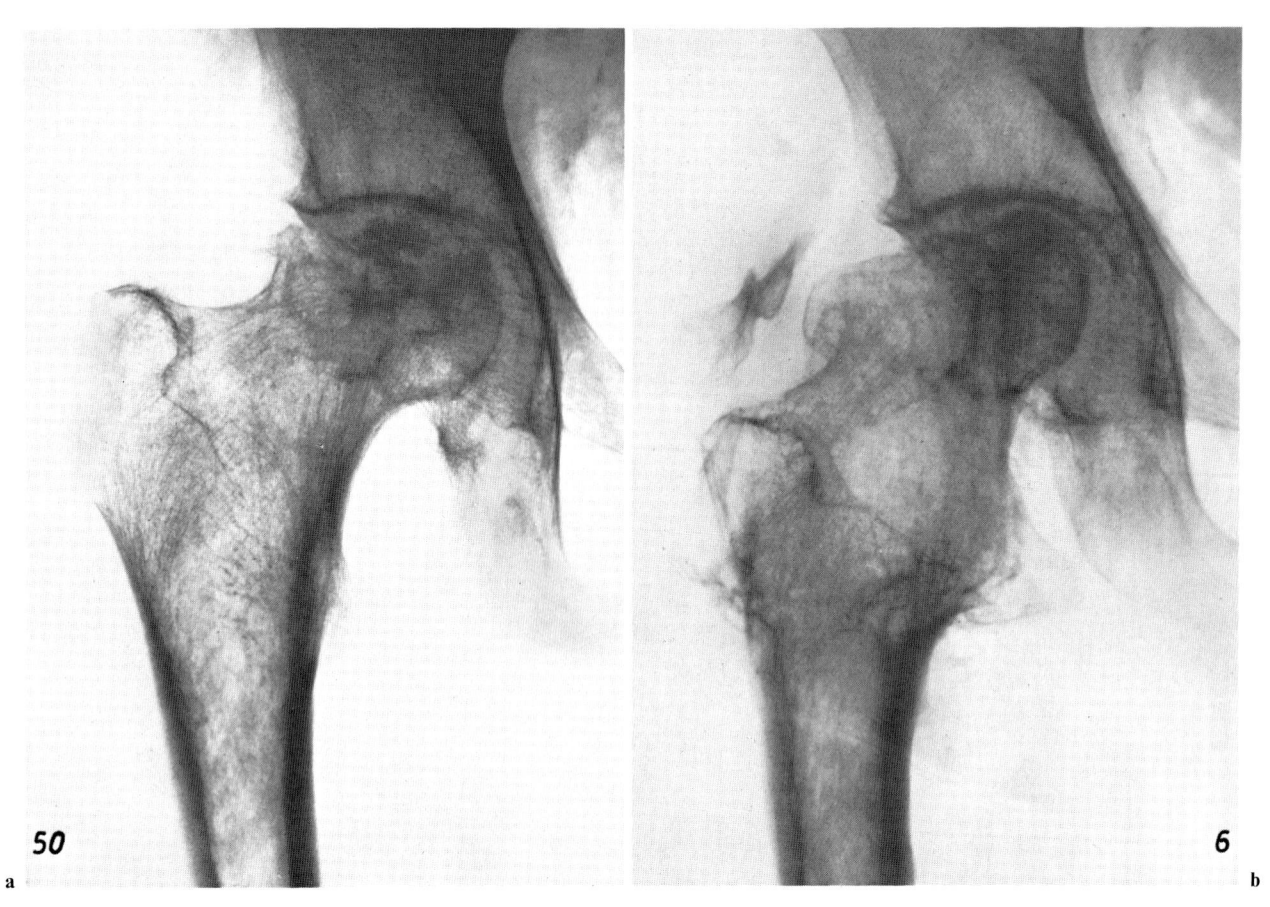

Fig. 236a, b. Same patient as in Fig. 235: opposite hip. **a** valgus intertrochanteric osteotomy and tenotomy at the age of 50; **b** 6-year follow-up

F. Conclusion

The same principles of treatment can be applied successfully in avascular necrosis of the femoral head as in osteoarthritis of the hip.

In children with a "hip at risk" in LEGG-CALVÉ-PERTHES' disease, the acetabulum will provide the weakened femoral head with as much congruent coverage as possible after a varus osteotomy. Simultaneously, the operation considerably reduces the articular pressure. This seems to enable the tissues to become revascularized without collapsing, in the spherical mould provided by the socket.

In avascular necrosis of the adult femoral head, a varus osteotomy can also result in a better coverage of the femoral head and, above all, in a significant reduction of the articular pressure. This occurs only if the articular surfaces remain congruent. However, in such cases a hanging-hip operation alone may be sufficient. Lateral displacement of the greater trochanter combined with tenotomy decreases the articular pressure by enlarging the weight-bearing surface of the joint and by reducing the load transmitted. Valgus intertrochanteric osteotomy combined with tenotomy pursues the same goal. It is recommended when the flattened articular surfaces tend to become congruent in full adduction.

Chapter VI. Dysplastic Hips

I. Introduction

Systematic examination at birth and treatment of newborn hips susceptible to subluxation, by abduction on an adequate pillow or splint, have considerably reduced the incidence of dislocated hips in children.

A child whose mother suffered from congenital hip dysplasia, was born with a bilateral dislocation (Fig. 237a). She was kept on an abduction splint for 12 months from the day of birth. The hips became relocated (Fig. 237b) and subsequently developed normally, as the X-ray taken 14 years later shows (Fig. 237c).

Orthopaedic surgeons, however, still encounter old dysplastic hips and even congenital hip dislocations. We shall consider congenital dislocation or subluxation of the hip in young children, in adolescents and in adults, and also untreated high congenital dislocation in adults. Treatment of the condition is based on a thorough knowledge of the mechanics of the hip as described in the preceding chapters and of the reaction of the tissues to mechanical stress.

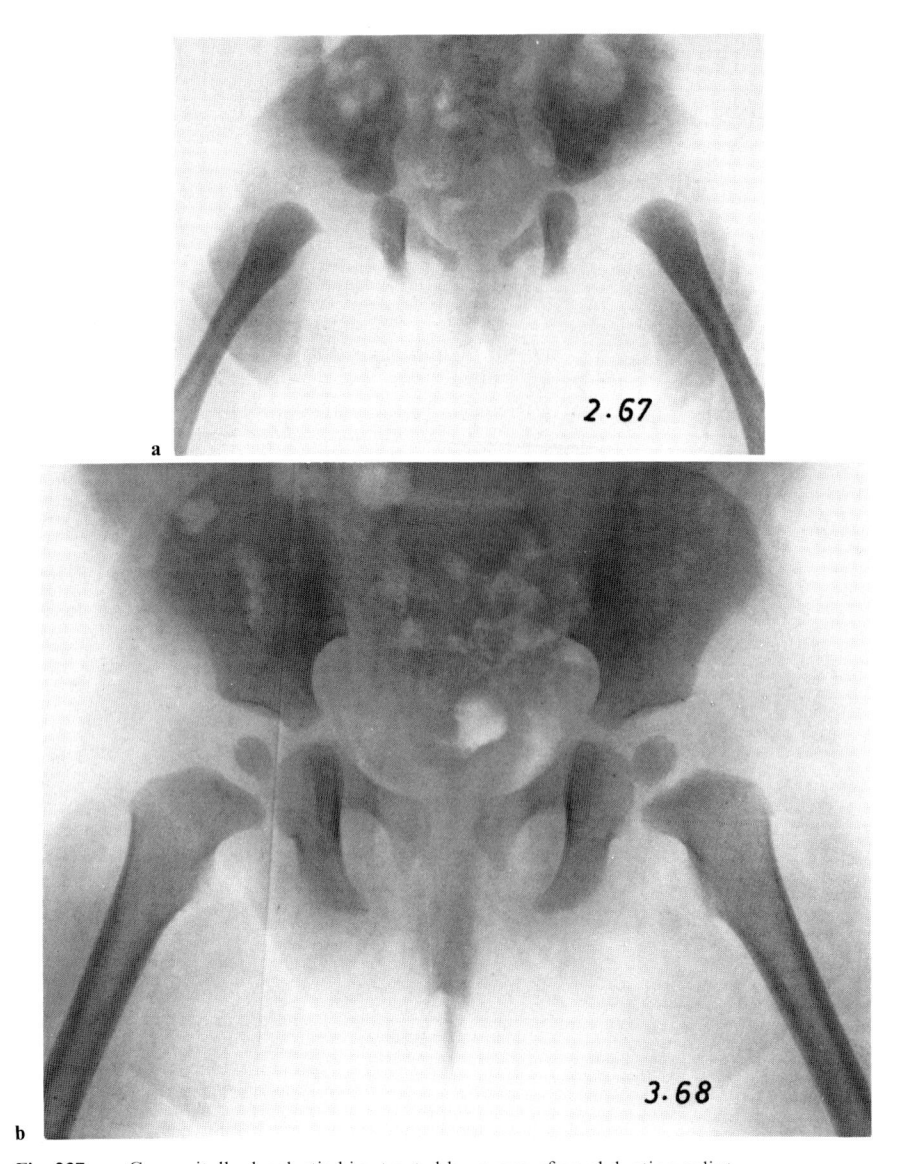

Fig. 237 a–c. Congenitally dysplastic hips treated by means of an abduction splint

254

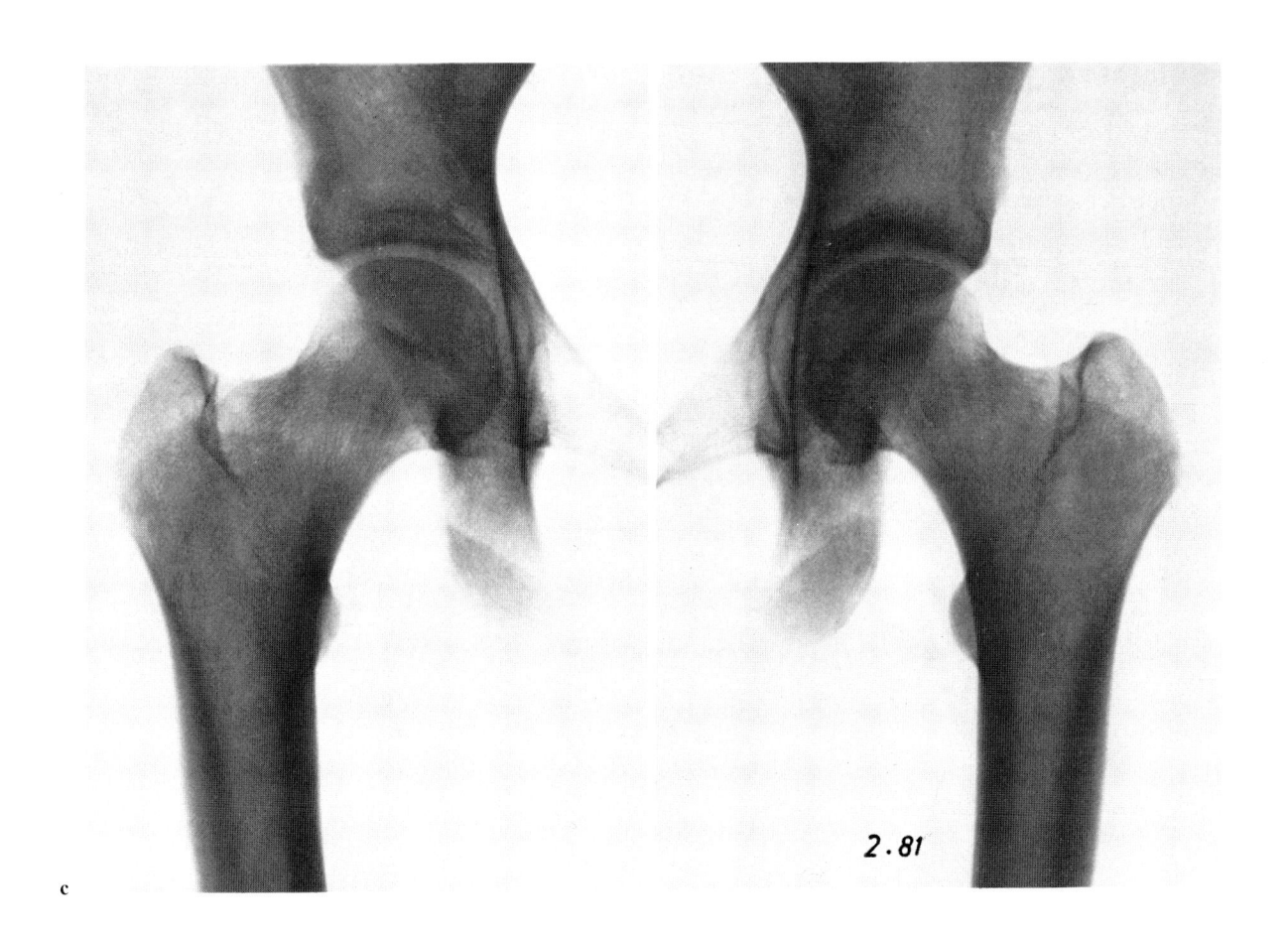

c

2.81

II. In Infants

In infancy, thanks to the plasticity of the tissues, an appropriate modification of the stresses in the hip can lead to considerable adaptation.

A. Innominate Osteotomy

A SALTER pelvic osteotomy ensures coverage of the femoral head and increases the weight-bearing area of the joint by tilting the acetabular contact surface laterally. The balance of forces is not or is only slightly modified, but the weight-bearing surface is increased. If subjected to tolerable stresses, the hip joint can develop further as long as the femoral epiphysis is not altered.

In a 7-year-old female patient with congenital dislocation of the hip (Fig. 238a), an open reduction of the femoral head was carried out and a SALTER osteotomy of the pelvis was performed. Six months later, remodelling was taking place (Fig. 238b). One and a half years after the procedure, the hip looked normal, with a subchondral sclerosis of uniform thickness throughout. The orientation of the epiphysial plate and the structure of the femoral neck demonstrated that the hip was stressed normally (Fig. 238c).

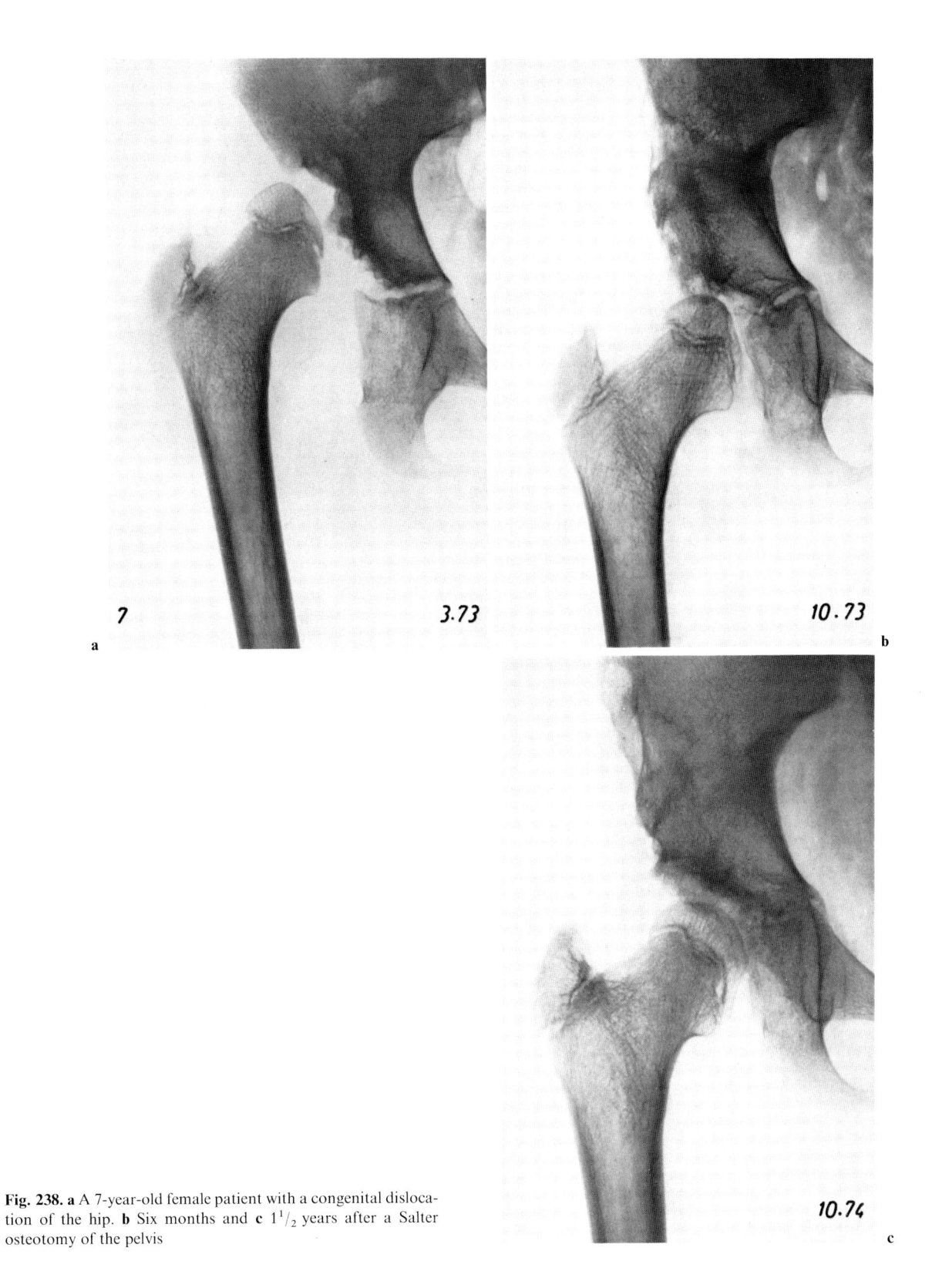

Fig. 238. a A 7-year-old female patient with a congenital dislocation of the hip. **b** Six months and **c** $1^1/_2$ years after a Salter osteotomy of the pelvis

B. Lowering the Lateral Aspect of the Acetabulum

Lowering the lateral aspect of the acetabulum as described by BERTRAND (1965) can have the same effect. The operation consists of an open reduction with resection of the limbus. Three thin osteotomes are introduced obliquely and concentrically above the socket and the handles are lowered together. Grafts are inserted into the gap thus created in order to maintain the lowered position of the articular margin (Fig. 239). This procedure may entail a risk of damaging the articular cartilage of the socket. Usually, however, it results in an acceptable hip which then develops normally, as illustrated in the X-rays (Fig. 240). A 3-year-old patient with a subluxated hip (Fig. 240a) underwent a lowering of the roof of the acetabulum with good results (Fig. 240b, c). When the patient was 14, the hip looked normal (Fig. 240d).

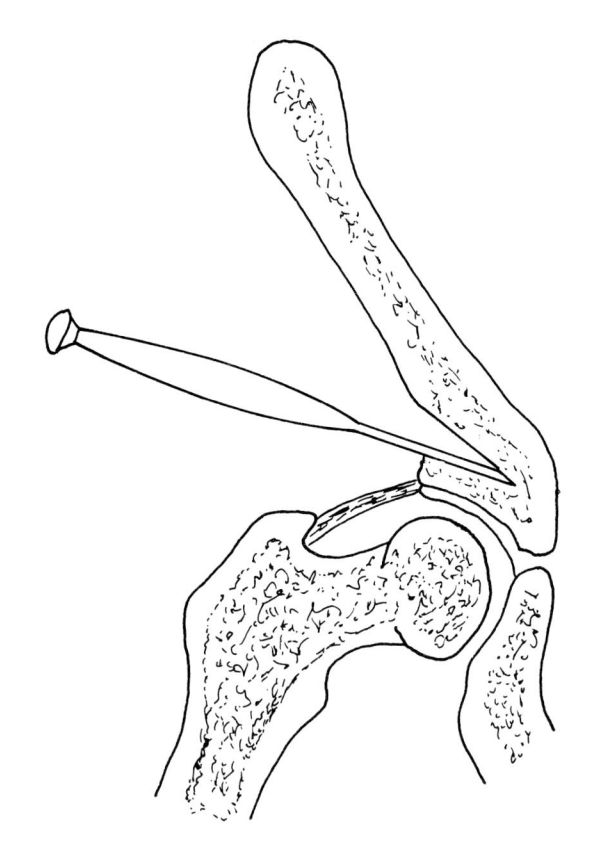

Fig. 239. Lowering the lateral aspect of the acetabulum. (After BERTRAND 1962)

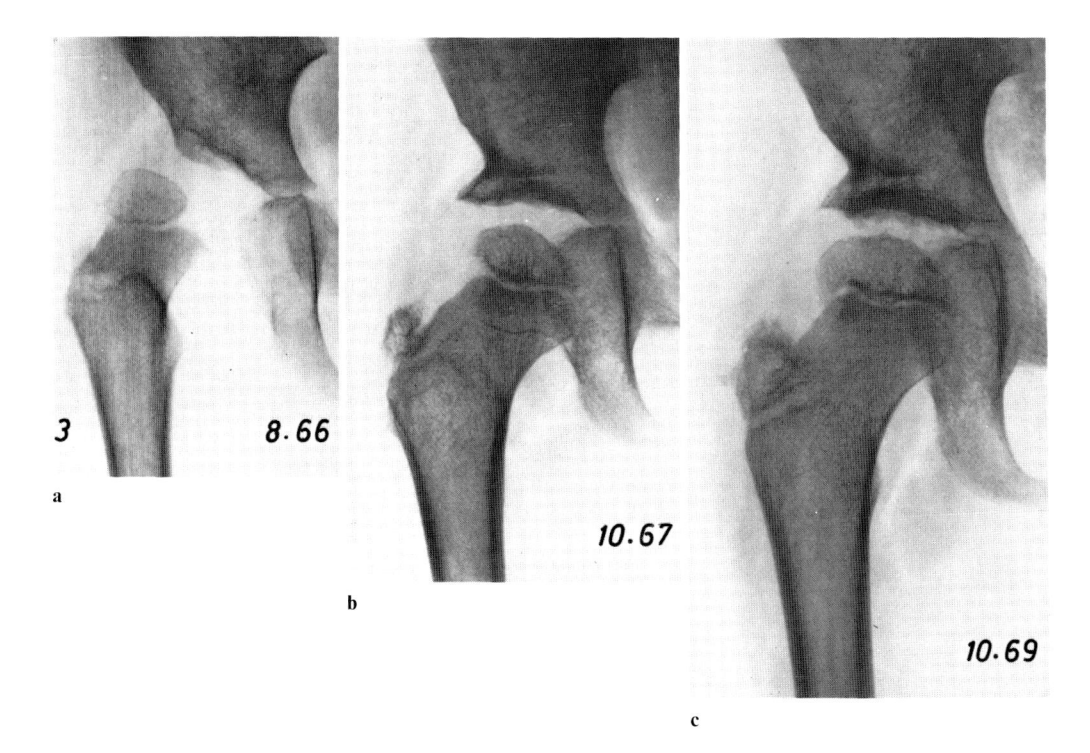

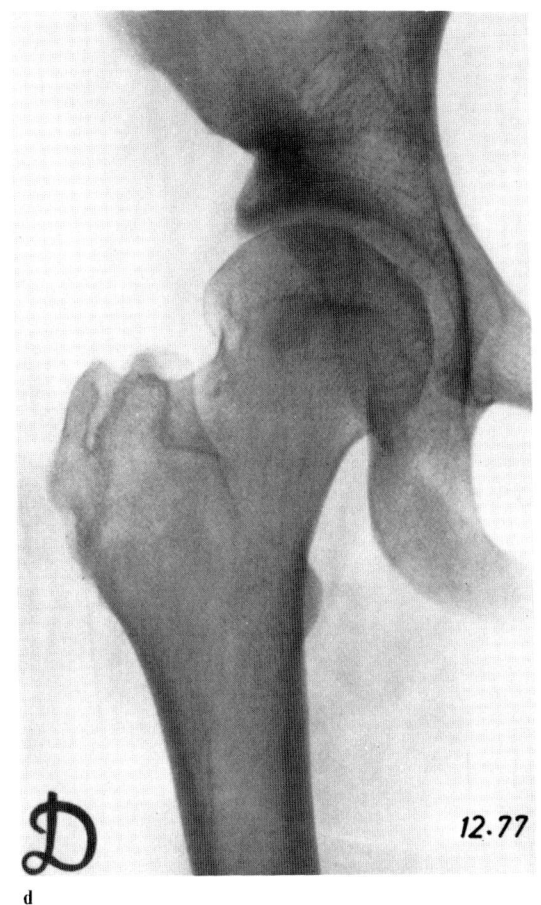

Fig. 240. a Subluxation of the hip in a 3-year-old female patient. **b, c** Evolution after a lowering of the lateral aspect of the socket. **d** 11-year follow-up

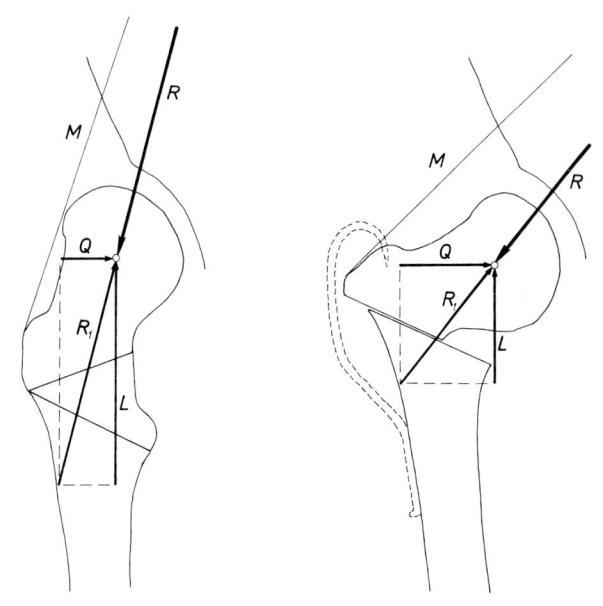

Fig. 241. Alteration in the balance of forces and increase in the transverse component Q resulting from correction of coxa valga by means of a varus osteotomy. L, longitudinal component; M, force exerted by the abductor muscles; R, resultant force; R_1, counter-force of R

C. Varus Intertrochanteric Osteotomy

When there is coxa valga subluxans, a varus osteotomy lengthens the lever arm of the abductor muscles and modifies their direction (Fig. 241). Changing the direction of M, the force exerted by the abductor muscles, lowers the intersection of the forces M and K. Consequently, the line of action of the resultant force R is displaced medially into the socket. This results in an increase in the weight-bearing surface of the joint. The procedure also considerably decreases the longitudinal component L of the resultant force R and increases its transverse component Q. This reduces the tendency to subluxation. Acting on the plastic articular tissues of an infant, the transverse force Q can deepen the acetabulum, as demonstrated by the evolution in a female patient operated on at the age of 5 (Fig. 242a) and reviewed 17 years later (Fig. 242b).

D. Combining Different Surgical Procedures

A varus intertrochanteric osteotomy may be carried out to complement the mechanical effect of an innominate osteotomy or of an open reduction with lowering of the rim of the acetabulum.

In a 3-year-old female patient with congenital bilateral dislocation (Fig. 243a), an innominate pelvic osteotomy was carried out on both sides. One year later the sockets seemed to be significantly deepened (Fig. 243b). On the left side, the upper epiphysis of the femur looked normal. On the right

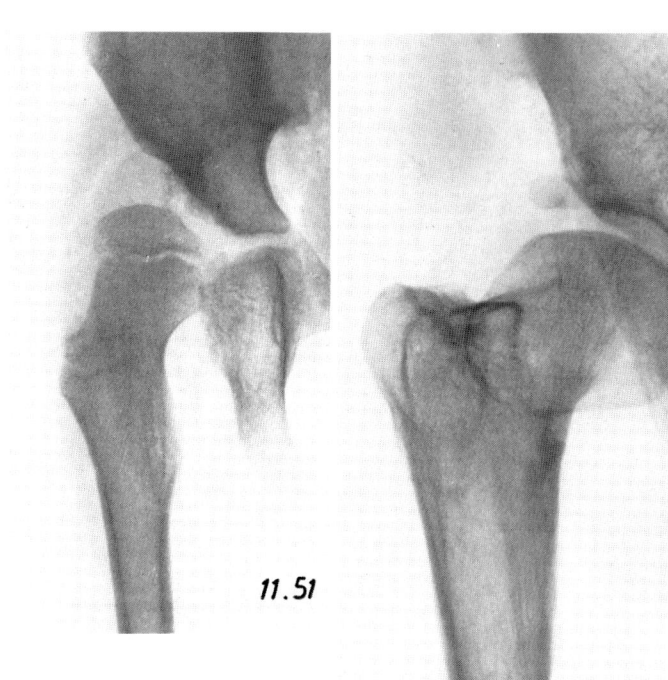

Fig. 242. a A 5-year-old female patient with a subluxated hip. **b** Seventeen years after a varus intertrochanteric osteotomy

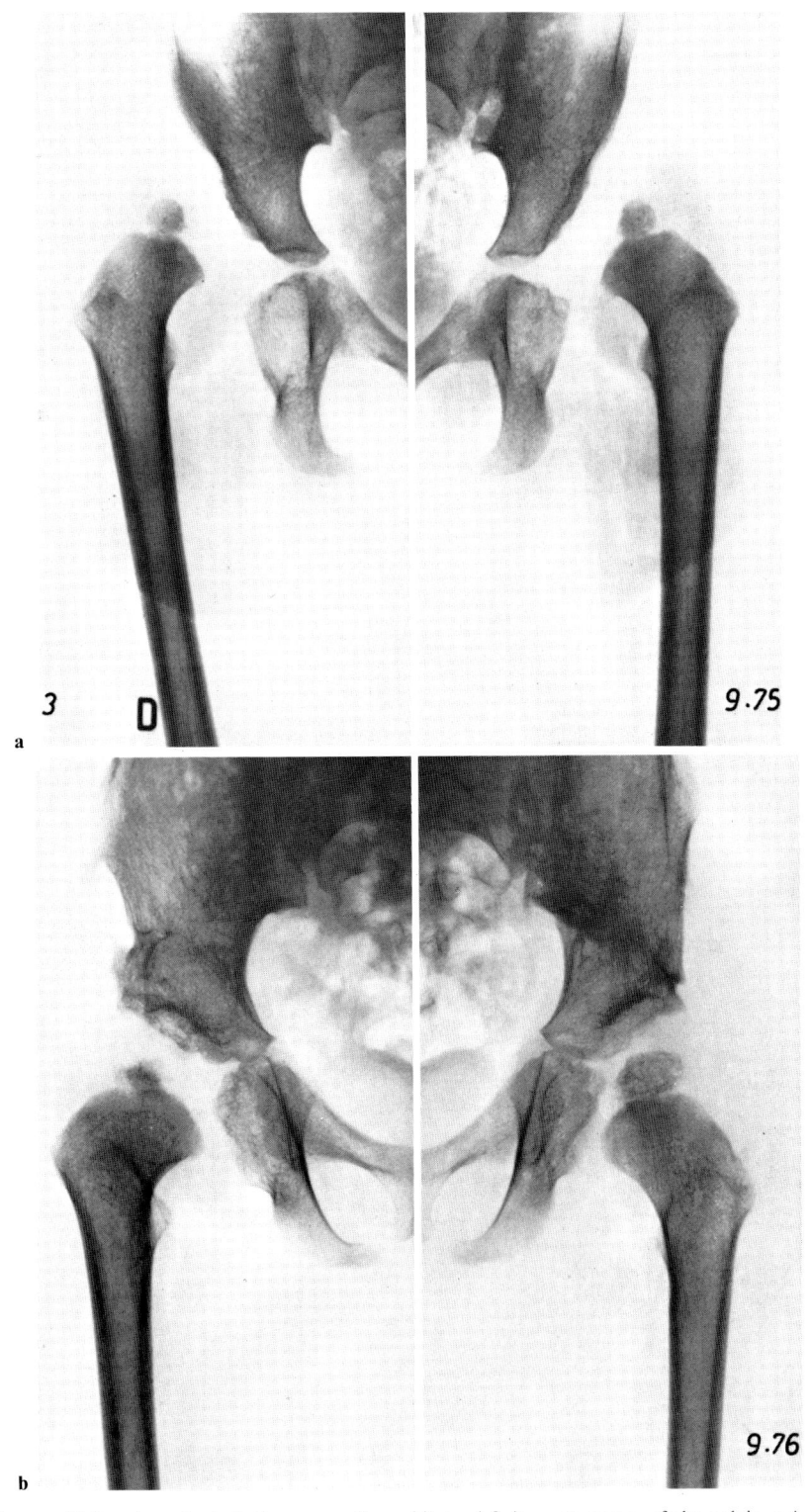

Fig. 243. a Bilateral dislocation in a 3-year-old female patient. **b** One year after a bilateral Salter osteotomy of the pelvis. **c** A varus intertrochanteric osteotomy was carried out on the right side. **d** Four-year and **e** 5-year follow-up. Fig. 243c–e see pages 262–263

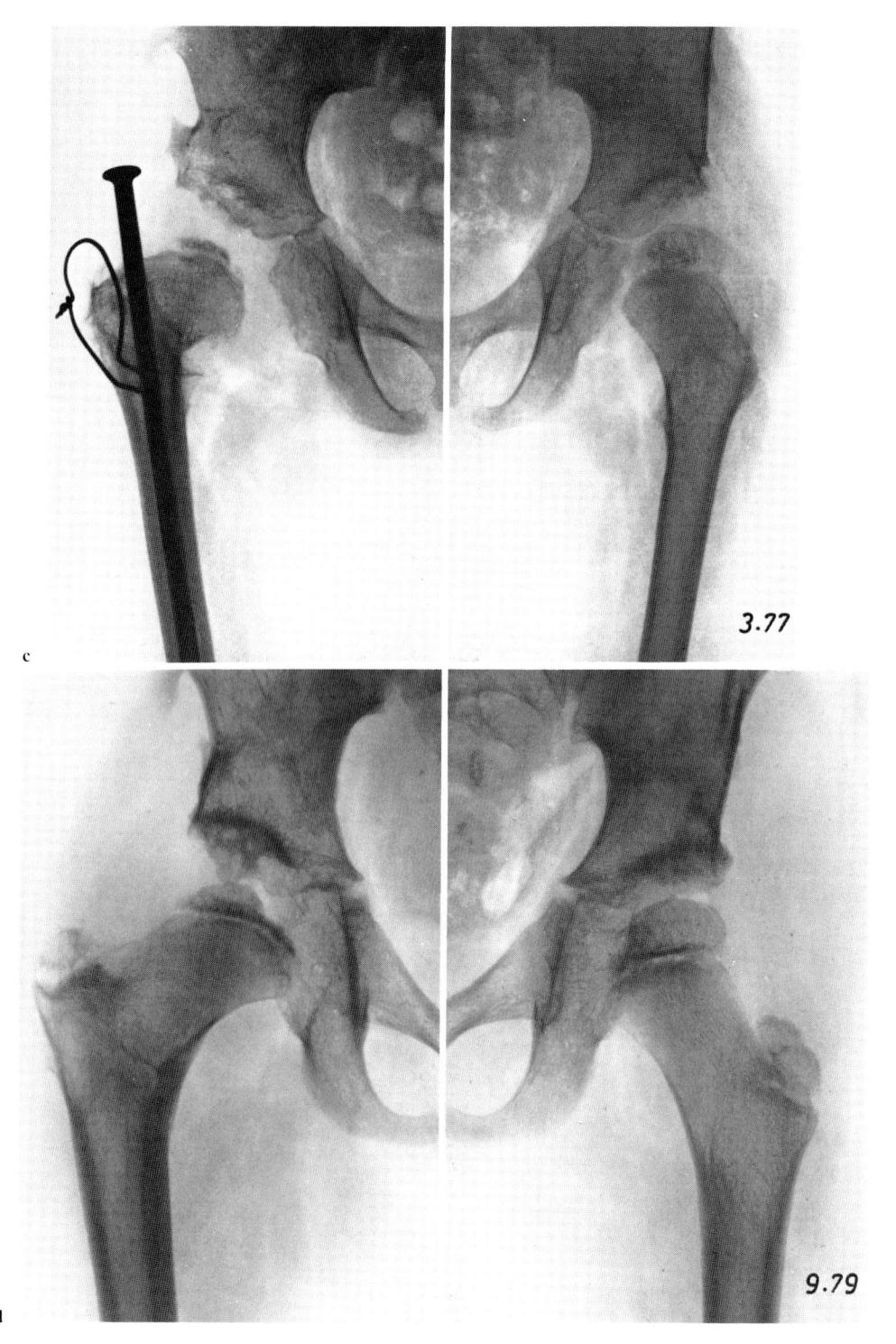

Fig. 243c, d

3.77

9.79

side, it was apparently small, fragmented and located at the edge of the socket. A varus intertrochanteric osteotomy was carried out on the right side, recentring the femoral head more deeply in the socket (Fig. 243c). It is interesting to observe the cancellous architecture in the femoral necks at the 4-year (Fig. 243d) and 5-year follow-ups (Fig. 243e). On the left side, all the trabeculae appeared nearly parallel to the axis of the neck. This is the typical structure in pure compressive stressing, the line of action of the resultant force R lying inside the core of the left femoral neck. On the right side, a bundle of trabeculae leaves the medial cortex of the shaft and spreads towards the upper part of the head. It intersects a bundle of trabeculae originating in the lateral cortex of the shaft,

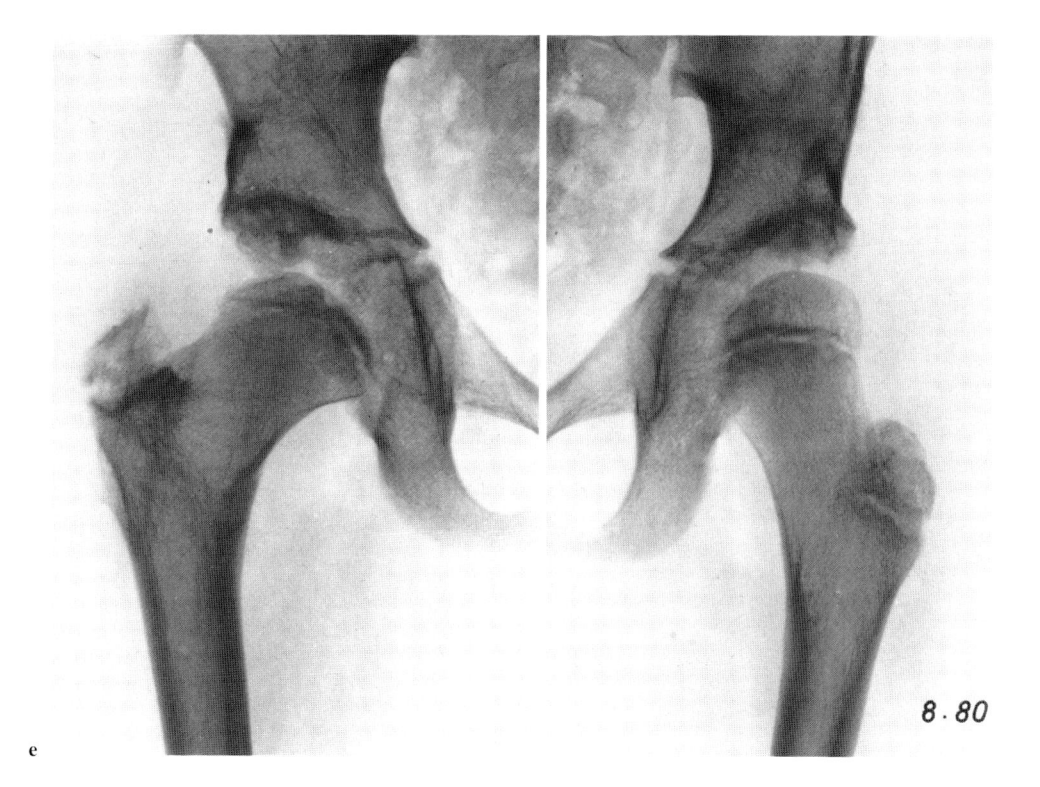

Fig. 243e

curving along the upper aspect of the neck and head. This is the typical structure in bending stress combined with shearing stress, that is to say, the line of action of the resultant R leaves the core of the right femoral neck, which is thus subjected to bending stress in addition to compression.

A 2-year-old female patient presented with a congenital unilateral hip dislocation (Fig. 244a). An open reduction was carried out and the lateral aspect of the acetabulum was lowered. After 6 weeks in a plaster spica, the patient was able to walk and lead a normal life. The X-ray taken 1 year after surgery showed a femoral head well-seated in the acetabulum, the roof of which was wide and nearly horizontal (Fig. 244b). The surgical procedure had restored the anatomical shape to normal. This represents the goal of classical orthopaedics.

The patient was followed-up regularly. Six years after the open reduction, the femoral head remained in a deep socket (Fig. 244c). The anatomical shape was still satisfactory. However, a dense triangle could be seen at the edge of the acetabulum. The triangular subchondral sclerosis pointed

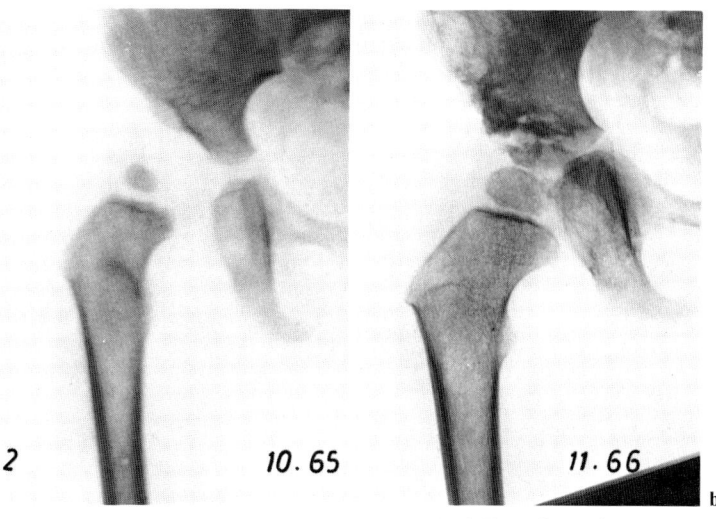

Fig. 244a, b. Legend see page 264

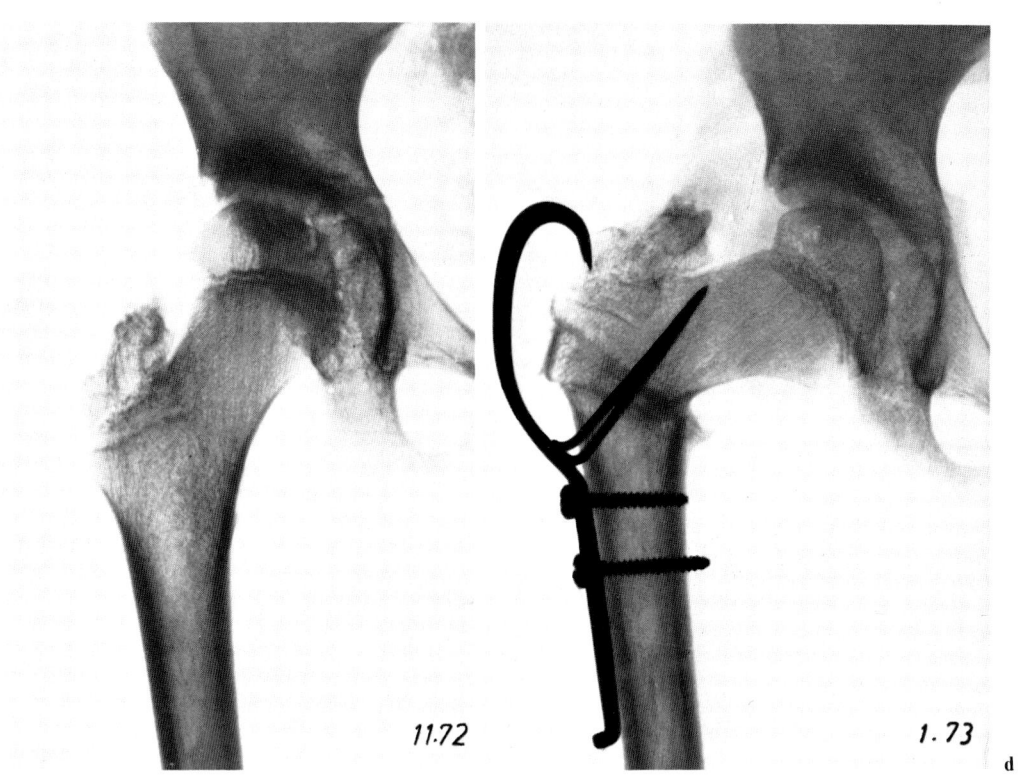

Fig. 244. a Congenital dislocation of the hip in a 2-year-old female patient. b One year after open reduction and lowering of the lateral aspect of the acetabulum. c At the age of 8 years the patient has a dense triangle in the roof of the acetabulum, a sign of abnormal stressing. The resultant force R acting on the hip is vertical. A *dotted line* inclined at 16° to the plumb-line indicates what the direction of force R should normally be. d After a varus intertrochanteric osteotomy. e One year after the varus osteotomy. f Two years after the varus osteotomy. g At the age of 16 years

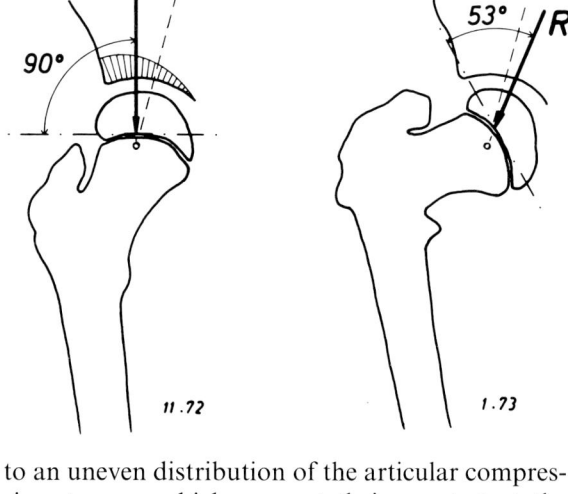

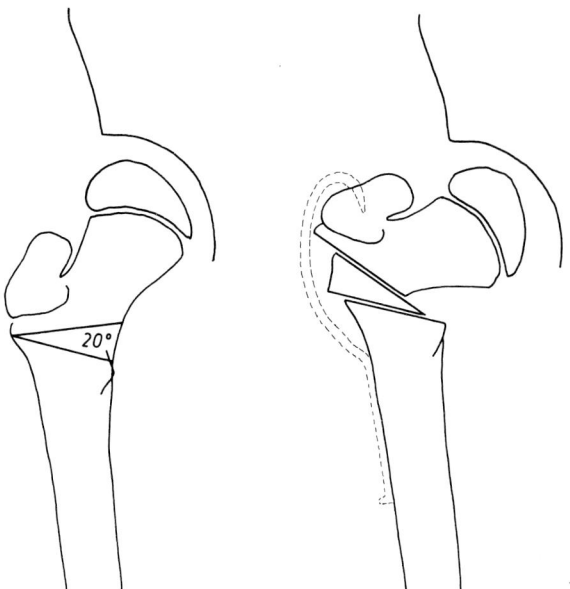

to an uneven distribution of the articular compressive stresses, which were at their greatest at the edge of the acetabulum and decreased towards its depths. Despite a normal anatomical shape, the mechanical stressing of the hip was pathological and would have inevitably led to osteoarthritis, as experience has shown. The triangular subchondral sclerosis constituted the first sign of osteoarthritis.

The line of action of the resultant force R acting on the hip passes through the centre of the femoral head and the point at the junction of the lateral

◄ Fig. 245. Planning the varus osteotomy carried out on the hip shown in Fig. 244

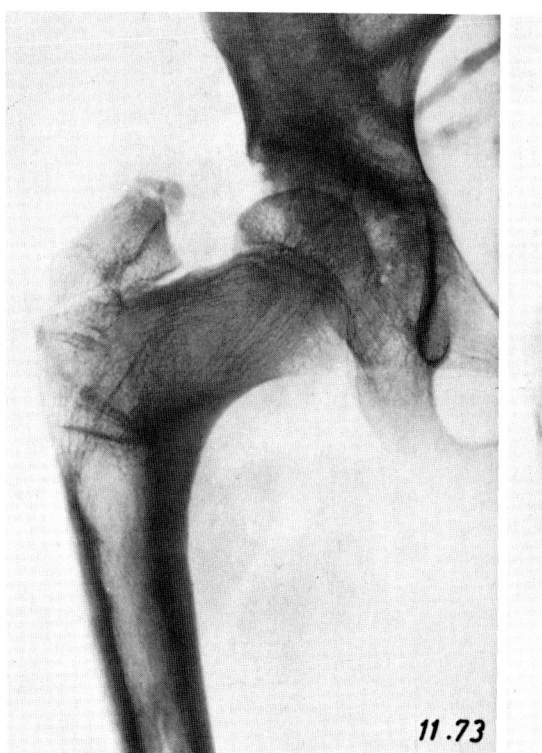

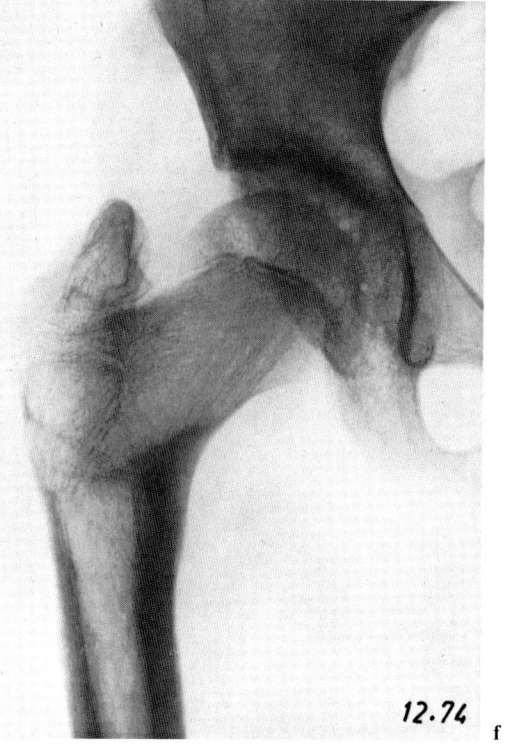

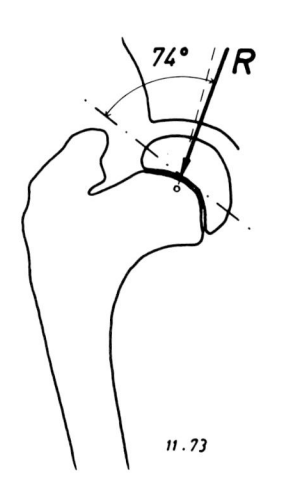

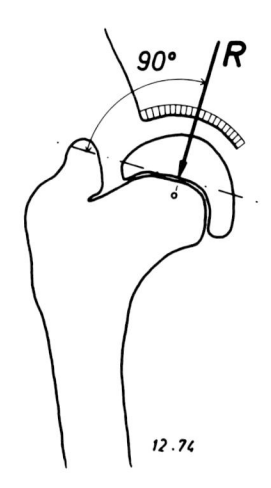

third and medial two-thirds of the triangular sub-chondral sclerosis (Pauwels 1976). The line of action of R can thus be determined. In the present case it was vertical. Its direction was confirmed by the orientation of the cancellous trabeculae in the femoral neck and that of the epiphysial plate. The cancellous trabeculae constituted one vertical bundle in the neck, which was thus subjected to pure compression. The resultant force acted within the core of the neck. The growth plate was horizontal. Physiologically, it is at right angles to the line of action of the resultant R (Pauwels 1973). R was thus vertical instead of being inclined at 16° to the perpendicular as normally (interrupted line).

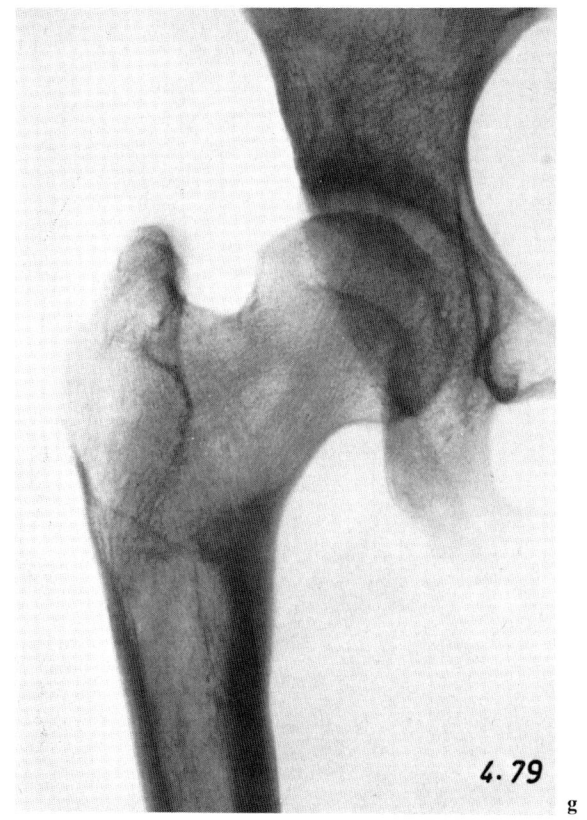

Fig. 244e–g

In order to complement the treatment, the mechanical stressing of the hip had to be altered and brought to normal. To this end, a 40° varus intertrochanteric osteotomy was planned and carried out. In order to avoid too much shortening, a 20° wedge with a medial base was removed, rotated and reinserted between the main fragments with its base lateral (Fig. 245). The varus osteotomy changed the direction of the abductor muscles and lengthened their lever arm. This resulted in a decrease in the magnitude of resultant R and in a medial displacement of its line of action into the socket (Fig. 244d). Thereafter, the angle formed by the line of action of force R with the perpendicular was greater than in a normal hip (interrupted line).

On the other hand, the varus intertrochanteric osteotomy tilted the growth plate (clockwise in our diagram). The growth plate now formed a 53° angle with the direction of force R. Consequently, the medial part of the growth plate was subjected to more compressive stress than its lateral part, which might even be subjected to slight tension. The cartilage reacted with increased growth where the compression was augmented (PAUWELS 1958). This uneven growth progressively reorientated the femoral neck, opening the neck-shaft angle. This reduced the inclination of the abductor muscles and, consequently, that of the resultant force R. The line of action of R came to lie closer and closer to the physiological 16° angle with the vertical, as represented by an interrupted line. At the same time, the opening of the neck-shaft angle modified the position of the growth plate, which 1 year after the varus osteotomy (Fig. 244e) formed an angle of 74° with the line of action of the resultant force R. Tensile trabeculae appeared in the upper aspect of the neck.

Two years after the varus osteotomy (Fig. 244f), the line of action of the resultant force was inclined at 16° to the perpendicular and intersected the centre of the weight-bearing surface of the hip joint, as in a normal hip. The compressive stresses were thus evenly distributed over the weight-bearing surface. The subchondral sclerosis, of even width throughout, demonstrates this. The resultant force R, which formed a 53° angle with the plane of the growth plate immediately after the osteotomy, had become normal to the epiphysial cartilage. In the femoral neck, two bundles of cancellous trabeculae could be seen (Fig. 244f). The medial bundle was under compression, the lateral under tension. The femoral neck was thus subjected to bending stress by the resultant force R, which acted outside the core.

In summary, the compressive force R, was now inclined at 16° to the perpendicular, and was distributed over a larger articular weight-bearing surface. It acted at right angles to the centre of the growth plate. Its line of action left the core of the femoral neck. Open reduction had restored a satisfactory anatomical shape, but the mechanical stressing remained pathological. The varus osteotomy restored the mechanical stresses to normal. As a consequence, the dense triangle at the edge of the acetabulum, the first sign of osteoarthritis, was replaced by a subchondral sclerosis of uniform width throughout, which demonstrates an even distribution of the compressive stresses in the joint. When the patient was aged 16 the hip was still normal (Fig. 244g).

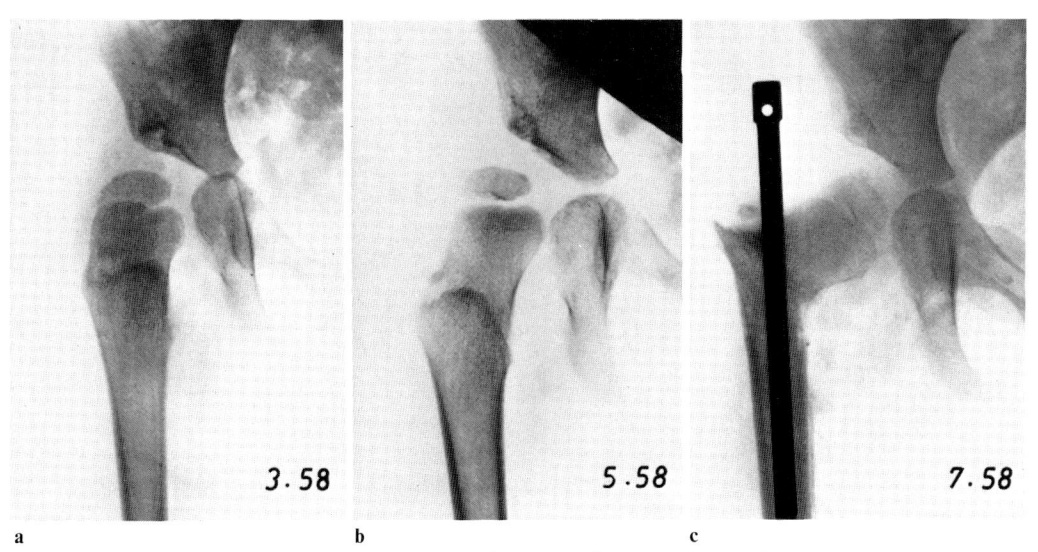

Fig. 246a–h. Evolution of the femoral neck requiring three successive varus osteotomies

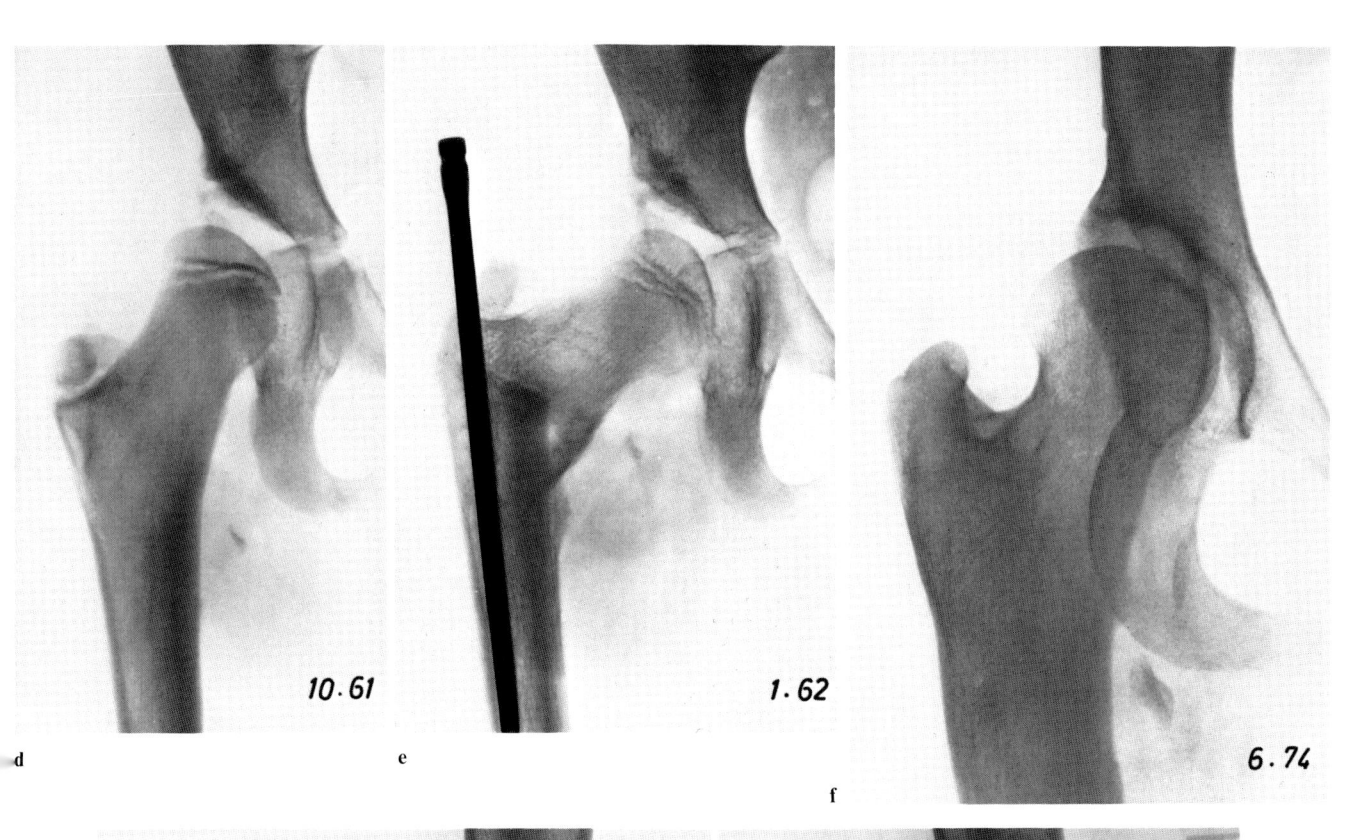

10.61

1.62

6.74

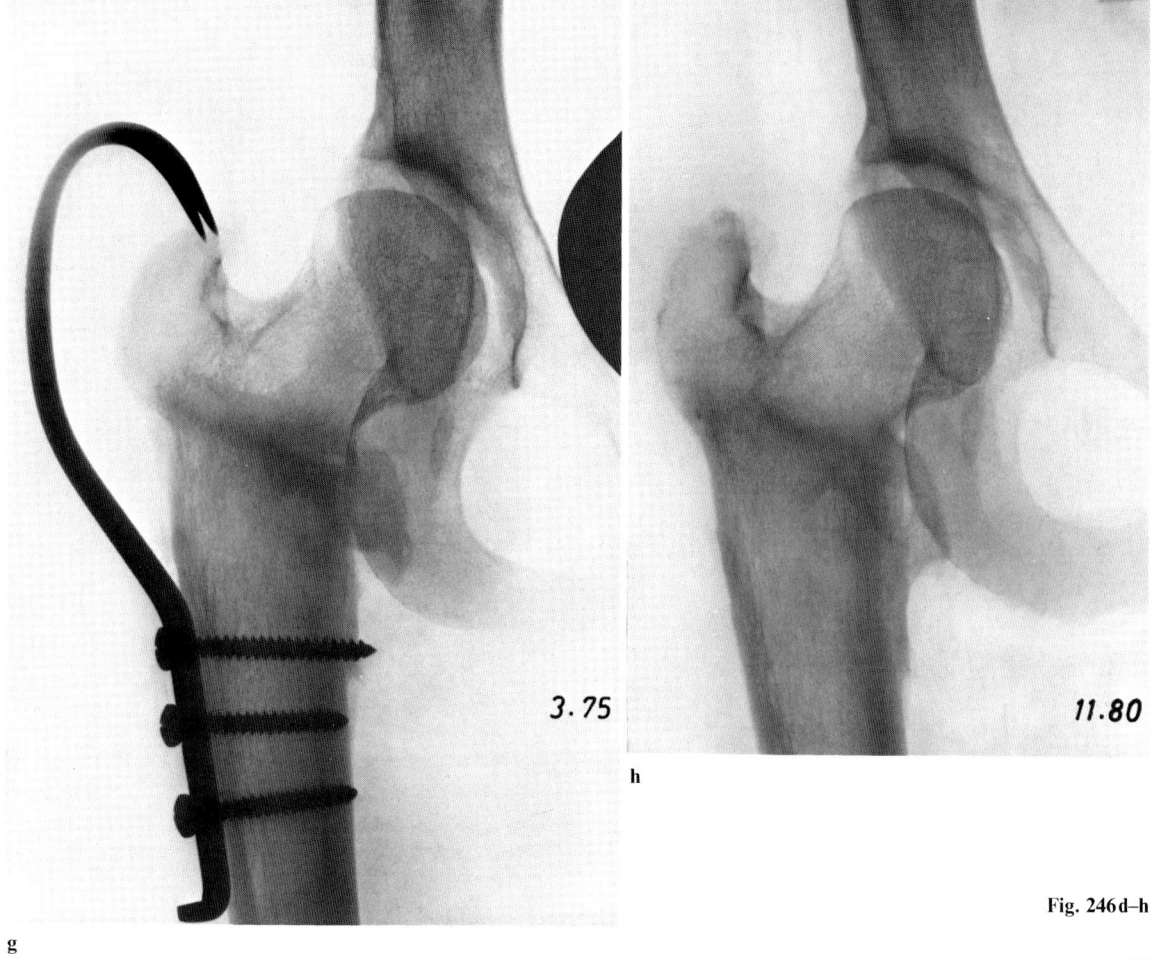

3.75

11.80

Fig. 246d–h

As shown by the analysis of this particular case, in dealing with a congenital hip dislocation or subluxation it is not sufficient to restore a normal anatomical shape by an open reduction. This is the aim of classical orthopaedics. However, it is also necessary to achieve an even distribution of the articular compressive stresses over as large a weight-bearing surface as possible. This is the important new concept introduced by PAUWELS.

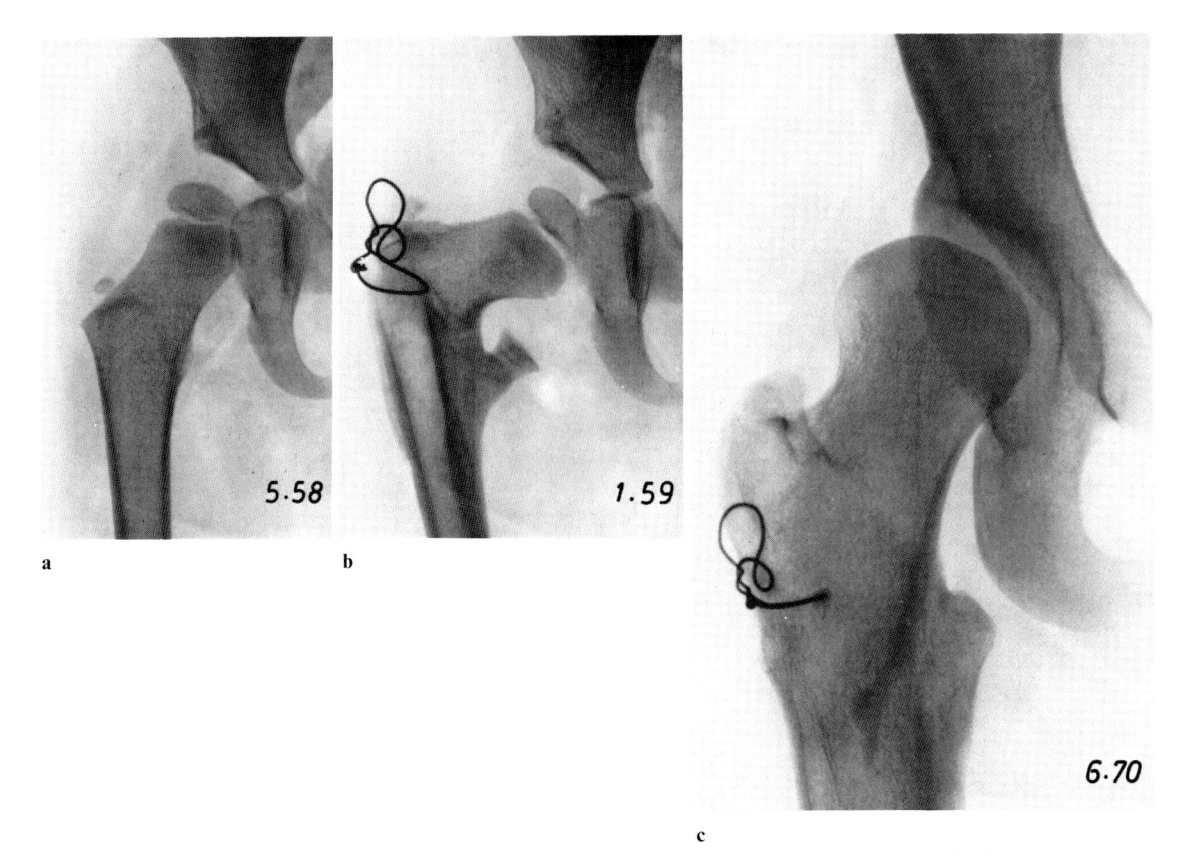

Fig. 247a–e. Same patient as in Fig. 245: opposite hip. Two varus osteotomies were carried out successively

E. Spontaneous Recurrence of the Valgus Deformity of the Femoral Neck

As already mentioned, a normal growth plate, when inclined to the plane at right angles to the line of action of the resultant force R, is stressed unevenly and reacts with increased growth where the compressive stresses are higher than normal (page 27). This may lead to recurrence of coxa valga.

A patient (Fig. 246a) was subjected to a varus osteotomy at the age of $2^1/_2$ years (Fig. 246c). The coxa valga recurred (Fig. 246d). The patient had to undergo a new varus osteotomy at the age of $5^1/_2$ years (Fig. 246e). The deformity recurred again (Fig. 246f). A third varus osteotomy was carried out when the patient was $18^1/_2$ (Fig. 246g). When she was 25 the result remained excellent (Fig. 246h). On the opposite side, two varus osteotomies had to be carried out successively at an interval of 13 years (Fig. 247).

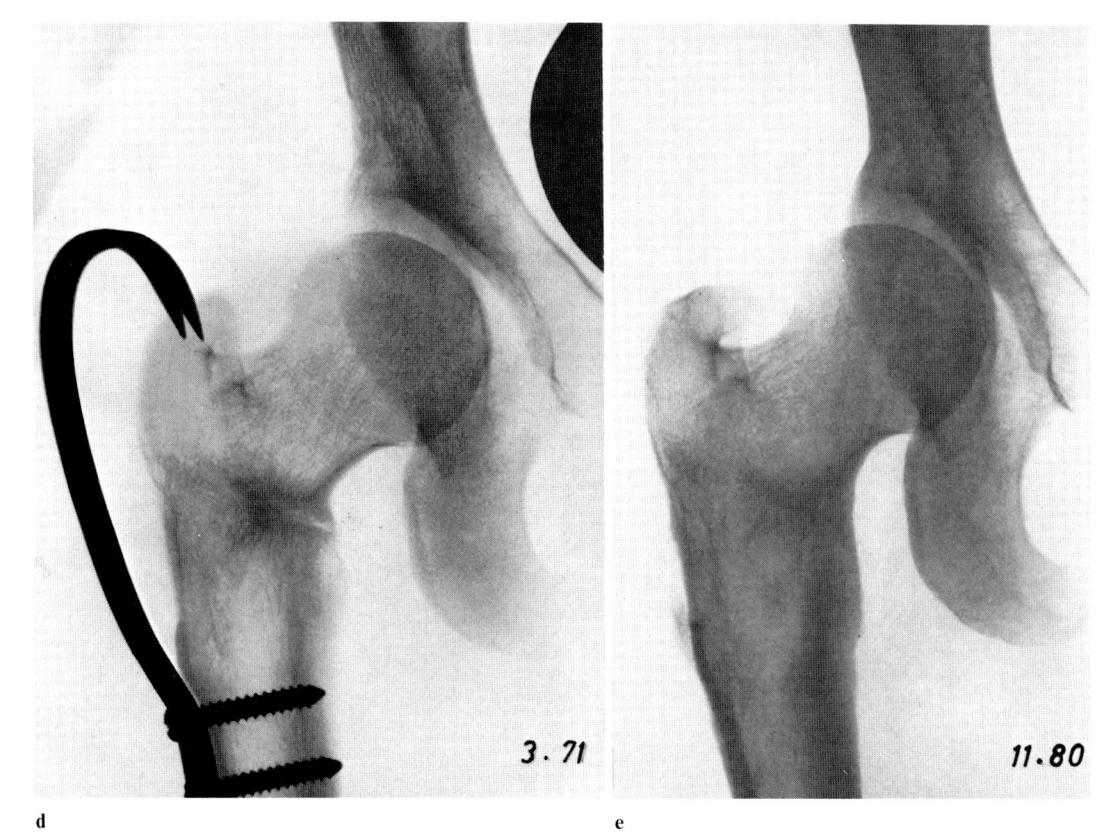

Fig. 247 d, e

III. In Children and Adolescents

After infancy, plasticity of the tissues can no longer be relied upon in attempts to deepen the acetabulum. However, the tissues continue to be capable of some adaptation.

A. Colonna Procedure

A dislocated or subluxated femoral head can be relocated after a socket has been dug with a reamer (COLONNA 1936). The results of the COLONNA procedure seem to have been disappointing and the procedure is no longer generally in use as far as we know, but it can give an occasional lasting good result after prolonged physiotherapy of the hip to prevent stiffness.

Both hips of a female patient were operated on successively when she was 10 years old (Figs. 248a and 249a). Thirteen years after the first operation (Figs. 248b and 249b) she was leading a normal life and was not limping, but the range of movement of her hips remained limited (Table 39).

Table 39. Range of movement of the hips (Figs. 248 and 249)

	Right hip (Fig. 248)	Left hip (Fig. 249)
Flexion	65	75
Extension	5	5
Adduction	25	35
Abduction	20	20
Internal rotation	5	5
External rotation	45	30

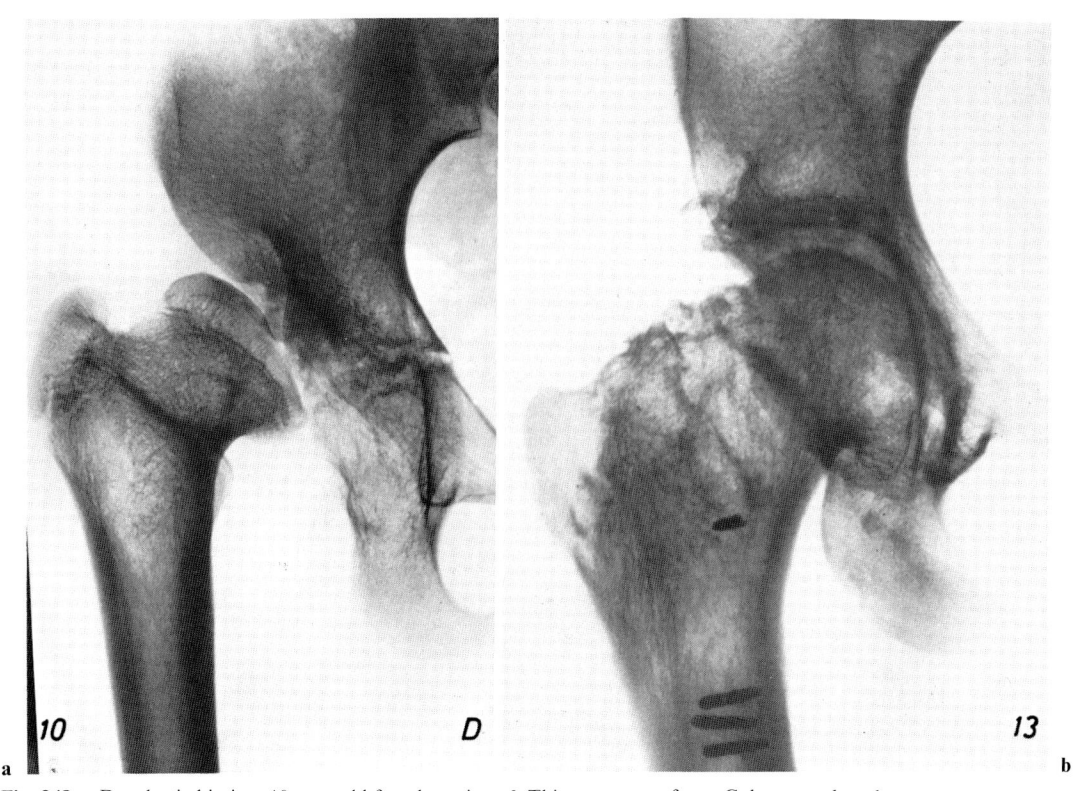

Fig. 248. a Dysplastic hip in a 10-year-old female patient. b Thirteen years after a Colonna arthroplasty

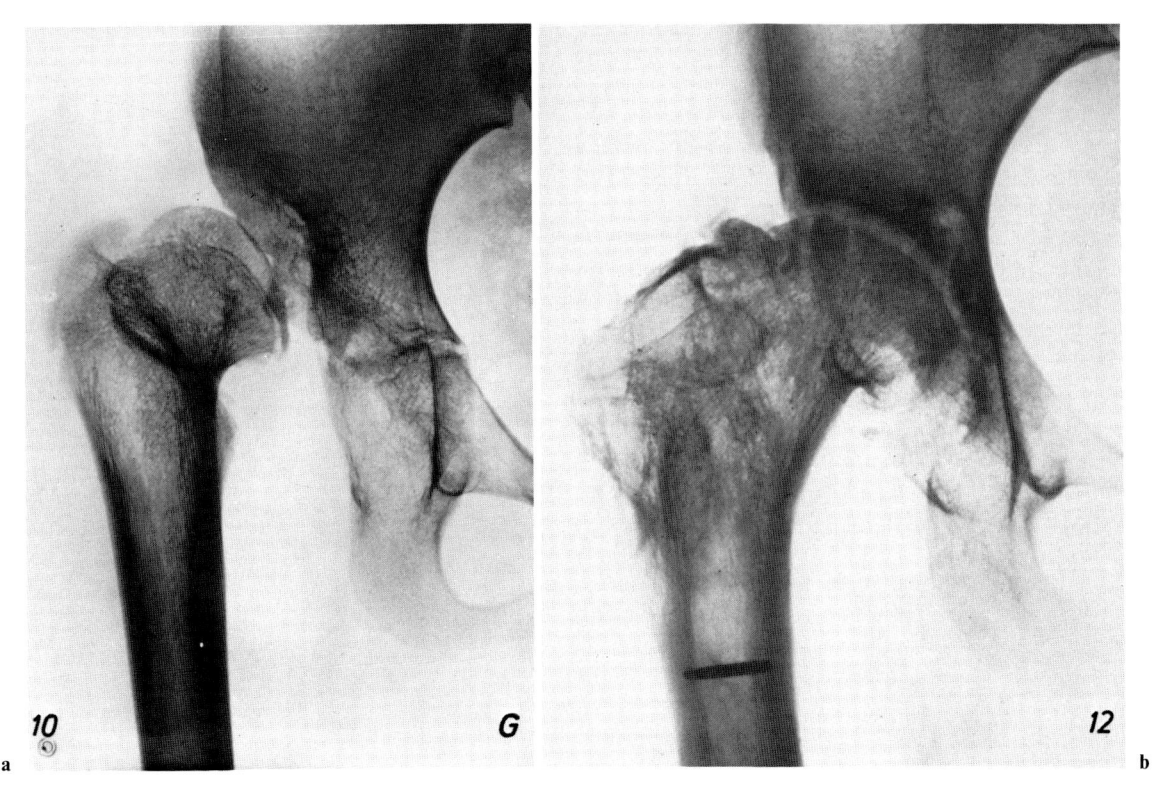

Fig. 249. a Same patient as in Fig. 248: opposite hip. Age at operation: 10 years. **b** Twelve-year follow-up

B. Varus Intertrochanteric Osteotomy

Whereas in infants and children we tend to relocate a dislocated or subluxated hip, in adolescents and adults we tend to operate only on painful subluxated hips, usually with a dense triangle manifesting an excess of pressure at the edge of the acetabulum. The goal of the treatment is to decrease the articular compressive stresses by enlarging the articular weight-bearing surface and by reducing the resultant force R transmitted across the joint. In coxa valga subluxans in the adolescent, the articular components usually remain spherical and a varus intertrochanteric osteotomy represents the method of choice to this end.

As in the adult, anteroposterior X-rays in the neutral position, in full abduction and in full adduction are required. The procedure is planned from a tracing of the X-ray in the neutral position. It is carried out as in the adult (see p. 84). When the anteversion of the neck is exaggerated, a derotation is carried out at osteotomy level. The leg is put into external rotation. The necessary degree of external rotation depends on the range of rotation available pre-operatively, and mainly on the degree of internal rotation of the leg when the greater trochanter is protruding laterally at its maximum. The greater trochanter is therefore palpated through the skin while the leg is internally rotated. When the greatest protrusio occurs, the degree of internal rotation is noted. During the osteotomy, the leg is brought to an equivalent degree of external rotation, that is to say, an equal and opposite position. After surgery, when the patient consciously corrects the external rotation, he also corrects the anteversion of the femoral neck and provides his abductor muscles with the longest possible lever arm.

A 13-year-old female patient (Fig. 250a) suffered pain in both hips and limped. On both sides, a dense triangle indicated that the pressure was abnormally increased at the edge of the socket. The trabeculae of cancellous bone were parallel to the axis of the femoral neck, which they completely filled. There was no WARD's triangle. The femoral neck was thus subjected to pure compressive stress.

A varus osteotomy was carried out successively on both sides. Five years later (Fig. 250b), the dense triangle at the edge of the socket had disappeared. There was now a subchondral sclerosis of uniform width throughout. This demonstrates an even distribution and a reduction of the articular compressive stresses. Two bundles of cancellous trabeculae intersect in the femoral neck just beneath the base of the head. They form the typical architecture of bending stress combined with shearing stress.

Fig. 250. a Dysplastic hips in a 13-year-old female patient. **b** Five years after bilateral varus intertrochanteric osteotomy

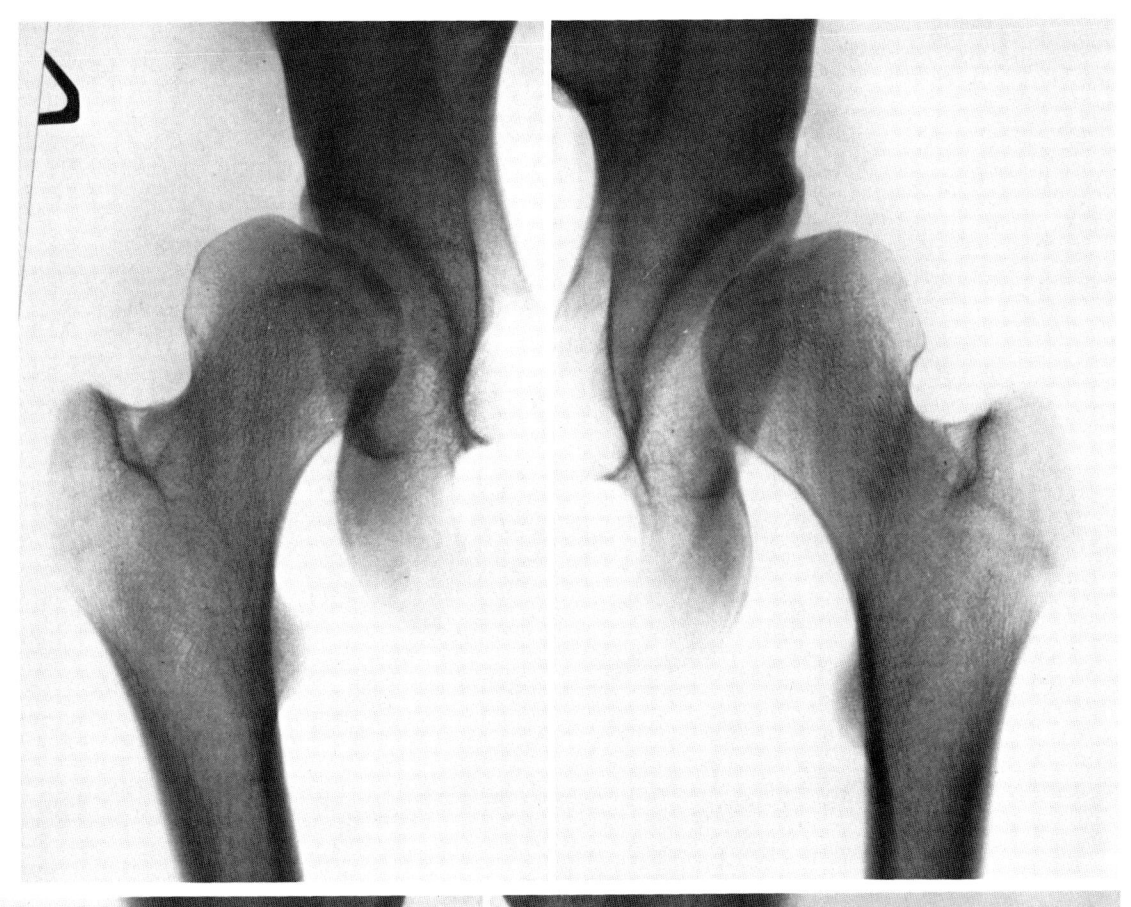

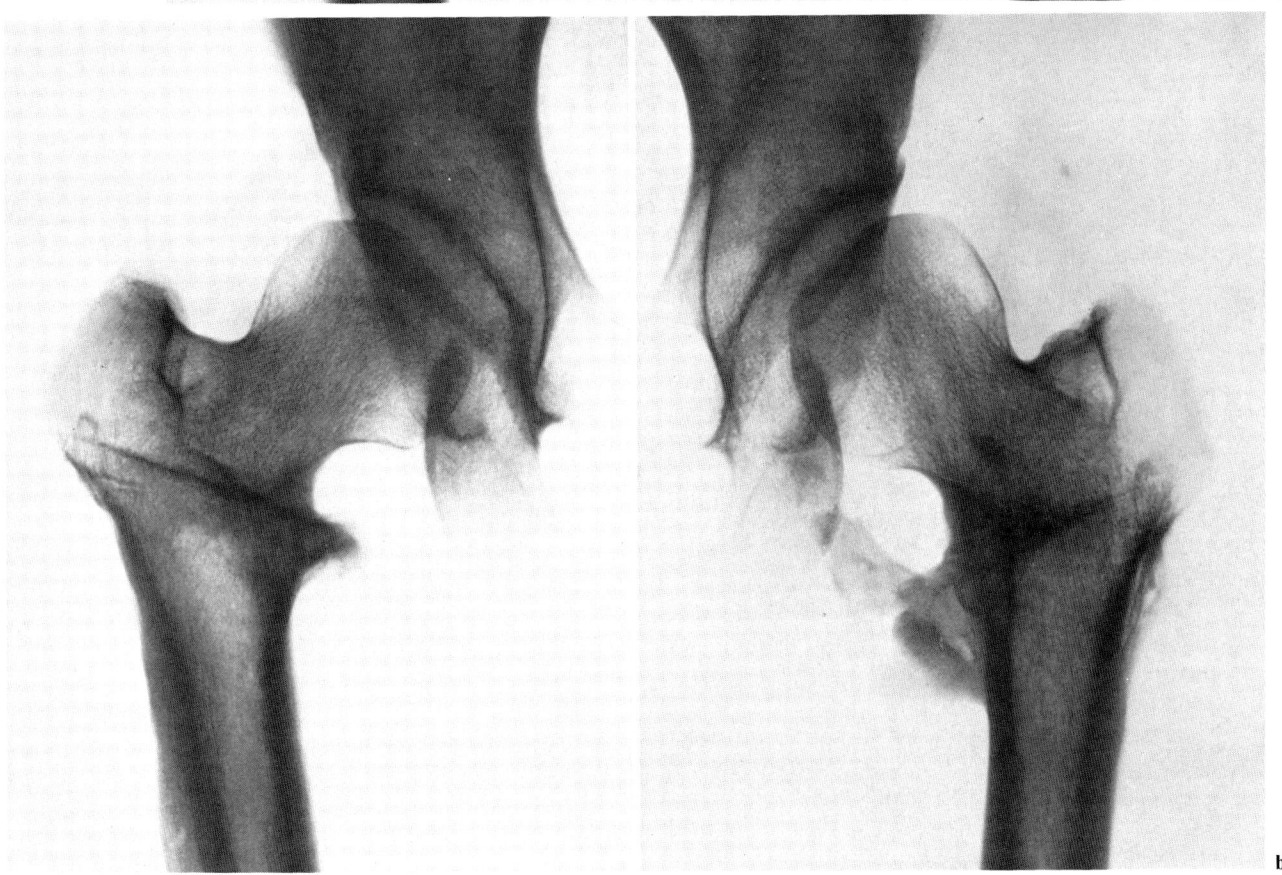

a

b

273

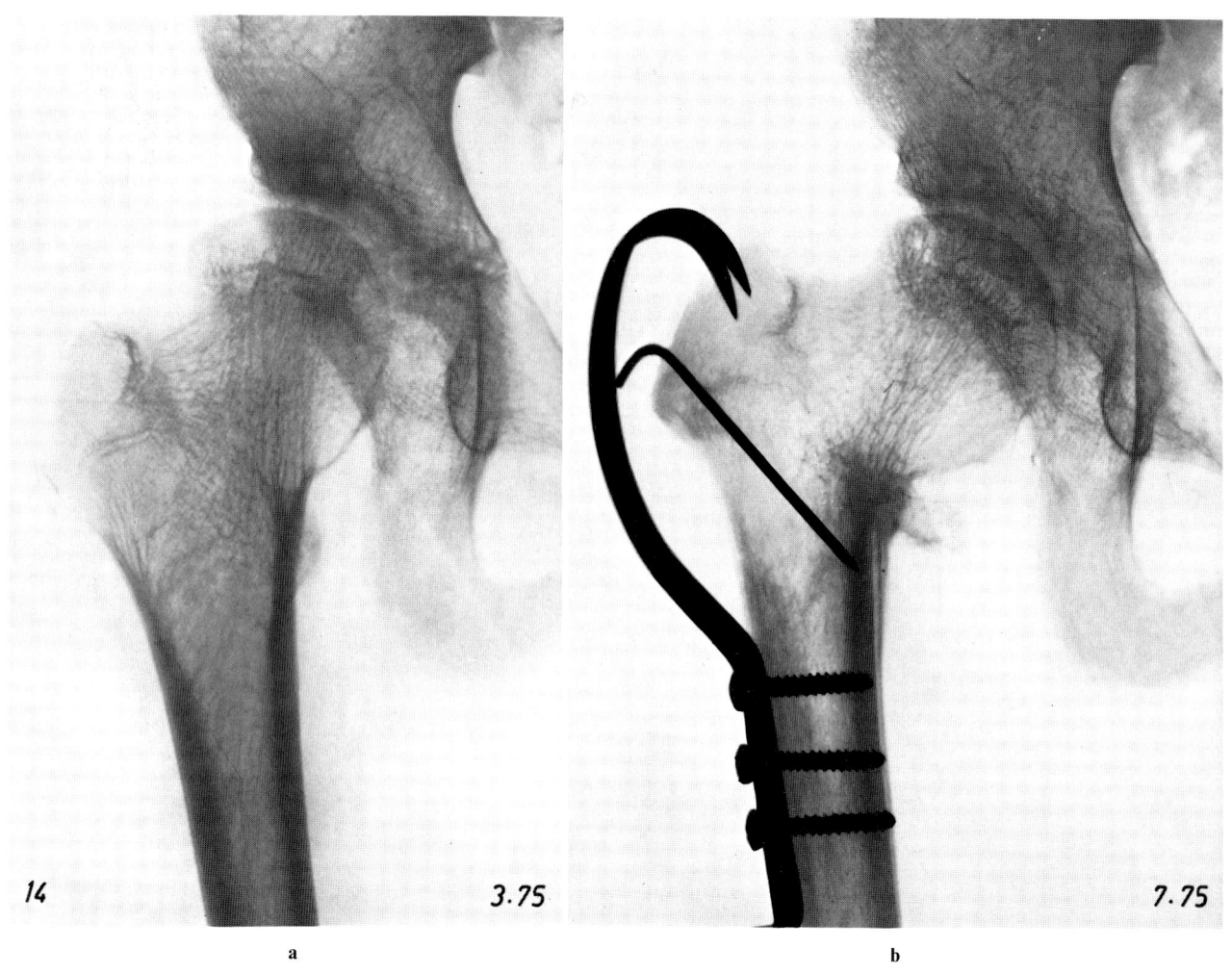

Fig. 251. a Dysplastic left hip in a 14-year-old male patient. **b** After a varus intertrochanteric osteotomy. **c** Lateral displacement of the greater trochanter. **d** Six-year follow-up

C. Varus Intertrochanteric Osteotomy Supplemented by Lateral Displacement of the Greater Trochanter

In patients with a short femoral neck and a relatively high greater trochanter, a varus intertrochanteric osteotomy is first carried out in order to relocate the femoral head in the socket in an attempt to deepen the latter. A lateral displacement of the greater trochanter performed at a second session supplements the mechanical effect of the varus osteotomy.

In a 14-year-old boy with a subluxation of both hips (Figs. 251a and 252a), a 25° varus osteotomy was carried out on the left side (Fig. 251b). Three months later, a similar operation was carried out on the right hip (Fig. 252b). At the same session the left greater trochanter was displaced laterally, making use of the wedge removed from the right intertrochanteric region (Fig. 251c). Five months later, the right greater trochanter was also displaced laterally (Fig. 252c). Six years after these procedures, the left hip was pain-free and had a full range of movement. The patient no longer limped. In the X-ray, the socket appeared deepened. A subchondral sclerosis of uniform width throughout delineated a wide joint space (Fig. 251d). The patient complained of some discomfort in the right hip, the range of movement of which was normal. In the X-ray, the socket appeared deepened but the joint surfaces were not congruent and a dense triangle persisted at the edge of the acetabulum (Fig. 252d). A valgus intertrochanteric osteotomy has been proposed and will very probably solve the problem.

c 8.75

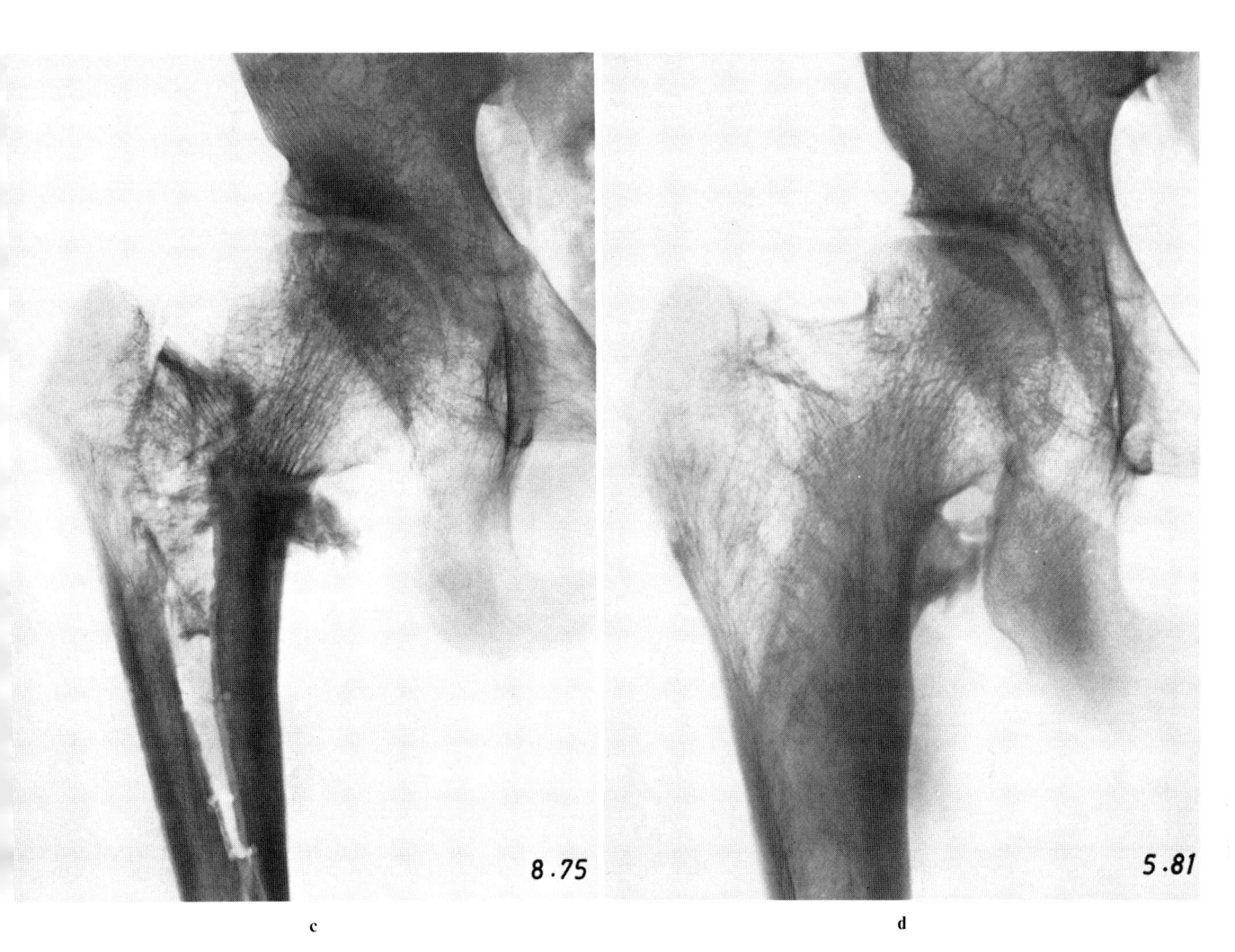

d 5.81

Fig. 251 c, d

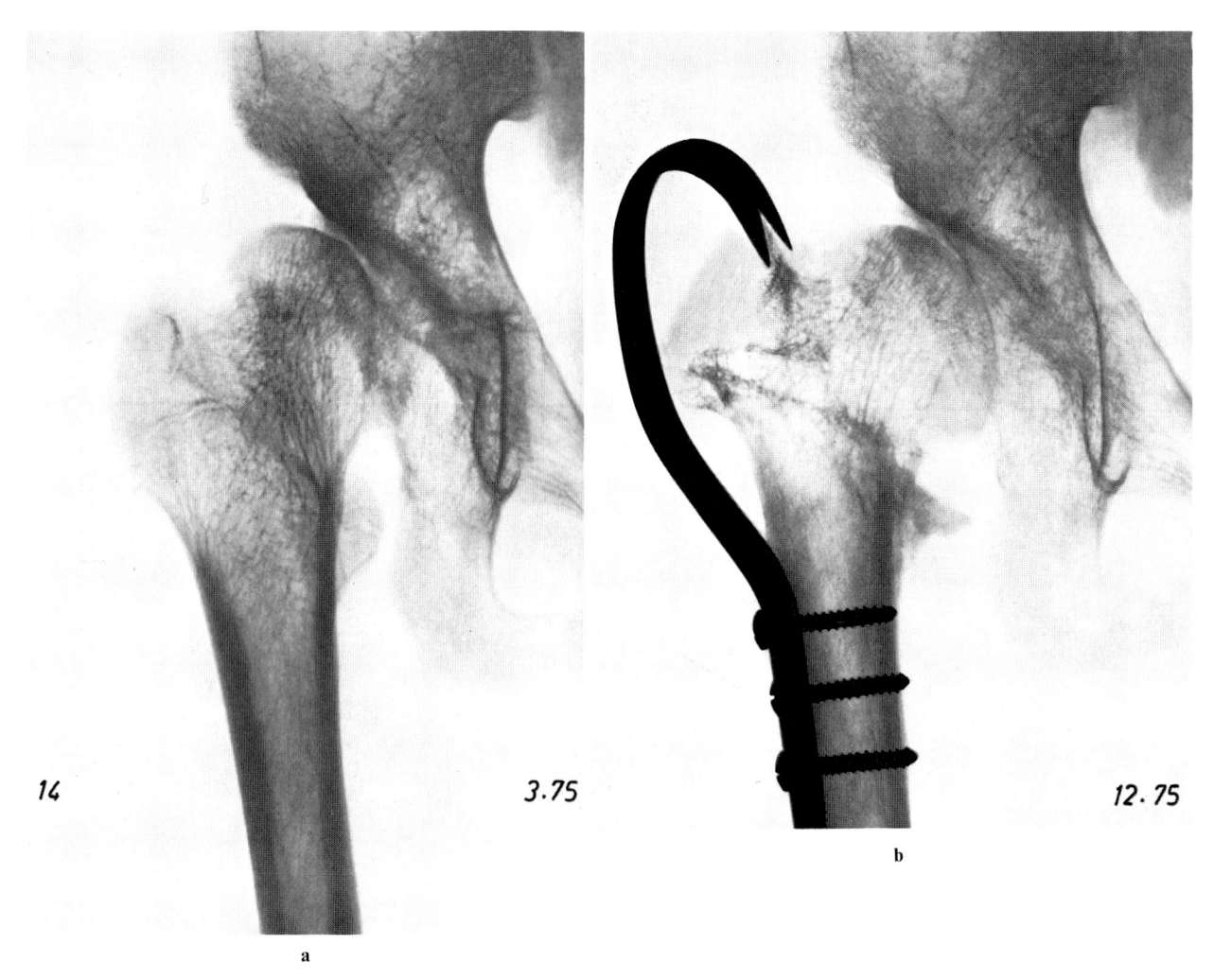

a

b

Fig. 252a–d. Same patient as in Fig. 251: **a** dysplastic right hip; **b** after a varus intertrochanteric osteotomy; **c** lateral displacement of the greater trochanter; **d** 6-year follow-up

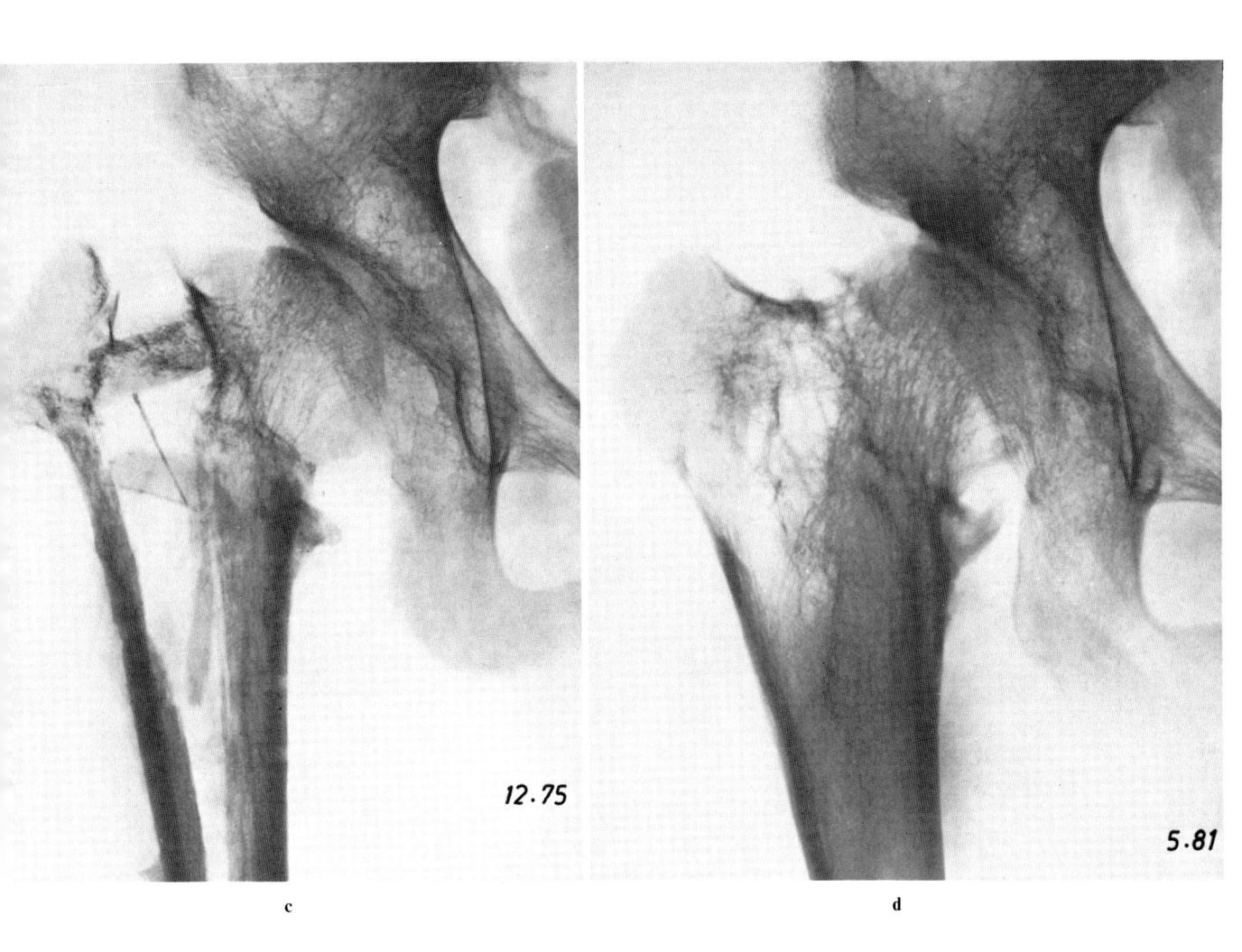

c

d

12.75

5.81

IV. In Adults

A. Dysplastic Hips with Osteoarthritis

In the adult, the dysplastic hip is operated on only if painful and osteoarthritic or if a shortening of the leg is desired. As long as turning the femoral head in the acetabulum by abduction ensures congruence of the joint surfaces, a varus osteotomy must be considered (page 76). This is true above all in the presence of coxa valga. However, if the greater trochanter lies relatively high, a lateral displacement of the greater trochanter combined with a tenotomy of the adductor and iliopsoas muscles often results in a more efficient mechanical effect than a varus intertrochanteric osteotomy (page 134).

When the articular components are deformed and particularly when the femoral head is pushed laterally in the socket by a medial osteophyte, congruence of the joint surfaces only occurs in adduction. Then a valgus osteotomy must be planned and carried out, combined with a tenotomy of the abductor, adductor and iliopsoas muscles (page 102). In some particular cases, a valgus osteotomy and a shortening on one side can result in a healing of both osteoarthritic hips. This occurs when, by chance, the rotation of the pelvis about the untreated femur due to the shortening of the opposite side is sufficient to ensure congruence of the articular surfaces and to enlarge the weight-bearing surface of the joint (page 150). Obviously, this occurs only exceptionally.

Sometimes, the acetabulum is so small that none of the aforementioned surgical procedures can enlarge the weight-bearing surface of the joint sufficiently. In such instances a pelvic osteotomy may have to be considered to provide the femoral head with more coverage.

The CHIARI osteotomy does not ensure sufficient articular congruence. It creates a bony step (Fig. 253) though this may disappear as a consequence of bony adaptation. The CHIARI osteotomy slightly shortens the lever arm h' of the force K exerted by the partial body mass by displacing the femoral head medially, due to the pivoting of the distal fragment about the pubis. But the muscular force M is made more vertical, since the origin of the abductor muscles on the ilium is displaced laterally in relation to their distal insertion. This tends to make the resultant force R more vertical. It may come to lie laterally to the original acetabulum. Finally, the result of the surgical procedure depends on a problematic functional adaptation of the bone. It does not seem to be completely reliable in severe osteoarthritis.

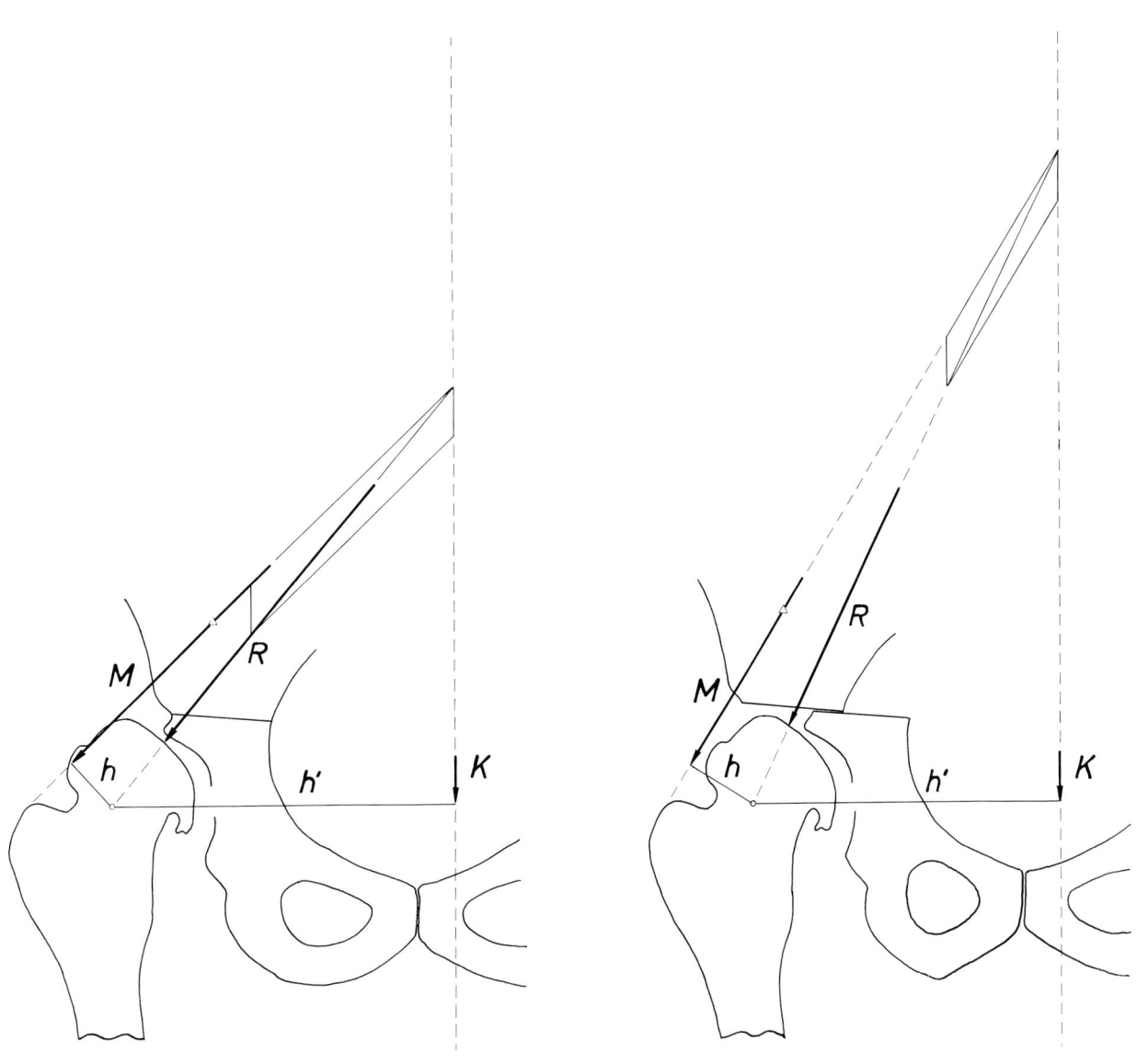

Fig. 253. Chiari osteotomy. M, force exerted by the abductor muscles; K, force exerted by that part of the body supported by the hip; h, lever arm of M; h', lever arm of K; R, resultant of forces M and K

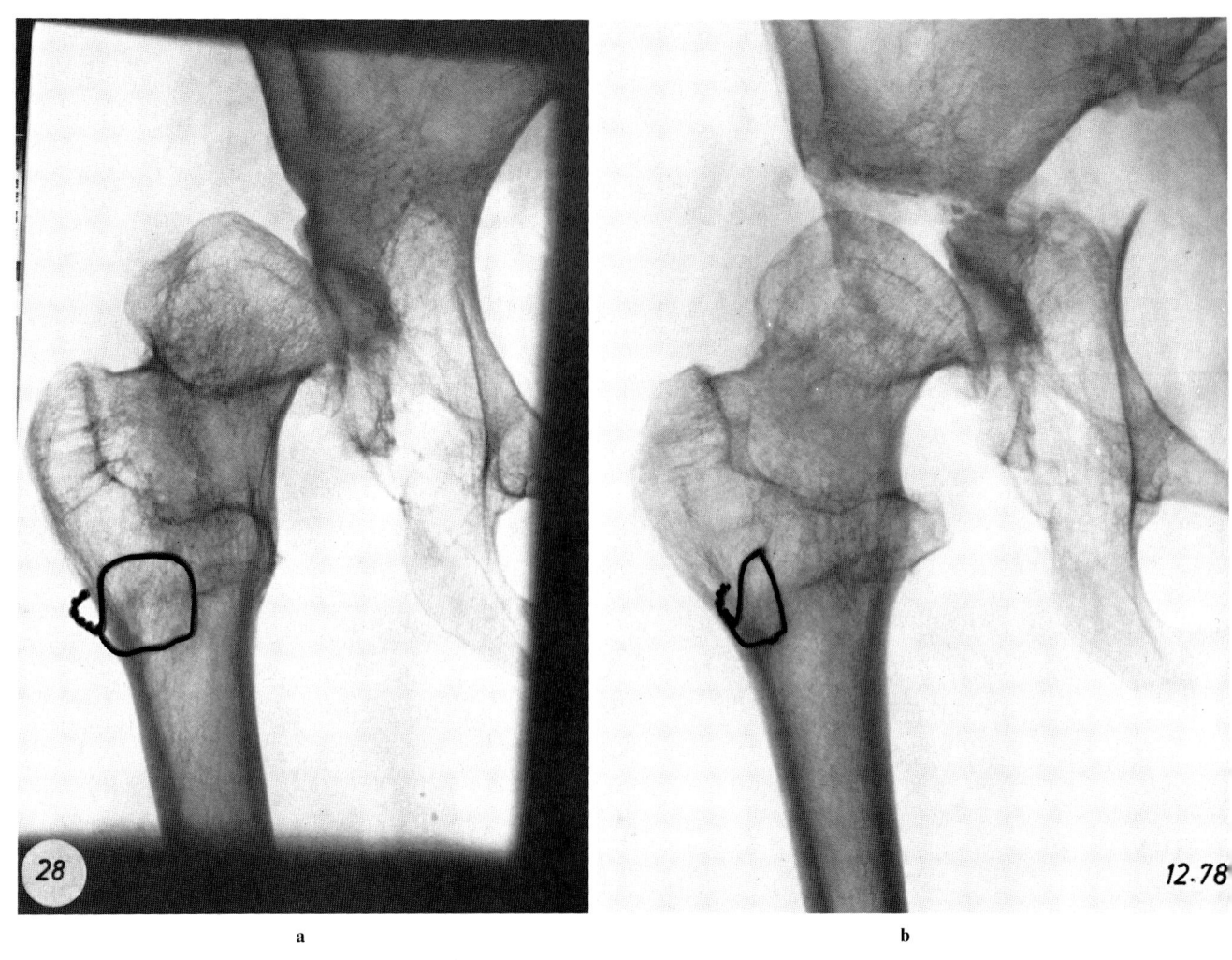

Fig. 254. a A 28-year-old female patient who had been subjected to several operations previously. b After a Chiari osteotomy. c Three-year follow-up. At this stage a lateral displacement of the greater trochanter was carried out. d Two years later

A 28-year-old female patient (Fig. 254a) had undergone several surgical operations for a dysplastic hip elsewhere, but the hip remained painful with a limited range of movement and the patient limped. The socket was very small and shallow. The opposite hip was also dysplastic, but with a larger acetabulum. A CHIARI osteotomy enabled us to bring the ilium above the femoral head. The conditions were thus created for the formation of an efficient acetabulum through functional adaptation (Fig. 254b), which is what in fact took place. At the 3-year follow-up, the new socket was underlined by a sclerosis of uniform width throughout (Fig. 254c). This points to an even distribution of the compressive stresses in the enlarged joint. At this stage, the hip was not causing pain and had a better range of movement. In order to improve the result and to eliminate limping, the greater trochanter was then displaced laterally.

The displacement was maintained by inserting the bony wedge removed from the opposite intertrochanteric region during a varus osteotomy. At the latest follow-up, the result was most satisfactory clinically (Table 40) and radiologically (Fig. 254d).

Table 40. Range of movement of the hip (Fig. 254)

	Before surgery	At the 3-year follow-up	Gain
Flexion	90°	95°	
Extension	5°	0°	0°
Adduction	50°	45°	
Abduction	20°	25°	0°
Int. rotation	40°	50°	
Ext. rotation	5°	25°	30°

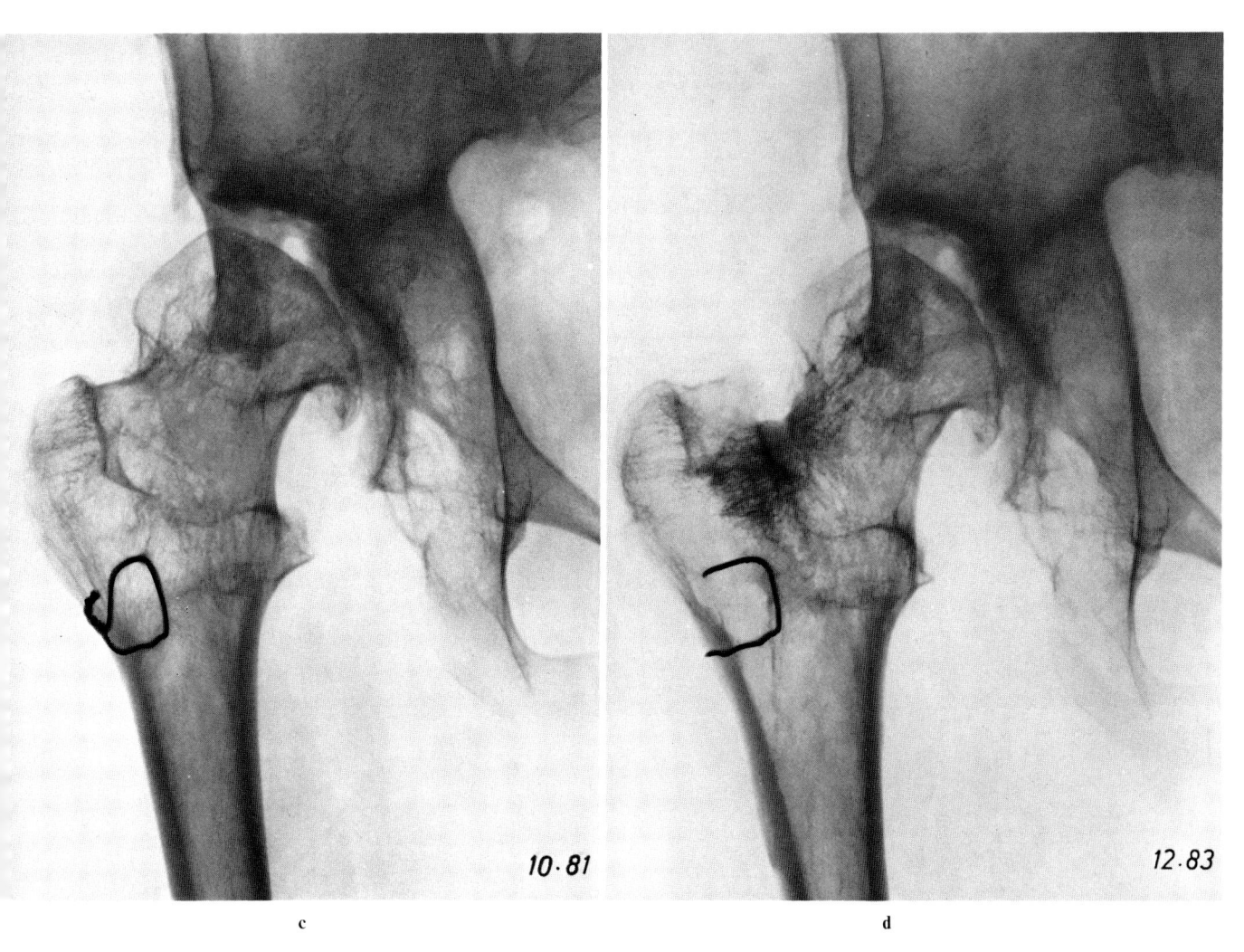

Fig. 254c, d.

B. Unreduced Congenital High Dislocation

As mentioned above, when an old unreduced congenital high dislocation of the hip becomes painful, a SCHANZ osteotomy should be considered (page 201). This procedure can lead to a valgus deformity of the knee and may have to be followed by a varus osteotomy of the ipsilateral supracondylar region. A shortening of the opposite femur may also be useful in making the pelvis level.

V. Conclusion

The surgical procedure required by a dysplastic hip differs according to the age of the patient and the particular configuration of the affected hip. In infants, we aim at relocating the femoral head properly in the acetabulum and at ensuring appropriate mechanical stressing of the joint.

In young children, a varus osteotomy of the femur may result in a deepening of the acetabulum through functional adaptation. A SALTER osteotomy of the pelvis or a lowering of the lateral aspect of the acetabulum according to BERTRAND may ensure that the femoral head is satisfactorily contained. A varus osteotomy may have to be carried out additionally in order to improve the mechanical stressing of the relocated hip.

In adolescents and, to an even greater extent, in adults, we aim rather at decreasing the articular pressure by enlarging the articular weight-bearing surface and by reducing the force transmitted across the joint. This is achieved either by means of a varus osteotomy, or a lateral displacement of the greater trochanter plus a tenotomy, or a valgus osteotomy plus a tenotomy, or a shortening of the opposite leg. In rare cases with a very small socket, a pelvic osteotomy may have to be considered.

In old unreduced congenital dislocations, the SCHANZ osteotomy constitutes a valuable salvage procedure.

Chapter VII. Results

In most hips, the tissues seem to react advantageously to adequate reduction of the articular compressive stresses. Long follow-up studies and a statistical analysis are necessary in order to find out whether this is the rule and whether this reaction is lasting. If it is, our approach to the problem of osteoarthritis makes practical sense.

I. Hanging-Hip Procedure

Between 1961 and 1979 we carried out 131 hanging-hip procedures, 94 of them for osteoarthritis of the hip or for necrosis of the femoral head, the others for rheumatoid or septic arthritis or miscellaneous conditions. Six of the patients operated on for osteoarthritis or necrosis of the femoral head died before the 3-year follow-up. We were able to review 52 of the remainder with at least a 3-year follow-up; 63.5% were female and 73.1% of the patients were 50 years old or more (Fig. 255). The right side was affected in 48.1%, the left in 51.9%. The follow-up period ranged from 3 to 18 years. About a third of the patients were followed-up for longer than 10 years (Fig. 256).

In 13 of the 52 hips reviewed, the hanging-hip procedure was carried out as a temporary measure aimed at relieving pain whilst waiting for the evolution of the disease to make the hip suitable for an osteotomy or a lateral displacement of the greater trochanter. In the other 39 hips the procedure was regarded as the appropriate definitive treatment. The results in this latter group are much better than in the former, as might be expected.

A. As Procedure of Choice

We shall deal in more detail with the 39 hips for which the hanging-hip procedure was considered to have been the treatment of choice. There was osteoarthritis of the concentric type in 56.4% of these hips, of the subluxating type in 25.6% and of the protrusive type in 17.9%.

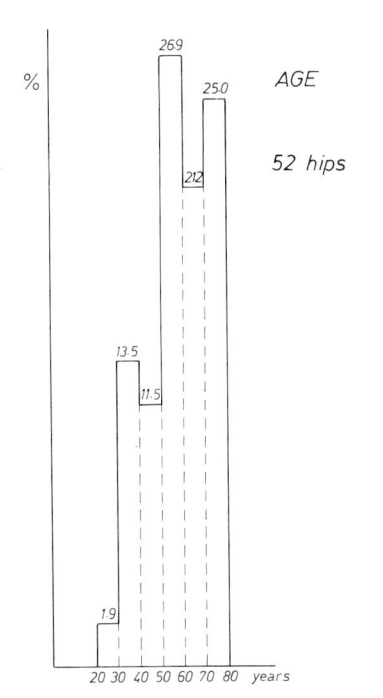

Fig. 255. Age distribution of patients in whom a hanging-hip procedure was carried out

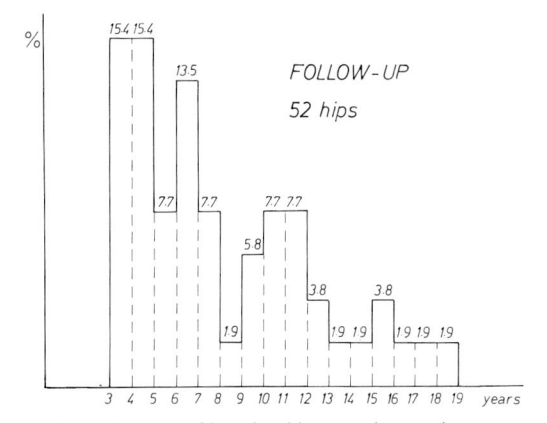

Fig. 256. Follow-up of hanging-hip procedure patients

The MERLE D'AUBIGNÉ rating, (Table 41), was used to evaluate the clinical picture before surgery and at the latest follow-up. According to this rating, pain, range of movement and gait are each marked on a scale from 6 to 0. Absence of pain, full range of movement and normal gait are rated 6. A normal hip thus scores $6+6+6=18$. 0 denotes permanent pain, a stiff hip in fixed deformity and inability to walk. The other figures represent intermediate stages.

The pain-relieving effect of the procedure was impressive and lasting (Fig. 257). At the latest follow-up, 53.8% of the patients did not complain at all, and an additional 23.1% mentioned occasional discomfort but only when starting to walk. The range of movement was increased, with 74.4% of the hips flexing beyond 60° and abducting beyond 15° at the latest follow-up, whilst only, 46.2% had a similar range before surgery. The gait was improved: 20.5% of the patients walked without limping and 38.5% limped only slightly; 92.3% of the patients regarded their walking distance as unlimited, although 33.3% used a walking-stick for walking long distances.

The TRENDELENBURG sign was positive in 74.4% of the hips before surgery and negative in 25.6%.

Table 41. Grading of functional value of the hip

	Pain	Range of movement	Gait
0	Pain intense and permanent	Ankylosis with bad position of the hip	Unable to walk
1	Pain severe at night	No movement with pain or slight deformity	Only with crutches
2	Pain severe when walking, preventing any activity	Flexion less than 40°	Only with two sticks
3	Pain tolerable with limited activity	Maximum flexion between 40° and 60°	With one stick, less than one hour, very difficult without stick
4	Pain mild when walking, disappearing with rest	Maximum flexion between 60° and 80°, can reach foot	A long time with a stick—a little without stick but with limp
5	Very mild and inconstant pain, permitting normal activity	Maximum flexion between 80° and 90°, abduction at least 25°	Without stick but with slight limp
6	No pain	Maximum flexion more than 90°, abduction to 40°	Normal

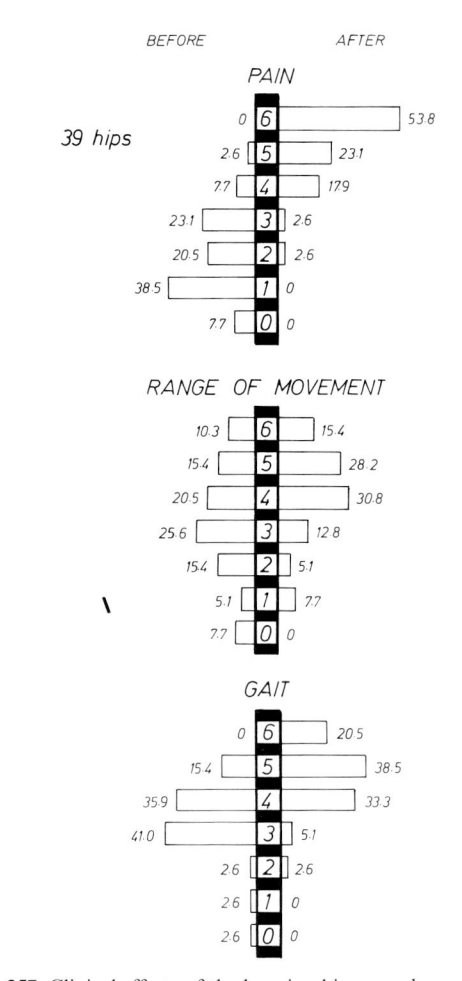

Fig. 257. Clinical effects of the hanging-hip procedure

At the latest follow-up it was negative in 61.5% and remained positive in 38.5%.

Most patients had gained between 1 and 14 points on the MERLE D'AUBIGNÉ rating. The average gain was 5.41 points. Only two patients lost points, one lost one point and the other 2 (Fig. 258). Before surgery the average rating was 8.79, with extremes of 1 and 14. at the latest follow-up the rating ranged between 7 and 18, with an average of 14.05; 53.9% of the hips scored more than 14 postoperatively, whereas none reached this level before (Table 42).

The subchondral sclerosis, which was abnormal in 64.2% of the hips before operation, appeared normal in 61.5% of the X-rays taken at the latest follow-up. It was cup-shaped in 25.6% (Fig. 259). The joint space was less than half the normal width in 61.5% before surgery. It appeared normal or greater than half the normal width in 82% at the latest follow-up. The cysts in the femoral head and in the acetabulum were numerous or large in 41% of the hips before the hanging-hip procedure. They

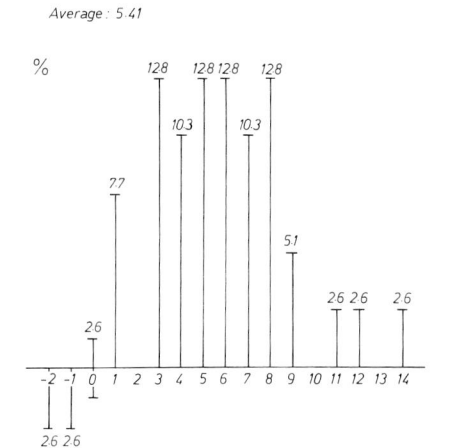

Fig. 258. Improvement in the Merle d'Aubigné rating following the hanging-hip procedure

Table 42. Effect of the hanging-hip operation on the total clinical rating · n = 39

Before[a] (% of total)	Rating	At latest follow-up[b] (% of total)		
0	18	7.7 }	18.0	Excellent
0	17	10.3 }		
0	16	7.7 }	35.9	Good
0	15	28.2 }		
10.3	14	5.1 }		
5.1	13	15.4 }	30.8	Fair
10.3	12	10.3 }		
2.6	11	7.7 }		
5.1	10	2.6 }		
15.4	9	2.6 }	15.5	Poor
20.5	8	0 }		
7.7	7	2.6 }		
10.3	6	0		
7.7	5	0		
0	4	0		
2.6	3	0		
0	2	0		
2.6	1	0		

[a] Average rating 8.79; [b] Average rating 14.05

remained so in 25.6% at the latest follow-up. Whereas only 5.1% of the hips were free from cysts before, 30.8% of the hips appeared without cysts afterwards.

Five (12.8%) of the 39 hips of this group deteriorated after 3, 3, 13, 15 and 16 years respectively. Three underwent a valgus intertrochanteric osteotomy, with excellent results and one a total replacement.

B. As Temporary Palliative Measure

Among the 13 hips of this group in which the hanging-hip procedure was carried out as a temporary measure, osteoarthritis was concentric in one instance, subluxating in 9 and protrusive in 3. Only 2 patients remained pain-free at the latest follow-up, and one experienced slight discomfort when starting to walk. No patient had a full range of movement, and all of them limped. In 11 patients the TRENDELENBURG sign was positive pre-operatively; it remained so in 8.

The total MERLE D'AUBERGNÉ rating score ranged between 3 and 14 both before surgery and at the latest follow-up. The average was 7.62 before and 9.23 after surgery. Only one hip gained more than 8 points. Four lost between 1 and 3 points.

The average gain was 1 point. The X-rays showed a lateral dense triangle in the roof of the socket in ten hips both before surgery and at the latest follow-up. Only one medial dense triangle (protrusio acetabuli) had changed into a normal subchondral sclerosis.

In none of the hips did the joint space look normal at the latest follow-up. In the nine in which

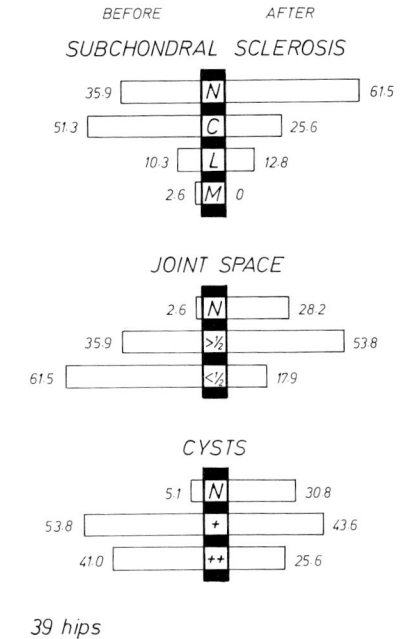

Fig. 259. Radiological changes following hanging-hip procedure. *Subchondral sclerosis*: N, normal subchondral sclerosis in the roof of the acetabulum; C, cup-shaped subchondral sclerosis; L, triangular sclerosis at the lateral edge of the acetabulum; M, medial sclerotic triangle in the depths of the acetabulum. *Joint space*: N, normal joint space; $>1/2$ joint space wider than half its normal width; $<1/2$ joint space narrower than half its normal width. *cysts*: N, no cysts; +, small cysts; ++, big cysts

the joint space had been less than half the normal width, this was still the case. The cysts had not disappeared.

C. Complications

There were no complications among the patients followed-up.

II. Varus and Valgus Intertrochanteric Osteotomy

A. Three-Year Follow-up

In 1976 we contributed to a review of hips in which osteotomy had been performed for severe osteoarthritis in different Belgian and French centres (WATILLON et al. 1978). Severe osteoarthritis meant that at least two of the following signs were present in the X-ray: (a) narrowing of the joint space to less than 50% of the normal width, (b) increased and uneven subchondral sclerosis in the roof of the acetabulum and (c) cysts.

Prior to 1973, we had carried out osteotomies in 540 hips for osteoarthritis or necrosis of the femoral head. Of these, we retained in the review those patients who had had severe osteoarthritis and had been followed-up for at least 3 years. We added the hips with a shorter follow-up in which early complications had impaired the outcome or which were seen to be failures before the 3-year follow-up. Discarding these hips because of the short follow-up would have distorted the picture and given a false impression of the complication rate. We thus reviewed 305 hips, 60% of which were right hips. The ages ranged from the second to the eight decade (Fig. 260); 79% of the patients were female.

In 284 of these 305 hips, the mechanical goal of surgery appeared to have been attained and the follow-up was at least 3 years. We used these 284 hips for analysis of the results. The other hips were taken into account when dealing with the complications, or with particular points, such as congruence of the articular surfaces. The follow-up ranged from 5 to 10 years in 55.2% of the hips (Fig. 261).

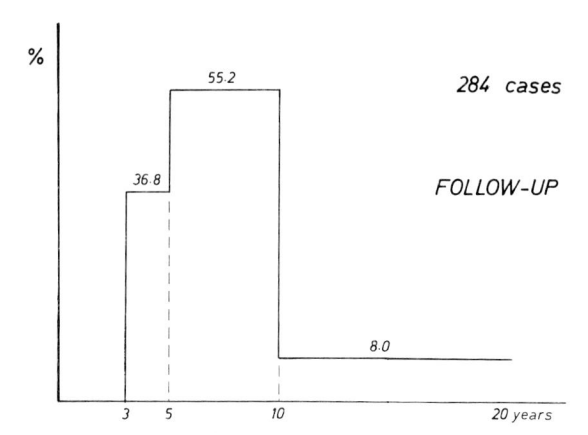

Fig. 261. Follow-up of Pauwels' intertrochanteric osteotomy patients

There was subluxating osteoarthritis in 62.2%, protrusive osteoarthritis in 11.5% and concentric osteoarthritis in 26.3%. The procedure was a varus osteotomy in 9.5% of the cases and a valgus osteotomy in 90.5%.

In most of the 284 cases in which the mechanical aim of surgery seemed to have been attained, the relief of pain was dramatic, the range of movement considerably increased and the gait significantly improved (Fig. 262). The final clinical picture (Fig. 263) is summarized in Table 43.

Table 43. Results of intertrochanteric osteotomy

Before (%)	Rating	At latest follow-up (%)
0	17–18	23.0
1.3	15–16	28.5
9.2	13–14	25.5
89.5	0–12	23.0

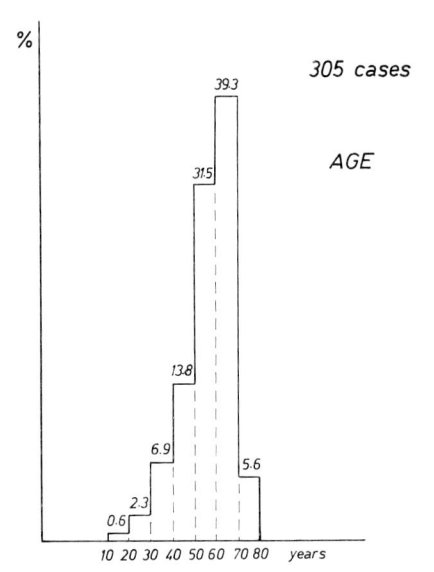

Fig. 260. Age distribution of patients subjected to a Pauwels' intertrochanteric osteotomy. Follow-up of 3 years and more

Fig. 262. Clinical effects of Pauwels' intertrochanteric osteotomy. Follow-up of 3 years and more

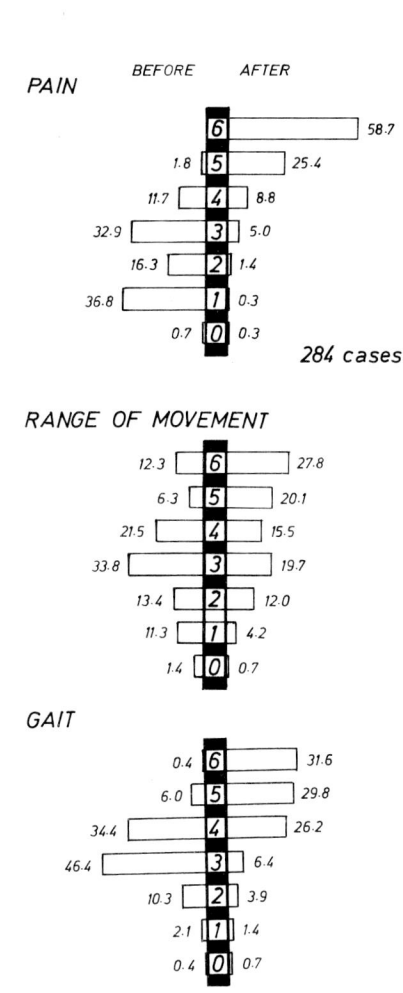

Fig. 263. Effect of Pauwels' intertrochanteric osteotomy on total clinical scores. Scores before (*left*) and afterwards (*right*). Follow-up of 3 years and more

The X-rays showed that the subchondral sclerosis had reverted to normal or improved considerably in 92% of the 284 hips. The joint space had become normal or widened in 85%. The cysts had filled up or decreased in volume and number in 97% (Fig. 264).

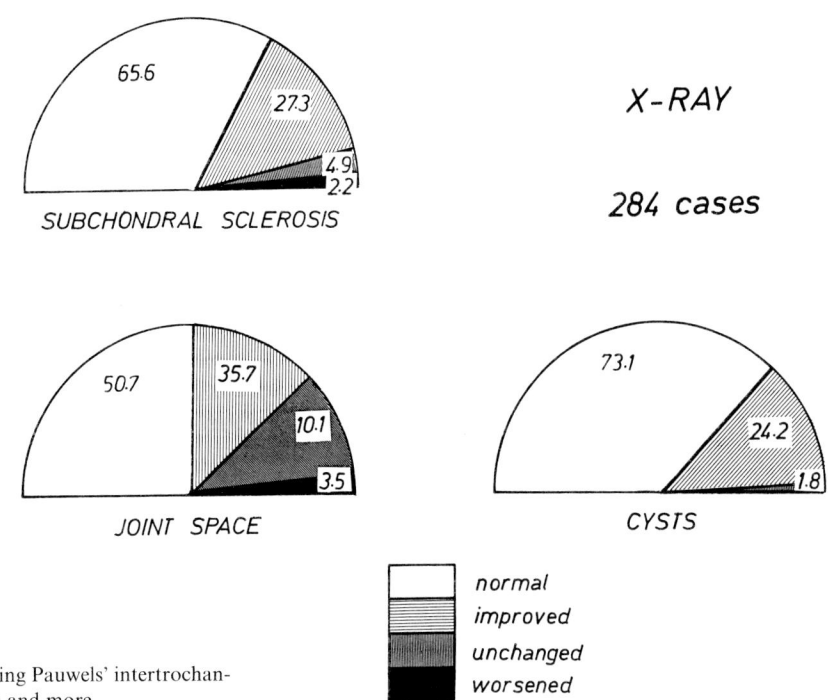

Fig. 264. Radiological changes following Pauwels' intertrochanteric osteotomy. Follow-up of 3 years and more

Table 44. Effect of Pauwels' intertrochanteric osteotomies on the total clinical rating (3-year follow-up). $n=284$

Before[a] (% of total)	Rating	At latest follow-up[b] (% of total)		
0	18	14.44		
0	17	17.25	31.69	Excellent
0	16	13.03		
1.06	15	14.44	27.47	Good
2.82	14	11.62		
4.93	13	9.86	29.58	Fair
5.28	12	8.10		
9.51	11	6.69		
12.32	10	3.52		
12.32	9	0	11.26	Poor
15.95	8	0.70		
11.62	7	0.35		
10.56	6			
9.15	5			
4.58	4			
0	3			
0	2			
0	1			
0	0			

[a] Average rating, 8.58; [b] Average rating, 14.81

We attempted to evaluate the overall results by comparing the hips before the osteotomy and at the latest follow-up (Table 44). This stresses the improvement thus obtained as well as the actual state of the hips. The results thus derived were correlated with different parameters.

Of the osteotomies carried out for osteoarthritis with a subluxation of the joint, 77.5% gave excellent or good results, as compared to 69.7% in protrusio acetabuli and 61.5% in concentric osteoarthritis (Fig. 265). The quality of the results depended on whether articular congruence had been improved or pre-existing incongruence had been worsened (Fig. 266). The longer the follow-up, the better were the results (Fig. 267). Improvement continues with time.

There were some complications (Table 45). As already mentioned, these complications were taken into account even if the follow-up was less than 3 years. The rate of fatal pulmonary embolism was almost prohibitively high in the first 200 hips which we operated on. Since we have been using the prophylactic means described above (p. 89),

Table 45. Complications (305 hips)

	Number	%
Pulmonary embolism (fatal in 7, 2.3%)	9	3.0
Phlebitis	8	2.7
Superficial sepsis	4	1.3
Deep sepsis	3	1
Breakdown of fixation	11	3.6
Non-union	2	0.6

Table 46. Deterioration (305 hips)

	None	1 year	2 years	3 years	4 years and more
Number	250	11	13	9	18
%	83	3	4	2	5

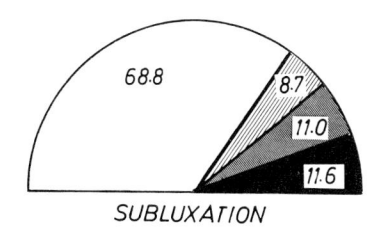

RESULTS

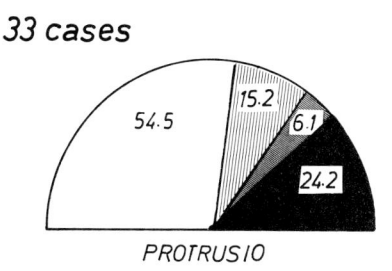

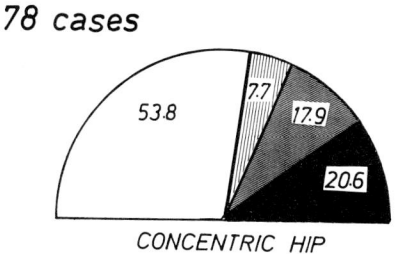

173 cases — SUBLUXATION: 68.8 / 8.7 / 11.0 / 11.6

33 cases — PROTRUSIO: 54.5 / 15.2 / 6.1 / 24.2

78 cases — CONCENTRIC HIP: 53.8 / 7.7 / 17.9 / 20.6

excellent / good / fair / poor

Fig. 265. Overall results of Pauwels' intertrochanteric osteotomy. Follow-up of 3 years and more

POSTOP. CONGRUENCE

BETTER

248 cases

- 70.2
- 10.1
- 11.3
- 7.7

WORSE

10 cases

- 70
- 20
- 10

Legend:
- excellent
- good
- fair
- poor

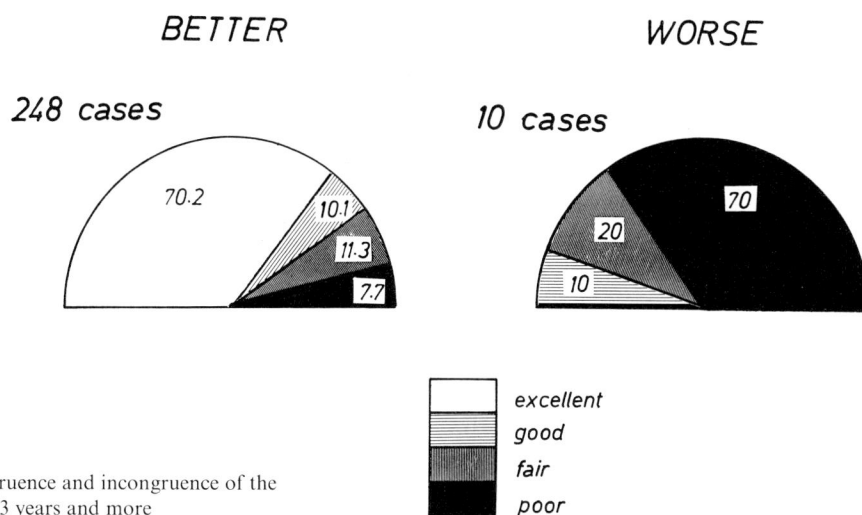

Fig. 266. Results related to congruence and incongruence of the articular surfaces. Follow-up of 3 years and more

some embolisms have still occurred following hip osteotomy but none has been fatal.

In the few instances where deep sepsis occurred, this healed when bony union had taken place and the implant had been removed. Breakdown of fixation occurred when too little of the greater trochanter had been left to provide the hook with a good hold. This is easily avoided by cutting the wedge more distally (p. 110).

Non-union was observed in adults in whom a wedge had been removed, rotated by 180° and reinserted between the main fragments in order to avoid too great a shortening (p. 89). This is not recommended in adults. The two cases of non-union were reoperated on and eventually healed.

Some patients enjoy a good result for some years and then the hip deteriorates again (Table 46). In these cases either a second osteotomy, can be carried out or the hip can be replaced by a prosthesis.

FOLLOW-UP

106 cases (3-5 years)
- 53.8
- 8.5
- 16.0
- 21.7

156 cases (6-10 years)
- 67.3
- 8.3
- 10.9
- 13.5

22 cases (11-20 years)
- 77.3
- 18.2
- 4.5

Legend:
- excellent
- good
- fair
- poor

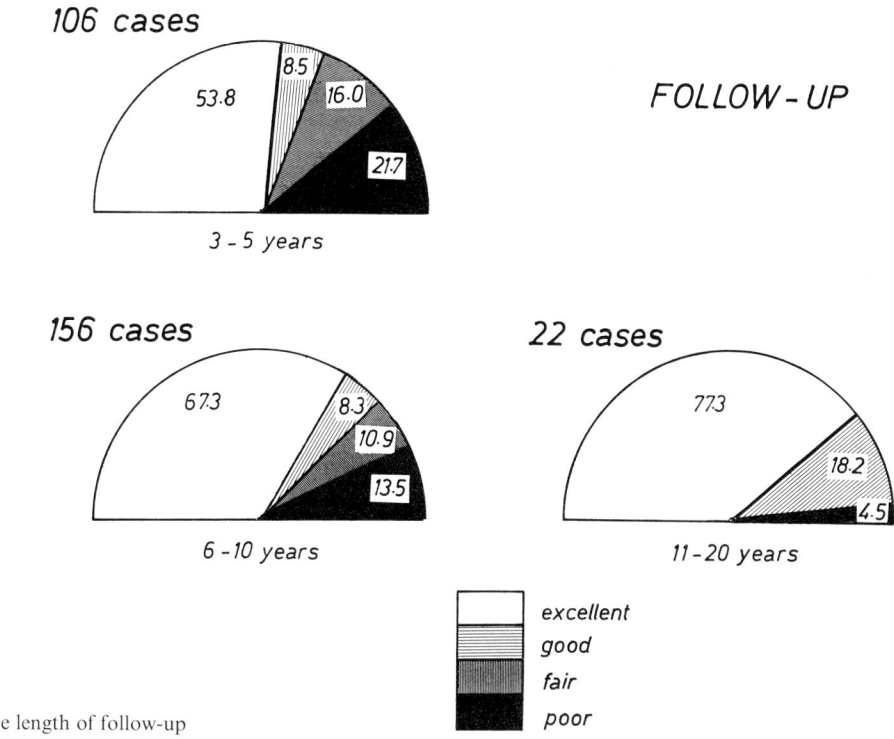

Fig. 267. Results related to the length of follow-up

B. Ten-Year Follow-up

More recently, we have reviewed 174 hips with a follow-up of at least 10 years after an intertrochanteric osteotomy. Most of them (160) were operated on for severe osteoarthritis as defined above (p. 286). The others (14) were dysplastic, with fewer than two of the three radiological signs mentioned above (p. 286). These 14 hips all underwent varus osteotomy. Many of the hips in this series were included in the previous analysis (WATILLON et al. 1978). Among the patients who could not be re-examined at 10 years, 64 were certainly dead. Some others expressed their satisfaction or dissatisfaction by mail. We heard from others through their families or general practitioners. However, 66 could not be traced (Table 47).

Table 47. Ten-year follow-up after Pauwels' intertrochanteric osteotomies

	Operations	Reviewed at 10 years	Not reviewed			
			Deaths	Good results	Poor results	Results unknown
PI	76	41	2	21	0	12
PII	464	133	62	146	69	54
Total	540	174	64	167	69	66

PI, Pauwels I; PII, Pauwels II

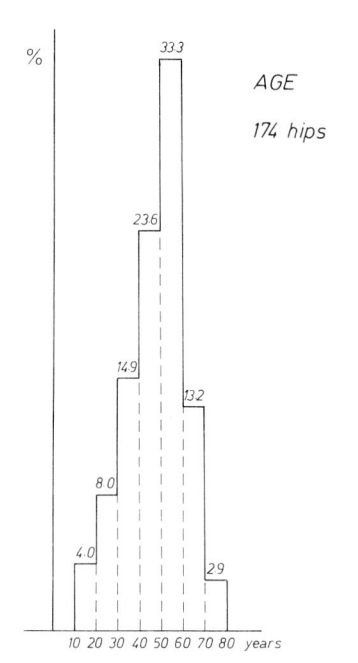

Fig. 268. Age distribution of patients in whom Pauwels' intertrochanteric osteotomy was performed. Follow-up of 10 years and more

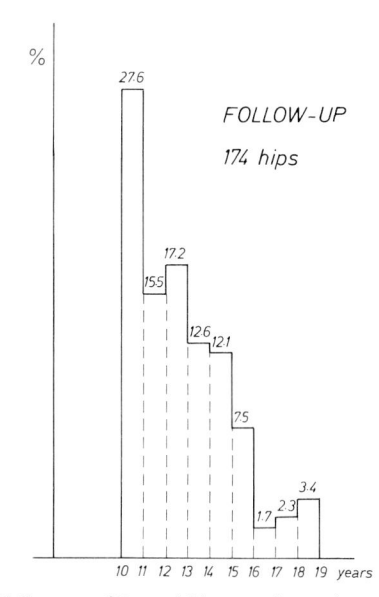

Fig. 269. Follow-up of Pauwels' intertrochanteric osteotomy patients

We thus personally examined and X-rayed 174 osteotomized hips with a follow-up of at least 10 years. The ages at operation ranged from 13 to 78 years (Fig. 268), and the follow-up periods from 10 to 18 years (Fig. 269). The right hip was affected in 60.9% of the cases and the left in 39.1%; 85.6% of the hips belonged to female patients and 14.4% to male patients. The results of valgus and varus intertrochanteric osteotomies were analysed separately.

1. Varus Intertrochanteric Osteotomy (Pauwels I)

Forty-one hips on which varus intertrochanteric osteotomies were carried out have been reviewed with a follow-up of at least 10 years. Among them, 27 were operated on for severe osteoarthritis as defined above (p. 286). The other 14 were dysplastic and exhibited fewer than two of the three radiological signs considered to indicate severe osteoarthritis. In nine of them the clinical symptoms associated with a dense triangle at the edge of the acetabulum prompted the operation. The other five patients had no clinical complaint, although in two of them a dense triangle was present at the edge of the acetabulum. In each of these five patients, a varus osteotomy was carried out as a means of shortening the leg to make the pelvis level. At the same time it was regarded as a prophylactic measure against osteoarthritis. These five hips causing no pre-operative complaint constitute 12.2% of the group of 41, and are represented by striped areas in Figs. 270 and 272.

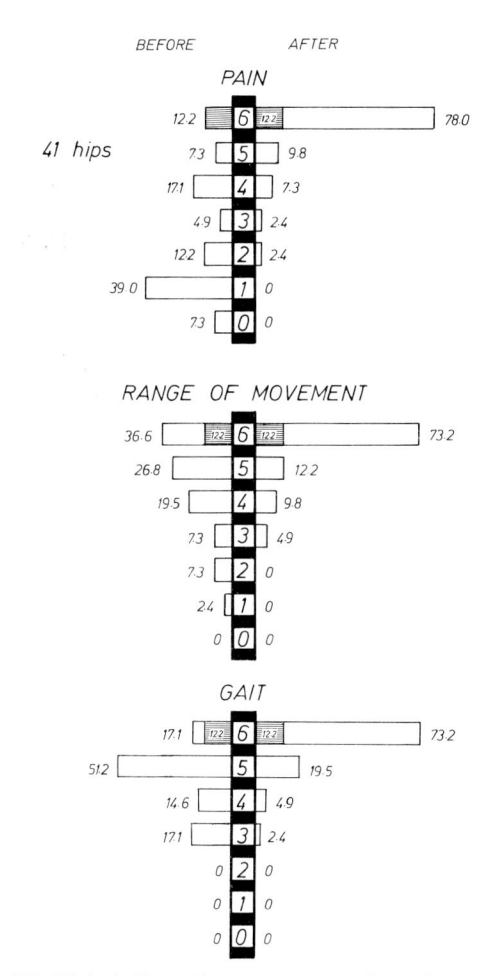

Fig. 270. Clinical effects of varus osteotomy. *Striped areas* represent the hips that were not showing clinical symptoms before operation. Follow-up of 10 years and more

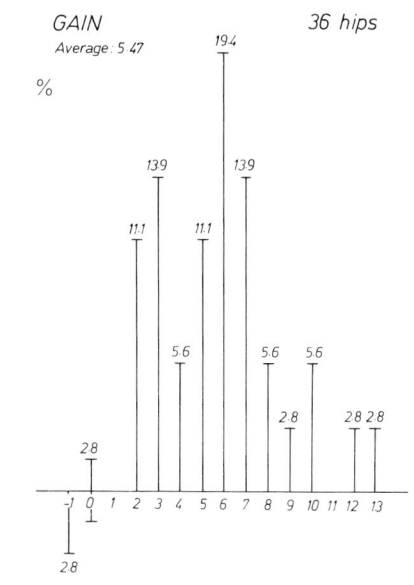

Fig. 271. Improvement in the Merle d'Aubigné rating following varus osteotomy. Follow-up of 10 years and more

The improvement in clinical rating has been calculated only for the 36 hips with clinical symptoms, since there was nothing to be gained clinically in the others (Fig. 271). The average gain was 5.47 points and 53.1% of the hips gained six points or more.

At the 10-year follow-up, 78% of the hips operated on were causing no pain at all; 9.8% were causing some discomfort, but only intermittently when the patient started walking (Fig. 270). The range of movement was improved, with 87.8% of the patients having a hip flexion range of at least 90° and abduction of at least 25°. The gait was normal in 73.2% and 19.5% had a slight limp. The TRENDELENBURG sign was positive in 43.9% of these patients before the operation and was negative in 85.4% at the latest follow-up.

The average total score was 11.95 (4–18) before the operation and 16.76 (8–18) at the latest follow-up (Table 48). At the latest follow-up 87.8% of the hips scored more than 14. These can be regarded as excellent or good clinical results.

Table 48. Effect of varus intertrochanteric osteotomy (Pauwels I) on the total clinical rating. $n = 41$

Before[a] (% of total)	Rating	At latest follow-up[b] (% of total)		
12.2	18	61.0 ⎫	73.2	Excellent
	17	12.2 ⎭		
4.9	16	7.3 ⎫	14.6	Good
9.8	15	7.3 ⎭		
4.9	14	2.4 ⎫		
9.8	13	2.4 ⎬	9.7	Fair
17.1	12	4.9 ⎭		
12.2	11	0 ⎫		
7.3	10	0 ⎬	2.4	Poor
4.9	9	0 ⎪		
	8	2.4 ⎭		
4.9	7	0		
7.3	6	0		
2.4	5	0		
2.4	4	0		

[a] Average rating 11.95; [b] average rating 16.76

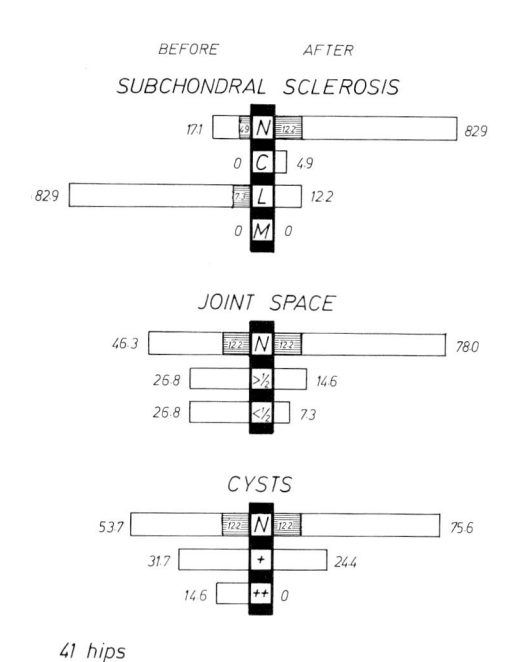

Fig. 272. Radiological changes following varus osteotomy. *Striped areas* represent the hips that were not showing clinical symptoms before operation. See Fig. 259 for abbreviations. Follow-up of 10 years and more

In the X-rays the subchondral sclerosis looked normal or cup-shaped in 87.8% of the hips, whereas it was normal in only 17.1% before operation (Fig. 272). The joint space had widened in most of the hips in which it was previously narrowed. The voluminous cysts had disappeared.

Five of the hips in this group deteriorated after delays varying between 7 and 16 years (Table 49). In one of these a valgus osteotomy was subsequently carried out; at the latest follow-up the result was excellent.

Table 49. Deterioration following varus intertrochanteric osteotomy (Pauwels I)

Delay (years)	No. of hips	Reoperation
16	1	
12	2	
10	1	PII
7	1	

PII, Pauwels II

The complications amounted to one pulmonary embolism (non-fatal) and one deep sepsis, which eventually healed after bony union had taken place and the metal had been removed.

We have attempted to rate the hips according to combined clinical and radiological criteria, as follows:

1. Excellent: scoring 17 or 18 *and* showing a subchondral sclerosis of even width throughout, a normal joint space and no cysts
2. Good: scoring 15 or 16 *and* showing at least two normal radiological signs (subchondral sclerosis, joint space, cysts)
3. Fair: scoring 12 to 14 *and* showing at least one normal radiological sign
4. Poor: the others

This rating is very severe. For instance, a hip scoring 18, although excellent clinically, will be rated as poor if it shows abnormal subchondral sclerosis, a joint space somewhat narrowed and some cysts. In other words, in order for the result to be regarded as excellent, a hip must be clinically *and* radiologically normal for all purposes. It is obvious that, according to these overall criteria, *no* total replacement would be rated as excellent or good since a replacement arthroplasty precludes the possibility of a normal or nearly normal radiological picture.

This rating is completely different from the one used in the previous analysis (p. 286). In this previous analysis the quality of the results was related to the clinical and radiological *improvement* of the hips after the operation rather than the *actual status*. The hips subjected to a varus intertrochanteric osteotomy were rated as shown in Table 50.

Table 50. Effect of varus intertrochanteric osteotomy on the overall rating

Before	Rating	At latest follow-up
0	Excellent	23 (56.1%)
8 (9.5%)	Good	10 (24.4%)
12 (29.3%)	Fair	3 (7.3%)
21 (51.2%)	Poor	5 (12.2%)

2. Valgus Intertrochanteric Osteotomy (Pauwels II)

One hundred and thirty-three hips on which we performed a valgus intertrochanteric osteotomy combined with a tenotomy of the abductor, adductor and iliopsoas muscles have been reviewed. In all of them there was severe osteoarthritis preoperatively. At the latest follow-up, 65.4% of these hips were giving absolutely no pain; 15.8% of the patients mentioned some intermittent discomfort when starting to walk (Fig. 273).

The range of movement was improved significantly, although it was complete only in 17.3% of the patients; 54.1% of the hips had flexion of more than 90° and abduction of more than 25°, whereas only 14.3% had that ability before the operation. The gait had become normal in 20.3% of the cases; 46.6% of the patients reported limping slightly when tired. However, 85.7% were able to walk for several hours, some of them (18.8%) with the aid of a walking stick. The TRENDELENBURG sign, which was positive in 88.7% of the hips before the operation, was negative in 74.4% at the latest follow-up.

Before the operation the total score ranged between 3 and 14, with an average of 7.88 (Table 51); at the latest follow-up it ranged between 5 and 18, with an average of 13.91, and 45.0% of the hips scored more than 14. The improvement in the clinical rating ranged from −3 (a loss of 3 points) to 13 (a gain of 13 points), with an average of 5.98 points (Fig. 274).

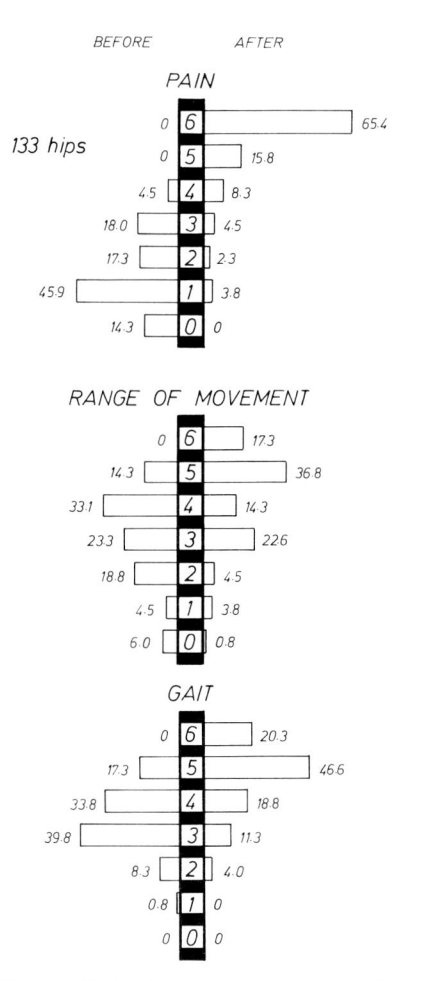

Fig. 273. Clinical effects of valgus osteotomy. Follow-up of 10 years and more

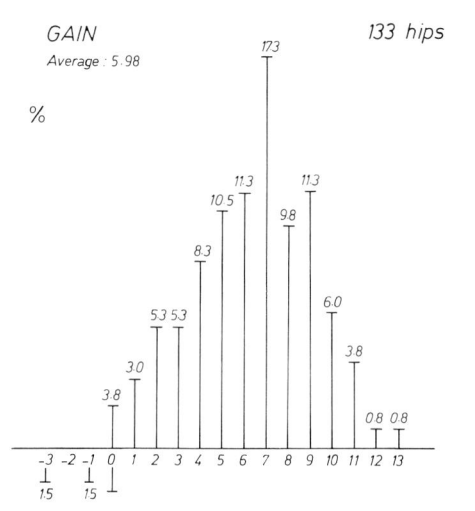

Fig. 274. Improvement in the Merle d'Aubigné rating following valgus osteotomy. Follow-up of 10 years and more

Table 51. Effect of valgus intertrochanteric osteotomy (Pauwels II) on the total clinical rating

Before[a] (% of total)	Rating	At latest follow-up[b] (% of total)		
0	18	6.0	19.5	Excellent
0	17	13.5		
0	16	15.0	25.5	Good
0	15	10.5		
1.5	14	21.1	37.7	Fair
1.5	13	11.3		
3.8	12	5.3		
7.5	11	5.3	17.4	Poor
12.8	10	2.3		
15.8	9	3.8		
14.3	8	1.5		
14.3	7	3.0		
13.5	6	0		
6.0	5	1.5		
4.5	4	0		
4.5	3	0		

[a] Average rating 7.88; [b] average rating 13.96

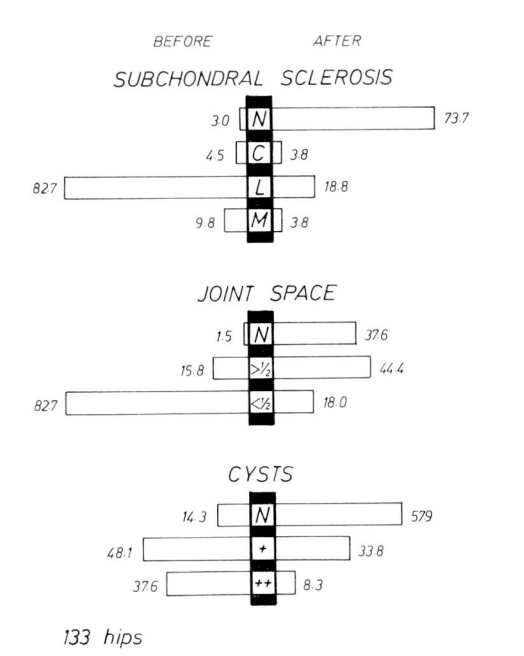

Fig. 275. Radiological changes following valgus osteotomy. Follow-up of 10 years and more. See Fig. 259 for abbreviations

The subchondral sclerosis was of even width throughout in the X-rays of 73.7% of the hips at the latest follow-up, whereas this was the case in only 3% before the operation (Fig. 275). There was no joint space in 82.7% of the hips before the operation. A joint space of normal width was present in 37.6% at the latest follow-up, and one of reduced width in 44.4% others. In only 18% did the joint space remain obliterated. The cysts disappeared or diminished in size and number in most of the hips. Large cysts remained in only 8.3%.

Deterioration occurred in 36 hips (27.1%) after periods varying from 4 to 18 years (Table 52). Six of these hips were reoperated on with good results.

The complications comprised one pulmonary embolism, one superficial sepsis, which eventually healed, and three breakdowns of fixation due to technical errors. These patients were reoperated on immediately and subsequently did well.

The hips have also been rated as explained on page 292 (Table 53). According to these very demanding criteria all the 133 hips were regarded as in poor condition before surgery, but in 36.1% of them the results were excellent − indicating a normal hip − or good at the latest follow-up.

Table 52. Deterioration following valgus intertrochanteric osteotomy (Pauwels II)

Delay (years)	No. of hips	%	Reoperation
18	2	1.5	
16	1	0.8	1 TP
15	1	0.8	
14	2	1.5	
13	3	2.3	
12	5	3.8	1 Arthrodesis
11	4	3.0	1 TP
10	7	5.3	2 TP
9	3	2.3	
8	4	3.0	
7	1	0.8	1 PII
6	1	0.8	
5	1	0.8	
4	1	0.8	

TP, total prosthesis; PII, Pauwels II

Table 53. Effect of valgus intertrochanteric osteotomy (Pauwels II) on the overall rating

Before	Rating	At latest follow-up
0	Excellent	18 (13.5%)
0	Good	30 (22.6%)
0	Fair	48 (36.1%)
133 (100%)	Poor	37 (27.8%)

3. Comment

The results of the varus osteotomy seem to be better than those of the valgus osteotomy. However, as shown by Figs. 270, 272, 273 and 275, a valgus osteotomy was generally carried out on hips in far worse condition than those undergoing a varus osteotomy. This results from the respective indications for the two types of osteotomy. Thus it appears that the sooner an osteoarthritic hip is operated on, the better is the outcome. But it is remarkable that so many joints which looked dismal both clinically and radiologically could recover a good and pain-free function and show a kind of regeneration in the X-ray after being operated on.

Only clinical considerations are usually taken into account in judging the outcome of a total replacement, since the X-ray pictures before and after the procedure are hardly comparable. Therefore, in order to compare the results of replacement arthroplasty with those of joint-preserving procedures reference must be made to Tables 42, 48, 51 and 54.

The early X-ray results in the majority of the hips seemed to imply that the mechanical aim of the intertrochanteric osteotomy had been achieved, so false indications were rare in this series. However, in some instances of late deterioration, it appeared that the congruence of the articular surfaces had never been ideal or that some mechanical defect, such as a very short lever arm of the abductor muscles, had not been corrected sufficiently. Other deteriorations can be explained only by metabolic disturbances.

III. Lateral Displacement of the Greater Trochanter

A. Single Procedure

Lateral displacement of the greater trochanter combined with a tenotomy of the adductor and iliopsoas muscles was carried out as the sole procedure for severe osteoarthritis or aseptic necrosis of the femoral head in 25 hips, with a follow-up of 1 year or more. These 25 hips have all been reviewed.

The ages at operation ranged from 21 to 73 years (Fig. 276), the follow-up from 1 to more than 6 years (Fig. 277). Except for one complete failure, which was followed by reoperation and total hip replacement, the pain relief was dramatic. The range of movement increased considerably and the gait improved (Fig. 278). The TRENDELENBURG

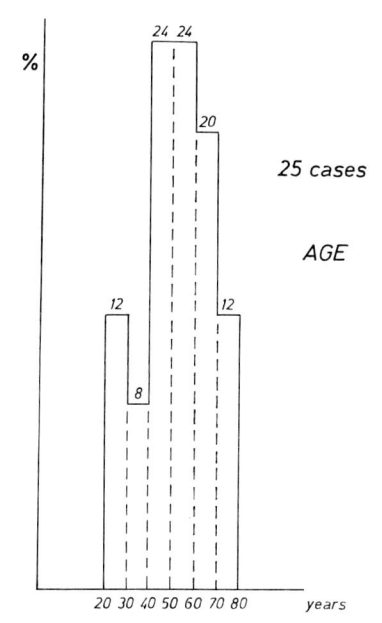

Fig. 276. Age distribution of patients in whom a lateral displacement of the greater trochanter was carried out

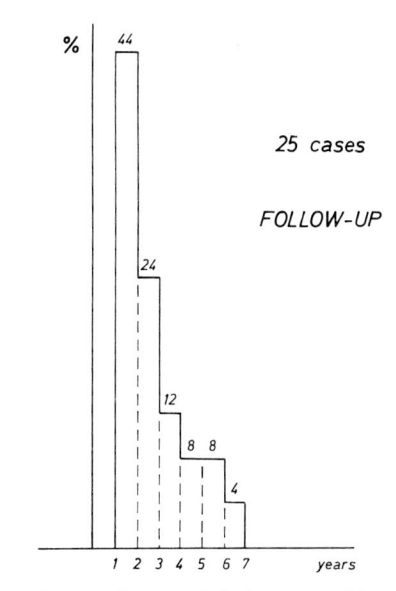

Fig. 277. Follow-up after lateral displacement of the greater trochanter

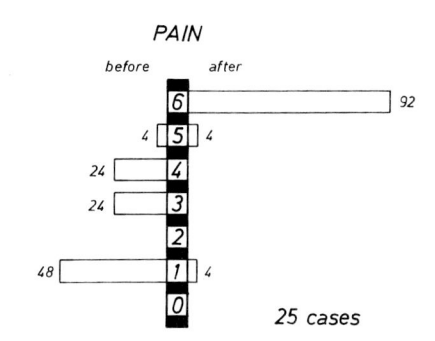

Fig. 278. Clinical effects of lateral displacement of the greater trochanter

sign was previously positive in three patients and it remained positive in 1.

The total clinical score ranged from 5 to 16, with an average of 10.60 before the operation; at the latest follow-up it ranged from 7 to 18, with an average of 16.44 (Table 54). The average gain was 5.84 points, with extremes of -1 and $+10$ (Fig. 279).

Table 54. Effect of lateral displacement of the greater trochanter on the total clinical rating

Before[a] (% of total)	Rating	At latest follow-up[b] (% of total)		
0	18	44.0	72.0	Excellent
0	17	28.0		
4.0	16	8.0	8.0	Good
4.0	15	0		
4.0	14	12.0		
12.0	13	4.0	16.0	Fair
16.0	12	0		
12.0	11	0		
16.0	10	0		
4.0	9	0		
20.0	8	0	4.0	Poor
0	7	4.0		
4.0	6	0		
4.0	5	0		

[a] Average rating 10.60;   [b] average rating 16.44

In the X-ray, the joint space had widened in most cases. The subchondral sclerosis had become normal or nearly normal except in the failed case. The cysts had filled up or were filling up (Fig. 280).

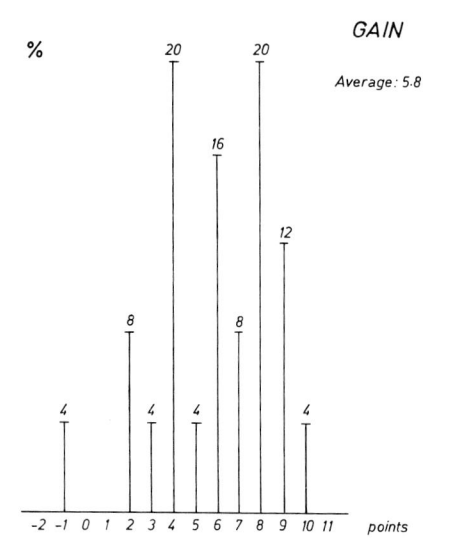

Fig. 279. Improvement in the Merle d'Aubigné rating following lateral displacement of the greater trochanter

The only complication in this series was fracture and displacement of the lateral fragment at its base, which occurred in five cases. These cases were reoperated on during the first postoperative days and the lateral fragment fixed with a screw. This complication is avoided by fixing the fragment systematically with a screw at operation. Its occurrence does not seem to have influenced the end result.

We have attempted to rate these hips by combining clinical *and* radiological criteria as described on page 292. Table 55 gives the overall results based on these very demanding criteria.

Table 55. Effect of lateral displacement of the greater trochanter on the overall rating

Before	Rating	At latest follow-up
0	Excellent	5 (20.0%)
0	Good	8 (32.0%)
4 (16.0%)	Fair	8 (32.0%)
21 (84.0%)	Poor	4 (16.0%)

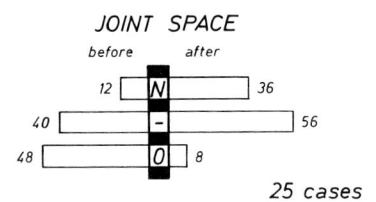

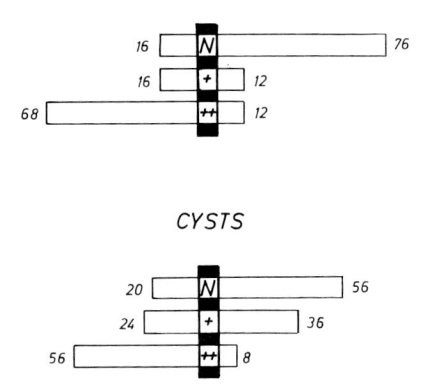

Fig. 280. Radiological changes following lateral displacement of the greater trochanter. *Subchondral sclerosis*: N, normal subchondral sclerosis in the roof of the acetabulum; C, cup-shaped subchondral sclerosis; L, triangular sclerosis at the lateral edge of the acetabulum; M, medial sclerotic triangle in the depths of the acetabulum. *Joint space*: N, normal joint space; $>1/2$ joint space wider than half its normal width; $<1/2$ joint space narrower than half its normal width. *Cysts*: N, no cysts; +, small cysts; + +, big cysts

B. As a Complement to an Intertrochanteric Osteotomy

Lateral displacement of the greater trochanter was also carried out in an additional series of 11 patients in whom previous intertrochanteric varus or valgus osteotomy had provided congruence of the articular surfaces. In these patients, the lateral displacement of the greater trochanter was intended further to improve the mechanical condition of the hip. These cases are not included in our review, since the contribution of each of the two successive operations in the overall regeneration of the joint is difficult to evaluate properly.

IV. Schanz Osteotomy

We carried out eight SCHANZ osteotomies for congenitally dislocated hips (painful in seven cases). In the eighth case, the purpose of the osteotomy was to eliminate a limp in a 12-year-old girl. This was the youngest patient of the series, which included only female patients. The oldest was 68 years (average age: 47.5 years). One of the patients had undergone, 22 and 20 years previously, a shelf operation and then an intertrochanteric osteotomy, the aim of which was not clear. This patient was the only one with bilateral dislocation. The others had been immobilized in a plaster spica, one at the age of 15 months, the other at the age of 3 years, probably after an attempt to reduce the congenital dislocation. The apparent discrepancy in length of the legs ranged from 0 (bilateral dislocation) to 7.5 cm. The discrepancy corresponds to the height of the support which had to be inserted under the foot of the affected side to make the pelvis level.

Except in the youngest patient, before operation the pain was excruciating and persisted at night. In six of the eight cases, the range of movement was satisfactory. Walking was limited in all cases.

The shortening resulting from surgery varied from 0 to 4.5 cm in our series. In four patients there was none. The apparent discrepancy in leg length after surgery ranged from 0 (bilateral dislocation) to 12 cm. Four patients requested and underwent shortening of the opposite femur to make the pelvis level (5, 6, 7 and 8 cm respectively). Two of these four patients and two others underwent supracondylar osteotomy of the femur on the dislocated side in order to correct a valgus deformity of the knee with overloading of the lateral plateau.

The patients were followed-up for periods between 3 years 8 months and 9 years 11 months after surgery, except for one who was reoperated on after 10 months because of early failure (Table 56). Six hips had become completely or almost completely pain-free. The range of movement had hardly changed, but the quality of gait had greatly improved (gain of 1 or 2 points). If we consider a total of 17–18 points an excellent result and a total of 14–16 points a good result, two of the eight patients had an excellent result and three a good result. Seven patients had resumed their previous occupation or had become more active. Six patients had improved by 5–10 points. One had not progressed as far as the rating was concerned. The patient with the poor result lost 2 points.

We have no personal experience of the LORENZ osteotomy.

Table 56. Schanz osteotomy. Ages and follow-ups

Age (years)	Follow-up (years–months)	
12	6	7
42	6	1
42	3	8
44	9	2
49	9	11
59	4	10
64	6	2
68	0	10

V. Conclusion

The results (and principally the long-term results) of these joint-preserving operations obviously justify the mechanical approach to the problem of osteoarthritis of the hip and emphasize its practical significance.

Chapter VIII. General Conclusions

In an attempt to assess the initial research of PAUWELS (1935), we have calculated the force transmitted across a normal hip joint when the subject is standing with the weight supported symmetrically, when the subject is standing on one leg and during the single-support period of gait. The normal hip of our study was that of the subject studied by BRAUNE and FISCHER (1895) and FISCHER (1899, 1900, 1901, 1903, 1904). Our results thus pertain to this particular individual, whose weight was 58.7 kg and whose height was 169 cm. They can be expressed conveniently in fractions or multiples of body weight. The force exerted on the hip joint attains more than four times body weight during the single-support period of gait at a velocity of 5.6 km/h, whereas while the subject is standing on both feet it reaches only 31% of body weight. This corresponds closely to the data collected by other authors dealing with other individuals. The resultant force thus calculated depends on the formularization of the mechanical conditions and must be regarded not as an exact figure but rather as an approximation of the force actually transmitted across the hip. This force may vary in different individuals. However, in view of the range of anatomical variations which is accepted as normal, the variations in this force between different individuals can only be small. Therefore, the results we achieved can be regarded as indicating the order of magnitude of the force exerted on the normal hip joint.

With respect to the weight-bearing surface of the joint we relied on the work of KUMMER (1968, 1978, 1979). Knowing the force exerted on the hip and the weight-bearing area, and assuming an even distribution of joint pressure over the weight-bearing surface, KUMMER deduced that the articular compressive stresses attain 16–20 kg/cm^2 during gait. This coincides with the value of the compressive stresses evoked in the knee joint under similar circumstances, as calculated in a previous work (MAQUET 1976).

According to PAUWELS' law, the quantity of bone present depends on the magnitude of the stresses to which it is subjected. Between certain limits, an increase in the compressive stresses in the joint leads to apposition of bone in the subchondral area of the joint, particularly in the roof of the acetabulum; a decrease in the articular compressive stresses causes resorption of bone. Actually, the subchondral sclerosis in the roof of the acetabulum displays the same shape as the outline of the diagram of the articular compressive stresses in a model. It was called "sourcil" by PAUWELS (Sourcil is a French word meaning eyebrow). In a normal hip, the sourcil appears as a thin ribbon of uniform width throughout. In subluxating osteoarthritis this thin ribbon is replaced by a dense triangle at the edge of the socket. In protrusive osteoarthritis, a dense triangle is observed in the depths of the acetabulum. A cup-shaped subchondral sclerosis, a sourcil thick in the middle and thinning towards its edges, implies a normal geometry of the forces but a biological deficiency of the tissues, which are no longer able to distribute the physiological pressure evenly over the weight-bearing surface of the joint. Secondarily, the cartilage disappears, subjected to articular compressive stresses which it is no longer able to withstand. *Osteoarthritis thus represents an imbalance between the resistance of the articular tissues and their mechanical stressing.* This is our working hypothesis.

We can hardly influence the resistance of the tissues, so *the only logical way of dealing with osteoarthritis is to decrease the compressive stresses in the joint* in an attempt to make them tolerable to the articular tissues, even if the resistance of the latter is lower than normal. As pointed out by PAUWELS, the compressive stresses in a joint can be decreased either by reducing the force transmitted across the joint or by enlarging the weight-bearing surface of the joint. The ideal solution would combine both possibilities.

Voss suggested the division of the tendons of the adductor and abductor muscles. PAUWELS also divided that of the iliopsoas. This multiple tenotomy (hanging-hip procedure) decreases the resultant force acting on the hip. It does not modify the weight-bearing surface of the joint. In properly selected hips it has given us amazing results clinically and radiologically: suppression of pain, improvement of the range of movement and of gait, regression of the signs of osteoarthritis and reappearance of a wide joint space in the X-rays. Such results are achieved only when the weight-bearing surface of the joint is not reduced. When it is reduced, it is imperative that it be enlarged.

The weight-bearing surface of the joint can be enlarged either by carrying out a varus intertrochanteric osteotomy, a valgus intertrochanteric osteotomy or a lateral displacement of the greater trochanter, or by shortening the opposite leg, thus simulating a valgus osteotomy. The varus intertrochanteric osteotomy and the lateral displacement of the greater trochanter also decrease the force transmitted across the joint by lengthening the lever arm of the muscular force. To the same end, that is the reduction or further reduction of the resultant force, a tenotomy of the abductor, adductor and iliopsoas muscles always complements the valgus intertrochanteric osteotomy, and a tenotomy of the adductor and iliopsoas muscles complements the lateral displacement of the greater trochanter.

As long as the indications are correct, these surgical procedures usually result in dramatic changes in the joint: replacement of the dense triangle at the edge or in the depths of the acetabulum by a subchondral sclerosis of uniform width throughout, filling in of the cysts and development of a wide joint space. These signs are concomitant with relief of pain and in most instances with an increase in the range of movement and an improvement in gait. The same impressive results are achieved by any of the aforementioned procedures, although some of them, such as the varus and the valgus osteotomies, seem to be exactly contrary to each other. The prerequisite for a good result is a sufficient enlargment of the weight-bearing surface of the joint. Conversely, when these same procedures fail to enlarge the weight-bearing surface of the joint because they were never truly indicated, they are usually followed by a poor clinical result and further deterioration of the joint. These facts actually make sense in the light of our working hypothesis.

Despite the biological effects of osteotomy, simply dividing the bone does not seem to be sufficient systematically to ensure satisfactory results. Careful planning and precise surgery are mandatory. Every case must be analysed individually. X-rays taken with the hip in different positions facilitate the choice of the proper operation. The procedure must be planned on paper from a tracing of an anteroposterior X-ray. The wedge to be resected, the magnitude of the lateral displacement of the greater trochanter or that of the shortening of the opposite leg must be determined accurately. Only then should the operation be carried out. It must be performed precisely, according to the pre-operative plan. Lack of planning or of operative accuracy both lead to failure.

Enthusiastic rehabilitation with forceful strengthening of the muscles will jeopardize the result. We do not want strong muscles, since we divide tendons in order to decrease the force exerted on the hip by the muscles. With gentle walking the muscles will strengthen sufficiently quite soon enough.

No standard procedure has been proposed. Each affected hip must be considered individually on the basis of its own mechanical conditions. This is, therefore, a demanding approach, although the procedures themselves are simple enough, once they have been correctly chosen and planned.

If the mechanical conditions are surgically improved to a significant extent at an early stage of the disease, when the original cartilage is not yet destroyed, the results are long-lasting. Not one secondary deterioration was observed among such cases in our series. It can be assumed that the articular tissues which are original retain their coefficient of safety. This coefficient of safety was estimated as 6–7 by PAUWELS. This means that the tissues can withstand stresses 6 or 7 times higher than normal for relatively long periods of time without yielding.

When appropriate surgery is carried out at a later stage of the disease, after cartilage has been destroyed and bone remodelled, the signs of osteoarthritis regress and a wide joint space develops. This joint space seems to be composed of fibrocartilage. This represents a healing process, a scar. It is reasonable to assume that the coefficient of safety of such tissue is lower than normal. It may vary from one patient to another. The healed hip would then be less resistant than normal to mechanical stressing. This would explain the recurrences occurring after 10 years or more. Some of these recurrences are concomitant with arterial occlusions in the lower limb or with a cerebral thrombosis. Some occur at the menopause. But many remain unexplained. Does the coefficient of safety of the healed tissues vary during the life of the individual, depending on hormonal or vascular circumstances? This question remains as yet unanswered. Most hips in which the condition recurs after a certain number of years remain clinically better than they were before the operation. This also remains to be explained.

In some of the hips with recurrent osteoarthritis a total replacement was eventually carried out without any difficulty. These patients had gained a certain number of years before having a prosthetic replacement. Some, mainly because of their age, underwent a further osteotomy and the process of healing was observed again. After such revisions, our results remained good at the 6- or 7-year follow-up. This demonstrates the continuous ability of the living tissues to react positively to improved mechanical conditions. The ability of the tissues to react persists to the last years of life, as demonstrated by our results in patients over 70 years old.

Most of the hips operated on, however, have remained pain-free and fully functional, with X-ray pictures which show the result of a healing process or the continuation of the healing process over many years. We cannot yet say whether or not these hips will remain in good condition indefinitely. However, some of our patients have walked on their healed joints for 15 years and more without any alteration. Except for the first postoperative months, their lives were active and practically without restriction. The result achieved by using living tissues thus seems to be satisfactory and far more stable than that following any prosthetic replacement.

The surgical procedures thus proposed, when properly indicated, lead to a true regression of the degenerative process which we call osteoarthritis. Therefore, they constitute a real treatment of the condition. They are hardly to be compared with any of the prosthetic arthroplasties which actually bypass the problem of osteoarthritis by extirpation of the affected joint.

Appendix: Fixation of the Fragments After Intertrochanteric Osteotomy

The fixation of the fragments after intertrochanteric osteotomy which we devised (MAQUET 1967) constitutes an application of the tension band principle. At the osteotomy level the femur is subjected to bending stress by a force acting medially and posteriorly in such a way that, after a fracture or an osteotomy, the fragments tend to open laterally and anteriorly (Fig. 281) (PAUWELS 1973).

The femur can be compared to a curved column supporting a load (Fig. 282a). If the column is broken at its mid-point its upper part and the load tip (Fig. 282b). A chain attached on the side of the convexity will hinder tipping of the load (Fig. 282c). Then the fragments are subjected to compressive stresses at fracture level, with a maximum at the concave margin. The chain can be replaced by a turn-buckle. Tightening of the turn-buckle produces compressive stresses between the fragments, with a maximum at the convex margin if the column is unloaded (Fig. 282d). This is called "prestressing". Loading the column creates compressive stresses with a maximum on the concave side. Following an appropriate tightening of the turn-buckle, the compressive stresses can become evenly distributed over the fracture surfaces of the loaded column (Fig. 282e).

The compression-hook acts on the fragments of the femur as does the turn-buckle on those of the column. During surgery the hook prestresses the osteotomy site (Fig. 283), producing compressive stresses which are at their greatest at its lateral margin and decrease medially.

As soon as the muscles and, eventually, the body weight act, they also produce compressive stresses, which are at their greatest in the medial aspect of the osteotomy site. From an appropriate prestressing of the hook, the compressive stresses are distributed over the whole osteotomy surfaces when muscles and body weight act (Fig. 284).

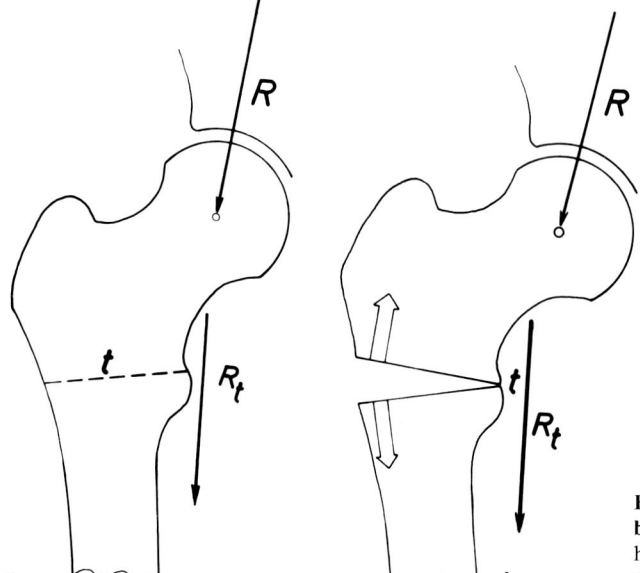

Fig. 281a, b. Force acting at osteotomy level: **a** intact hip, **b** after osteotomy. R, resultant of the forces acting on the hip; R_t, resultant of the forces acting on the femur at osteotomy level t

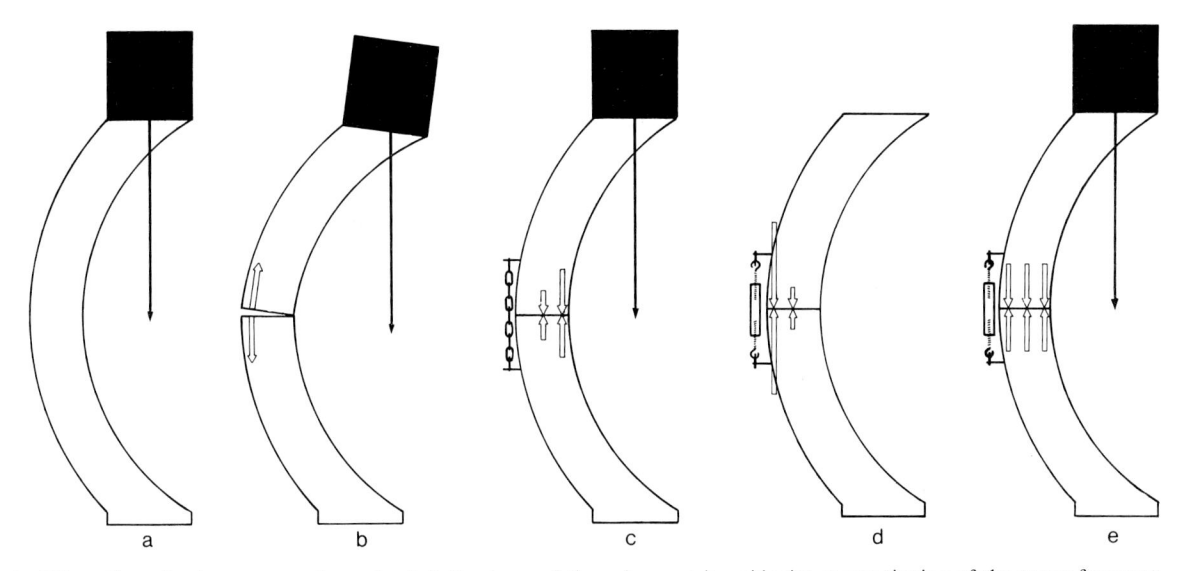

Fig. 282. a Curved column supporting a load. **b** Breakage of the column at its midpoint causes tipping of the upper fragment with the load. **c** A tension band attached to the convex side hinders tipping. **d** Turn-buckle prestressing the column. **e** Combined action of the load and turn-buckle

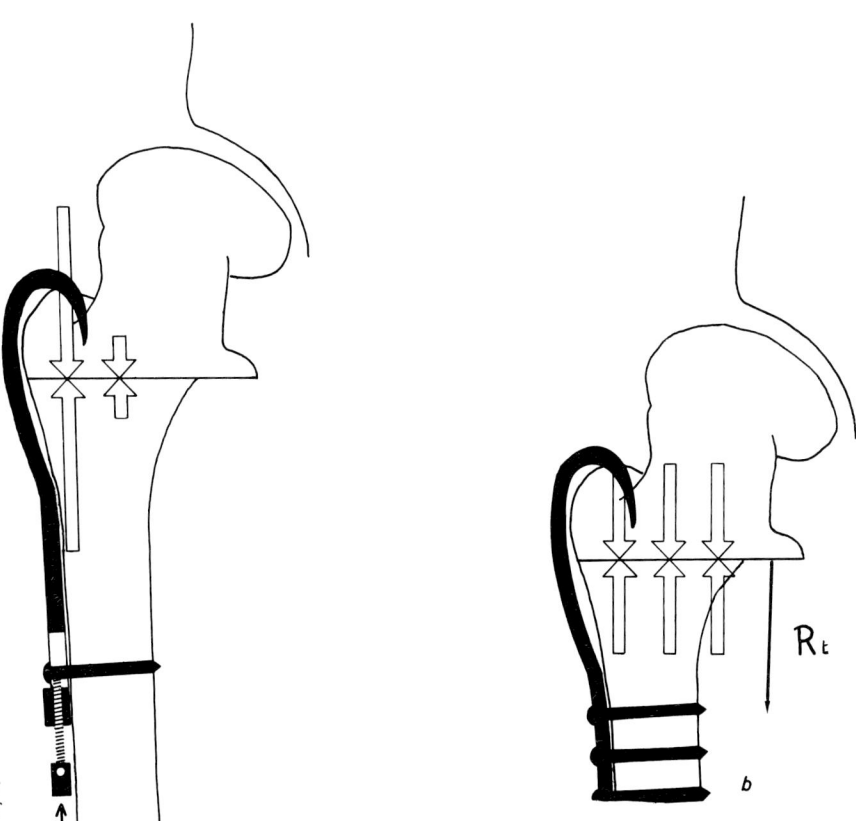

Fig. 283. Prestressing of the femur after osteotomy and tigthening of the compression-hook

Fig. 284. Combined action of the load and compression-hook

We illustrated the action of the compression-hook in a photoelastic model of the upper end of the femur, transversely divided at the level of the lesser trochanter. The fragments were fixed by a compression-hook. When the hook is tightened, isochromatics appear in the lateral aspect of the model, attaining the fringe order 6 (Fig. 285a).

The model is then loaded medially by a cable pulling downwards from the medial aspect of the femoral head. Isochromatics appear all over the fracture site. They attain the order 4 in its centre (Fig. 285b). Our hook thus acts as a prestressing tension band and ensures solid fixation of the fragments under compression.

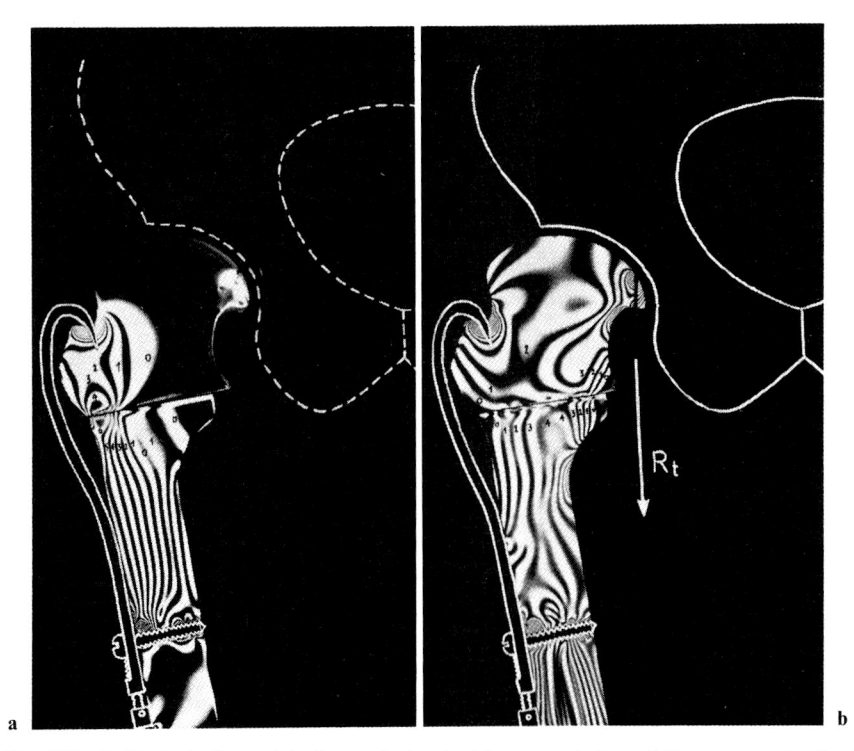

Fig. 285a, b. Photoelastic model of an osteotomized femur. **a** Action of the compression-hook; **b** combined action of the load and compression-hook

References

Amtmann E, Kummer B (1968) Die Beanspruchung des menschlichen Hüftgelenks II. Größe und Richtung der Hüftgelenkresultierenden in der Frontalebene. Anat Embryol (Berl) 127:286–314

Banks SW, Laufman H (1958) An atlas of surgical exposures of the extremities. Saunders, Philadelphia

Bertrand P (1962) Malformations luxantes de la hanche. Doin, Paris

Bertrand P, Guias H, Benard HM (1964) Réflexions sur les butées dans les subluxations de la hanche. Rev Chir Orthop 50:123–131

Bertrand P, Benard HM, Chassagne A, Havret P (1966) Notre expérience de la résection cervico-diaphysaire du fémur avec ostéotomie d'angulation. Rev Chir Orthop 52:121–135

Bombelli R (1976) Osteoarthritis of the hip. Springer, Berlin Heidelberg New York

Boppe (1936) Bull méd 281

Braune W, Fischer O (1889) Über den Schwerpunkt des menschlichen Körpers mit Rücksicht auf die Ausrüstung des Deutschen Infanteristen. Abhandl der math-phys Cl d k Sächs Ges der Wissensch XV:560–672

Braune W, Fischer O (1895) Der Gang des Menschen. I Teil. Versuche am unbelasteten und belasteten Menschen. Abhandl d Math-Phys Cl d k Sächs Ges. der Wissensch 21:153–322

Byers PD (1974) The effect of high osteotomy on osteoarthritis of the hip: an anatomical study of six hip joints. J Bone Joint Surg [Br] 56:279–290

Camera U (1954) Ostéoplasties articulaires et juxta-articulaires comme traitement complémentaire de l'arthroplastie biologique de la hanche. SICOT 6th Congress, Bern. Imprimerie des Sciences, Bruxelles, pp 531–539

Camera U (1956) Le traitement opératoire biologique de certaines affections osseuses et ostéo-articulaires. Lyon Chir 51:73–83

Carlson CJ (1969) Healing of cartilage defects. Clin Orthop 64:45

Carstens C (1982) Untersuchungen zur mechanischen Beanspruchung der Osteophyten des arthrotischen Femurkopfes. Z Orthop 120:698–701

Chiari K (1955) Ergebnisse mit der Beckenosteotomie als Pfannendachplastik. Z Orthop 87:14

Chiari K (1970) Die Beckenosteotomie (Kongress Wien, Sept. 1969) F. Enke Stuttgart

Colonna PC (1936) An arthroplastic operation for congenital dislocation of the hip — a two stage procedure. Surg Gynecol Obstet 63:777

Colonna PC (1947) Arthroplasty of the hip for congenital dislocation in children. J Bone Joint Surg 29:711

Delchef J, Delchef J, Falla G (1959) L'utilisation de la peau en chirurgie orthopédique. Acta Orthop Belg 25:1–84

Doliveux P (1966) Proposition de définition de l'opération de Mc Murray. Rev Chir Orthop 52:561–563

Endler F (1972) Traitement biomécanique chirurgical de la nécrose avasculaire de la tête fémorale. Acta Orthop Belg 38:537–545

Fick A (1860) Über die Längenverhältnisse der Skeletmuskeln; Moleschotts Untersuchungen zur Naturlehre, vol 7

Fick A (1879) Handbuch der Physiologie, vol 1. Hermann, Leipzig

Fischer O (1899) Der Gang des Menschen. II Teil. Die Bewegung des Gesammtschwerpunktes und die äußeren Kräfte. Abhandl d Math-Phys Cl d k Sächs Ges der Wissensch 25:1–163

Fischer O (1900) Der Gang des Menschen. III Teil. Betrachtungen über die weiteren Ziele der Untersuchung und Überblick über die Bewegung der unteren Extremitäten. Abhandl Math-Phys Cl Sächs Ges der Wissensch 26:87–185

Fischer O (1901) Der Gang des Menschen. IV Teil. Über die Bewegung des Fußes und die auf denselben einwirkenden Kräfte. Abhandl d Math-Phys Cl d k Sächs Ges der Wissensch 26:471–569

Fischer O (1903) Der Gang des Menschen. V Teil. Die Kinematik des Beinschwingens. Abhandl d Math-Phys Cl d k Sächs Ges. der Wissensch 28:321–428

Fischer O (1904) Der Gang des Menschen. VI Teil. Über den Einfluß der Schwere und der Muskeln auf die Schwingungsbewegung des Beins. Abhandl d Math-Phys Cl d k Sächs Ges. der Wissensch 28:533–623

Föppl L, Mönch E (1959) Praktische Spannungsoptik. Springer, Berlin Göttingen Heidelberg

Fujisawa Y, Masuhara K, Matsumoto N, Mil N, Fujihara H, Yamaguchi T, Shomi S (1976) The effect of high tibial osteotomy on osteoarthritis of the knee. An arthroscopic study of 26 knee joints. Clin Orthop Surg (Jpn) 11:576–590

Gardner DL (1983) The nature and cause of osteoarthrosis. Br Med J 286:418–424

Grasset EJ (1960) La coxarthrose. Georg, Genève, Masson, Paris

Greenwald AS, O'Connor JJ (1971) The transmission of load through the human hip joint. J Biomech 4:507–528

Greenwald AS, Haynes DW (1972) Weight bearing areas in the human hip joint. J Bone Joint Surg 54:157–163

Hamacher P, Roesler H (1971) Die Berechnung von Größe und Richtung der Hüftgelenksresultierenden im Einzelfall. Arch Orthop Trauma Surg, 70:26–35

Hamacher P, Roesler H (1972) Ergebnisse der Berechnung von Größe und Richtung der Hüftgelenksresultierenden im Einzelfall. Arch Orthop Trauma Surg 72:94–106

Herbert JJ (1950) Chirurgie et orthopédie du rhumatisme. Masson, Paris

Kettunen KO (1958) Skin arthroplasty. Acta Orthop Scand [Suppl] 29:9

Kiaer S (1950) Afferent pain paths in man running from the spongiosa in the femoral head and running through the lumbar sympathetic ganglion. Acta Orthop Scand 19:383–390

Knief JJ (1967) Materialverteilung und Beanspruchungsverteilung im coxalen Femurende. Densitometrische und spannungsoptische Untersuchungen. Anat Embryol (Berl) 126:81–116

Kummer B (1956) Eine vereinfachte Methode zur Darstellung von Spannungstrajektorien, gleichzeitig ein Modellversuch in den Gelenkenden der Röhrenknochen. Anat Embryol (Berl) 119:223–234

Kummer B (1959) Bauprinzipien des Säugerskelets. Thieme, Stuttgart

Kummer B (1963) Principles of the biomechanics of the human supporting and locomotor system SICOT IXe Congres. Postgraduate course. Verlag der Wiener Medizinische Akademie, Vienna, pp 60–80

Kummer B (1968) Die Beanspruchung des menschlichen Hüftgelenks. I. Allgemeine Problematik. Anat Embryol (Berl) 127:277–285

Kummer B (1969) Die Beanspruchung der Gelenke, dargestellt am Beispiel des menschlichen Hüftgelenks. Verhandlungen der Deutschen Gesellschaft für Orthopädie und Traumatologie 55th Congress, Kassel, 1968. Enke, Stuttgart

Kummer B (1972) Biomechanics of bone: mechanical properties, functional structure, functional adaptation. In: Fung YC, Perone N, Anliker M (eds) Biomechanics: its function and objectives. Prentice-Hall, Englewood Cliffs

Kummer B (1973) Bone remodeling as a function of mechanical stress. Jugosl Akad Znanosti Umjetnosti 5–20

Kummer B (1974) Biomechanik der Gelenke (Diarthrosen). Die Beanspruchung des Gelenkknorpels. Biopolymere und Biomechanik von Bindegewebssystemen. 7. Wiss Konf Dtsch Nat-Forsch. Ärzte. Springer, Berlin, Heidelberg New York

Kummer B (1978) Anatomie fonctionnelle et biomécanique de la hanche. Acta Orthop Belg 44:94–104

Kummer B (1979) Die Tragfläche des Hüftgelenks. Z Orthop 117:411–712

Kurrat HJ (1977) Die Beanspruchung des menschlichen Hüftgelenks. VI. Eine funktionelle Analyse der Knorpeldickenverteilung am menschlichen Femurkopf. Anat Embryol (Berl) 150:129–140

Langlais F, Roure JL, Maquet P (1978) L'ostéotomie de valgisation dans les coxarthroses évoluées. Indications et résultats de 150 interventions consécutives. Rev Chir Orthop 64:607–623

Langlais F, Roure JL, Maquet P (1979) Valgus osteotomy in severe osteoarthritis of the hip. J Bone Joint Surg [Br] 61:424–431

Leriche R, Jung A (1933) Essais de traitement de la polyarthrite chronique par des opérations sympathiques. Presse Méd 41:66

Lorenz A (1919) Über die Behandlung der irreponiblen angeborenen Hüftluxationen und der Schenkelhalspseudarthrosen mittels Gabelung (Bifurkation des oberen Femurendes). Wien Klin Wochenschr 14

Maquet P (1966) Ostéotomie de Mc Murray. Rev Chir Orthop 52:526–532

Maquet P (1967) La fixation des fragments fémoraux après ostéotomie intertrochantérienne Acta Orthop Belg 33:57–66

Maquet P (1970) Biomechanics and osteoarthritis of the hip. SICOT XIe Congrès, Mexico 1969. Imprimerie des Sciences, Bruxelles, pp 317–357

Maquet P (1971) A biomechanical approach to the surgical treatment of osteoarthritis of the hip. Am Dig foreign Orthop Lit 1:16–20

Maquet P (1971) Le principe de Pauwels dans le traitement de la coxarthrose. Acta Orthop Belg 37:477–487

Maquet P (1971) Le coapteur à griffes pour ostéotomie intertrochantérienne. Acta Orthop Belg 37:495–504

Maquet P (1972) Traitement biomécanique de la nécrose ischémique de la tête du fémur. Acta Orthop Belg 38:526–536

Maquet P (1973) Coxarthrose protrusive: bases biomécaniques et résultat du traitement chirurgical. Proceedings of the 12th Congress of the SICOT, Tel Aviv, 1972. Excerpta Medica, Amsterdam, p 424

Maquet P (1974) Le sourcil cotyloïdien, matérialisation du diagramme des contraintes dans l'articulation de la hanche. Acta Orthop Belg 40:150–165

Maquet P (1974) Coxarthrose protrusive. Etude biomécanique et traitement. Acta Orthop Belg 40:166–171

Maquet P (1975) Traitement de la coxarthrose: de la chirurgie de la forme anatomique à la chirurgie des contraintes mécaniques. Rev Med Liège 30:196–202

Maquet P (1975) Traitement rationnel d'une luxation congénitale de la hanche. Acta Orthop Belg 41:575–582

Maquet P (1976a) Biomécanique de la hanche et traitement chirurgical conservateur de la coxarthrose. Cahiers d'enseignement de la SOFCOT. 4. Conférences d'enseignement 1975 – Expansion Scientifique Française, Paris, pp 95–125

Maquet P (1976b) Réduction de la pression articulaire de la hanche par latéralisation chirurgicale du grand trochanter. Acta Orthop Belg 42:266–271

Maquet P (1976c) Biomechanics of the knee with application to the pathogenesis and treatment of osteoarthritis. Springer, Berlin Heidelberg New York

Maquet P, Radin EL (1977) Osteotomy as an alternative to total hip replacement in young adults. Clin Orthop 123:138–142

Maquet P (1977) Techniques orthopédiques 1977. II. Ostéotomie intertrochantérienne valgisante (Pauwels II). Expansion Scientifique Française, Paris

Maquet P (1978a) Différents moyens de réduire les contraintes de compression dans l'articulation de la hanche. Acta Orthop Belg 44:115–131

Maquet P (1978b) La latéralisation chirurgicale du grand trochanter. Acta Orthop Belg 44:192–196

Maquet P (1978c) Les ostéotomies. Indications et résultats. In: La coxarthrose et son traitement. J Med Strasbourg (Europa Medica) 9:331–336

Maquet P (1980a) Surgical treatment of painful congenital dislocation of the hip. Arch Orthop Trauma Surg 96:1–4

Maquet P (1980b) Traitement chirurgical de la luxation congénitale de hanche haute invétérée devenue douloureuse. Acta Orthop Belg 46:18–27

Maquet P (1980c) Results of biomechanical surgery. Biology of the articular cartilage in health and disease. Shattauer, Stuttgart

Maquet P (1980d) Analyse mécanique de l'ostéosynthèse des fractures basi-cervicales, per- et sous-trochantériennes. Acta Orthop Belg 46:28–43

Maquet P, Vu Anh Tuan (1981) Des forces exercées sur la hanche durant la marche. Acta Orthop Belg 47:5–11

Maquet P, Vu Anh Tuan (1981) On the forces exerted on the hip during gait. Arch Orthop Traum Surg 99:53–58

Marneffe R de, Duchesne L, Blaimont P, Bonte J, Collet J (1965) Le traitement chirurgical de la coxarthrose. Acta Orthop Belg 31:101–440

McMurray TP (1935) Osteoarthritis of the hip joint. Br J Surg 22:716

McMurray TP (1939) Osteoarthritis of the hip joint. J Bone Joint Surg 21:1–11

Merle d'Aubigné R (1970) Cotation chiffrée de la fonction de la hanche. Rev Chir Orthop 56:481

Milch H (1944) The post-osteotomy angle. J Bone Joint Surg 26:394–400

Milch H (1955) The resection-angulation operation for the hip joint disabilities. J Bone Joint Surg 37:699–711

Molzberger H (1973) Die Beanspruchung des menschlichen Hüftgelenks. IV. Analyse der funktionellen Struktur der Tangentialfaserschicht des Hüftpfannenknorpels. Anat Embryol (Berl) 139:283–306

Nissen K (1960) The arrest of primary osteoarthritis of the hip. J Bone Joint Surg 42B:423–424

Nissen K (1963) The arrest of early primary osteoarthritis of the hip by osteotomy. Proc R Soc Med 56:1051–1060

Nissen K (1964) Un cas d'ostéoarthrite primitive débutante de la hanche traité par ostéotomie avec déplacement minime. Acta Orthop Belg 30:651–662

Nissen K (1971) The rationale of early osteotomy for idiopathic coxarthrosis (epichondral-osteoarthrosis) of the hip. Clin Orthop 77:98

Oberländer W (1973) Die Beanspruchung des menschlichen Hüftgelenks. V. Die Verteilung der Knochendichte im Acetabulum. Anat Embryol (Berl) 140:307–384

Oberländer W (1977) Die Beanspruchung des menschlichen Hüftgelenks. VII. Die Verteilung der Knorpeldicke im Acetabulum und ihre funktionelle Deutung. Anat Embryol (Berl) 150:141–153

Osborne GV, Fahrni WH (1950) Oblique displacement osteotomy for osteoarthritis of the hip joint. J Bone Joint Surg 32B:148–160

Palazzi AS (1958) On the operative treatment of arthritis deformans of the hip joint. Acta Orthop Scand 27:291–301

Paul JP (1966) The biomechanics of the hip joint and its clinical relevance. Proc R Soc Med 59:943–948

Paul JP, Poulson J (1974) The analysis of forces transmitted by joints in the human body. Proceedings of the fifth international conference on experimental stress analysis. Paper 32. Udine 1974

Pauwels F (1935) Der Schenkelhalsbruch, ein mechanisches Problem. Z Orthop Chir 63 (suppl)

Pauwels F (1956) La sollicitation de l'extrémité supérieure de fémur et son importance clinique. Proceedings of 3rd Conférence internationale des maladies rhumatismales. Aix-les-Bains, pp 9–35

Pauwels F (1958) Funktionelle Anpassung des Knochens durch Längenwachstum. Proc Dtsch Orthop Ges, 45th Congress

Pauwels F (1959) Directives nouvelles pour le traitement chirurgical de la coxarthrose. Rev Chir Orthop 45:681–702

Pauwels F (1961) Neue Richtlinien für die operative Behandlung der Koxarthrose. Verhandlungen der Deutschen Orthopädischen Gesellschaft, 48th Congress. Enke, Stuttgart

Pauwels F (1963a) Basis and results of an etiological therapy of osteoarthritis of the hip joint. SICOT, 9th Congress, Postgraduate course. Verlag der Wiener Medizinischen Akademie. Vienna, pp 32–50

Pauwels F (1963b) The importance of biomechanics in Orthopaedics. SICOT, 9th Congress, Postgraduate course. Verlag der Wiener Medizinischen Akademie. Vienna, pp 1–30

Pauwels F (1963c) Grundsätzliches zur kausalen Behandlung der Coxarthrose. Méd Hyg 21:363–367

Pauwels F (1965) Gesammelte Abhandlungen zur funktionellen Anatomie des Bewegungsapparates. Springer, Berlin Heidelberg New York

Pauwels F (1966) Über die Bedeutung einer Zuggurtung für die Beanspruchung des Röhrenknochens und ihre Verwendung zur Druckosteosynthese. Verhandlungen der Deutschen Orthopädischen Gesellschaft 52nd Congress. Enke, Stuttgart

Pauwels F (1973a) Atlas zur Biomechanik der gesunden und kranken Hüfte. Springer, Berlin Heidelberg New-York

Pauwels F (1973b) Kurzer Überblick über die mechanische Beanspruchung des Knochens und ihre Bedeutung für die funktionelle Anpassung. Z Orthop 2:681–705

Pauwels F (1976) Biomechanics of the normal and diseased hip. Springer, Berlin Heidelberg New York

Pauwels F (1980) Biomechanics of the locomotor apparatus. Springer, Berlin Heidelberg New York

Pirard A (1960) Notes du cours de photoélasticité. Laboratoire de Photoélasticité Univ. Liège

Radin EL, Paul IL, Pollock D (1970) Animal joint behaviour under excessive loading. Nature 226:554–555

Radin EL, Maquet P, Parker H (1975) Rationale and indications of the "hanging hip" procedure. Clin Orthop 112:221–230

Rosen S von (1962) Diagnosis and treatment of congenital dislocation of the hip joint in the newborn. J Bone Joint Surg [Br] 44:284

Rowntree LG, Adson AN (1927) Bilateral lumbar sympathectomy for polyarthritis in lower extremities. J A M A 88:694

Salter R (1961) Innominate osteotomy in the treatment of congenital dislocation and subluxation of the hip. J Bone Joint Surg [Br] 43:518

Scaglietti O (1964) Crisi vascolare chirurgica. Congrès Soc Ital orthop e traumatol Venice, 1964

Schanz A (1922) Zur Behandlung der veralteten angeborenen Hüftverrenkung. Verh Dtsch Orthop Ges Berlin 1921. Z Orthop 42 (Suppl) 442–444

Schanz A (1922) Zur Behandlung der veralteten angeborenen Hüftverrenkung. Münch med Wschr 69:930–931

Sugioka Y (1978) Transtrochanteric anterior rotational osteotomy of the femoral head in the treatment of osteonecrosis affecting the hip. Clin Orthop 130:191–201

Tillmann B (1969) Die Beanspruchung des menschlichen Hüftgelenks II. Die Form des Facies lunata. Anat Embryol (Berl) 128:329–349

Tillmann B (1973) Zur Lokalisation von degenerativen Veränderungen am Femurkopf bei der Coxarthrose. Z Orthop 3:23–27

Tillmann B (1978) A contribution to the functional morphology of articular surfaces. Thieme Stuttgart

Tillmann B, Konermann H (1979) Zur Tragfunktion der Gelenkkapsel bei der Hüftluxation. Funktionelle und morphologische Untersuchungen. Orthop Praxis XV:288–294

Venable, Stuck (1956) Ann Chir 123:

Voss C (1956) Die temporäre Hangenhüfte. Münch med Wschr 98:1

Voychenkova A (1972) Combined surgical management of degenerative hip disease. Am Dig Foreign Orthop Lit 3:151–152

Watillon M, Hoet F, Maquet P (1978) Analyse de 804 cas d'ostéotomies provenant des services de H. Benard, R. de Marneffe, R. Litt, P. Maquet, A. Vincent et du Club Orthopédique de Charleroi. Acta Orthop Belg 44:248–279

Wolff J (1892) Das Gesetz der Transformation der Knochen. Hirschwald, Berlin

Subject Index

Abduction contracture of the hip 218
Acceleration 1
   curve of 3
Adduction contracture of the hip 57, 117

Body weight 1

Cartilage 22
   epiphysial 27
Centre of gravity S_5 1, 2
Centre of gravity S_6 2
Coefficient of friction of cartilage 2, 51
Congenital coxa vara 29
Congruence
   articular 58, 288
Co-ordinates of centre of gravity S_5 3
Core of the femoral neck 16, 30
Coxa valga 25, 30
Coxa vara 25, 30, 34
Cysts 39, 71

Deepening of acetabulum 260, 270
Directional cosines 11
Discrepancy in leg length 60, 151
Displacement of greater trochanter
   distal 135
   lateral 58, 78, 134
Displacement of femoral shaft, lateral 78, 109
   medial 48, 78, 209

Exercises 70, 89, 118, 141

Fascia lata 69
Femoral head 16
Femoral neck 16, 25
Flattening of the acetabulum and femoral head 163
Flexion contracture 117
Force
   acting on the hip 1
   compressive 14
   exerted on the foot 1
   line of action of 2
   plane of 6
   reaction 4, 76, 213
Force plate 1

Girdlestone operation 205
Gothic arches 34

Hammering 15, 52
Histology 51, 64
Holography 19

Incongruence, articular 60, 288
Isochromatics 17
Isoclinics 17, 19
Isopachics 17
Isostatics 17, 19

Judet prosthesis of femoral head 208

Legg-Calvé-Perthes' disease 221
Lever arm
   of body weight 2, 102, 202, 279
   of abductor muscles 2, 76, 102, 104, 134, 202, 279
Load 50
Lowering the acetabulum 258
Lumbar sympathectomy 47

Merle d'Aubigné rating 284
Moment of inertia 1
Muscles
   abductor 1, 2, 17, 76, 102, 104, 134, 279
   adductor 64
   external rotator 1
   gluteus maximus 17
   gluteus medius 17, 69
   gluteus minimus 17, 69

Neck of the femur 30
Neck-shaft angle 25
Necrosis of the femoral head 238
Nerve
   obturator 69
Network of tridimensional co-ordinates 1
Neutral fibre 16

Osteoarthritis 45, 299
   atrophic 42
   hypertrophic 42
   primary 37
   rapidly destructive 44
   secondary 39
Osteophyte
   medial 39, 51, 102
Osteotomy
   Bombelli 50
   Chiari 278
   Lorenz 201, 202
   Mc Murray 47
   Milch 201, 205
   Salter or innominate 256
   Schanz 201, 204
   valgus intertrochanteric (Pauwels I) 76
   varus intertrochanteric (Pauwels II) 102
   without displacement (Nissen) 47

Photoelasticity 17
Physiotherapist 89
Poliomyelitis 138
Protrusio acetabuli 37, 213

Resultant force 1, 12, 25, 64, 76, 102, 134, 202

Shallow acetabulum 131, 132
Shearing component 17
Shelf operation 50, 133, 167
Shortening of the leg 115, 150
Skin arthroplasty 47
Straight leg raising 70
Stress trajectories 31
Stresses
   bending 21
   compressive 16, 50
   distribution of 23, 37
   maximum 19
   minimum 19
   normal 19
   shearing 17, 19
   tensile 16
Subchondral sclerosis 23, 37, 58
   cup-shaped 37, 71
   triangular, lateral 39, 78
   triangular, medial 41, 213
Support area 54

Tenotomy
   multiple 50, 64, 214, 240
Thrombo-embolism 70
Total hip arthroplasty 92, 192, 194, 301
Trabeculae (of cancellous bone) 30
Trajectorial architecture of cancellous bone 17, 22, 30, 263
Trendelenburg sign 70, 89, 202, 291, 293, 295

Velocity
   curve of 3

Weight-bearing surface of the joint 16, 22, 76, 102, 134, 151
Ward's triangle 22
Working hypothesis 299

The Intertrochanteric Osteotomy

Edited by **J. Schatzker**
1984. 204 figures. VII, 205 pages. ISBN 3-540-10719-3

Contents: *J. Schatzker:* Introduction. – *F. Pauwels:* Biomechanical Principles of Varus/Valgus Intertrochanteric Osteotomy (Pauwels I and II) in the Treatment of Osteoarthritis of the Hip. – *M. E. Müller:* Intertrochanteric Osteotomy: Indication, Preoperative Planning, Technique. – *R. Bombelli, J. Aronson:* Biomechanical Classification of Osteoarthritis of the Hip with Special Reference to Treatment Techniques and Results. – *R. Schneider:* Intertrochanteric Osteotomy in Osteoarthritis of the Hip Joint. – *E. Morscher, R. Feinstein:* Results of Intertrochanteric Osteotomy in the Treatment of Osteoarthritis of the Hip. – *H. Wagner, J. Holder:* Treatment of Osteoarthritis of the Hip by Corrective Osteotomy of the Greater Trochanter. – Subject Index.

The Cementless Fixation of Hip Endoprostheses

Edited by **E. Morscher**
1984. 230 figures. XV, 284 pages. ISBN 3-540-12254-0

This book examines the problems associated with hip endoprostheses, emphasizing the possibilities and limitations of cementless fixation.
It surveys the biomechanics of prosthetic loosening, the biochemistry of implants, and the choice of implant material. Special consideration is also given to the design of acetabular prostheses, the character of the prosthetic surface, and the elastic and mechanical properties of the implant.
The volume comprises the papers presented at a symposium on cementless hip endoprostheses, held in Basle in June, 1982. This was the first symposium ever held which dealt exclusively with this topic. There were presentations on various methods of hip endoprosthetic attachment used at present, as well as those still being tested and assessed. This is the first comprehensive account of cementless hip prostheses and provides on overview of the special problems in this field. It summarizes the current state of knowledge and indicates the direction of future developments.

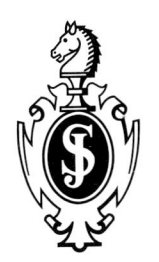

Springer-Verlag
Berlin
Heidelberg
New York
Tokyo

The Dynamic Hip Screw Implant System

By **P. Regazzoni, T. Rüedi, R. Winquist, M. Allgöwer**
1984. 45 figures in 119 separate illustrations.
Approx. 60 pages. ISBN 3-540-13668-1

Surgery of the Hip Joint

Volume 1
Editor: **R. G. Tronzo**
2nd edition. 1984. 609 figures. XV, 428 pages. ISBN 3-540-90922-2

R. Bombelli

Osteoarthritis of the Hip

Classification and Pathogenesis
The Role of Osteotomy as a Consequent Therapy

With a Foreword by M. E. Müller
2nd, revised and enlarged edition. 1983. 374 figures (partly in colour).
XVIII, 386 pages. ISBN 3-540-11422-X

E. W. Somerville

Displacement of the Hip in Childhood

Aetiology, Management and Sequelae
1982. 262 figures. XIII, 200 pages. ISBN 3-540-10936-6

J. Charnley

Low Friction Arthroplasty of the Hip

Theory and Practice
1979. 440 figures, 205 in colour, 22 tables. X, 376 pages
ISBN 3-540-08893-8

R. Liechti

Hip Arthrodesis and Associated Problems

Foreword by M. E. Müller, B. G. Weber
Translated from the German edition by P. A. Casey
1978. 266 figures, 35 tables. XII, 269 pages. ISBN 3-540-08614-5

F. Pauwels

Biomechanics of the Normal and Diseased Hip

Theoretical Foundation, Technique and Results of Treatment
An Atlas

Translated from the German by R. J. Furlong, P. Maquet
1976. 305 figures, in 853 separate illustrations, VII, 276 pages
ISBN 3-540-07428-7

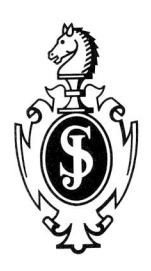

Springer-Verlag
Berlin
Heidelberg
New York
Tokyo